Death, Dying, and Bereavement

Judith M. Stillion, PhD, CT, is professor emerita of psychology and currently serves as a consultant on a variety of issues, including end-of-life issues, meaningful aging, positive psychology applied to grieving and dying, and strategic planning and facilitation of grief groups. Her varied career includes teaching and counseling in the public schools and at the university level. She began teaching the psychology of death and dying in 1975 and continued for more than 20 years. She also served as associate and vice chancellor for academic affairs at Western Carolina University, associate vice president for academic affairs in the University of North Carolina system, and founding director of the Institute for Leadership, Ethics & Character at Kennesaw State University. She is a past president of the Association for Death Education and Counseling and recipient of both their Death Educator and Contributions to the Field awards. She has written three books and numerous chapters and articles in her field of expertise, which includes suicide across the life span, aging, positive psychology applied to grief groups, and gender issues in death and grief.

Thomas Attig, PhD, is the author of *Catching Your Breath in Grief . . . and Grace Will Lead You Home* (2012), *The Heart of Grief: Death and the Search for Lasting Love* (2000), *How We Grieve: Relearning the World* (2011), and numerous articles and reviews on grief and loss, care of the dying, suicide intervention, death education, expert witnessing in wrongful death cases, the ethics of interactions with the dying, and the nature of applied philosophy. He spent the greater part of his career (1972–1995) as professor of philosophy (now emeritus) at Bowling Green State University, where he served as department chair for 11 years and established the first PhD in applied philosophy in the world in 1987. A past president of the Association for Death Education and Counseling, he has also served as vice chair of the board of directors of the International Work Group on Death, Dying, and Bereavement. He holds degrees in philosophy from Northwestern University (BA) and Washington University in St. Louis (MA and PhD). He currently resides in Victoria, British Columbia, Canada, and devotes his time to writing and speaking. He invites you to visit his web site at www.griefsheart.com.

Springer Publishing Company, LLC
11 West 42nd Street
New York, NY 10036
www.springerpub.com

Acquisitions Editor: Sheri W. Sussman
Production Editor: Brian Black
Composition: S4Carlisle Publishing Services

ISBN: 978-0-8261-7141-2
e-book ISBN: 978-0-8261-7142-9

14 15 16 17 / 5 4 3 2 1

The author and the publisher of this Work have made every effort to use sources believed to be reliable to provide information that is accurate and compatible with the standards generally accepted at the time of publication. The author and publisher shall not be liable for any special, consequential, or exemplary damages resulting, in whole or in part, from the readers' use of, or reliance on, the information contained in this book. The publisher has no responsibility for the persistence or accuracy of URLs for external or third-party Internet websites referred to in this publication and does not guarantee that any content on such websites is, or will remain, accurate or appropriate.

Library of Congress Cataloging-in-Publication Data

Stillion, Judith M., 1937–
    Death, dying, and bereavement : contemporary perspectives, institutions, and practices / Judith M. Stillion, PhD and Thomas Attig, PhD.
        pages cm.
        ISBN 978-0-8261-7141-2—ISBN 978-0-8261-7142-9 (e-book) 1. Death—Psychological aspects. 2. Death—Social aspects. 3. Bereavement—Social aspects. I. Title.
        BF789.D4S754 2015
        306.9—dc23
                                                                    2014020866

Special discounts on bulk quantities of our books are available to corporations, professional associations, pharmaceutical companies, health care organizations, and other qualifying groups. If you are interested in a custom book, including chapters from more than one of our titles, we can provide that service as well.

For details, please contact:
Special Sales Department, Springer Publishing Company, LLC
11 West 42nd Street, 15th Floor, New York, NY 10036-8002
Phone: 877-687-7476 or 212-431-4370; Fax: 212-941-7842
E-mail: sales@springerpub.com

Printed in the United States of America by McNaughton & Gunn.

Death, Dying, and Bereavement

Contemporary Perspectives, Institutions, and Practices

Judith M. Stillion, PhD, CT, and Thomas Attig, PhD

Editors

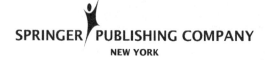

SPRINGER PUBLISHING COMPANY
NEW YORK

*For Glenn, John William, Bethany Dawn, and Daniel James, who
form the core of meaning in my life; and for all those who are courageous
enough to serve the dying and bereaved.*

—JMS

*For Betty, Julie, Ty, Jamie, Sher, Skyler, and Dan, the loves
of my life, and for all who take seriously the stories of love and sorrow
the dying and bereaved have to tell.*

—TWA

CONTENTS

PART III: PRACTICE DEVELOPMENTS

CONTRIBUTORS

Dawn Allen, PhD, Associate Director, Palliative Care McGill, McGill University, Montreal, Quebec, Canada

Thomas Attig, PhD, Professor Emeritus, Department of Philosophy, Bowling Green State University, Bowling Green, Ohio

Sandra Bertman, PhD, Distinguished Professor (retired), Thanatology and Arts, National Center for Death Education, Newton, Massachusetts; Good Shepherd Community Care Hospice & Institute, Newton, Massachusetts

David Clark, PhD, Professor of Medical Sociology, School of Interdisciplinary Studies, Institute of Health and Wellbeing, University of Glasgow, Glasgow, Scotland

Stephen Connor, PhD, International Palliative Care Consultant, Open Society Foundations, New York, New York; Senior Fellow, Worldwide Hospice Palliative Care Alliance, London, England; Senior Research Fellow, Capital Caring, Washington, DC

Inge B. Corless, PhD, RN, FAAN, Professor, MGH Institute of Health Professions, School of Nursing, Boston, Massachusetts

Charles A. Corr, PhD, Member, Board of Directors, Suncoast Hospice Institute, Clearwater, Florida

Betty Davies, RN, CT, PhD, FAAN, Professor Emerita, Family Health Care Nursing, University of California San Francisco, San Francisco, California; Adjunct Professor and Senior Scholar, School of Nursing, University of Victoria, Victoria, British Columbia

Kenneth J. Doka, PhD, Professor, The Graduate School, The College of New Rochelle, New Rochelle, New York; Senior Consultant, The Hospice Foundation of America, Washington, DC

Linda Goldman, MS, FT, LCPC, Adjunct Professor of Graduate Counseling, School of Education, Johns Hopkins University, Baltimore, Maryland

Leeat Granek, PhD, Assistant Professor, Department of Public Health, Faculty of Health Sciences, Ben Gurion University of the Negev, Beer Sheva, Israel

John R. Jordan, PhD, Private Practice, Pawtucket, Rhode Island

Allan Kellehear, PhD, AcSS, Professor of Community Health, School of Health & Education, Middlesex University, London, England

David W. Kissane, MB, BS, MPM, MD, FRANZCP, FAChPM, Professor of Psychiatry and Head of Discipline, Chairman, Department of Psychiatry, Monash University and Monash Medical Centre, Victoria, Australia; Professor of Psychiatry, Weill Cornell Medical College and Memorial Sloan-Kettering Cancer Center, New York, New York

Bernard J. Lapointe, MD, Eric M. Flanders Chair in Palliative Medicine, Director, Palliative Care McGill, McGill University, Montreal, Quebec, Canada

Judith L. M. McCoyd, PhD, LCSW (PA), QCSW, Associate Professor, Rutgers University School of Social Work, Camden and New Brunswick, New Jersey

Robert A. Neimeyer, PhD, Professor of Psychology, Department of Psychology, University of Memphis, Memphis, Tennessee

Colin Murray Parkes, OBE, MD, FRCPsych, DL, Consultant Psychiatrist Emeritus, St Christopher's Hospice, Sydenham, London, England

Vanderlyn R. Pine, PhD, Professor Emeritus, Department of Sociology, State University of New York at New Paltz, New Paltz, New York

Therese A. Rando, PhD, BCETS, BCBT, Clinical Director, The Institute for the Study and Treatment of Loss, Warwick, Rhode Island

Phyllis R. Silverman, PhD, Resident Scholar, Women's Studies Research Center, Brandeis University, Waltham, Massachusetts

Judith M. Stillion, PhD, CT, Professor Emerita, Psychology, Stillion Consulting Services, Ormond Beach, Florida

Mary L. S. Vachon, PhD, RN, Private Practice; Professor, Department of Psychiatry and Dalla Lana School of Public Health, University of Toronto; Clinical Consultant, Wellspring, Toronto, Canada

Carolyn A. Walter, PhD, LCSW, Professor Emerita, Center for Social Work Education, Widener University, Chester, Pennsylvania

Tony Walter, PhD, Professor of Death Studies, Centre for Death & Society, University of Bath, Bath, England

James L. Werth Jr., PhD, ABPP, Director, Behavioral Health and Wellness Services, Stone Mountain Health Services, Pennington Gap, Virginia

Diana J. Wilkie, PhD, RN, FAAN, Professor, Harriet H. Werley Endowed Chair for Nursing Research, and Director of the Center of Excellence for End-of-Life Transition Research, Department of Biobehavioral Health Science, College of Nursing, University of Illinois at Chicago, Chicago, Illinois

J. William Worden, PhD, ABPP, Clinical Psychologist, Harvard Medical School, Massachusetts General Hospital, Boston, Massachusetts

PREFACE

The two of us met in 1979 at one of the early conferences sponsored by the then newly formed Forum for Death Education and Counseling, each having already devoted several years to work in the emerging contemporary death, dying, and bereavement movement. It was so good to gather with others from such diverse backgrounds in teaching, research, health care, counseling professions, and volunteer service. We were not alone in sensing the excitement of meeting others who were passionate about learning from one another and about changing ways of understanding, living with, and caring for others facing death, dying, and bereavement.

We were privileged then, and have been in the years since, to learn from, work with, and in many cases befriend pioneers and major contributors in the field. Two years ago, while looking back at how remarkably far the movement has come, we realized how many leading figures and friends have died. We saw an opportunity to capture the collective wisdom of living pioneers, major contributors, and participant witnesses to the founding and evolution of the movement before more voices were lost. We would bring those voices together in a book that would be a testament to and celebration of the work of all those who have led us to where we are today. We are excited to have gathered together an extraordinary team of 28 authors with nearly a millennium of experience in the field to tell stories that only they can tell about unprecedented changes that have been unfolding since the movement began in the middle of the 20th century. We are grateful that our editor at Springer Publishing Company, Sheri W. Sussman, endorsed our idea enthusiastically and helped us so ably to bring it into reality. We are also so grateful for the opportunity to work together again on this volume, work that has deepened both our knowledge and friendship.

We asked all of our authors to describe what drew them into the field, discuss the most important strands of early development in the area of their chapters that they consider to be foundational and not to be forgotten, review the most valuable current work in the area, and assess major challenges and hopes for future developments. Although we hope that all will live long and continue to prosper, we wanted to harvest the insights of these seminal figures before it became too late to do so.

We are amazed and enormously grateful for the foundational and revolutionary efforts of the thought leaders, institutional innovators, imaginative practitioners, and concerned citizens whose stories our authors tell. As their informative and often provocative chapters came flooding in and we began the editorial review and polishing process, we realized how collectively they were expanding our own understanding and appreciation of how rich and varied the contributions of the death, dying, and bereavement movement are. Taken together, we believe these writers have created a unique and lasting contribution to the growing body of work that is defining a new discipline: thanatology.

We bring this book to you out of the following shared convictions. First, we pay too high a price individually and collectively in missing what matters most in life if we persistently turn away from and remain silent about the realities of mortality that are so intimately interwoven in the fabric of our being. Everyone can benefit from development and dissemination of better understanding the meanings of death, dying, and bereavement for individuals, families, and communities and of their implications for how we live. We do well to counter tendencies to isolate the dying and bereaved that increase their dependence on professionals. We believe there is a deep human need to come together as family and community while loved ones are dying, grieving, traumatized, or contemplating suicide to hear their stories, bear witness to their suffering, and offer support and compassion. We endorse efforts to reach past the limitations of disease-focused medical care and pathology-focused bereavement support to recognize and respond more effectively to the multidimensional needs of whole persons living with disease and relearning the world in grief. We affirm and call for increased understanding and support of the resilience and capacities for overcoming suffering and finding healing that are inherent in the human spirit. We heartily support revival of the art of medicine as at least coequal with the science and value team-based and volunteer-based approaches to end-of-life care. We applaud resistance to professional paternalism in favor of informed consent; respect for human dignity; attunement through dialogue to the particularities of individual, family, and community experiences and needs; and affirmation of their freedom to shape their own experiences. We seek to enable families and communities to reclaim responsibilities for death education and care and support of those who are dying, bereaved, traumatized, or suicidal. We eagerly await the day when death education will be integrated into schooling at all levels to prepare citizens for those responsibilities, for scholars to deepen their understanding, and professional caregivers to use the best of what is known wisely.

We intend this book for all who have been interested or actively engaged in the movement through the years, and especially for those relatively new to the field as students or practitioners who share these convictions and passions and will carry on, extend, and creatively transform the efforts discussed here. Our authors trace the development of thanatology as an interdisciplinary field of study (in Part I) and organizational and practice developments in response to the diverse needs of dying, bereaved, suicidal, and traumatized individuals, families, and communities (in Parts II and III). A unique feature of this book is a detailed chronology that includes many, though of course not all, of the most important milestones of the last 60 years. It is intended to serve as an overview as well as the foundation for understanding this burgeoning field and as a guide for readers who wish to understand in detail its short, but rich, history.

Robert Kastenbaum often casually defined the emerging academic field of thanatology as "the study of life with death left in." Clearly, we have in this book stretched beyond the study of death, dying, and bereavement to encompass institutional and practice developments in response to these universal human experiences. Gandhi charged us to "be the change you want to see in the world." The pioneers and major contributors to the movement (including our authors) have done that and in so doing crafted better, more humane ways to conceptualize and cope with the many faces of death, dying, and bereavement in our times. We invite you to join them and learn from them as we move forward together.

Judith M. Stillion and Thomas Attig

Thomas Attig

INTRODUCTION: CHRONOLOGY OF DEVELOPMENTS IN THE MOVEMENT

It is impossible to capture all of the events, strains of thought, organizational developments, and changes in practice that have shaped the study of death, dying, and bereavement and transformed contemporary responses to them. However, this chronology captures many of the most important influences on and milestones in the evolution of contemporary responses to death, dying, and bereavement as we, after consultation with our authors, see them. We know of nothing else like it in the literature.

We invite you to peruse this chronology (1) as a broadly based introduction to work in the death-and-dying field; (2) as an organizing framework for reading the chapters that follow, enabling you to see where the works described in them fit in this larger context; (3) as a review to return to when you've finished reading the book; and (4) as a detailed guide to further, in-depth reading in the field.

1955   Robert W. Habenstein and William Lamers author *The History of American Funeral Directing*, helping to solidify understanding of the role of the funeral director as a professional.

*   Geoffrey Gorer publishes "The Pornography of Death," an early study of reasons why society at that time tended to ignore or deny death.

1958   William Faunce and Robert Fulton write "The Sociology of Death: A Neglected Area of Research," the first call for systematic investigation of the subject of death following the Second World War.

*   Edwin Shneidman, Norman Farberow, and Robert Litman found the Los Angeles Suicide Prevention Center, the first of its kind.

1959   Herman Feifel publishes *The Meaning of Death*, promoting establishment of death studies as an interdisciplinary academic field.

*   Renée C. Fox writes *Experiment Perilous: Physicians and Patients Facing the Unknown* on conflicting responsibilities of caring for incurably ill men and conducting research on them.

*   Margaret Torrie founds Cruse Clubs for Widows, subsequently developed by Colin M. Parkes and Derek Nuttall into Cruse Bereavement Care, for all bereaved persons in the United Kingdom.

1960   Robert Habenstein and William Lamers publish *Funeral Customs the World Over*, a comprehensive overview of ritual responses to death.

1961   Robert Fulton writes "The Clergyman and the Funeral Director: A Study in Role Conflict," about the two primary functionaries associated with burial of the dead.

*   C. S. Lewis's *A Grief Observed* appears, a singularly memorable grief journal by a leading religious thinker describing his spiritual struggles after the death of his wife.

1962   Ernest Morgan publishes *A Manual of Death Education and Simple Burial*, used widely by memorial societies in North America.

1963   Jessica Mitford authors *The American Way of Death*, raising public awareness of ethical issues surrounding American funeral practices.

*   Jeanne Quint Benoliel's report, "The Impact of Mastectomy," in *American Journal of Nursing*, is the first in nursing to focus on issues of dying and catapults her research in death and dying.

1965   Barney Glaser and Anselm Strauss write *Awareness of Dying* about communication patterns between the dying and their caregivers.

*   Robert Fulton edits *Death and Identity*, calling for the scientific study of attitudes and reactions toward grief, bereavement, and human mortality.

1967   Dame Cicely Saunders founds the first modern hospice, St Christopher's in London, England, marking a revolutionary turn in care of the dying and their families.

*   Jeanne Quint Benoliel authors *The Nurse and the Dying Patient*, the first systematic study of the role of nurses in caring for the dying.

*   David Sudnow writes *Passing On: The Social Organization of Dying* on how presumed social value of dying patients determined treatment and information exchange in hospitals.

*   Phyllis Silverman begins the Widow-to-Widow Project through Harvard Medical School, which has served as a basis for mutual-help programs for widows in the United States and other countries.

*   The Euthanasia Society of America (Concern for Dying after 1978) introduces the "Living Will" to specify desires concerning cessation of end-of-life treatment.

*   Robert Fulton establishes the Center for Thanatological Studies at the University of Minnesota (the Center for Death Education and Research in 1969), sponsor of early conferences bringing together scholars from many fields.

*   Austin Kutscher founds the Foundation of Thanatology, sponsor of multidisciplinary symposia and publisher of the first journal in the field, *The Journal of Thanatology*. This work continues in the Columbia University Seminar on Death.

*   John Bowlby releases *Attachment*, followed by *Separation* (1973) and *Loss* (1980), a cornerstone trilogy in contemporary thinking about grief and loss.

*   John Fryer founds Ars Moriendi, publishing a newsletter and bibliographies and sponsoring symposia.

1968   Edwin Shneidman founds the American Association of Suicidology and the first American journal in the study of suicide, *Suicide and Life Threatening Behavior*.

1969   Elizabeth Kübler-Ross publishes *On Death and Dying*, bringing death out of the shadows into public discourse, urging acceptance of the reality of death.

*   Robert Kastenbaum establishes the Center for Dying, Death, Suicide and Lethal Behavior at Wayne State University.

1970   Richard Kalish, Robert Kastenbaum, and Robert Fulton found *Omega: Journal of Death and Dying*, which continues to publish thinking and research in death, dying, and bereavement.

*   Colin Murray Parkes starts the first hospice-based bereavement service using carefully selected, trained, and supervised volunteers at St Christopher's Hospice.

1971   *The Hastings Center Report* begins publication, a journal devoted to ethical, legal, and social issues in medicine, including end-of-life ethics.

1972   Colin Murray Parkes authors *Bereavement: Studies of Grief in Adult Life* on potentially detrimental effects of bereavement and typical manifestations of grief.

*   Avery Weisman publishes *On Dying and Denying*, a psychiatric study of living with terminality and introducing the idea of "appropriate death," a death one would choose.

*   Robert Kastenbaum and Ruth Eisenberg release *The Psychology of Death*, a treatment of our construction of death from a developmental perspective.

*   A. Alvarez authors *The Savage God*, a review of attitudes toward suicide and death through history and literature.

*   Albert Cain writes *Survivors of Suicide*, the first clinically oriented volume to describe problematic reactions to a suicide experienced by many survivors.

1974   Florence Wald (Dean of the Yale School of Nursing) and her colleagues cofound the first hospice in North America in Branford, Connecticut.

*   Ars Moriendi sponsors the International Convocation of Leaders in the Field of Death and Dying, centering on dialogue rather than paper presentations, prefiguring the International Work Group on Death, Dying, and Bereavement.

*   The first hospital-based hospice programs are established at the Royal Victoria Hospital in Montreal and St. Boniface General Hospital in Winnipeg. Dr. Balfour Mount first uses the term "palliative care" in the name of the Royal Victoria program.

*   Ernest Becker publishes *The Denial of Death*, a sustained reflection on how human refusal to face mortality shapes culture in wide-ranging and unexpected ways.

*   Lily Pincus authors *Death and the Family*, a social worker's perspective on understanding and working therapeutically with grieving families.

1975   Hannelore Wass convenes the first American conference that brings together academics and practitioners in Orlando, Florida, inspiring the founding of the Forum on Death Education and Counseling.

*   Karen Ann Quinlan falls into a permanent vegetative state. Her parents' request that she be removed from life support rouses controversy that leads to establishment of hospital, hospice, and nursing home ethics committees and wider use of advanced directives.

*   Raymond Moody publishes *Life After Life*, the first book devoted to the modern study of near-death experiences.

1976   The Forum on Death Education and Counseling (now the Association for Death Education and Counseling: The Thanatology Association [ADEC]) first meets in Washington, DC. The original name is retained in ADEC's publication, *The Forum.*

*   The Royal Victoria Hospital in Montreal sponsors the first biennial International Congress on Care of the Terminally Ill (later the International Congress on Palliative Care), bringing together clinicians and scholars from around the world.

*   William Worden authors *PDA: Personal Death Awareness* on the fear of death.

1977   The National Hospice Organization (NHO) is founded to support the spread of hospice in the United States (The National Hospice and Palliative Care Organization [NHPCO] since 2000).

*   Herman Feifel publishes *New Meanings of Death*, a second interdisciplinary anthology featuring many of the early thinkers in the field.

* Phillipe Aries authors *L'Homme devant la mort*, an amateur social-historian's review of a thousand years of Western responses to death, translated as *The Hour of Our Death* in 1981.
* Hannelore Wass founds *The Journal of Death Education*, dedicated to death education in schools and universities. As *Death Studies*, it is a major outlet for researchers and theorists.
* The International Work Group on Death, Dying, and Bereavement (IWG) incorporates, fostering interdisciplinary group discussion and occasional publications.

1978 The Society for Compassionate Friends, a support group providing friendship, understanding, and hope for bereaved parents, incorporates.

* Myra Bluebond-Langner releases *The Private Worlds of Dying Children*, an anthropological study of the experiences of and communication with dying children.
* The International Symposium on the Dying Human, held in Tel Aviv, Israel, brings together scholars and practitioners from around the world.

1979 Robert Fulton coordinates Courses by Newspaper: Death & Dying, a 15-part series on death in American culture, published in more than 400 newspapers with a readership of 12 million and offered in more than 300 colleges and universities, with a student enrollment of more than 12,000.

* Robert Lifton publishes *The Broken Connection*, about immortality (literal and symbolic) in an era of declining traditional belief and possible nuclear annihilation.

1980 Dr. Josefina Magno founds the International Association of Hospice and Palliative Care (IAHPC), initially as the International Hospice Institute, later the American Academy of Hospice and Palliative Medicine and the International Hospice Institute and College (IHIC).

* Ida Martinson demonstrates that it is possible to care for children dying of cancer at home.

1981 Simon Shimshon Rubin introduces his two-track model of bereavement in the *American Journal of Orthopsychiatry*.

* Harold Kushner authors *When Bad Things Happen to Good People*, reflecting compassionately on spiritual doubts and fears that surface when loved ones die.

1982 William Worden writes *Grief Counseling and Grief Therapy*, urging that grieving is not only reactive but also actively responsive, and providing guidance for grief counselors and therapists.

* Beverly Chappell founds the Dougy Center for Grieving Children in Portland, Oregon.
* The Hospice Foundation of America is established to raise funds for South Florida hospices but later to provide leadership on a broad spectrum of end-of-life issues.
* The Medicare hospice benefit is approved by Congress, providing coverage for hospice care for the elderly and the poor in the United States.
* Sister Francis Dominica and her colleagues open Helen House, the world's first free-standing hospice for children in Oxford, England.
* The journal *Bereavement Care* begins, edited by Colin Murray Parkes and Dora Black.
* Lynne DeSpelder and Albert Strickland publish *The Last Dance: Encountering Death and Dying*, destined to become the best-selling textbook in the field.

1983 Ann Armstrong-Dailey starts Children's Hospice International (CHI), with the objective of providing education, legislation, and support for families of children with terminal illness.

* The first annual King's College International Conference on Death and Bereavement is held in London, Ontario (in LaCrosse, Wisconsin since 2006).

* Colin Murray Parkes and Robert Weiss author *Recovery From Bereavement*, the main account of the *Harvard Bereavement Project*, a study that facilitated bereavement risk assessment.

1984 Beverley Raphael offers *The Anatomy of Bereavement*, showing how the dynamics of grief and recovery vary from infancy through old age.

1985 The first triennial International Conference on Grief and Bereavement in Contemporary Society is held in Jerusalem, Israel, bringing together scholars, researchers, and clinicians.

* *The Journal of Palliative Care*, edited by David Roy, begins publication.

* Thomas Beauchamp and James Childress write *Principles of Biomedical Ethics* on core principles of beneficence, nonmaleficence, personal autonomy, and justice in medical ethics.

* Therese Rando edits *Loss and Anticipatory Grief*, followed in 2000 by *Clinical Dimensions of Anticipatory Mourning* on grieving as death approaches.

* Betty Rollin releases *Last Wish*, a poignant account of her response to her mother's plea for assistance in killing herself while facing terminal illness.

1986 The Hospice and Palliative Nurses Association is founded, dedicated to promoting excellence in hospice and palliative care nursing.

* Beverley Raphael writes *When Disaster Strikes: How Individuals and Communities Cope With Catastrophe*, on the psychological consequences of disasters.

* Thomas Beauchamp and Ruth Faden author *A History and Theory of Informed Consent*, a comprehensive treatment of its subject.

* Arthur Kleinman publishes *The Illness Narratives: Suffering, Healing, and the Human Condition*, a groundbreaking work in development of a narrative approach to end-of-life ethics.

* Judith M. Stillion authors *Death and the Sexes*, the first book on gender issues in death and grief.

1987 The Royal College of Physicians (Great Britain) is the first to recognize palliative care as an official subspecialty in medicine.

* Mary Vachon writes *Occupational Stress in the Care of the Critically Ill, Dying and Bereaved*, a international interview study of 581 professional caregivers.

* Randy Shilts authors *And the Band Played On*, a searing critique of institutional failure in response to the early stages of the AIDS epidemic.

1988 The Academy of Hospice Physicians is founded (later the American Academy of Hospice and Palliative Medicine).

* The European Association for Palliative Care (EAPC) is founded. EAPC now consists of 55 associations in 32 countries.

* Dennis Klass writes *Parental Grief: Solace and Resolution* on the basis of his work with bereaved parents in Compassionate Friends.

1989 Kenneth J. Doka edits *Disenfranchised Grief: Recognizing Hidden Sorrow* on the range of loss experiences not acknowledged by the larger society (followed in 2002 by *Disenfranchised Grief: New Directions, Challenges and Strategies for Practice*).

* Judith M. Stillion and Eugene McDowell author *Suicide Across the Lifespan: Premature Exits*, offering a developmental perspective on suicide.

* Michael Kearl writes *Endings: A Sociology of Death and Dying*, arguing that death is the central force shaping our social life and order.

1991 The Association for Children With Life Threatening or Terminal Conditions and Their Families (ACT), now known as Together for Short Lives, is formed in the United Kingdom.

* The Canadian Palliative Care Association is established (now the Canadian Hospice and Palliative Care Association [CHPCA]).
* The journal *Illness, Crisis & Loss* is established, a reflective forum for practitioners, researchers, leaders, and students, linking theory, research, and practice.
* Eric Cassell authors *The Nature of Suffering and the Goals of Medicine*, describing how persons suffer in all dimensions of their being, not just physically.
* Sandra Bertman writes *Facing Death: Images, Insights and Interventions*, sensitizing readers via the arts to universal issues confronting the dying and those who care for them.
* Derek Humphry publishes *Final Exit*, a how-to guide to suicide at the end of life, arousing great controversy about issues in end-of-life ethics.

1992 Ronnie Janoff-Bulman authors *Shattered Assumptions: Towards a New Psychology of Trauma*, focusing on the loss of the assumptive world in bereavement.

1993 Oxford University Press releases *The Oxford Textbook of Palliative Medicine*, the first comprehensive textbook on the subject, now in its fourth edition.

* Timothy Quill writes *Death and Dignity*, for physicians and their terminally ill patients about the active role the dying should take in end-of-life decisions.
* Edwin Shneidman publishes *Suicide as Psychache*, a collection and reworking of his seminal papers on suicide from 1971 to 1993.
* Therese Rando authors *Treatment of Complicated Mourning* about working therapeutically with individuals for whom standard counseling techniques do not suffice.
* Margaret Stroebe, Wofgang Stroebe, and Robert Hannson edit the *Handbook of Bereavement*, featuring essays covering a broad range of research and clinical practice.
* Kenneth J. Doka publishes *Living With Life-Threatening Illness: A Guide for Patients, Their Families, and Caregivers*, tracing prediagnostic, diagnostic, and terminal phases of dying.

1994 Genocide kills about 700,000 in Rwanda. Leila Gupta, assisted by Colin Murray Parkes, sets up a Trauma Recovery Program for UNICEF.

* The Hospice Foundation of America broadcasts its first teleconference, an event that has become the single largest annual death education experience in the United States.
* The Project on Death in America begins funding initiatives in education, the arts, research, clinical care, and public policy to transform the culture of dying and bereavement.
* Robert Neimeyer edits the *Death Anxiety Handbook: Research, Instrumentation & Application*, a comprehensive treatment of research on its subject.

1995 Sherwin Nuland writes *How We Die*, about the biological and clinical realities of dying from cancer, heart attack, AIDS, Alzheimer's disease, trauma, and old age.

* Margaret Pabst Battin publishes *The Least Worst Death: Essays in Bioethics on the End of Life*, featuring reflections on withdrawal of treatment, euthanasia, and suicide.
* Brian L. Mishara writes *The Impact of Suicide*, examining the impact of suicide on individuals, families, helping professionals, and society as a whole.
* Betty Davies, Brenda Eng, and their colleagues cofound Canuck Place, the first free-standing hospice for children in North America in Vancouver, British Columbia.

1996   Thomas Attig authors *How We Grieve*, an all-encompassing phenomenology of grieving as a process of relearning how to be and act in a world transformed by loss.

*   Dennis Klass, Phyllis Silverman, and Steven Nickman publish *Continuing Bonds*, reporting on research indicating that grievers maintain connections with the dead.

*   William Worden releases *Children & Grief: When a Parent Dies* on the basis of his work with Phyllis Silverman on the Harvard Child Bereavement Study.

*   Colin Murray Parkes, Pittu Laungani, and Bill Young edit *Death and Bereavement Across Cultures*, about major world systems of belief and ritual and their practical implications.

*   Allan Kellehear writes *Experiences Near Death: Beyond Medicine and Religion*, a sociological study of what near-death experiences (NDEs) look like in diverse cultural contexts.

1997   The Education in Palliative Care and End-of-Life Care (EPEC) program, sited within the American Medical Association and sponsored by the Robert Wood Johnson Foundation, begins training trainers of national and international physicians in palliative care.

*   Oregon enacts its Death with Dignity Act, authorizing physician-assisted suicide for the first time in the United States.

*   *Mortality*, an English publication (now the official journal of the Association for the Study of Death and Society), is first published and is devoted to the interdisciplinary study of death and dying.

*   Mitch Albom authors *Tuesdays With Morrie: An Old Man, A Young Man, and Life's Greatest Lesson*, a memoir of sessions with his former professor, who is dying of ALS.

1998   Ira Byock writes *Dying Well*, containing poignant and instructive accounts of a hospice team attending to the whole person of those in their care.

*   Janice Winchester Nadeau publishes *Families Making Sense of Death*, an exploration of meaning reconstruction from a familial perspective.

*   Kathleen Dowling Singh authors *The Grace of Dying*, an account of psychological and spiritual transformation as we surrender our egos and bodies to death.

*   Stephen Connor publishes *Hospice: Practice, Pitfalls, and Promise* chronicling the growth of hospice (second edition entitled *Hospice & Palliative Care: The Essential Guide*, 2009).

1999   Margaret Stroebe and Henk Schut introduce the dual-process model of coping with bereavement in *Death Studies*.

*   Pauline Boss writes *Ambiguous Loss* on grieving when there is no direct confirmation of death—used widely after the 9/11 terrorist attacks.

*   Betty Davies authors *Shadows in the Sun: The Experience of Sibling Bereavement in Childhood*, about childhood experiences of and lifelong consequences of sibling loss.

*   Tony Walter writes *On Bereavement: The Culture of Grief*, a study of the sociological and cultural dimensions of and influences on grieving.

2000   The End-of-Life Nursing Education Consortium (ELNEC), a train-the-trainer initiative sponsored by the Robert Wood Johnson Foundation and administered by the American Association of Colleges of Nursing and the City of Hope, begin training nurses and other health care providers the world over.

*   Terry L. Martin and Kenneth J. Doka author *Men Don't Cry . . . Women Do: Transcending Gender Stereotypes of Grief*, contrasting intuitive and instrumental styles in grieving.

*   Phyllis Silverman publishes *Never Too Young to Know: Death in Children's Lives*, based on her work with William Worden on the Harvard Child Bereavement Study.

*   *On Our Own Terms: Moyers on Dying*, a four-part series on efforts to improve how we die, produced by Public Affairs Television, airs on PBS, reaching millions.

2001   Terrorist attacks kill 2,981 in the United States on 9/11, sparking the "War on Terror."

*   The Latin American Association for Palliative Care is founded (Asociación Latino Americana de Cuidado Paliativo [ALCP]).

*   The Asia Pacific Hospice Palliative Care Network (APHN) is founded.

*   Robert Neimeyer edits *Meaning Reconstruction and the Experience of Loss*, underscoring the place of meaning-making in grieving.

*   Edward Rynearson authors *Retelling Violent Death*, for those bereaved through suicide, homicide, or accident and those who work with them.

*   Routledge publishes *The Encyclopedia of Death and Dying*, the first volume of its kind.

*   *Finding Our Way: Living and Dying in America*, a 15-part newspaper series is published in 161 newspapers, reaching an audience of more than 7 million.

2002   Susan Roos writes *Chronic Sorrow: A Living Loss*, sensitizing counselors to issues that arise when individuals cope with ongoing loss.

*   David Kissane and Sidney Bloch publish *Family Focused Grief Therapy: A Model of Family-Centred Care During Palliative Care and Bereavement*.

2003   Kathleen Nicholson Hull, Barbara Beach, and their colleagues cofound George Mark House, the first free-standing children's hospice in the United States in San Leandro, California.

2004   The African Palliative Care Association (APCA) is founded.

2005   The International Children's Palliative Care Network (ICPCN) is founded to achieve the best quality in living with life-threatening conditions for children and young people, their families, and carers worldwide.

*   Oxford University Press releases the *Oxford Textbook on Palliative Nursing*, the first comprehensive textbook on the subject, now in its third edition.

*   Allan Kellehear authors *Compassionate Cities: Public Health and End-of-Life Care*, a vision of whole communities adopting a compassionate approach to dying, death, and loss.

*   Sharon Kaufman writes *... And a Time to Die: How American Hospitals Shape the End of Life*, an anthropical examination of dying within the medical culture in American hospitals.

2006   The posthumous publication of *Cicely Saunders: Selected Writings 1958–2004* provides key references for historians and Dame Cicely's personal influence on hospice/palliative care.

*   Oxford University Press releases the *Oxford Textbook on Palliative Care for Children*, the first comprehensive textbook on the subject, now in its second edition.

*   Edward Rynearson edits *Violent Death: Resilience and Intervention Beyond the Crisis* for those planning clinical and spiritual services following violent death.

*   Colin Murray Parkes publishes *Love and Loss: The Roots of Grief and Its Complications*, an interpretation based in attachment theory.

*   Lawrence Calhoun and Richard Tedeschi author the *Handbook of Posttraumatic Growth: Research and Practice* about possible growth following bereavement.

2007 Alan Horwitz and Jerome Wakefield write *The Loss of Sadness: How Psychiatry Transformed Normal Sorrow Into Depressive Behavior*, distinguishing abnormal reactions due to internal dysfunction and normal sadness brought on by external circumstances.

* ADEC publishes the *Handbook of Thanatology: The Essential Body of Knowledge for the Study of Death, Dying, and Bereavement*, edited by David Balk.

* Allan Kellehear writes *A Social History of Dying*, a historical review of the human and clinical sciences literature about human dying through the ages.

2008 Rita Charon publishes *Narrative Medicine: Honoring the Stories of Illness* on using techniques of literary interpretation to understand the stories the ill and dying have to tell.

* Irvin Yalom writes *Staring at the Sun: Overcoming the Terror of Death*, an existentialist interpretation of the fear of death.

* The Worldwide Palliative Care Alliance is incorporated in the United Kingdom as a global alliance of all the hospice and palliative care associations to advocate for palliative care.

2009 SAGE publishes the *Encyclopedia of Death and the Human Experience*.

* Carolyn Walter and Judith McCoyd author *Grief and Loss Across the Lifespan: A Biopsychosocial Perspective* about maturational losses and losses through death.

* George Bonanno writes *The Other Side of Sadness* about our resilience and innate ability to thrive in life after loss.

2011 Robert Neimeyer, Darcy Harris, Howard Winokuer, and Gordon Thornton edit *Grief and Bereavement in Contemporary Society: Bridging Research and Practice*, pairing pieces by researchers and clinicians who use the research in their counseling practice.

* Jack Jordan and John McIntosh edit *Grief After Suicide: Understanding the Consequences and Caring for the Survivors*, covering impacts on survivors, helping survivors, and support programs in the United States and internationally.

2012 Harvey Chochinov writes *Dignity Therapy: Final Words for Final Days* about a program to help the dying say what they need to say.

* Robert Neimeyer edits *Techniques of Grief Therapy: Creative Practices for Counseling the Bereaved*, featuring a broad range of case studies and useful counseling techniques.

2013 William G. Hoy writes *Do Funerals Matter? The Purposes and Practices of Death Rituals in Global Perspective* on the value of death rituals for individuals, families, and communities.

2014 Laurie Ann Pearlman, Camille Wortman, Catherine A. Feuer, Christine Farber, and Therese Rando publish *Treating Traumatic Bereavement: A Practitioner's Guide*, providing conceptual and clinical guidance for reconstructing a world transformed by trauma and loss.

* Barbara E. Thompson and Robert Neimeyer edit *Grief and the Expressive Arts: Practices for Creating Meaning*, about what art therapy techniques to use when in counseling with the bereaved.

* David Kissane and Francine Parnes edit *Bereavement Care for Families*, covering conceptual frameworks, practical approaches, and particularly challenging circumstances.

* Stephen R. Connor and Maria Cecilia Sepulveda release *The Global Atlas of Palliative Care at the End of Life*, painting a picture of palliative care worldwide.

Thomas Attig

1

SEEKING WISDOM ABOUT MORTALITY, DYING, AND BEREAVEMENT

Philosophy means, literally, the "love of wisdom." The disciplines of the philosopher are thought to be worth cultivating because, as Socrates said, "The unexamined life is not worth living." Philosophy takes root in this conviction that living wisely is preferable to not doing so. This chapter begins with a brief description of my being attracted to philosophy by a hunger for wisdom. It then expands on the nature of wisdom and its value for guiding (a) a search for truth and understanding and (b) the pursuit of living well or meaningfully. It is not possible in a single chapter to cover the full history of what philosophers have said about death and dying across several millennia (Chapter 6 is devoted to philosophical perspectives on ethics at the end of life). Hence, this chapter focuses on the contributions of phenomenology and existentialism to recent developments in the death and dying field: Phenomenology calls for descriptive and interpretive analyses of experiences of facing mortality, dying, and grieving as foundations for all theories about them. Existentialism stresses the importance for caregiving of attuning to the singularities of the lived experiences of unique individuals living near the boundaries of life and death. Together these perspectives provide means for evaluating representative theories in these areas in (a) enriching general understanding of lived experience or (b) providing caregivers with entrée into effective dialogue with those in their care to learn about and respond appropriately to their unique needs and experiences.

PERSONAL HISTORY

When my Dad died more than 40 years ago, my young head filled with wonder. Where had the forces that animated his life gone? Where had they come from? What was it like for him to realize that his life would soon end? What did the flow of life through his 73 years mean to him, at the peaks and in the valleys? Why was I still alive and he not? How had sharing 24 years changed us? What would my life mean to me without his presence? What would carry me through sorrow and crisis? What would dying be like for me one day? Why do any of us ever come to life? Where does any single life fit in the vastness of the universe?

I knew I was not alone in wondering about such matters. We humans have been wondering about them since we first began to care about and love one another; experience brokenness and sorrow coming over us; express ourselves in tears, gestures, words, actions, art, and ritual; struggle to overcome suffering; and engage with the mysteries of life. It is said that the search for wisdom begins in wonder, and when my father died, I longed for wisdom in the depth of my being. I have carried such wonder and longing with me ever since.

As I was returning to graduate school after Dad's funeral, I wanted to share my wondering with and seek wisdom from my graduate school philosophy professors. But sadly (and possibly quite mistakenly) I did not feel confident in approaching any of them about matters then so vital to me. Silently, I vowed to myself that I would do my best to become the kind of philosopher that others would want to approach with wonder and invite to join them in seeking wisdom about such things as the meanings of life, love, death, and suffering.

Eventually, my wondering moved me to introduce a course on death and dying for students entering helping professions. I knew they would want wisdom about being with and supporting the dying and the bereaved and about coming to terms with their own mortality. I knew I did not have such wisdom, but I knew we could search together.

Over years of reflecting on my own experiences, hearing and reading stories of literally thousands of others, and wondering with so many students, survivors, family members, friends, teachers, researchers, and caregivers, I've become well acquainted with the contour and depth, poignancy and power of the challenges in facing personal mortality, living while dying, and living meaningfully in the aftermath of loss.

PHILOSOPHY AS LOVE OF WISDOM

It is easy to read Socrates's call for the examined life as an affirmation of the value of wisdom. Plato's dialogues portray Socrates as regularly undermining pretention in knowing and affirming the wisdom of (1) recognizing the limits of one's knowing and (2) reflecting carefully about the challenges of living virtuously and meaningfully, especially in the shadows of uncertainty.

Wise persons weigh *ideas* mindfully, concerning themselves with their truth value and applicability to the realities they encounter. They cultivate understanding of how to refine and adapt ideas to changing experiences that call them into question. They acknowledge the limits of their perspectives and ways of knowing, what they know, and what they can know. Wise persons also evaluate *ways of living* mindfully, concerning themselves with their practical value and appropriateness in their particular embodied, social, and cultural life circumstances. They cultivate understanding of how to adapt and refine ways of living to changing experiences that call them into question. They acknowledge the limits of (1) their habitual ways of living, (2) their control in the responsible exercise of freedom, and (3) what they've learned about how to live. Wise persons remain ever aware of the limits of the application of static ideas, plans, and principles to flowing experiences of dynamic realities. Ultimately, wisdom is a virtue of humility, discernment, imagination, and adaptability in making claims to truth and seeking value and meaning in living.

There is nothing boastful in claiming to be a seeker of wisdom. It is a noble aspiration. Most who so aspire sense that growth in wisdom is incremental, hard-won, worth the trouble, and never finished. Few, if any, are consummately wise, and none would ever claim to be so. Seeking wisdom is not the exclusive province of professional philosophers. Many across the broad spectrum of other disciplines and professions have been driven in wonder to seek wisdom. Because wonder and the impulse to seek wisdom are common human experiences, it is no stretch to say that all conscious and mindful persons are philosophical to some degree.

EXISTENTIAL PHENOMENOLOGY

Life can only be understood backwards; but it must be lived forwards.
—Søren Kierkegaard

Existential philosophers (including Friedrich Nietzsche, Søren Kierkegaard, Martin Heidegger, Karl Jaspers, Jean-Paul Sartre, Simone deBeauvoir, Albert Camus, Gabriel Marcel, Maurice Merleau-Ponty) wonder about what it is to exist as a singular and irreplaceable human being. They seek wisdom about *how to live* given that each of us is a conscious subject at the center of a unique world of experience. We are born into unique life circumstances not of our own choosing. We are grounded in, consciously aware of, and engaged with the world in and through our bodies. We are historical and temporal beings who exist in time, emerging from the past, through the present, and into the future. We find and make meaning in our lives (*lived meaning*) in practical, caring interactions with the world, including our physical surroundings, social surroundings, and selves. We find our identities in the particularities of our unique daily life patterns and life histories of caring interaction with the world. We are social beings, challenged to live meaningfully and with integrity through the responsible exercise of our freedom in the world around us, especially, but not only, with our fellow humans. We are multidimensional beings, at once biological, cognitive, emotional, psychological, behavioral, social, soulful, and spiritual. We are finite beings: small, transitory, vulnerable, uncertain, and fallible. We first *learn how to live* in the world prereflectively, as we seek what we need and desire, acquire abilities, form habits and dispositions, shape life patterns, and move through the days of our lives. Typically, we purposefully reflect, seek knowledge *about* the world, develop theories, make plans, and the like only in extraordinary experiences or when life proves challenging. Most of the time we live unselfconsciously in straightforward engagement with the world.

Phenomenological philosophers, beginning with Edmund Husserl (Spiegelberg, 1960), wonder about the essential features of the experiences within which we encounter and interact with the world. They seek wisdom about how, within experiences appropriate to their objects, we come to *know about the world* and all that is in it, including logical relationships, mathematics, the physical world, the biosphere, our selves, other persons and the social world, relationships, systems, histories, and cultures. In his call, "to the things themselves," Husserl urges that good thinking about anything requires a firm understanding of just what the thing is. Because it is through experiences that we come to know anything, describing and analyzing experiences is crucial for understanding and building the foundations of knowledge, the evidential ground of theory in experience. Intent on capturing the subtlety and nuance of experiences and the richness of what they are about, phenomenologists resist reductionism, or thinking that any experiencing process *has to unfold in a certain way* or that anything experienced *amounts to nothing more than* but one aspect of what it is, or even something else entirely. Phenomenologists would insist that theories *about* death, dying, and bereavement must be grounded in understanding of the distinctive combinations of experiences within which we become familiar with them. They view the stories of those who have the experiences as the heart of the matter in building such theories.

Existential phenomenologists (prominently Heidegger, Sartre, deBeauvoir, Merleau-Ponty, and Paul Ricoeur) add to accurate description and analysis the element of *interpretation* of the lived meanings of experiences. Less interested in experiences of coming to *know about the world* for their own sake, they wonder about experiences of coming to *know how to live* in the world. They extend the use of phenomenological methods to exploration of not only cognitive experiences but also the full ranges of our physical, emotional, psychological, behavioral, social, soulful, and spiritual experiences. They pay special attention to how experiences come to have meaning for us as they shape our daily life patterns, affect the unfolding of our life histories, and contribute to our becoming the individuals we are. Existential phenomenologists seek wisdom about *how to live* with personal mortality, dying, and bereavement. They would insist that counseling with persons facing mortality, dying, or grieving requires attending to the singularities of their experiences and the meanings they find and make in them. The stories they tell, then, are the heart of the matter in fostering self-discovery and mutual understanding among the story-tellers, their caregivers, and members of their families and friendship circles.

FACING PERSONAL MORTALITY

Without death men would scarcely philosophize.
— Arthur Schopenhauer

Experiences of Death and Mortality

We do not experience our own *deaths* directly. One of my professors, William Earle, described our situation with regard to death as like standing in a small pool of light surrounded by vast darkness. If someone were to call attention to the darkness and we to turn flashlights onto it, we would not see darkness but rather more illuminated areas. We know the dark only as the limit of, or background condition of, our light; we cannot *see* it, but we are aware that it is there. We know death itself only as the limit of life as we know it. Those among us who have near-death experiences (Moody, 2001), by no means only in clinical contexts, or extraordinary encounters with those who have died (LaGrand, 1999), experience and interpret them as experiences of a possible afterlife beyond life as we know it rather than as experiences of death or being dead.

We are more directly aware of our own *mortality*, our vulnerability to dying. We may be immediately aware in, for example, experiences of life-threatening illness, serious accidents, disasters, armed conflict, or life under oppressive regimes. Less directly, we may be reminded of our mortality in midlife crises, witnessing the dying and deaths of loved ones, or caring for the dying and bereaved. Such encounters remind us of how attached we are to our bodies, how small and vulnerable we are, and how short our time on Earth is.

Existentialists on Mortality

Jaspers, Kierkegaard, and Heidegger wonder and seek wisdom about death, viewing it as an irreducible limit to our possibilities in living. Jaspers (1969) writes of death as one of the "boundary situations" that define life in the human condition, along with such things as chance and suffering. Although other animals are also mortal, only we humans are capable of knowing our mortality and taking it into account as we exercise our freedom and shape and direct our lives.

Kierkegaard stresses the vital difference between objective and subjective experiences of human mortality (Kierkegaard, 1941). In *objective* experience, we remain at an intellectually safe distance from mortality, focusing on facts, ideas, and theories about it in general. We can recognize that all persons are mortal but not grasp that this means, "I must one day die." In a *subjective* experience, we appropriate the truth of our personal mortality, allowing it to inform our self-understanding, values, and decisions about how to live. Mortality is a defining feature of personal existence that we can either accept and affirm or treat with indifference. Not merely a biological fact about us, its significance permeates all dimensions of our experience. We are not safe and distant from our mortality, even if we ignore it. It is in us as a condition of our existence, part of our present reality. Kierkegaard holds that the seeker of wisdom will attend to how awareness of mortality can affect and transform an entire life as it confers seriousness, urgency, and passion on choice among possible ways of living.

Heidegger (1962) distinguishes between inauthentic and authentic experiences of mortality. In *inauthentic* experience, I remain at a safe, objective distance from death, as if it happens to everyone but has no particular significance for me or for how I live my life. He observes that many of us live in retreat from acknowledging death as something that involves us personally until the end of life is clearly approaching, distracting ourselves in diversions, keeping busy, or investing in unexamined efforts. In *authentic* experiences of mortality, we understand our being as a being-unto-death and acknowledge and accept responsibility for achieving honesty, genuineness, integrity, individuality, and meaning in life in the finite time available.

Heidegger describes five signature characteristics of authentic experience of mortality: (1) It is *unique* among all of the possibilities in living. Authentically embracing this singular possibility grounds and focuses our concern, or care, about all other possibilities, our purpose in living, our individual destiny. (2) It is *nonrelative*. Acknowledging it brings us back to appreciation of how irreplaceable our individual life is. We cannot transfer to another responsibility for living and dying the uniquely mortal life that is ours alone to live. (3) It *cannot be outstripped*. Unlike other possibilities, it is permanent. In authentic experience, facing the possibility of dying frees us for it and the possibility of affirming the whole of our existence before it ends. (4) It is *certain*. In authentic experience, we courageously face the certainty of personal death and recognize its relevance in every moment of life-altering decision. (5) Its *timing is indefinite*. In authentic experience, we are aware that as soon as we are born, we are old enough to die. This awareness awakens in us a constructive anxiety about losing all other possibilities for being in the world. Authentically embracing mortality frees us to evaluate and decide with the whole of our being what matters most to us in living a finite life.

Existential Suffering

Each of us is susceptible to existential suffering that may be defined as "the distress and anguish we experience when limitation, change, loss, brokenness, and sorrow lead us to question our very existence, the value and meaning of our lives" (Attig, 2011a). We may suffer existentially as we wonder what mortality means for who we are and can become, why we are living, what our lives mean or might mean, and whether it is worth continuing to live.

We may recoil in fear before the prospect of dying. Ernest Becker writes as if we can only flee in terror in response to personal mortality and interprets virtually all individual and cultural efforts and achievements as nothing but expressions or manifestations of the fear of death (Becker, 1973). Although there may be elements of fear in what motivates some effort and achievement, this interpretation is decidedly reductionist as it flies in the face of experiences of nearly all of these *as* affirmations of the value and meaning of living. William Worden writes of the possibility of taking the measure of whatever fear of death may come over us, cautioning against both (1) overestimating the extent to which mortality threatens living meaningfully and allowing fear to grip and paralyze us and (2) underestimating the threat and allowing ourselves to live carelessly, without due caution (Worden, 1976). I have described how we struggle to come to terms with the meaning of our own mortality in all dimensions of our being at once, not simply in fear (Attig, 1989). Rachel Naomi Remen writes of mortality and suffering as mysteries rather than everyday problems. As constants in living, we cannot change, control, manage, eliminate them from our experience, or fully understand their meanings. We can only change how we live in response to them. Instead of facing mortality alone, she urges that:

> Perhaps real wisdom lies in not seeking answers at all. Any answer we find will not be true for long. An answer is a place where we can fall asleep as life moves past us to its next question. After all these years I have begun to wonder if the secret of living well is not in having all the answers but in pursuing unanswerable questions in good company. (Remen, 2000, p. 338)

Frankl (1959), writing out of his suffering in Auschwitz says, "Everything can be taken from a man but one thing; the last of human freedoms—to choose one's attitude in any given circumstance, to choose one's own way" (p. 86). This is the freedom the existentialists say comes to light as we suffer existentially and authentically embrace our mortality.

Existentialism Versus Stoicism

Stoicism, ancient and contemporary, promotes one form of authentic response to personal mortality. It recognizes that human life is finite, that all beginnings have endings, all attachments bring eventual separations, and all commitments come with attendant risks. Finding these human limitations to be tragic flaws, stoicism advises that we rein in our passions and hold back from entanglements that will inevitably bring us pain and unhappiness. It sees wisdom in resolving to begin little, minimize attachment, and avoid commitment. Such emotional disengagement from the world leads to peace of mind and a tempered human happiness.

Existentialism promotes an alternative authentic response to personal mortality. It urges acceptance of the finiteness and fragility of human existence and embraces limited opportunities for meaning and fulfillment as fortuitous and precious. It advises persevering in our vulnerability and accepting the hurts and disappointments that come with mortality as the price of realizing the values that beginnings, attachments, and commitments can bring. It sees wisdom in embracing the possibilities of living a finite life meaningfully with the whole of our freedom and passion.

We can see this existential wisdom in response to mortality in Kierkegaard's description of three ways of living in the world: (1) *aesthetic* investment in what interests us; (2) *ethical* adherence to moral principles, making commitments, and taking on responsibilities; and (3) *religious* appreciation of wonder and awe before the mystery, presence, and transcendence of eternal meanings that cannot be touched by death in others, nature, and the divine (Kierkegaard, 1940). We see this wisdom in

Nietzsche's (1999) urging that we should live our lives creatively, as works of art. We see it in deBeauvoir's (2000) urging that we embrace the potential of living ethically and politically with integrity in the face of ineradicable uncertainty and ambiguity.

LIVING WHILE DYING

In my first death and dying classes, I invited a university colleague, Dorothy Hamilton, to come to discuss her experiences of living with terminal cancer. She invariably came around to saying the equivalent of, "I wish I could look each of you in the eye and tell you that we are not so very different. I'm living with cancer, but we are all going to die some day. The only difference is that someone has told me that I am likely to die before you do. But he could be wrong." She reminded us that we are all eligible to die from the moment of birth whether we make that truth our own or not. She urged us not to wait for terminal illness to awaken from indifference to, or avoidance of, mortality and begin living now in terms of what matters most to us.

Coming to Know That We Are Dying

Phenomenologically, the inherent indefiniteness of the time of our dying makes it difficult for anyone to know when death is approaching. Dying most often begins to show itself in our bodies. At first, we may mistake physical changes and symptoms for signs that we are ill, as we have been before and recovered. As they persist or worsen, and often as we experience companion emotional, behavioral, social, or spiritual distress, we commonly turn to physicians. Few of us know enough to tell that we are seriously ill or even dying without expert opinion. If our primary physician cannot, or will not, tell us we may be dying, we will be sent to a specialist.

Nuland (1993, pp. 248–261) describes how the primary focus of specialized medicine falls on the dual challenges in "The Riddle" of (1) coming to a correct diagnosis of life-threatening illness and (2) discerning the most effective ways to cure it. Knowing what is happening in our bodies is often difficult for experts. Diagnosis is often tentative and prognosis more difficult, given wide variation in individual responses to illness, treatments, and procedures. On the way to our physician's solving (or not solving) The Riddle, we may come to know all too well the unpredictable progression of our illness or life-threatening condition, its implications for the quality of our living, medical personnel and institutions, invasive and physically challenging procedures, and their independent serious consequences for our bodies and overall well-being. Doka (1993) describes prediagnostic, diagnostic, chronic, and terminal phases of living with life-threatening illness with uncertainty a near constant companion in all but the last, terminal phase. Glaser and Strauss (1966) describe how, even when others know "the truth" about our dying, we may be kept in uncertainty or not acknowledge it openly as others withhold it, decline to confirm our suspicions, or join us in mutually pretending that matters are not as serious as they are.

In the most well-known account of living while dying, Kübler-Ross (1969) describes it as unfolding in five stages. They are most aptly read as aspects of resistance to recognizing the growing certainty that we are dying, a struggle that often continues long after a serious diagnosis is given. She describes ego fight/flight defenses against the harshness of realities of dying as in *denial* we retreat from persistent reality, with *anger* we try to control the uncontrollable, or in *bargaining* we attempt to negotiate the nonnegotiable. In *depression* we concede the futility of these efforts. We can die at any time before reaching the last stage, *acceptance,* when we acknowledge that we are dying. It is a reductionist mistake to claim that these stages are the sum of "how we cope with dying." *Coming to know that we are dying* is by no means the same as, but can only be the beginning of, learning *how to live while dying.*

When we acknowledge that we are dying, we realize *that* our physical distress, the progress of our illness or condition, and whatever emotional, behavioral, social, and spiritual distress have arisen from it, are all aspects of living while dying. We experience our dying against the horizon of memories of prior illnesses and brushes with mortality, experiences of others that we have witnessed, and social and cultural expectations and understandings that shape and color our present experiences. We also experience our dying against the horizon of often uncertain anticipations of possible challenges and difficulties ahead, approaching the end of life, letting go of goals and aspirations, and parting from those we love.

Meanings in Living While Dying

Meanings in what happens to us

Existential phenomenologists are interested in what dying means, *how we live* while dying. Many experiences of living while dying are *passive*. Physically, taken-for-granted health maintenance and immune systems in our bodies begin to give way beneath our awareness and beyond our control. Others too often treat us as if we are the disease or condition we have rather than the whole persons we are living with the disease or condition. Both Cicely Saunders, founder of the modern hospice movement, and Balfour Mount, founder of hospital-based palliative care, devoted their lives to countering this tendency and wisely promoting whole-person care. Frank (1991) reminds us that we cannot simply drop off our bodies for repairs. Our whole conscious being is *embodied*; we live "at the will of the body." We are consciously aware of and engage with the world through our bodies. Things that happen in our bodies limit what we can do and experience in the rest of our lives. Intense physical suffering makes it nearly impossible to attend to or care about anything else. The progress of disease or a life-limiting condition, treatments and procedures, or their consequences can affect our access to and abilities to move about within our environment, limit our interactions with familiar things and places, undermine our abilities to do things or enjoy doing them, reduce the range and variety of our experiences and activities, compromise our acting on our decisions, distort or undermine our abilities to express ourselves, alter our interactions with others, make us increasingly dependent, distort our awareness of the world around us, and even undermine our capacities to orient ourselves cognitively in reality.

Eric Cassell writes of how we suffer in living while dying as the whole persons we are, from both disease and its treatment (Cassell, 1991). We can define *suffering* as the experiences of loss of wholeness (brokenness) and pain and anguish that come over us. Our suffering may include helplessness before what we cannot control, fear of being overwhelmed, shame in dependence or loss of appearance, longing for life as it was, sensing we do not belong where we are, anguish over connections with those we hold dear, feeling distant from the ground of our being in the divine or the sacred, fear that the world is chaotic or unfair, feeling deserted by faith, doubting our abilities to persevere, fear that joy and laughter are no longer possible, longing for hope and courage to face and venture into the unknown, anguish over what is to become of our loved ones, or doubting the value and meaning of our lives as already lived or as they remain to be lived. Rando's works on "anticipatory mourning" (Rando, 1985, 2000) vividly describe experiences of loss and grief reactions to them as well as the suffering that accompanies anticipation of leaving behind everyone and everything we have cared about in the finite life we know.

We are often gripped, even stopped, by *emotions* as we live while dying. As the etymology of the word "emotion" (attachment of the prefix "e" to "motion") tells us that it literally means "without motion," it captures this aspect of our emotional experiences. It is a mistake to interpret emotions as *nothing but* the physical sensations we associate with them. Judgments about reality and some of our deepest desires and needs are inherent in them (Solomon, 1983). Many interpret emotions as crying for expression to dissipate their energy and power. I prefer to read them (Attig, 2012, p. 40) as like physical pains calling us to attend to things that give rise to them and have serious implications for how we live. Like physical pains, they persist and intensify until we give them and their underlying causes appropriate attention.

Meanings in what we do

Many experiences of living while dying are *active*. As life-threatening illness and life-limiting conditions come into our lives, much of what we do in their shadows involves learning *how to live* within a changing life environment, in relationships with others, and within our own skins, as we reshape our daily life patterns, learn to carry elements of brokenness and sorrow, and focus on what is most important to us in what may be the last chapter or chapters of our life stories. These engagements with major change are active aspects of anticipatory mourning strongly analogous to my interpretation below of grieving response as the active aspect of *relearning the world*.

How much more valuable and urgent is the existentialist wisdom in authentically facing our mortality when we see that our life possibilities are rapidly diminishing! Tragically, many of us become caught up in increasingly futile attempts to find a cure, experience suffering that spirals out of control, or die suddenly without realizing genuine possibilities for living meaningfully while dying. As Weisman and Worden describe the possibility of dying an *appropriate death* (Worden, 2000) and Corr (1992) writes of *task work* in actively coping with dying, they focus of how we can do what matters most to us while dying.

Frankl (1959) describes three possible sources of meaning in living. We can reach for meaning in *achievement values* as we attend to unfinished business, contribute in small ways at home or in community, or put our affairs in order. We can teach others important lessons in how to live through telling or showing the way in what we do (Albom, 1997; Kübler-Ross, 1969). We can help loved ones prepare for living in separation from us (Attig, 2000b); write ethical wills to pass on values, beliefs, and blessings (Baines, 2006); or, in dignity therapy, say what we need to before we die (Chochinov, 2012).

We can reach for meaning in *experiential values* as we savor happenings and encounters in everyday life we may have taken for granted or reach for joy, excitement, awe, and wonder in the extraordinary in events we do not want to miss: nature, the arts, or items on a "bucket list." Many of us treasure experiences in loving relationships most of all.

Finally, we can reach for meaning in *suffering* and attempts to overcome or transcend it. Balfour Mount speaks often of the possibility of *healing* when physical healing is no longer possible, asserting boldly that "a person can die healed."

Defining "healing" as turning *from* suffering *toward* experiences of integrity, wholeness, and inner peace, he believes that deep within we all tend, in hope, toward healing in connections with our deep selves, others, the world perceived through our senses (in nature or music), and ultimate meaning as variously conceived.

Byock (2004) describes how we and our survivors can complete or heal our relationships as we express our love for one another, say thank-you for what we treasure most about each other and our lives together, forgive and ask for forgiveness, and find meaningful ways to say good-bye. He tells compelling stories of interactions among his dying patients and their families that vividly illustrate these healing possibilities (Byock, 1997).

Singh (1998) describes engagement with mystery at the end of life unfolding in three stages. *Chaos* includes letting go of ego defenses and dread of being engulfed or overwhelmed. We sense we are entering unknown depths that appear at first to be dark, mysterious, and "other." In *surrender* we can open to and find healing connection with deeper aspects of ourselves (soul and spirit); review our whole lives with forgiveness, gratitude, and compassion; let go of our sense of separateness; begin to sense that the power our ego had been resisting is a higher power within us; and come to a deep stillness. In *transcendence* we can experience ourselves expanding into a spiritual connection with the most subtle and sacred dimensions of being, the divine or the surrounding mystery that holds us all, and experience the ground of our being as love itself. Singh reports that many dying persons say they have never felt so truly alive; have tears of joy, awe, and gratitude; feel spirit pouring into them; sense the presence of God; and feel that they are "entering into something vast."

BEREAVEMENT AND GRIEVING

Her absence is like the sky, spread over everything.
—C. S. Lewis

Experiences of bereavement and grieving, like C. S. Lewis's when his wife died, are about matters of the heart. They invariably include losing an irreplaceable loved one through death (bereavement); reacting to loss in brokenness and sorrow (suffering); and responding to loss and suffering in a process I have called relearning the world that includes *learning how* to live in a world transformed by loss, carry the pain of missing our loved one, and love in separation.

As perhaps the only existential phenomenologist work in the field, I wrote *How We Grieve: Relearning the World* (Attig, 1996) to capture what I had learned about the general contours and singularities of bereavement and grieving. I describe grieving as relearning *how to live* in the world, including our physical and social surroundings, spiritual place in the world, selves, and ties with the deceased. Where others have described, more or less well, particular dimensions of bereavement and grieving (organic/biological, psychological, cognitive, familial, and social), to my knowledge *How We Grieve* remains the only comprehensive phenomenology of these experiences. The Introduction to the revised edition (Attig, 2011b) explores extensively the view in relation to other writings that I cannot repeat here in detail.

I wrote *The Heart of Grief: Death and the Search for Lasting Love* (Attig, 2000a) to describe more of what I had learned about how love in separation is both possible and desirable and to discuss what I found missing in descriptions of love and lasting connection in other works (Klass, Silverman, & Nickman, 1996). Too often authors, following John Bowlby, write as if attachment were *all there is* to love. Attachment involves holding on to relationships for the security and safety in them. Although there may be elements of attachment in many relationships, it is central in few mature ones, and rarely their most valued aspect. Attachment may sometimes provide a means of staying alive, but rarely if ever a reason for living. Love includes experiences of mutual respect, valuing, caring, generosity, receptivity, and reciprocity. In love we commit to a different way of being with and for others, as we let go of attempts to hold or control and instead engage in soul and spirit with the vitality, depths, and mystery of another.

Coming to Know That a Loved One Has Died

Usually we come to *know that* we have lost a loved one far more directly than we come to know that we are mortal or dying. Most of our loved ones die anticipated deaths from illness. We have contacted or visited them in hospitals, nursing homes, hospices, or at home. Some die suddenly from acute illness, in accidents or disasters, or at the hands of others. Often we see for ourselves that they have died, though if death has been horrible and away from home, some may try to prevent our doing so. In rare and excruciating instances, we do not know with certainty that a loved one has died because their body has not been or cannot be recovered.

Meanings in Bereavement and Grieving

Meanings in what happens to us
Existential phenomenologists are interested in what bereavement and grieving mean *in the living* of them. Many experiences of loss and grief are *passive*. Deaths of our loved ones happen, and we find ourselves in *bereavement*, a state of having lost, or deprivation. Loss brings unwelcome changes into the world of our experience, undermining the rhythm and disrupting the momentum of the flow of our lives. It takes our breath away (Attig, 2012).

In *grief reactions*, brokenness and sorrow *come over us* as we experience the emotional, psychological, physical, behavioral, social, cognitive, soulful, and spiritual impacts of bereavement. We *relearn the world* in reaction as we absorb, or take in, the realities of loss in our individual, family, and community experiences. We experience *brokenness* in shattered illusions of control, invulnerability, and separateness; unraveled individual, familial, and communal daily life patterns; and disrupted individual and collective life stories taken into unanticipated next chapters. Bereavement leaves us still poised in needs, wants, emotions, motivations, habits, dispositions, interaction patterns, expectations, and hopes that shaped *how* we lived when our loved ones were alive that now may no longer find their objects in a world where they have died. Bereavement renders useless all of what we and our families and communities have assumed, or taken for granted, about *how to live* in the presence of our loved one. It undermines our egos' practical functioning and self-confidence, uproots our souls, and shakes our spirits. It often undermines beliefs *about* the world as being more or less safe and just and our place in it secure (Janoff-Bulman, 1992). For most of us this cognitive disenchantment, painful though it may be, is not the most important aspect of the loss of the assumptive world in bereavement. The visceral unsettling losses of the sense that we are safe, the feeling that there is a place where we belong in the great scheme of things, and so much of what we have taken for granted about *how to live* are far more daunting (Attig, 2002).

Our *sorrows* (Attig, 2001b) may include pain that comes when we meet with something that reminds us of separation, or as memories spontaneously surface from within or in conversation among us. This is only rarely the pain of separation anxiety (as attachment theory would have it) but rather the pain of *missing* someone we love. We may experience *ego pain* in helplessness, frustration, disillusionment about fight/flight defenses, or fear of being overwhelmed. We may feel *soul pain* in sadness; longing for the presence of our loved one and all it made possible; homesickness for the familiar, guilt or anger about ties with the deceased; isolation or alienation from others; doubt about caring deeply again; or abandonment by, or loss of trust in, God. We may experience *spirit pain* in despair, discouragement, fear that life is meaningless or joyless, or doubt that we can overcome suffering, face unwelcome change, or open to an unknown future. We may feel *family and community pain* in missing an irreplaceable character in our lives, feeling for others' grieving, or dread for our futures together.

Meanings in what we do

Many experiences in bereavement and grieving are *active*. In *grieving responses*, we invest time and effort in coming to terms with what happens to us in bereavement and grief reactions. We *relearn the world* not by cognitively mastering information but instead by learning *how to live* in all dimensions of our being with our brokenness and sorrow, in our physical surroundings, with those who survive with us, in our place in the great scheme of things, within ourselves, and in our relationship with the one who died.

The labors of relearning the world (labors of love; Attig, 2001a, 2012) are as richly varied as are those of learning how to live from birth. Most often without thinking and in styles uniquely our own, we straightforwardly engage in ways of living we already know well. Sometimes, we self-consciously solve problems. Often we complete relatively small bits of work, or tasks properly so-called. We undertake life long projects of adapting our understandings (sometimes deliberately changing our life narratives), emotions, behavior patterns, and relationships as we meet with new aspects and implications of our losses, what Worden (2009) calls "tasks." In encounters with mysteries of finiteness, change, uncertainty, life, love, suffering, and death inherent in our human condition, we change ourselves and how we live. We do these things in contexts in which we are vulnerable (Attig, 1996) to anguish over unfinished business with the deceased, trauma, disenfranchised grieving (Attig, 2004; Doka, 2002), other challenging social circumstances, and limits of our coping capacities.

We relearn the world as we engage with our sorrows. Sometimes from past experience we sense what our reactions and the needs reflected in them are, are guided in usual ways by them, and feel no need to dwell in or express them. It is only human to experience sorrowful emotions as things we would like to avoid or overcome quickly if possible. So we may respond to them in ego fight/flight defenses (Kübler-Ross & Kessler, 2007) in attempts to control reactions we may experience as threats, failings, or weaknesses (Greenspan, 2003). As they persist and grip us more tightly, we can experience our grief reactions as crying more for attention and understanding than expression. We can reflect on them self-consciously alone or with others. We can use sorrow-friendly practices to befriend our sorrows: to make ourselves at home in our deep selves, dwell compassionately with our suffering, and venture beneath life's surface to discover our deepest needs and capacities to meet them (Attig, 2012). Attending to and learning from sorrows loosens their grip. We can learn to carry sorrow as, through our tears, we meet with and welcome our loved one's soul and spirit in the world around or within us in lasting differences he or she has made. Experiencing the pain of missing them after they've died can then become more and more like the pain of missing them in separation when they lived.

We relearn the world as we draw on our *resilience*, or what is not broken within us (Attig, 2012). Our breath animates our bodies. Our egos, humbled by mysteries, return to practical functioning, dealing with threats, controlling appropriately, solving problems, and fixing when possible. Our souls find sustenance in our surroundings, draw from roots in family and community, and still care and love deeply. Our spirits find hope and courage to rise above suffering, venture into the new, change and grow, know joy again, and seek transcendent understanding. Our love cherishes precious memories and legacies, revives connections with fellow survivors, and opens to new relationships. As we do these things, we revive ourselves, weave a web of old and new cares and loves into our daily lives, and give new direction and meaning to our life stories.

We relearn the world as we learn *how* to love in separation (Attig, 2000a, 2012). We continue loving while apart in ways familiar from when we were apart when our loved ones lived. We find renewed wholeness as we weave threads of enduring connection into our daily life patterns, develop themes of lasting love in next chapters of our lives, and sustain movements of loving and being loved in next figures of the dances of our lives. We "let go" of the living presence of our loved ones and all it made possible and of troubles in ties with them that may cause separation anxiety, anger, or guilt. We forgive our loved ones or ourselves in order to reach through trouble to enduring value and meaning. When we meet with painful reminders of separation, we can reach through the hurt and attend to how the reminders also hold something touched by our loved ones or from our lives together. In such experiences, and through deliberately remembering, we reconnect with some of the best in life (not "inner representations" as some in the field would have it), attend to and are moved by our loved ones here and now, feel the warmth of our love for them, sense their love for us, and enjoy them again in praise and gratitude. We embrace their legacies: material things and genetic inheritances; interests and ways of doing things; ways of making ourselves at home in the familiar, caring, and loving; and ways of reaching for the extraordinary, changing, growing, striving, overcoming, and searching for understanding. We appreciate how our families, our communities, and we are indelibly different because they lived and how we have become, in part, their living legacies.

As we relearn the world in these ways, we can sense that we are returning home in the universe (Attig, 2012). We can draw on belief, trust, and loyalty to life; engage in spiritual practices; pour our souls and spirits into living well again; make ourselves at home in the world around us; give places in our hearts to all of our loved ones as well as to the full range of cares, loves, hopes, and aspirations that make us who we are; acknowledge our good fortune in loving and being loved by the deceased; sense that, in the end, courage, hope, and joy outweigh fear, despair, and sorrow; and live more fully when we are grateful.

LOOKING TO THE FUTURE

The phenomenologist in me appreciates the wonder in efforts to learn about all aspects (physical, emotional, psychological, cognitive, behavioral, social, or spiritual) of lived experiences of facing mortality, living while dying, and grieving. When done well they enable us to be more mindful of these ongoing, primarily prereflective experiences and of the hazards of imposing inapt conceptual frameworks on them. We experience mortality, dying, and grieving in all dimensions of our being at once. It can be useful, but it is inevitably limiting and can be distorting to focus on only one dimension of any of these experiences for research purposes. Good studies have and will continue to shed light on particular aspects of them, but it is wise to be clear about their limited scope. I worry about all-too-prevalent reductionist tendencies to read facing mortality as nothing but fear or terror, to overly medicalize dying, and to pathologize or overly intellectualize grieving. I hope for broader recognition that "the things themselves" to be studied here are the experiences themselves and that the best available evidence, or foundation, for theories about them is in the stories those having them have to tell. Pressures to study only what can be counted or measured should be resisted and more qualitative studies undertaken.

The existentialist in me appreciates the wisdom of recognizing the limited usefulness of generalizations of even the most acutely sensitive phenomenologist in meaningfully informing the singular experiences of individuals in facing mortality, living while dying, or grieving. Although it is safe to say that the generalizations offered here are not irrelevant to the experiences of individuals, we must be clear that they do not, and can never in principle, capture all that is important in their singular experiences. It can be wise to cultivate such insights so we can know what it is reasonable to expect in interacting with or counseling persons having the experiences and become more empathetic. Rather than expressing the insights all too knowingly in interactions with persons caught up in the experiences, it would be wiser to use the insights as mind frames for attuning to the specific details of the lives of the individuals having them. It turns out, paradoxically, that they want both reassurance that their experiences are not outliers, that they are not alone in having them, and empathy and full appreciation of how fresh and unprecedented the experiences are in their lives.

REFERENCES

Albom, M. (1997). *Tuesdays with Morrie: An old man, a young man, and life's greatest lesson*. New York, NY: Doubleday.

Attig, T. (1989). Coping with mortality: An essay on self-mourning. *Death Studies, 13*(4), 361–370.

Attig, T. (1996). *How we grieve: Relearning the world*. New York, NY: Oxford University Press.

Attig, T. (2000a). *The heart of grief: Death and the search for lasting love*. New York, NY: Oxford University Press.

Attig, T. (2000b). Anticipating the transition to loving in absence. In T. A. Rando (Ed.), *Clinical dimensions of anticipatory mourning: Theory and practice* (pp. 115–133). Champaign, IL: Research Press.

Attig, T. (2001a). Relearning the world: Making and finding meanings. In R. Neimeyer (Ed.), *Meaning reconstruction and the experience of loss* (pp. 33–54). Washington, DC: American Psychological Association.

Attig, T. (2001b). Relearning the world: Always complicated, sometimes more than others. In G. R. Cox, R. A. Bendiksen, & R. G. Stevenson (Eds.), *Complicated grieving and bereavement: Understanding and treating people experiencing loss* (pp. 7–19). Amityville, NY: Baywood.

Attig, T. (2002). Questionable assumptions about assumptive worlds. In J. Kaufman (Ed.), *Loss of the assumptive world: A theory of traumatic loss* (pp. 55–70). Washington, DC: Brunner-Routledge.

Attig, T. (2004). Disenfranchised grief revisited: Discounting hope and love. *Omega, 49*(3), 197–215.

Attig, T. (2011a). Existential suffering; Anguish over our human condition. In D. Harris (Ed.), *Counting our losses: Reflecting on change, loss, and transition in everyday life* (pp. 119–125). New York, NY: Taylor and Francis.

Attig, T. (2011b). Introduction. In *How we grieve: Relearning the world* (rev. ed., pp. xxi–lvii). New York, NY: Oxford University Press.

Attig, T. (2012). *Catching your breath in grief . . . and grace will lead you home*. Victoria, British Columbia, Canada: Breath of Life.

Baines, B. (2006). *Ethical wills: Putting your values on paper*. Boston, MA: Da Capo.

Becker, E. (1973). *The denial of death*. New York, NY: Simon and Schuster.

Byock, I. (1997). *Dying well: The prospect for growth at the end of life*. New York, NY: Putnam.

Byock, I. (2004). *The four things that matter most: A book about living*. New York, NY: Simon and Schuster.

Cassell, E. J. (1991). *The nature of suffering and the goals of medicine*. New York, NY: Oxford University Press.

Chochinov, H. M. (2012). *Dignity therapy: Final words for final days*. New York, NY: Oxford University Press.

Corr, C. A. (1992). A task-based approach to coping with dying. *Omega, 24*, 81–94.

deBeauvoir, S. (2000). *The ethics of ambiguity*. New York, NY: Citadel.

Doka, K. J. (1993). *Living with life-threatening illness*. Lexington, MA: Lexington Books.

Doka, K. J. (Ed.). (2002). *Disenfranchised grief: New directions, challenges, and strategies for practice*. Champaign, IL: Research Press.

Frank, A. W. (1991, 2002). *At the will of the body: Reflections on illness*. Boston, MA: Houghton Mifflin.

Frankl, V. (1959). *Man's search for meaning*. New York, NY: Simon and Schuster.

Glaser, B. G., & Strauss, A. (1966). *Awareness of dying*. Chicago, IL: Aldine.

Greenspan, M. (2003). *Healing through the dark emotions: The wisdom of grief, fear, and despair*. Boston, MA: Shambhala.

Heidegger, M. (1962). *Being and time* (J. Macquarrie & J. M. Robinson, Trans.). New York, NY: Harper & Row.

Janoff-Bulman, R. (1992). *Shattered assumptions: Towards a new psychology of trauma*. New York, NY: Free Press.

Jaspers, K. (1969). *Philosophy* (E. B. Ashton, Trans.). Chicago, IL: University of Chicago Press.

Kierkegaard, S. (1940). *Stages on life's way (1845)* (W. Lowrie, Trans.). Princeton, NJ: Princeton University Press.

Kierkegaard, S. (1941). *Concluding unscientific postscript (1846)* (D. Swenson, Trans.). Princeton, NJ: Princeton University Press.

Klass, D., Silverman, P., & Nickman, S. (Eds.). (1996). *Continuing bonds: New understandings of grief*. Washington, DC: Taylor and Francis.

Kübler-Ross, E. (1969). *On death and dying*. New York, NY: Macmillan.

Kübler-Ross, E., & Kessler, D. (2007). *On grief and grieving: Finding the meaning of grief through the five stages of loss*. New York, NY: Scribner's.

LaGrand, L. (1999). *Messages and miracles: Extraordinary experiences of the bereaved*. Woodbury, MN: Llewellyn.

Lewis, C. S. (1976). *A grief observed*. New York, NY: Bantam. Original work published 1961.

Moody, R. A., Jr. (2001). *Life after life*. San Francisco, CA: Harper San Francisco.

Nietzsche, F. (1999). *The birth of tragedy*. Cambridge, UK: Cambridge University Press.

Nuland, S. (1993). *How we die: Reflections on life's final chapter*. New York, NY: Alfred A. Knopf.

Rando, T. A. (Ed.). (1985). *Loss and anticipatory grief*. Lexington, MA: Lexington Books.

Rando, T. A. (Ed.). (2000). *Clinical dimensions of anticipatory mourning: Theory and practice in working with the dying, their loved ones, and their caregivers*. Champaign, IL: Research Press.

Remen, R. N. (2000). *My grandfather's blessings: Stories of strength, refuge, and belonging*. New York, NY: Riverhead Books.

Singh, K. D. (1998). *The grace in dying: How we are transformed spiritually as we die*. San Francisco, CA: HarperCollins.

Solomon, R. (1983). *The passions: The myth and nature of human emotions*. South Bend, IN: University of Notre Dame.

Spiegelberg, H. (1960). *The phenomenological movement: An historical introduction* (Vol. 2). The Hague, Netherlands: Nijhoff.

Worden, J. W. (1976). *PDA: Personal death awareness*. Englewood Cliffs, NJ: Prentice-Hall.

Worden, J. W. (2000). Towards an appropriate death. In T. A. Rando (Ed.), *Clinical dimensions of anticipatory mourning* (pp. 267–277). Champaign, IL: Research Press.

Worden, J. W. (2009). *Grief counseling and grief therapy: A handbook for the mental health practitioner*. New York, NY: Springer Publishing Company.

Judith M. Stillion 2

KNOW THYSELF: PSYCHOLOGY'S CONTRIBUTIONS TO THANATOLOGY

Know then thyself, presume not God to scan
The proper study of Mankind is Man.
—Alexander Pope (1734)

MY ENTRY INTO THE FIELD

The year was 1975. I had completed my doctorate in psychology 2 years before, was teaching a sequence of life-span development courses in psychology at Western Carolina University, and my father was dying. The subject of death rarely, if ever, appeared in the texts I was using. However, I identified myself as a phenomenological/existential psychologist and so had always studied and thought about the search for meaning. It seemed to me at that time, and still does, that awareness of death is intimately attached to questions of meaning. I asked for and received permission to offer a 2-week seminar in the psychology of death and loss. Permission was given with great reluctance and the question, "Who would ever sign up for such a seminar?" The question was answered soundly when we had to close out enrollment at 25 in order to keep it a seminar, rather than a lecture course. I expected that many of the students would have enrolled in order to get an elective out of the way in a 2-week period. To my delight, I found a group of serious students, somewhat older than the usual undergraduate, who read the few materials I had marshaled and went far beyond my expectations in their discussions of the subject matter.

That winter, I attended a national conference on death education, the first of its kind, chaired by Dr. Hannelore Wass in Orlando, Florida. There I found other people who were teaching courses like mine although in many different formats. We had one thing in common. We felt alone at our various institutions in proposing this subject for the curriculum. We decided then that we would share our sources, our class notes, and our syllabi through a forum, which later became the Association for Death Education and Counseling (ADEC). That was the beginning for me of a 40-year study in the psychology of death and dying. When my father died in 1976, my quiet grief was supported by insights gained from my teaching and study.

This chapter will summarize the major strains of psychology that were important in setting the foundation for death studies by psychologists, highlighting some of the most important contributions made by psychology to the field.

The chapter will purposely exclude elements of psychological thinking that are covered in other chapters of this book (e.g., grief theory, suicide prevention and intervention, developmental perspectives, and clinical practice).

EARLY PSYCHOLOGY

In the mid-20th century, the discipline of psychology was less than 100 years old. In those years, it had had little to say about death. Psychology, often regarded as an offshoot of philosophy and biology, traces its origin to Wilhelm Wundt (1897) who was what we today would call an experimental psychologist. Using methods drawn from experimental science, he wrote the first textbook in psychology in 1874 and opened the first laboratory dedicated to the scientific study of the workings of the mind in 1879. Thus began an approach in psychology, still in existence today, that emulates the "hard" sciences in its approach to gaining knowledge. Its insistence on applying the scientific method and its use of ever more complex statistical analyses has led to far greater understanding of such concepts as death anxiety, attitudes toward death and suicide, generational and age-related attitudes, patterns in grief, and many other constructs. It is beyond the scope of this chapter to review the hundreds of studies on death anxiety and death attitudes. For a comprehensive review of the first 40 years of research on death anxiety, see Neimeyer (1994). For an overview of the research on death attitudes, see Neimeyer, Wittkowski, and Moser (2004).

THE PSYCHOANALYTIC MOVEMENT

A parallel track to that of experimental psychology is the development of the psychodynamic approach led by Sigmund Freud. Freud was the first to hypothesize that many of the roots of individual behavior lay unseen and unknown, even to the individual. His well-known concept of the topography of the mind included three levels of individual awareness, which he called the conscious, preconscious, and unconscious. Conscious material made up the majority of our awareness. The preconscious material could be made conscious with appropriate stimuli, whereas unconscious material was beyond the ability of the person to realize without expert probing or hypnosis. This marked the beginning of the practice of psychoanalysis, sometimes called depth psychology. Freud's concept of the unconscious has penetrated Western thought completely and has influenced literature, painting, and therapeutic approaches throughout the past century. It has also been extremely important in the development of the death awareness movement.

In the early 1920s, Freud proposed that the goal of all life is death or a return to the inorganic state (Freud, 1922). He was elaborating on his earlier conception that human energy (or libido) is invested in seeking pleasure and avoiding pain. In this treatise, however, he theorized that libidinal energy may also be devoted to a death instinct. The juxtaposition of one's life instinct (eros) with the death instinct (later called "thanatos") became a central postulate of Freudian psychoanalysis and has led to much research, notably that of Orbach (1988), who wrote about attraction to and repulsion from life among suicidal children.

Most relevant to the field of death and grief were Freud's works *Totem and Taboo* (1913/1956) and *Mourning and Melancholia* (1917/1957). In the first work, Freud explained the ambivalence mourners might feel toward the deceased. He suggested that people in many cultures fail to recognize their relief and unresolved negative feelings toward the deceased. They therefore employ the defense mechanism of projection, which results in their fearing reprisal from the dead person. In this way, Freud explained many of the taboos he found in multiple cultures against speaking the name of the deceased, using their possessions, and so forth, lest the deceased person return to do them harm.

In the second work, Freud expanded on both mourning and melancholia. He described the physical and psychological features of both, noting that they are very similar. He specifically stated that in mourning "it never occurs to us to regard it as a pathological condition and to refer it to treatment (Freud, 1917/1957, p. 243) Melancholia, though, is a different story. It results in a dissolution of the ego as well as the other negative consequences that naturally occur when a close family member or friend dies. "In melancholia, dissatisfaction with the ego on moral grounds is the most outstanding feature" (Freud, 1917/1957, p. 248). Although Freud made the distinction between normal grieving (mourning) and the type of reaction that might need professional support or counseling (melancholia), that distinction has been lost to many who now practice in the counseling arena. At least one current author credits Freud with establishing grief as a "psychological object of study" (Granek, 2010, p. 51).

Freud proposed defense mechanisms that protected the ego. Among them was sublimation, which permitted people to avoid anxiety or other negative emotions by turning them into something positive and approved by society. This ego defense mechanism, coupled with total acceptance of Freud's topography of the mind, became important in understanding such writers as Ernest Becker, who popularized the role of the unconscious in our everyday life. His work *The Denial of Death* (1973) has been influential in many areas. He maintained that all of human endeavors—for example, child bearing and rearing, architecture and art, writing and cooking, farming and building roads—are done in defiance of death.

Lifton (1979) elaborated on this theory. He accepted that fear of death is universal and suggested that well-adjusted people come to grips with that fear by aspiring to a form of symbolic immortality. He suggested five forms of symbolic immortality. The first, biological, is realized through procreation and the bonds of family. The second, creative, is realized through leaving something of value in art, music, or literature or adding to the cumulative knowledge of humankind. The third, transcendental, refers to the power of religion or spirituality to moderate fear of death. The fourth, natural, refers to the belief that we are connected to all that is in nature and will go on being a part of that oneness even after death as the elements that make up the body become a part of the natural world. The fifth, experiential, can be achieved while living. For example, he pointed to the immediacy and depth of emotion experienced in orgasmic ecstasy as a form of stepping outside of time and therefore experiencing a piece of immortality. Lifton also suggested that the fear and denial of death may be channeled into violence toward others who disagree with those values we identify with. Protecting our own worldviews, which are extensions of our desire to avoid death, may lead to scapegoating and even to war.

Although Lifton acknowledged an intellectual debt to Becker, other social psychologists have attempted to operationalize and test some of Becker's assertions regarding denial of death. This has led to the theory of terror management (Greenberg, Pyszczynski, & Solomon, 1986). Basically, this theory accepts the notion that death anxiety is present in all humans and that the ways people cope with such deep awareness of their own mortality is by accepting and dedicating themselves to worldviews that make meaning in their lives. The theory has generated a great deal of research across four decades, much of which indicates that when subjects are reminded of their mortality, they judge people differently from those who do not receive mortality prompts. For example, when reminded of their mortality, subjects judge social deviants more harshly and heroic people less harshly than subjects who have not received mortality prompts. These studies seem to show that consciousness of our own mortality affects our attitudes, strengthening both negative and positive reactions toward others who either deviate from or support our own worldviews (e.g., Rosenblatt, Greenberg, Solomon, Pyszczynski, & Lyon, 1989).

Other notable psychologists of the psychoanalytic school include Alfred Adler and Carl Jung. Both of these practitioners eventually broke with Freud. Jung (1917, 1928) went on to found his own approach to analysis, which he called analytical psychology. His work was wide ranging, including typologies (e.g., extraversion/introversion), the study of symbols in many cultures and the coining of the term *collective unconscious*. Jung accepted Freud's view of the personal unconscious but he believed there was also a collective unconscious, which contained memories of the human species (Jung, 1934, 1954). Within the collective unconscious were universal symbols, one of which was death. He discovered that all of the cultures he studied had images of death deeply imbedded within them and concluded that the species memory of death was universal. This observation served to strengthen the notion that human life in all its aspects is influenced by our recognition of death. Although his work on this subject did not inspire empirical study, it has been largely accepted within the general culture.

Adler (1927/1954), who was greatly influenced by the philosophies of Immanuel Kant, Fredrich Nietzsche, and Karl Marx, founded his own school, which he called individual psychology. It differed from the Freudian approach in that it considered the person as the proper focus of study, rather than some subcomponent, such as the id, ego, or superego. Adler believed the person could best be studied within his or her environmental conditions. Unlike Freud, who believed in the pleasure principle, Adler, following Nietzsche, hypothesized that much of human behavior could be explained by the power principle, which he envisioned as the need to grow toward the ideal. He coined the term "inferiority complex," because he believed that all people strove to move from a position of inferiority to one of superiority, later called self-fulfillment. Although his roots lay in Freudian psychology, his readings in existentialism and his firm belief in moving beyond one's present position to something higher and better qualified him to be considered among the founders of the humanistic/existential school of psychology. His reasoning about the need for power also led later writers to suggest that such a need was present because life is finite. We seek power because of our fear of extinction.

One of the most prominent theorists coming from the psychoanalytic school was Erikson (1959). Although he never studied directly with Freud, he did accept much of Freudian theory. However, he de-emphasized the part that libido plays in life and emphasized psychosocial developmental tasks that must be mastered in each stage or phase of life in order to realize positive mental health. Erikson's stages appear in Table 2.1.

As is true of all the psychological theories explored in the first 100 years of psychology, Erikson's theory reflects his understanding of his own time and place. If he were writing today, there is little doubt that the age ranges for some of the tasks would change even if the tasks themselves remained in the order presented. It is noteworthy that Erikson moved beyond adolescence, suggesting that growth

TABLE 2.1 Erikson's Stages of Psychosocial Development

DEVELOPMENTAL TASK	AGE RANGE
Trust vs. mistrust	0–2
Autonomy vs. shame, doubt	2–4
Initiative vs. guilt	4–6
Industry vs. inferiority	6–12
Identity vs. role diffusion	12–18
Intimacy vs. isolation	18–30
Generativity vs. stagnation	30–65
Ego integrity vs. despair, disgust	65+

occurs throughout the life span. He also taught that individuals can become fixated in or regress to any of these stages depending on their life circumstances and coping abilities. However, it is only in the final stage, that of ego integrity, that he addresses death. Erikson believed that the mentally healthy adult above age 65 was capable of attaining wisdom. He believed the developmental task of that phase of life is coming to grips with the meaning of one's individual life and thereby coming to terms with the end of life. Persons who achieve ego integrity should show little fear of death. Put another way, the well-adjusted elder should have high death acceptance or at least lower death anxiety. Much of the research of the 20th century supports this observation (e.g., Bengston, Curllar, & Ragan, 1977; Kalish & Johnson, 1972; Templer, 1971).

HUMANISTIC/EXISTENTIAL PSYCHOLOGY

A third school of 20th-century psychology is humanistic/existential psychology. Influenced greatly by existential philosophy, this school of thought was led by such luminaries as Abraham Maslow, Viktor Frankl, and Irvin Yalom. Largely a reaction to both experimental and psychoanalytic thought, this school emphasized individual human responsibility. It also focused on the ability of the human being to mature and develop his or her own positive mental health. It illuminated human potential, stressing the positive growth that was possible for human beings to attain and thus could be conceptualized as height psychology. The most widely used concept from this school of thought was Maslow's hierarchy of needs (Maslow, 1954). This construct came to be taught in all introductory psychology courses as well as in business schools, nursing education, criminal justice, and many other disciplines. It described a ladder-like progression by which humans could move from meeting basic physical and safety needs through love and esteem to a state of self-actualization. At the base are physiological needs like water, food, sex, sleep, and so forth. The second level involves safety needs and includes security of the body, employment, resources, health, and so forth. At the third level are needs for love and belonging evidenced by friendship, family, and sexual intimacy. The fourth level consists of esteem needs, including self-esteem, confidence, achievement, and respect of self and others. The fifth level is what Maslow called self-actualization. It is marked by such elements as lack of prejudice, morality, creativity, problem solving, and acceptance of facts. In later years, Maslow extended his hierarchy to include cognitive and aesthetic needs (Maslow, 1970a) and transcendence needs (Maslow, 1970b).

Frankl (1963) developed his own form of existential therapy called logotherapy. In his influential book, *Man's Search for Meaning*, he proposed that the main motivation in living is our desire to find meaning in life. He believed that life has meaning no matter what the circumstances and that humans always have the freedom to find meaning in what we do or create, what we experience and learn from experiencing, or at the very least in the stance we take in the face of unchangeable suffering. Logotherapy has been used with the dying, and at least one study (Zuehlkke & Watkins, 1977) found it to be useful in reducing the anxiety of dying patients.

Of all the existential psychologists, Irvin Yalom wrote most directly about the fear of death as it related to seeking meaning (Yalom, 1980). In addition to writing explicitly about existential psychotherapy, he wrote a popular book about the human fear of death and the multiple ways we try to disguise it, transcend it, or deny it (Yalom, 2008). He defined existential psychotherapy as "a dynamic approach to therapy which focuses on concerns that are rooted in the individual's existence" (Yalom, 1980, p. 5). His approach to therapy involves helping individuals become aware of the role that death anxiety has played and is playing in their lives. Working with dying people, he wrote lucidly about ways to find meaning in the face of death: altruism (leaving the world a better place in which to live, serving other people, dedicating oneself to a larger purpose) and creativity in self-expression that may be a gift to the world or lead to self-actualization or self-transcendence by moving beyond self-absorption to true caring for others or for larger causes. Yalom believes that the key processes of therapeutic change lie in such psychic phenomena as "willing (openness to change), assuming responsibility, relating to the therapist, and engaging in life" (Yalom, 1980, p. 485). Providing a therapeutic environment that fosters the growth of such abilities can alleviate the existential anxiety that results from being aware of one's mortality.

COGNITIVE PSYCHOLOGY AND COGNITIVE BEHAVIORISM

A fourth major 20th-century approach to human behavior is the study of cognition, led by Piaget (1926, 1969) whose methods differed from the experimentalists in that he used small samples of children and studied them in depth and longitudinally. He began by studying his own children but soon was able to describe the pattern of stages in the cognitive reasoning of children. In the first stage, sensorimotor, Piaget hypothesized that the child comes to know his world through his senses, particularly his oral sense. The two preconventional stages (ages 2–7) are marked by growing capabilities to conserve number, mass, and volume. The conventional stage, from about 7 until 11 years of age, is the age of the scientist as children explore their world using developing cognitive skills and come to understand the natural world around them. The final stage in Piaget's theory, which begins around age 12, is that of formal operations, sometimes conceived as the age of the philosopher. With the changes that occur in puberty flooding the developing brain, children develop the ability to ask meaningful questions, such as "Why is there injustice in the world?" These questions also include, "What is the meaning of life when its end is always death?"

One of the earliest studies using Piaget's theory showed that children's concepts of death followed the Piagetian structure (Schilder & Wechsler, 1934). Another classical study suggested that a firm understanding of death's permanence, universality, and irreversibility was not present in children before the age of 10 or 12 (Nagy, 1948). By 1994, there were more than 100 studies concerning children's understanding of death (Speece, 1995). Subsequent studies have lowered the age at which children attain mature understandings of death. Indeed, depending on life circumstances and their exposure to death, children as young as 5 years old have evidenced a real understanding of death (Speece & Brent, 1984). Piaget gave us a glimpse into how such age differences can be found by different researchers at different times. He postulated that humans create schemas (structures) in their minds. As they learn new material, they either assimilate it (add it to existing schemas) or accommodate it (change existing structures to integrate new material). In this way, children exposed to death and grief at earlier ages would change their schema concerning the meaning of death toward a more mature construct than would same-age children who had little or no experience of death.

Other cognitively oriented psychologists formulated the cognitive–behaviorist school of psychology. Among the best known are Albert Ellis and Aaron Beck. Ellis created an approach known as rational-emotive therapy (RET), later called rational-emotive behavioral therapy (REBT), which taught people to cope by using a four-step approach (ABCD) to problems (Ellis, 1963, 1977). The first step, he taught, was to identify the problem facing you, the **A**ntecedent (A) condition or **A**ctivating event. The next step was to identify your feelings about the problem—the **C**onsequences of A. Then, the most important step came into play; the identification of the belief system (**B**). Contrary to most people's understandings, it is what comes between the antecedent condition and its consequences that is most important and is often not consciously considered. For example, grieving people can easily identify the A in this formula as the death of a loved one. They can also recognize their feelings of loneliness and isolation, depression, and even some physical sequelae caused by the loss. But a rational-emotive-behavioral therapist would challenge the person to pause, go back, and uncover his/her belief system surrounding the death (e.g., I'll never be loved by anyone else again; I'll never be happy again; I can't go on without him/her; it's unfair that my child should have died so young; this loss will kill me, etc.). Having identified the specific beliefs, the therapist would explore ways to dispute (D) each of them. An example of disputation would be to challenge the belief that a particular person believes he or she cannot go on after loss. Ellis would call this a neurotic fallacy and would point out that the choice to go on is his or hers to make. Further, Ellis would probe to see what remains worthwhile in his or her life and what new avenues he or she could explore that would enable him or her to go on.

Aaron Beck, sometimes called the father of cognitive therapy, contributed prolifically to research on depression and suicide in such works as *the Diagnosis of Depression* (1967) and *Depression: Causes and Treatment* (1972). Today, the Beck Depression Inventory, the Beck Hopelessness Scale, and the Beck Anxiety Inventory are widely used in research on clinical depression. His approach to therapy is similar to that of Ellis in that he advocates that therapists help clients develop skills to test and modify beliefs as well as to recognize distorted thinking and identify behavior patterns that are nonproductive and plot ways to change them. Cognitive therapy has become a major approach for dealing with grieving, depressed, and suicidal persons. The major criticism of the practice is that it is too cognitive in nature, depending on the rational mind to address situations that are more holistic in nature.

POSITIVE PSYCHOLOGY

In 1998, a new approach to understanding human beings burst upon the scene (Seligman & Csikszentmihaly, (2000)). It is eclectic in nature and has its roots in all the schools of psychology discussed earlier. From the experimental school, it takes its emphasis on using the scientific method to study human behavior. Indeed, this approach was founded by Martin Seligman, whose previous work was grounded in experimental psychology. He is well known for his operant conditioning of dogs, which induced learned helplessness after multiple inescapable shocks. His model of learned helplessness became the model for human depression in those who could not escape their life circumstances and has great relevance for treating depression and suicidal behavior. However, after several decades of dealing with the depressed and people with other types of mental illnesses, Seligman decided to focus on the positive aspects of the human condition. From the psychoanalytic school, positive psychology takes permission to study unseen behavior. It accepts the notions of the unconscious and the use of ego defense mechanisms. It perhaps owes its greatest debt to the humanistic/ existential school of psychology in that it stresses the human potential for growth.

Proponents of positive psychology celebrate what the discipline has achieved during its first century of existence (e.g., treatments for depression, psychosis, schizophrenia, etc.; testing methods for personality and many kinds of intelligences; classification systems for mental illnesses, etc.). However, they criticize the discipline for dealing mainly with mental illness, emotional deficiencies, and crisis situations. They believe it is important to include the study of the strengths inherent in the human condition and proclaim that the psychology of the 21st century will help people move beyond "normal" adjustment into a realm where they can flourish (Seligman, 2011).

In order to fully understand what this approach brings to the study of death, dying, grief, and loss, it is necessary to understand its general structure and mission. Briefly, the founders of positive psychology aim to move the discipline of psychology into the study of happiness and well-being. They seek also to develop a data-based and replicable body of work that can be shown to produce positive well-being in non–mentally-ill people. They have produced a volume that defines and classifies characteristics of healthy functioning in much the same way that the *Diagnostic and Statistical Manual of Mental Disorders* (*DSM-5*; American Psychiatric Association, 2013) used by the social sciences does for mental illness (Peterson & Seligman, 2004). Focusing on the ways in which humans can flourish, proponents reject the idea that constructs, such as human strengths, happiness, and optimism, cannot be measured using experimental methods as well as qualitative and case study approaches, thus combining both the humanist and the experimental schools of the 20th century. Using newly available technology, the founders of positive psychology adopt the attitude that their exercises and experiments should be available to all people to use with others and on themselves. In other words, the findings of positive psychology are to be shared broadly, rather than used to enrich a few practitioners in the field.

At the core of positive psychology is the acknowledgment that six ancient virtues promoted in oral traditions as well as sacred religious and classical philosophical texts are universal across time and across cultures. Each virtue is made up of several strengths as seen in Table 2.2.

Although the virtues are general categories of positive behavior, the strengths are the hallmarks of positive mental health. Specific exercises for developing the strengths exist, permitting people to practice, increasing their current levels of the strength, and becoming ever healthier. Researchers in positive psychology have been collecting data on the efficacy of these exercises for more than a decade.

TABLE 2.2 Virtues and Strengths as Defined in Positive Psychology

VIRTUES	STRENGTHS
Transcendence—beliefs and practices that are grounded in the conviction that there is a transcendent (nonphysical) dimension of life; the opposite of nihilism	Appreciation of beauty and excellence, gratitude, hope, humor, spirituality
Wisdom and Knowledge—a noble form of intelligence; knowledge hard fought for and then used for good	Creativity, curiosity, open-mindedness, love of learning, perspective (wisdom)
Courage—includes physical, moral, and psychological bravery; composed of not just observable acts but of the cognitions, emotions, motivations, and decisions that bring them about	Bravery (valor), persistence (perseverance, industriousness), integrity, vitality
Humanity and Love—interpersonal strengths; altruistic or prosocial behavior	Love, kindness, social intelligence
Justice—refers generally to what makes life fair; fairness of opportunity	Citizenship, fairness, leadership
Temperance—control over excess; a form of self-denial that is ultimately generous to the self or others	Forgiveness and mercy, humility, prudence, self-regulation (self-control)

One of the major benefits of using this approach is that it does not assume that grief is an illness. Rather, it takes people where they are in grieving their loss, whether the death of a loved one or the imminent death of self, and gives them specific types of support, companioning them while offering specific tools for their use. I have written elsewhere about the use of positive psychology with grievers (Stillion, 2013) and space does not permit an exploration of each virtue here. Suffice it to say that both attitudes and behaviors change as grieving people understand their strengths and follow the exercises that have been shown to be effective in promoting positive mental health. All of the virtues and their accompanying strengths hold promise for grieving people, but the one virtue that I have found most useful to consider both with dying and grieving people is transcendence.

From its inception, the founders of this approach have believed that transcendence, defined as the belief that there is some larger meaning or purpose in life, is an innate component of the human condition. Facing one's own death or the death of a beloved person often challenges such a belief. The five strengths that fit under transcendence are able to take us outside our self-concerns. Gratitude, especially, if practiced regularly, broadens our appreciation of life even in the face of death. Appreciating the beauty around us gives us a brief vacation from the depths of grieving, while seeking out and responding to humor can buffer even our deepest sadness. It is a gift in that it enables us to experience joy even when faced with adversity. Hope, of course, brings with it the ability to envision positive aspects of a future without a loved one that we would welcome or even to face our own death in a more positive frame of mind. We can hope for a pain-free day or for good things for our loved ones or, if our faith permits, for a better life after death.

Finally, humans are programmed for spirituality of some sort. Indeed, research on brain activity is accumulating that shows that when people meditate or pray, there are accompanying changes in brain activity that promote a feeling of universality or oneness with all that is (Newberg, D'Aquili, & Rouse, 2001). There have even been suggestions that part of our brain is specifically formed to worship something greater than ourselves (The Dana Foundation, 2009). Whatever the situation, tapping into the spiritual nature of dying or grieving people can lend support to them in periods of crisis.

Proponents of positive psychology have also attempted to define what is meant by the "full life" (Seligman, 2002). An understanding of this concept may help grief counselors and therapists to help their clients find balance in their grief. To experience the full life, one must exercise at least three approaches.

The first approach is that of pleasure. Grief often undermines this dimension. In grief, we find ourselves experiencing the opposite of pleasure. Even if grieving people should find pleasure in some activity or occurrence, they often experience guilt for having experienced that pleasure and find themselves back in the depths of grief once again. A positive psychology approach gives permission to once again find pleasure even in the midst of grief. Stressing the need for finding something that gives physical pleasure (e.g., getting a massage, savoring a good meal) is a routine practice of positive psychologists working with grieving people.

The second approach is called engagement. Fully functioning people experience engagement often. They find themselves losing track of time and their surroundings as they work on a special project, meditate deeply, read a good book, paint or sculpt, write a poem or article, and so forth. Csikszentmihalyi (1990) refers to this experience as "flow." For grievers, this type of engagement can be regarded as "taking a mini-vacation from grief." Such short respites fit well within the dual-process theory of grieving, which suggests that normal grievers move between confronting and avoiding the difficult work of grief (Stroebe & Shut, 1999; for a full review, see Richardson, 2010).

The third approach to a full life is finding meaning. As we grieve or face our own mortality, we often have to reevaluate our purpose in life. It has been suggested that life review is a natural practice among aging people. Butler (1963) defined the concept as follows:

> A naturally occurring, universal mental process characterized by the progressive return to consciousness of past experience, and particularly, the resurgence of unresolved conflicts; simultaneously, and normally, these revived experiences and conflicts can be surveyed and reintegrated . . . prompted by the realization of approaching dissolution and death, and the inability to maintain one's sense of personal invulnerability. (p. 66)

Concerned caregivers and/or friends can help grievers recognize the values that have guided and may still guide their lives. Arriving at an understanding that one's life has had meaning or determining to seek such meaning in the time remaining challenges both grievers and those who are facing death to make the most of life.

ECLECTIC THINKERS

Some contemporary thinkers who have contributed greatly to psychology's view of death and dying cannot be fitted into any one school. They are highly creative people who have mastered other schools of thought but have gone on to create their own gifts to the field. There is room here only to speak about three of them: Robert Kastenbaum, William Worden, and Robert Neimeyer.

Some of the most original and compelling work in psychology was done by Robert Kastenbaum. A Renaissance man who wrote plays, books, and poetry, Kastenbaum studied many cultures and his work has broadened the minds of students for 50 years. He was a founding editor (with Robert Fulton and Richard Kalish) of the journal, *Omega: Journal of Death and Dying*, and he introduced the idea of a "death system" that each society develops in order to interpret death for its citizens. He defined the death system as "the interpersonal, sociocultural, and symbolic network through which an individual's relationship to mortality is mediated by his or her society" (Kastenbaum, 2001, p. 66). It includes roles (e.g., coroners, funeral directors), places (e.g., hospitals, hospices), times (e.g., Day of the Dead, in Mexican culture), objects (e.g., caskets, skull and crossbones), and rituals (e.g., funeral, "last rites").

In the third edition of his book, *Psychology of Death* (2000), Kastenbaum took a modified life-span approach to understanding death and examined Freud's concept of thanatos versus eros in a chapter entitled, "A Will to Live and an Instinct to Die?" Although he had criticized mainstream psychology for turning a blind eye to the importance of death, dying, and grief until quite late in the 20th century, he summarized psychology's growing interest in the field in a chapter entitled "Dying: Toward a Psychological Perspective." He was open to new information throughout his life and raised issues and questions, rather than settling for pat answers. In this way, he served as a model to psychologists who want to share their knowledge while continuing to grow throughout their lifetimes.

William Worden is the first clinical psychologist to differentiate between counseling and therapy early in the development of the field of thanatology. His book, *Grief Counseling and Grief Therapy* (2008), is now in its fourth edition and should be required reading for all psychologists, whether they want to work in end-of-life situations or not because of its thorough differentiation between the type of grief that can benefit from a counseling approach as opposed to the type of grief that needs extended and/or longer and deeper therapy. In the fourth edition of his book, he has revised his earlier discussion of the four tasks of grieving in order to recognize new thinking and research in the field, including meaning making, resilience, and continuing bonds. His continuous studying and clinical experience ensures that his work will remain useful and inspiring.

Robert Neimeyer, whose work appears in this volume, has been a prolific and original thinker in the developing field of thanatology. He succeeded Hannelore Wass as the editor of the journal *Death Studies* and has blended his interest in personal construct theory with his approach to grief in his writing, teaching, and clinical work. His voice continues to be heard worldwide within the area of psychological approaches to death and grief.

FACING THE FUTURE

Psychology is not a unitary discipline. It is made up of developmental, experimental, social, clinical, counseling, cognitive, and many other areas that defy simple classifications. That is both its strength and its challenge. How will the many dimensions of psychology begin to come together to develop a coherent body of knowledge concerning death and grief across the life span? Kastenbaum (2000) began the conversation, but it will take many voices from the many areas in psychology to develop a truly comprehensive psychology of death, dying, and bereavement.

A second challenge for psychologists lies in finding ways to marry research and clinical practice. Even now workgroups in the Association for Death Education and Counselin: the Thanatolgy Association (ADEC) and International Work Group on Death, Dying and Bereavement (IWG) are leading the way in this effort. This trend will undoubtedly increase in the future, providing a tested base for new students entering psychology.

A third major issue for psychology is finding ways to integrate the study of death, dying, and grief into both the undergraduate and graduate curricula. This is especially important for those who are entering counseling or clinical psychology. Without such exposure, new professionals will not be willing or able to confront the existential issues that may lie behind many of their clients' problems. Indeed, examining their own personal understandings and attitudes toward death, dying, and grief in order to be prepared to recognize and respond to their clients would advantage students as well as practitioners in every helping profession.

A fourth challenge for current and future psychologists lies in mastering the growing literature in the field. When I entered the field in 1975, one could read everything that was available in a few weeks' time. Today, the task is daunting and becoming more so with every passing year. However, it is essential that psychologists understand past theories and research as well as those that are current. We all stand on the shoulders of giants who came before us. For those psychologists who choose to center their research or practice on end-of-life issues, the task will be to create their own approaches based on familiarity with the work of the past augmented by understanding of the current rich interdisciplinary work that is the promise of the future.

Perhaps the most promising development for psychologists lies in the growing understanding of the interface between biology and psychology. The mind–body dualism of Descartes is well behind us now. It is clear that the mind and the body are one. Some dying people need psychological as well as medical treatment. Some grieving people need to be able to use both physical (e.g., exercise and nutritional resources) and psychological (e.g., counseling or therapy if and when needed). Both grieving and dying people will be ever more advantaged by the growing recognition that mind–body approaches are more effective than either approach alone. A fuller understanding of the brain as it interacts with emotions and attitudes should advantage those who are counseling with dying and bereaved people as they work alongside medical doctors to reduce the pain and suffering experienced by those dying or bereaved. New understandings being promulgated by neuroscientists will certainly expand treatment approaches in this century, and psychologists will need to be able to incorporate such approaches into their practices.

Psychology has come a long way in recognizing and incorporating the study of death, dying, and grief into its mainstream in the past three quarters of a century. The remainder of the 21st century should see full integration as researchers and practitioners respond to the challenges presented above.

REFERENCES

Adler, A. (1954). The practice and theory of individual psychology. In H. L. Ansbacher & R. R. Ansbacher (Eds.), *The individual psychology of Alfred Adler*. New York, NY: Basic Books. (Reprinted from *The practice and theory of individual psychology* by A. Adler, 1927, Totowa, NJ: Rowman & Allanheid)

American Psychiatric Association. (2013). *Diagnostic and statistical manual of mental disorders* (5th ed.). Arlington, VA: American Psychiatric Press.

Beck, A. (1967). *The diagnosis and management of depression*. Philadelphia, PA: University of Pennsylvania Press.

Beck, A. (1972). *Depression: Causes and treatment*. Philadelphia, PA: University of Pennsylvania Press.

Becker, E. (1973). *The denial of death*. New York, NY: Free Press.

Bengston, V., Cuellar, J., & Ragan, P. (1977). Stratum contrasts and similarities in attitudes toward death. *Journal of Gerontology, 32*, 76–88.

Butler, R. (1963). The life review: An interpretation of reminiscence in the aged. *Psychiatry, 26*, 65–76.

Csikszentmihalyi, M. (1990). *Flow: the psychology of optimal experience*. NY: Harper and Row

The Dana Foundation. (2009, December 1). *Religion and the brain: A debate*. Retrieved from http://www.Dana.org/news/cerebrum/detail.aspx?id=24068

Ellis, A. (1963). *Reason and emotion in psychotherapy*. New York, NY: Lyle Stuart.

Ellis, A. & Greiger, R. (1977). *Handbook of rational-emotive therapy*. New York, NY: Springer Publishing Company.

Erikson, E. H. (1959). *Identity and the life cycle*. New York, NY: International Universities Press.

Frankl, V. (1963). *Man's search for meaning: An introduction to logotherapy* (I. Lasch, Trans.). New York, NY: Washington Square Press.

Freud, S. (1956). Totem and taboo: Resemblances between the psychic lives of savages and neurotics. In J. Strachey (Ed. & Trans.), *The standard edition of the complete psychological works of Sigmund Freud* (Vol. XIII, pp. 1–161). London, UK: The Hogarth Press and the Institute of Psycho-analysis. (Original work published 1913).

Freud, S. (1957). Mourning and melancholia. In J. Strachey (Ed. & Trans.), *The standard edition of the complete works of Sigmund Freud* (Vol. XIV, pp. 239–260). London, UK: The Hogarth Press and the Institute of Psycho-analysis. (Original work published 1917)

Freud, S. (1922). *Beyond the pleasure principle*. (trans. C. Hubback) London: International Psycho-analytic Press.

Granek, L. (2010). Grief as pathology: The evolution of grief theory in psychology from Freud to the present. *History of Psychology, 13*(1), 46–73.

Greenberg, J., Pyszczynski, T., & Solomon, S. (1986). The causes and consequences of a need for self-esteem: A terror management theory. In R. F. Baumeister (Ed.), *Public self and private self* (pp. 189–212). New York, NY: Springer-Verlag.

Jung, C. (1917, 1928) Two essays on Analytic Psychology (1966 revised second edition, Collected Works, Vol 7, London: UK: Routledge.

Jung, C. (1934, 1954). The archetypes and the collective unconscious. (1981) 2nd edition Collected Works, Vol 9, part 1, Princeton, NJ: Bollingen

Kalish, R., & Johnson, A. (1972). Value similarities and differences in three generations of women. *Journal of Marriage and the Family, 34*, 49–54.

Kastenbaum, R. (2000). *The psychology of death* (3rd ed.). New York, NY: Springer Publishing Company.

Kastenbaum, R. (2001). *Death, society and human experience* (7th ed.). Englewood Cliffs, NJ: Prentice-Hall.

Lifton, R. (1979). *The broken connection: On death and the continuity of life*. New York, NY: Simon and Schuster.

Maslow, A. (1954) *Motivation and personality*. New York: Harper

Maslow, A. H. (1970a). *Motivation and personality*. New York, NY: Harper & Row.

Maslow, A. H. (1970b). *Religions, values, and peak experiences*. New York, NY: Penguin. (Original work published 1964)

Nagy, M. (1948). The child's theories concerning death. *Journal of Genetic Psychology, 73*, 3–27.

Neimeyer, R. (1994). *Death anxiety handbook: Research, instrumentation & application*. Washington, DC: Taylor & Francis.

Neimeyer, R., Wittkowski, J., & Moser, R. (2004). Psychological research on death attitudes: An overview and evaluation. *Death Studies, 28*(4), 309–340.

Newberg, A., D'Aquili, E., & Rouse, V. (2001). *Why God won't go away: Brains, science and the biology of belief*. New York, NY: Ballantine Books.

Orbach, I. (1988). *Children who don't want to live: Understanding and treating the suicidal child*. San Francisco, CA: Jossey-Bass.

Piaget, J. (1926). *The language and thought of the child*. New York, NY: Harcourt Brace.

Piaget, J., & Inhelder, B. (1969). *The psychology of the child*. New York, NY: Basic Books.

Peterson, C., & Seligman, M. E. P. (2004). *Character strengths and virtues: A handbook and classification*. New York, NY: Oxford University Press.

Richardson, V. E. (2010). The dual process model of coping with bereavement: A decade later. *Omega: Journal of Death and Dying, 61*(4), 269–371.

Rosenblatt, A., Greenberg, J., Solomon, S., Pyszczynski, T., & Lyon, D. (1989). Evidence for terror management theory: I. The effects of mortality salience on reactions to those who violate or uphold cultural values. *Journal of Personality and Social Psychology, 57*(4), 681–690.

Seligman, M. E. P. (2002). *Authentic happiness*. New York, NY: Free Press.

Seligman, M. E. P. (2011). *Flourish: A visionary new understanding of happiness and well-being*. New York, NY: Free Press.

Seligman, M. E. P., & Csikszentmihalyi, M. (2000). Positive psychology: An introduction. *American Psychologist, 55*, 5–14.

Schilder, P., & Wechsler, D. (1934). The attitude of children towards death. *Journal of Genetic Psychology, 45*, 406–451.

Speece, M. (1995). Children's concepts of death. *Michigan Family Review, 1*(1), 57–69.

Speece, M., & Brent, S. (1984). Children's understanding of death: A review of three components of a death concept. *Child Development, 55*, 1671–1656.

Stillion, J. (2013). Accentuate the positive: The use of positive psychology with grief groups. In H. Shanun-Klein (Ed.), *Studies of grief and bereavement* (pp. 19–34). New York, NY: Nova.

Stroebe, M. & Schut, H. (1999). The dual process model of coping with bereavement: Rationale and description. *Death Studies, 23*, 197–224.

Templer, D. I. (1971). Death anxiety as related to depression and health of retired persons. *Journal of Gerontology, 26*, 521–523.

Worden, J. W. (2008). *Grief counseling and grief therapy: A handbook for the mental health practitioner*. New York, NY: Springer Publishing Company.

Wundt, W. (1897). *Grundriss der Psychologie*. Leipzig, Germany: Engelmann. (Revised editions in 1897, 1898, 1901, 1902, 1904, 1905, 1907, 1909, 1911, followed by five unaltered editions)

Yalom, I. (1980). *Existential psycholtherapy*. New York, NY: Basic Books.

Yalom, I. (2008). *Staring at the sun: Overcoming the terror of death*. San Francisco, CA: Jossey-Bass.

Zuehke, T & Watkins, J. (1977) Psychotherapy with terminally ill cancer patients. *Psychotherapy Theory Research & Practice, 14* (4), 403–410.

Tony Walter

3

SOCIOLOGICAL PERSPECTIVES ON DEATH, DYING, AND BEREAVEMENT

WHAT DRAWS A SOCIOLOGIST TO STUDY DEATH?

First Stirrings

As an English sociologist, my motivation to study death and society has two roots: intellectual and practical. In the 1970s, I was fascinated by American sociologist Peter Berger's (1969) statement that "Every human society is, in the last resort, men banded together in the face of death" (p. 52); social order staves off the chaos brought by death. Culture provides a canopy, and religion a sacred canopy, that outlasts the individual and protects us from the meaninglessness implied by mortality. In this view, death, far from being just a minor subfield within sociology, becomes central to any understanding of society and of culture. In practice, it has not proved central to sociology, including Berger's. My own research and teaching, too, have proved more modest, contributing to the sociology of death as a subfield within sociology, particularly British sociology. So much for youthful ambitions!

Although I wrote a couple of early pieces (one on culture and the other on an Alpine mountaineering museum) in which death was central to the analysis, it was not until my father died in 1985 that I concentrated on researching, writing, and teaching about death and society, which I have done ever since. He gave his body to the local medical school, and without a body there is no need for a funeral or a funeral director; if the family wish to have some kind of ceremony, they have to create it themselves. This we did. At just this time I had been asked to teach a course on the sociology of religion, so my explorations of how ritual is constructed were intellectual as well as practical. I then found myself comparing my father's memorial ceremony positively against a number of funerals I had recently attended, which had not, I felt, done justice to the deceased's rich life. Thus I came to research and write *Funerals—And How to Improve Them* (Walter, 1990), one of many such books that came to be published in the United Kingdom in the 1990s campaigning for more personal, meaningful funerals with more family involvement. I soon found myself being asked to help train clergy in funeral ministry, and since the early 2000s, I have regularly trained civil funeral celebrants.[1] So improving funeral rites formed the initial practical motivation for studying and teaching death and society.[2]

Later Developments

Over time, my practical concerns extended beyond funerals. I have urged therapists to attend not only to their bereaved clients' feelings but also to what their clients say about the dead. I am concerned that neighborhoods engage more with their dying and bereaved members (hence the need to research social networks), and that the United Kingdom become a more friendly place for those dying in frail old age or with dementia—they have received barely a fraction of the research, support, and attention paid to those dying "out of time" from cancer, in childhood, or from suicide. Yet it is the fear of being abandoned in deep old age, unable to communicate after stroke or dementia, becoming no longer a person but just a body to be fed and watered, that haunts so many members of advanced industrial societies.

Intellectually, it has proved fascinating to work in a subfield of sociology that, in the United Kingdom at least, was new; it was possible to explore many different aspects, rather than getting hyperspecialized as happens in more mature academic fields. To research various aspects of death and society, I have had to get acquainted with sociological approaches to not only religion, but also medicine, the media, the body, social networks, and collective memory. And because death and society are the province not solely of sociologists, I have collaborated with scholars in religious studies, history, archaeology, anthropology, folklore, geography, linguistics, social work, psychology, medicine, and computer science, not to mention practitioners of medicine, nursing, social work, museum curation, and chaplaincy. Teaching sociology of death on bachelor's degrees in sociology has also proved stimulating, as death relates to so many aspects of society. All this keeps the intellectual juices flowing. An attempt in the mid-2000s to move into another (more mature) subfield of sociology was quickly abandoned: It was simply too boring!

This chapter is therefore written from the perspective not of an American thanatologist but of a British sociologist. What follows is my sketch from the United Kingdom of the most significant sociological perspectives for understanding death, dying, and bereavement within the English-speaking world and Europe. In no way do I claim my sketch to be comprehensive, and I apologize to any scholar offended by his or her omission. More comprehensive though now somewhat dated reviews from the United States, revealing how much I have left out, are Fulton and Bendiksen (1994); Owen, Markusen, and Fulton (1994); and Riley (1983); students will profit from Kearl's textbook (1989) and website.[3]

FOUNDATIONS

Durkheim, Weber, and Marx

Though not central to their work, foundations for a sociology of death may be discerned in sociology's three European "founding fathers," Emile Durkheim, Max Weber, and Karl Marx.

Durkheim's book *The Elementary Forms of the Religious Life* is famous for arguing that religion enables groups to gather together and symbolize their collective identity. What is often forgotten is that many of the rites discussed by Durkheim were funeral rites. Durkheim (1915) therefore provides the basis for a sociology of death: "When someone dies, the group to which he belongs feels itself lessened and, to react against this loss, it assembles. . . . Collective sentiments are renewed which then lead men to seek one another and to assemble together" (p. 339). Death prompts social solidarity. A graphic example of this is the immediate response to 9/11, with newspapers depicting suburban front lawns flying the stars and stripes: several thousands are dead, but America lives on and will not be defeated. It is precisely when groups—from families to nations—are depleted by death that they reconstitute themselves, symbolically and practically. Of course, the long-term social responses to death, as after 9/11, are complex, with anger, power, and conflict trumping social solidarity.

Another famous essay, Max Weber's *The Protestant Ethic and the Spirit of Capitalism* (1930), first published in 1904, analyzed the long-term consequences of one particular response to human mortality, namely, the 17th-century Puritan belief in predestination, which he argued was one key to the development of capitalism. Thus for both Durkheim and Weber, death may be the end of an individual, but its associated rites and beliefs can be at the heart of the formation or development of society.

Writing rather earlier, in 1844, Karl Marx introduced a critical edge to the social role of death rites and afterlife beliefs: they were the "opium of the people," an ideological superstructure produced by capitalist interests to keep its oppressed workers quiet. If Durkheim saw funeral rites and beliefs as socially functional, a view reflected in some mid-20th-century American sociological studies of funerals, a neo-Marxist approach might suggest not only that funeral rites promote false consciousness, but also that they exploit mourners. Marxist approaches have been rare in the sociology of death (Lofland, 1976), but resonate with historical studies of how churches have exploited fear of death to instill religious conformity and also with Mitford's (1963) best-selling polemic against the American funeral. People can have personal, religious, existential, and status anxieties around death, so are ripe for exploitation by purveyors of salvation, social respectability, or, nowadays in America, "closure" (Berns, 2011).

These examples show how fear, anxiety, and beliefs around death help shape society, but another of Durkheim's books shows how society can be a cause, rather than an effect, of mortality. *Suicide* (2002), published in 1897, is famous for showing how the most individual of acts, killing oneself, is shaped by social factors, revealed through statistical analysis of suicide rates between different social groups. That society affects mortality rates is at the heart of epidemiology, which shows how death and sickness from various causes are in part socially caused. Society also shapes *responses* to death. This insight is at the core of the sociology of death, which shows how social factors drive all manner of death practices, from palliative care, to funerals, to grief norms, to collective remembrance of the dead (not least within nationalism), to the politics and ethics of managing ancient human remains.

Anthropology

Durkheim was part sociologist, part anthropologist. His students Hertz (1960) and Van Gennep (1960) wrote in the early 20th century about funeral rites, their works not being translated into English until 1960. Since then, they have greatly influenced anthropological research into ritual. Bloch and Parry (1982) argue, contra Durkheim, that society does not automatically recreate itself after death; rather, postdeath rites provide an opportunity for people actively to create society as an apparently external force; change and development are thus possible. Applying such insights to contemporary society, Árnarson (2007) has argued that bereavement counseling functions to regenerate the autonomous individual who is at the heart of today's neoliberal political order, thus regenerating not only individuals but also the social order.

Like Durkheim, most anthropological studies have supposed death rites and practices to be socially functional. A major challenge comes from Holst-Warhaft

(2000), not a social scientist but a scholar of comparative and classical literature. She argues that the passion of grief can be so powerful as to destabilize the social order; political establishments therefore fear grief and do their best to turn it into something dull and depressive. One might add that, even within families, grief is suppressed in order to keep the family on an even keel; depression within grief, felt psychologically, can thus be caused by the exercise of power. Holst-Warhaft provides examples, such as Chile's Mothers of the Disappeared and the AIDS quilt, in which the power of grief drove successful challenges to the established sociopolitical order. We have here, then, an embryonic politics of grief that takes conflict and power seriously.

The 1960s

Sociology developed rapidly in the 1960s, in part due to the Civil Rights Movement and the counterculture, both of which prompted reflection on the nature of society. French theorist Foucault's (1973) concept of "the gaze" (first published 1963), especially the medical gaze, explored the dictum that knowledge is power. Thus medical knowledge gives doctors authority over patients' bodies; this includes the right to excavate the dead body through anatomy classes and autopsies, the knowledge gained therein further confirming medical authority. So knowledge and power mutually create each other; medical mystique derives in part from the doctor's privileged knowledge of, and occasional excursions into, our insides. Laypeople generally welcome the medical gaze, thus legitimating it further. They even use it to inspect themselves and those they love, for example, by using medical language to answer a well-wisher's inquiry about a sick family member; moreover, laypeople are disturbed if a medical cause of death cannot be ascertained. We *want* to explain our misfortunes medically.

Applying this to the end of life, American sociologists Arney and Bergen (1984) noted how holistic palliative care allows the doctor to gaze not only into the patient's body but also into their very soul, not to mention their family's. This gaze is one-way: the patient cannot ask the doctor "And how are you, in yourself?" or inquire into the doctor's love life. Spiritual and existential concerns have now come within palliative care's multidisciplinary professional domain. Dying has become a complex matter, requiring management via diverse professional knowledge and skills, which may empower, but may also disempower, patients, families, and communities.

Foucault linked macro and micro levels, showing how power is exercised in face-to-face interaction. The 1960s also saw two landmark studies examine the micro level in Californian hospitals. In their seminal study of awareness of, and communication about, dying, Glaser and Strauss (1965) held up a mirror to existing hospital practices, prompting readers to question and subsequently change institutional practice. Anglophone societies have consequently seen a dramatic shift, with doctors becoming much more open with cancer patients about their terminal condition. (Those suffering from other terminal conditions remain less likely to have such frank conversations with their doctors; as are those in less individualistic societies in the Mediterranean, Africa, and the Far East, where individual rights traditionally take second place to social, and particularly family, relationships.)

Sudnow's research (1967) demonstrated that the definition and moment of death are not entirely natural, but are socially produced through hospital routines, a perspective becoming increasingly relevant as health care bureaucracies become more complex and new technologies not only enable death to be both hastened and prolonged, but also cause its definition to become ever more obviously problematic. If, for Durkheim, death creates social order, for Sudnow death is produced through routine social practices. This perspective influenced Kaufman's (2005) more recent American hospital study which shows that, even in freedom-loving America, choices at the end of life (not only for patients and families but also for doctors) are profoundly constrained by largely invisible institutional structures.

CURRENT THEMES

I now sketch some themes in research since the 1980s that illustrate sociological perspectives on how modern societies engage with dying people, with mourners, and with the dead.

Social Death

Humans are born as primarily physical beings who in the ensuing years are shaped by culture. Dying entails a reversal of this process as the dying person "falls" from culture back into nature (Seale, 1998). "Much of the time I feel I'm just a body to be fed, watered and toileted," a friend, once vibrant but now in frail old age, told me a few weeks before she died, at home. For those dying in frail old age as institutionalized hospital patients, the feeding, watering, and toileting may be done automatically through tubes and pumps; their days are never again to be punctuated by the social rite, and social interaction, of meal times.

Thus the end of a person's social life and social identity may precede the end of his or her physical life: sociologists term this "social death" (Mulkay & Ernst, 1991). The person in a coma, or with advanced dementia, may no longer be related to as a person with agency; thus relatives may feel that the person has "already died." In the West, bad deaths comprise either a too early social death, the fate of many housebound or institutionalized elderly; or a too early physical death, the fate of those who die tragically young while in the full social engagement of youth or middle age. "Good deaths" are when physical and social death coincide. Euthanasia and hospice care—though ideologically opposed—each attempt to produce the good death, but by opposite means: euthanasia by bringing physical death forward, hospice care by enabling the person to live as a full social being until the body finally gives up. In some oppressive situations, such as slavery, social identity may be assaulted long before the body dies (Patterson, 1982); in genocide, stripping a person of social identity, for example, through rape, is a deliberately dehumanizing prelude to physical killing (Card, 2007).

The concept of social death illuminates what happens after, as well as before, physical death. A person's social identity—and arguably also his or her agency—may continue after, even long after, physical death. Thus Princess Diana, socially present in life largely through the mass media, was equally present in the media for another year after her untimely death in 1997. In relation to more personal bereavement, theories of "continuing bonds" show how mourners continue to relate to their beloved dead (Klass, Silverman, & Nickman, 1996), while Unruh (1983) has identified strategies Americans use to preserve identity each side of the grave. Ancestor rites in tribal and Far Eastern societies prescribe rites that construct postmortem agency.

Social death—the extinction of social identity—shows that death and dying are not just physical and that loss is not just psychological; both are inherently social.

Grief

Bereavement research on both sides of the Atlantic has been preponderantly psychiatric and psychological, but sociology also provides useful perspectives.

American sociology in the 1930s researched role reallocation within families, that is, how families restabilize themselves after a death (Owen et al., 1994); more recently, Nadeau (1998) has shown how meaning-making in bereavement is a familial as well as an individual process. The sociology of emotion has also offered insights. Hochschild's (1983) research with flight attendants developed the concepts of "feeling rules" and "feeling work": every group has norms as to what feelings are appropriately displayed by whom and in what situations; some occupations (typically female and low paid) are paid to manage people's feelings. Thus, for example, a hospice may have different feeling rules from a general hospital. Ken Doka (2002) examined feelings rules through the concept of "disenfranchised grief." His outline of the situations in which a person's grief might not be socially acknowledged has been influential within the American death awareness movement. His work brings to the fore a more sociological understanding of grief, but not yet a fully sociological understanding as "disenfranchisement" implies that all grief should be "enfranchised," that is, not socially regulated. Yet there is no society in history in which grief has not been socially regulated and informally policed—more sociological questions might be: Who makes the rules? For whom? Are they reasonable? Are they liberatory or oppressive (Fowlkes, 1990; Walter, 1999)?

Denial, Sequestration, or Exposure?

That death is denied, or taboo, in modern society is a cliché still regularly heard in journalism and in everyday language; it is also a rhetorical device used by the death awareness movement in its efforts to get society talking about death (Lofland, 1978). The notion of death having replaced sex as the taboo of the 20th century goes back to Gorer (1955); the notion of 20th-century death as at best hidden, at worst forbidden, was suggested by historian Ariès (1974); and the notion of death denial is rooted in psychoanalysis, popularized by Becker (1973) and Kübler-Ross (1970). These notions have been interrogated by sociologists wishing to develop more structural understandings of the position in society of death, the dying, and the grieving. Talcott Parsons observed that the division of labor in all modern countries has produced specialist occupations claiming rational authority over the management of death; specifically, American orientations to death are characterized by a typically American practical activism rather than denial (Parsons & Lidz, 1963). Others point specifically to death's medicalization, arguably part of a process of secularization that has eroded/replaced/supplemented the religious frame within which death was previously seen. Elias (1982) grounds avoidance of the dying or dead body within a historical process observable over several centuries in which Western bodies and emotions have been progressively regulated or "civilized."

Mellor and Shilling (1993) follow Anthony Giddens in suggesting that death, like madness and other fateful moments, has been sequestrated, and pushed to the margins, to protect modern society. With the dying hidden away in hospital and the bereaved no longer wearing visible signs of mourning, death is hidden in public, though very much present in private. Walter (1994), however, sees it somewhat differently, arguing that public discourses, notably that of medicine, cannot easily articulate private discourses of personal pain, spiritual anguish, or family dynamics—though holistic palliative care attempts to do just that. Noys (2005) argues that modernity produces a drastic and naked *exposure* to death. His empirical evidence rests on extreme cases, such as the Holocaust, HIV, refugees, and confrontational avant-garde art; Noys stands as a corrective to sequestration and medicalization theorists who have ignored the many millions who face extinction unprotected by medicine or even citizenship. Noys updates the observations of some American sociologists in the Cold War era when death had seemingly been banished by modern medicine, yet fear of the bomb hung over everyone (Fulton & Owen, 1987–1988). Today, it is fear of global warming, terrorism, and the dementia brought on by our medically induced long lives that concern even the affluent.

We should, however, note Pinker's (2012) well-evidenced argument that violent death as a *proportion* of all deaths has steadily declined from prehistory to the present. This has perhaps produced an increasing gap between the emotionally expressive values of secure "postmaterialists" (Inglehart, 2008) who populate the death awareness movement in developed societies and the concern with physical survival of those in poorer countries whose encounter with death is direct, unpredictable, and unprotected.

Death and Media

Death is increasingly visible in the mass media, from movies, to soaps, to the news (Kitch & Hume, 2008). Fulton and Geis (1962), in their argument that America was a death-avoidant society, cited a 1950 study of American movies; these "characteristically refused to allow the audience to build up any emotional identification with a character who would subsequently die or be killed" (p. 14). Within just a few years, that changed, with the leads in box-office hits *Bonnie and Clyde* (1967), *Butch Cassidy and the Sundance Kid* (1969), and *Easy Rider* (1969) all being gunned down in the final scene. A study in the mid-1990s found that half of all British national newspapers published over a 3-month period included death stories or pictures on their front pages. Although medicine may be the practical tool for staving off death, and psychology the increasingly approved tool for managing grief, it is the media that have replaced (or in the United States, augmented) religious attempts to construct meaning in death.

Much research, notably by English sociologist Clive Seale, has examined the dominant scripts used by the media to represent death, though it has proved much easier to analyze the scripts than to investigate empirically how they are produced or received. And though media deaths do not reflect everyday deaths, recent doctoral research by Sarah Coombs has shown how British teenagers creatively (and not uncritically) use media scripts to explore the kinds of death their own parents and grandparents are likely to encounter.

Dark tourism
Watching a television documentary about Auschwitz or Ground Zero, and going there as a tourist, are not the same but are clearly related. Dark tourism "is the act of travel and visitation to sites, attractions and exhibitions which has real or recreated death, suffering or the seemingly macabre as a main theme"[4] and ranges from exhibited human remains; to battlefield, cemetery, and Holocaust tourism; to the slavery heritage industry (Sharpley & Stone, 2009). Dark tourism as a research field is largely populated by British tourism academics, and more input from scholars from other disciplines and countries would be of mutual benefit.

Spontaneous shrines
Also intertwined with the media, and with dark tourism, is the rise of spontaneous shrines—a term coined by American folklorist Santino (2006)—found after road accidents, murder, disaster, and celebrity deaths. As with media studies in general, researchers have adopted two very different approaches. On the one hand is the careful collection of empirical data, documenting how the phenomenon is

changing; this is the approach of folklorists and several sociologists. On the other hand are cultural theorists who emphasize the cultural significance of the one mourned, along with psychoanalytic interpretations of how and why mourners may identify with the newsworthy deceased. The first, empirical, approach can be narrowly sociological, not recognizing emotional dynamics within individuals; the second, analytic, approach sometimes draws more on the cultural or psychoanalyst's pet theories than on empirical data.

The Internet

Since the mid-2000s, social media have radically altered the media scene, with millions of people inputting digital data and communicating with each other online, not least before and after a death (Sofka, Cupit, & Gilbert, 2012). This tends to undo death's sequestration. Like deaths that appear unasked on our television screens, so memorial posts pop up unasked on our mobile devices; this contrasts with both offline cemeteries and 1990s Internet cemeteries, which you had to choose to enter (Walter, Hourizi, Moncur, & Pitsillides, 2011–2012). Social media may also be eroding death's secularization. Even in secular countries, such as Britain and Germany, mourners seem more likely online than offline to use spiritual language, referring to the dead as in heaven or as an angel. It is as though heaven, deemed by many a nonplace once modern astronomy had charted the skies, becomes plausible again—as cyberspace, a mystical, incomprehensible intermediary between here and there, between now and then, between the living and the dead. Maybe this is why the online dead tend to be addressed not as souls, cut off in heaven from the living, but as angels maintaining some kind of ongoing relationship with the living (Walter, 2011). New media connect us to the dead as well as to the living.

The Living and the Dead

As well as mass media, dark tourism, spontaneous shrines, and social media just discussed, the living relate to the dead in many other ways. Ancestral cultures place great importance on guidance from, and placation of, the ancestral dead. Nineteenth-century sociologist Herbert Spencer thought this restricted a society's social and economic development, but evidence has since accumulated of dynamic individuals, families, groups, and societies needing to stay connected to their pasts, that is, to their dead, if they are to feel secure enough to face the future. Japan, for example, combines widespread ancestral veneration with economic dynamism and hypermodernity. Many modern nations, not least the United States, base their sense of national identity on the sacrifice of those who died for their country (Marvin & Ingle, 1999). Israel's identity is based on death awareness—specifically the 6 million Holocaust dead—and a significant proportion of Israeli youth, even those whose genetic ancestors were not European, are taken on pilgrimage to Auschwitz so each new generation can relearn this identity (Feldman, 2008).

Sociologists have been prominent in researching collective memory (Olick, 1999), not least after traumatic events, including war. It is, however, a challenge to link the mountain of psychological research into personal loss and grief with sociopolitical research into communal loss and grief, to link continuing bonds (how deceased individuals become part of personal or family ancestry) with collective memory (how previous generations become part of national identity).

If the living need the dead, American anthropologist Becker (1973) and psychiatrist Lifton (1979) have argued that the dead also need the living. Each author in his own way combined psychoanalysis with cultural analysis, arguing that humans deal with death anxiety by creating ways to live on after death, which Lifton termed "symbolic immortality." This might entail religious afterlife beliefs, children and grandchildren, or material and cultural products (homes, books, movies, etc.) that outlive the individual. (We are now back in the expansive how-death-molds-society territory with which this chapter began.) More recently, sociologist Kearl (2010) has shown how celebrities, such as Elvis Presley and Marilyn Monroe, may contribute even more to the American economy in death than in life; they remain highly potent economic actors. And since the 1990s, Becker's work has been reconceptualized as "terror management theory," a psychological theory with social, cultural, and political implications, currently being tested through a whole raft of experimental research into individual attitudes about, for example, racial prejudice (Pszczynski, Solomon, & Greenberg, 2003).

Demography

Blauner (1966) cogently argued that the impact made by a death depends on the deceased's social status and social involvement. The typical modern death, of an old person no longer centrally involved in the key institutions of work or child-rearing, fails to disrupt the social and economic order, however great its psychological impact on a few close kin. Retirement thus functions to limit death's economic and social impact.

Blauner's observation illuminates why, as the chapters in this book show, there has been so much research and practice development around untimely deaths—from cancer or suicide, and in the young. These deaths are socially and economically disruptive, necessitating policy initiatives and interventions. There is therefore a disjuncture between this social, political, and research agenda, and the underresearched, underresourced deaths that millions of people fear: a lingering social death through frailty, stroke, or dementia. Another disjuncture is that much gerontology (both in terms of practice and research) still avoids the reality that old age ends in death—despite the important work of sociologist Marshall (1991) on old age as a status passage toward death in which individuals "write" the last chapter of their lives.

CONTEMPORARY CHALLENGES

Differences Between Societies

All the sociological themes discussed in the previous section help us understand the ways that modern societies engage—and disengage—with death, with dying people, with mourners, and with the dead. These diverse and changing forms of engagement are not easily captured in simple catchwords such as "taboo," "denial," or "awareness"—however polemically powerful such catchwords are.

Nor are deathways the same in each modern society. There is a popular and often academic assumption that modern ways of death may be contrasted with those of traditional societies, but in fact there are wide variations in how all kinds of societies deal with the deaths of their members. In the modern urbanized world, for example, Americans, Irish, and Japanese regularly view human corpses at the wakes of colleagues and neighbors; the English do not. Southern Europe does not have the Anglo gothic fear of graveyards. Palliative care, premised on open communication between autonomous individuals, finds fertile soil in the English-speaking world, but struggles to take root in family-centered societies such as Italy or collectivist societies such as Japan. Grief norms vary widely by generation, gender, and class. Dying in many modern countries is largely medicalized, but 6 million Jews and up to 60 million Russians died in the 20th century as a result of state action. Deaths from alcohol afflict post-Communist Russia like no other nation. Thus, particular nations have particular histories and cultures of death.

Such differences, however, need thorough scrutiny. On the one hand, too many sociological and historical studies refer simply to America, England, or Australia, with no interest in other societies. Consequently, we do not know whether the data and processes discussed are specific to that nation, or to modernity, or to cities, or what. On the other hand, too many sociological studies refer to "modern society," as though all modern societies are the same, which in the area of death they manifestly are not. Anthropologists, along with several global encyclopedias, describe death practices and beliefs in different societies and religions, but rarely ask comparative questions as to why these might differ or how religion and culture interact to create variation—a welcome exception being Wikan (1988). A number of researchers have compared different ethnic groups within the United States (Kalish & Reynolds, 1981), which tends to reduce intergroup differences to culture. The only way, however, to find out whether any particular response to death is Western, modern, urban, middle class, globalized, or specific to a particular ethnicity, nation, or cluster of nations (whether Anglophone, Scandinavian, or ex-Soviet) is—as Fulton and Geis (1962) recommended 50 years ago—sustained comparative analysis. Comparative research remains rare, but see Goody and Poppi (1994) and Walter (2005, 2012).

Textbooks
All this reflects sociology in general, which in Bryan Turner's words has long been caught "between a science of particular nation-states and a science of global or universal processes" Turner (1990, p. 343). It is confusing for teachers and students alike that thanatology textbooks, whether emanating from the United States or from Europe, do not always make clear which sections, paragraphs, or even sentences apply to all modern societies, and which to their country of origin; apart from the potential to mislead students, the opportunity for comparative analysis, arguably at the heart of sociology, is missed. American students, for example, end up not knowing which of their own death practices are uniquely American, which are Western, and which are global.

Some light is shed by textbooks emanating from countries or regions with small populations dominated by more powerful neighbors, from which authors seek to differentiate their own country. Examples include Northcott and Wilson's (2008) Canadian text and Bleyen's (2005) Flemish text, along with McManus's (2013) text that focuses on neither modernity nor the author's own country but on the globalization of death practices; McManus, significantly, is a New Zealander with family origins in Scotland.

Social Change

Our sociological excursion started with Durkheim's insights about how death undergirds social order. Sociologists have been more challenged to understand how and why death practices change. Here we can identify idealist, structural, demographic, and materialist theories of change. Ariès's (1974) history of mentalities (an idealist approach) has been highly influential, but sociological analysis needs to ground the evolution of ideas in social structure. Blauner (1966) pointed to the importance of the demographic shift from death as the province of childhood to the province of old age, whereas Walter (1994) rooted mentalities in social structure, the body, and systems of authority, but it was not until Kellehear's *Social History of Dying* (2007) that an explicitly materialist sociological theory of dying emerged. For Kellehear, how we die depends, ultimately, on the dominant mode of production—not an unreasonable assumption, given the materiality of dying. Key to his analysis of dying, from the Stone Age to the globalized present, is urbanization in the ancient world, leading as we have seen to the division of labor, including specialists who manage death on behalf of everyone else. In this long-term perspective, the professionalization of death and dying goes back way beyond 19th-century doctors and undertakers to the ancient world's first priests.

Disadvantaged Dying

An estimated 100 million people died of state-sponsored deprivation and violence in the first half of the 20th century (Elliot, 1972; Pinker, 2012), yet they are at best marginalized, at worst ignored, by sociologists of death and dying who have generally failed to connect with studies of poverty, war, and the environment. Other kinds of death are also distinctly underresearched. We know far more about communication with middle-aged cancer patients than with old people suffering from dementia; far more about midlife bereavement than elderly bereavement; far more about counseling services frequented by middle-class clients than about working-class styles of coping; far more about adjustment to death and loss by privileged Westerners than by sub-Saharan Africans. Such are the biases that have dominated death studies. With a few notable exceptions (e.g., Moller, 2004), social scientists, like Western societies at large, have ignored their own elderly, their own poor, the poor half of the world, and those made stateless by exile or war—all of whom experience death and loss disproportionately often (Howarth, 2007). Scholars have theorized the consequences of the Holocaust for Jewish people today, but much less so the destruction of lives, homes, and communities by terror, war, civil war, and AIDS in the Middle East, sub-Saharan Africa, or parts of Asia. Just as palliative care has made dying a less terrifying event for Westerners dying of cancer but has made rather little impact outside the English-speaking world or with other diseases, so sociological knowledge of death and dying has focused on first-world cancer dying. Too much sociology of death has reflected parochial trends in palliative medicine, rather than offering a mirror to global society. Extending its vision, along with sustained comparative and historical research, is essential if the sociology of death is to retain both intellectual vibrancy and policy relevance in the coming decades.

NOTES

1. http://www.civilceremonies.co.uk/ceremonies/civil-funerals
2. Funeral reform was central to the American death awareness movement in the 1960s, but reformers' concerns then differed from those of 1990s British reformers (Mitford, 1963; Parsons & Lidz, 1963; Walter, 2005).
3. http://www.trinity.edu/mkearl/death.html; see also http://what-when-how.com/sociology/death-and-dying/
4. http://www.dark-tourism.org.uk/

REFERENCES

Ariès, P. (1974). *Western attitudes toward death: From the Middle Ages to the present*. Baltimore, MD: Johns Hopkins University Press.

Árnason, A. (2007). "Fall apart and put yourself together again": The anthropology of death and bereavement counselling in Britain. *Mortality*, 12(1), 48–65.

Arney, W. R., & Bergen, B. J. (1984). *Medicine and the management of living*. Chicago, IL: University of Chicago Press.

Becker, E. (1973). *The denial of death*. New York, NY: Free Press.

Berger, P. (1969). *The social reality of religion*. London, UK: Faber.

Berns, N. (2011). *Closure: The rush to end grief and what it costs us*. Philadelphia, PA: Temple University Press.

Blauner, R. (1966). Death and social structure. *Psychiatry, 29*, 378–394.

Bleyen, J. (2005). *De Dood in Vlaanderen* [Death in Flanders]. Leuven, Belgium: Davidsfonds.

Bloch, M., & Parry, J. K. (Eds.). (1982). *Death and the regeneration of life*. Cambridge, UK: Cambridge University Press.

Card, C. (2007). Genocide and social death. In C. Card & A. T. Marsoobian (Eds.), *Genocide's aftermath: Responsibility and repair*. Oxford, UK: Blackwell.

Doka, K. J. (Ed.). (2002). *Disenfranchised grief: New directions, challenges, and strategies for practice*. Champaign, IL: Research Press.

Durkheim, E. (1915). *The elementary forms of the religious life*. London, UK: Unwin.

Durkheim, E. (2002). *Suicide*. London, UK: Routledge. (First published 1897)

Elias, N. (1982). *The civilising process* (Vol. 2). Oxford, UK: Blackwell.

Elliot, G. (1972). *The twentieth century book of the dead*. Harmondsworth, UK: Penguin.

Feldman, J. (2008). *Above the death pits, beneath the flag: Youth voyages to Poland and the performance of Israeli national identity*. New York, NY: Berghahn.

Foucault, M. (1973). *The birth of the clinic: An archaeology of medical perception*. London, UK: Tavistock.

Fowlkes, M. R. (1990). The social regulation of grief. *Sociological Forum, 5*(4), 635–653.

Fulton, R., & Bendiksen, R. (1994). *Death and identity* (3rd ed.). Philadelphia, PA: Charles Press.

Fulton, R., & Geis, G. (1962). Death and social values. *Indian Journal of Social Research, 3*, 7–14.

Fulton, R., & Owen, G. (1987–1988). Death and society in twentieth-century America. *Omega, 18*(4), 379–395.

Glaser, B., & Strauss, A. (1965). *Awareness of dying*. London, UK: Penguin.

Goody, J., & Poppi, C. (1994). Flowers and bones: Approaches to the dead in Anglo and Italian cemeteries. *Comparative Studies in Society & History, 36*, 146–175.

Gorer, G. (1955, October). The pornography of death. *Encounter*, pp. 49–52.

Hertz, R. (1960). *Death and the right hand*. London, UK: Cohen & West.

Hochschild, A. (1983). *The managed heart: Commercialization of human feeling*. Berkeley, CA: University of California Press.

Holst-Warhaft, G. (2000). *The cue for passion: Grief and its political uses*. Cambridge, MA: Harvard University Press.

Howarth, G. (2007). Whatever happened to social class? An examination of the neglect of working class cultures in the sociology of death. *Health Sociology Review, 16*(5), 425–435.

Inglehart, R. (2008). Changing values among western publics from 1970 to 2006. *West European Politics, 31*(1–2), 130–146.

Kalish, R., & Reynolds, D. (1981). *Death and ethnicity: A psychocultural study*. Farmingdale, NY: Baywood.

Kaufman, S. (2005). *And a time to die: How American hospitals shape the end of life*. Chicago, IL: University of Chicago Press.

Kearl, M. C. (1989). *Endings: A sociology of death and dying*. Oxford, UK: Oxford University Press.

Kearl, M. C. (2010). *The proliferation of postselves in American civic and popular cultures. Mortality, 15*(1), 47–63.

Kellehear, A. (2007). *A social history of dying*. Cambridge, UK: Cambridge University Press.

Kitch, C., & Hume, J. (2008). *Journalism in a culture of grief*. New York, NY: Routledge.

Klass, D., Silverman, P. R., & Nickman, S. L. (Eds.). (1996). *Continuing bonds: New understandings of grief*. Bristol, PA: Taylor & Francis.

Kübler-Ross, E. (1970). *On Death and Dying*. London: Tavistock.

Lifton, R. J. (1979). *The broken connection: On death and the continuity of life*. New York, NY: Simon & Schuster.

Lofland, L. (Ed.). (1976). *Toward a sociology of death and dying*. Beverly Hills, CA: SAGE.

Lofland, L. (1978). *The craft of dying: The modern face of death*. Beverly Hills, CA: SAGE.

Marshall, M. (1991). *Last chapters: A sociology of ageing and dying*. Monterey, CA: Brooks/Cole.

Marvin, C., & Ingle, D. (1999). *Blood sacrifice and the nation: Totem rituals and the American flag*. Cambridge, UK: Cambridge University Press.

McManus, R. (2013). *Death in a global age*. Basingstoke, England: Palgrave Macmillan.

Mellor, P., & Shilling, C. (1993). Modernity, self-identity and the sequestration of death. *Sociology, 27*(3), 411–432.

Mitford, J. (1963). *The American way of death*. London, UK: Hutchinson.

Moller, D. W. (2004). *Dancing with broken bones: Portraits of death and dying among inner-city poor*. Oxford, UK: Oxford University Press.

Mulkay, M., & Ernst, J. (1991). The changing profile of social death. *Archives Europeennes De Sociologie, 32*(1), 172–196.

Nadeau, J. W. (1998). *Families making sense of death*. London, UK: SAGE.

Northcott, H. C., & Wilson, D. M. (2008). *Dying and death in Canada* (2nd ed.). Toronto, Ontario, Canada: University of Toronto Press.

Noys, B. (2005). *The culture of death*. Oxford, UK: Berg.

Olick, J. (1999). Collective memory: The two cultures. *Sociological Theory, 17*(3), 333–348.

Owen, G., Markusen, E., & Fulton, R. (1994). The sociology of death: A historical overview 1875–1985. In R. Fulton & R. Bendiksen (Eds.), *Death and identity* (3rd ed., pp. 80–102). Philadelphia, PA: Charles Press.

Parsons, T., & Lidz, V. (1963). Death in American society. In E. Shneidman (Ed.), *Essays in self-destruction* (pp. 133–170). New York, NY: Science House.

Patterson, O. (1982). *Slavery and social death: A comparative study*. Cambridge, MA: Harvard University Press.

Pinker, S. (2012). *The better angels of our nature: Why violence has declined*. New York, NY: Viking.

Pszczynski, T., Solomon, S., & Greenberg, J. (2003). *In the wake of 9/11: The psychology of terror*. Washington, DC: American Psychological Association.

Riley, J. W. J. (1983). Dying and the meanings of death: Sociological inquiries. *Annual Review of Sociology, 9*, 191–216.

Santino, J. (Ed.). (2006). *Spontaneous shrines and the public memorialization of death*. Basingstoke, UK: Palgrave Macmillan.

Seale, C. (1998). *Constructing death: The sociology of dying and bereavement*. Cambridge, UK: Cambridge University Press.

Sharpley, R., & Stone, P. (Eds.). (2009). *The darker side of travel: The theory and practice of dark tourism*. Bristol, England: Channel View.

Sofka, C., Cupit, I. N., & Gilbert, K. (2012). *Dying, death, and grief in an online universe: For counselors and educators*. New York, NY: Springer Publishing Company.

Sudnow, D. (1967). *Passing on: The social organization of dying*. Englewood Cliffs, NJ: Prentice Hall.

Turner, B. (1990). The two faces of sociology: global or national? In M. Featherstone (Ed.), *Global culture: Nationalism, globalization and modernity* (pp. 343–358). London: Sage, 343–358.

Unruh, D. (1983). Death and personal history: Strategies of identity preservation. *Social Problems, 30*(3), 340–351.

Van Gennep, A. (1960). *The rites of passage*. Chicago, IL: University of Chicago Press.

Walter, T. (1990). *Funerals—And how to improve them*. London, UK: Hodder Headline.

Walter, T. (1994). *The revival of death*. London, UK: Routledge.

Walter, T. (1999). *On bereavement: The culture of grief*. Buckingham, UK: Open University Press.

Walter, T. (2005). Three ways to arrange a funeral: Mortuary variation in the modern West. *Mortality, 10*(3), 173–192.

Walter, T. (2011). Angels not souls: Popular religion in the online mourning for British celebrity Jade Goody. *Religion, 41*(1), 29–51.

Walter, T. (2012). Why different countries manage death differently: A comparative analysis of modern urban societies. *British Journal of Sociology, 63*(1), 123–145.

Walter, T., Hourizi, R., Moncur, W., & Pitsillides, S. (2011–2012). Does the Internet change how we die and mourn? *Omega, 64*(4), 275–302.

Weber, M. (1930). *The protestant ethic and the spirit of capitalism*. London, UK: Allen & Unwin.

Wikan, U. (1988). Bereavement and loss in two Muslim communities: Egypt and Bali compared. *Social Science & Medicine, 27*(5), 451–460.

Diana J. Wilkie and Inge B. Corless   4

SCIENCE AND PRACTICE: CONTRIBUTIONS OF NURSES TO END-OF-LIFE AND PALLIATIVE CARE

Over the years, health care professionals from many disciplines have contributed to the knowledge base supporting palliative and end-of-life care. Nurses were early contributors to care of the dying as well as the scientific discoveries regarding end-of-life issues. Nurses then championed the translation of the innovations into practice as they cared for dying pediatric and adult patients and their families. These discoveries and innovations are the focus of this chapter. Adequately profiling all nurse leaders' impacts on the science and practice of end-of-life care, however, requires more space than is available for this chapter. We opted, therefore, to profile a number of nurse leaders whose sustained work influenced end-of-life care in seven major areas: (1) uncovering and combating the conspiracy of silence, (2) making meaning for children and adults as they live with the chronicity of a life-threatening illness, (3) promoting team-based collaborative approaches to care, (4) managing pain and symptoms of children and adults, (5) integrating bereavement as part of patient-centered and family-focused dying care, (6) conducting research, and (7) educating nurses to improve care of people at the end of life. These subjects represent only a fraction, but an important fraction, of those topics to which nurses have contributed. First, though, we share a brief description of our own backgrounds and the nurses who led the development of nursing as a profession as a context for other nursing leaders who contributed to the science and practice of palliative and end-of-life care.

PALLIATIVE AND END-OF-LIFE CARE JOURNEYS

The authors of this chapter both have a long history of contributions to palliative and end-of-life care. The impetus for Dr. Diana Wilkie's career in palliative care was the agony of two patients with cancer. In 1981, she became a volunteer hospice nurse to allow one of these patients to achieve his goal—dying comfortably at home surrounded by his family. Entering graduate school in 1982 afforded her the opportunity to study with world-renowned pain scientists and to learn how cancer pain could be relieved with further research on ways to improve practice. Ever since, the pain-relief needs of patients with advanced cancer or sickle cell disease motivated her efforts to implement innovative technology-based interventions that amplify the patients' voices about their pain and translate pain science to the point of care—in patients' homes, the clinic, emergency department, or hospital. She also founded and continues to direct the Center of Excellence for End-of-Life Transition Research, whose mission is to advance the science for palliative and end-of-life care worldwide.

Dr. Inge Corless had the experience of caring for family members with advanced illness in the home. Given this experience, she was interested in and chronicled hospice as a social movement. She subsequently helped develop a hospice program and engaged in research, in particular, on persons living with HIV. Recently, she has focused on the relationship of grief and depression in chronic disease. Both authors' work evolved from their personal and professional experiences, much like early nurse leaders who, two centuries ago, fought to reduce the suffering of war and disease.

Nursing Becomes a Profession

Early nursing care was provided by both the religious and others, including Clara Barton and Walt Whitman during the Civil War in the United States. The beginnings of nursing as a profession, however, are inevitably associated with Florence Nightingale and her work during the Crimean War. The "Lady with a Lamp" may be as well known for making rounds each evening to say "good night" to each patient as she was for relocating patients in the Scutari Barracks to prevent their exposure to the malodorous smells of decomposing horses buried beneath the barracks. Nightingale's *Notes on Nursing* (Nightingale, 1860/1969) detail her innovative commitment to creating an environment in which healing could occur. Nightingale is also known for her emphasis on the use of statistics and a variant of the pie chart, the polar area diagram, to illustrate data concerning the causes of mortality in the British Army.

Nightingale founded the St. Thomas' Training School in 1860 at St. Thomas' Hospital in London. A decade later, her approaches to education were the models for nursing education at the Bellevue Training School for Nurses in New York, which opened in May 1873, the Connecticut Training School in New Haven, Connecticut, which opened in October 1873, and the Massachusetts General Hospital Training School for Nurses in Boston, which opened 1 month later in November 1873 (Dock & Stewart, 1925).

One of the graduates of the Bellevue Schools of Nursing in 1886, Lavinia Dock, a nursing educator and author of nursing text books, including one on *materia medica* (pharmacology), was also active in national and international nursing organizations; she co-founded the International Council of Nurses. Dock is known widely for her work with Lillian Wald at the Henry Street Settlement. Dock, however, was equally active in fighting for women's suffrage. She was a woman for all seasons and fought for the health of immigrants and people with low incomes as well as for women's rights and the development of the nursing profession.

Lillian Wald, who founded the Henry Street Settlement in 1893 and established the first visiting nursing association, also founded the National League for Public Health Nursing in 1912, serving as its first president. She coined the term "public health nurse" (Fee & Bu, 2010, p. 1206). Wald's efforts extended to the development of the first university course on public health nursing at Columbia University to educate public health nurses; she also was involved in conceiving the federal Children's Bureau in Washington, DC.

Another nurse concerned with the welfare of her patients, Mary Breckinridge, founded the Frontier Nursing Service (FNS) in Kentucky in 1928. She and her nursing colleagues, midwives on horseback, strove to safeguard the health of women from pregnancy through delivery. Their efforts reduced the maternal mortality rates for women receiving their services. Safeguarding the health of women, Margaret Sanger (1879–1966) attributed multiple pregnancies particularly in women of restricted economic means as the cause of their early demise. Sanger's efforts in developing clinics and access to birth control methods are a case study in framing issues so as to engage advocates with allied interests. In 1952, with other like-minded individuals, she co-founded the International Planned Parenthood Federation.

This proud heritage of dedication to the welfare of patients, and the population at large, is the basis of the perspective that motivates the work of nurses who have contributed to palliative and end-of-life care and is the focus of the remainder of this chapter. The omission of commentary about the formidable scholarship of Dr. Mary Vachon and Dr. Betty Davies is with the happy acknowledgement of their contribution as authors of other chapters in this book.

UNCOVERING AND COMBATING THE CONSPIRACY OF SILENCE ABOUT DEATH AND DYING

One of the earliest nurse pioneers with a focus on end of life, Dr. Jeanne Quint Benoliel was an amazing thinker, scholar, and scientist who championed discourse on a range of topics, including the conspiracy of silence surrounding death and dying. Six years before Kübler-Ross (1969) published her book, Benoliel's insights from her research with women who had a mastectomy for breast cancer highlighted the societal taboo of talking about dying, showing that the women, when given an opportunity to tell their stories, spoke of their fears of death (Quint, 1963). Benoliel was sensitive to the conspiracy of silence as she encouraged educating nurses to engage patients in a dialogue to combat the taboo. Benoliel (1970, 1971) began a long, successful career of research focused not only on death awareness issues but also on improving care for the dying (Quint & Strauss, 1964). She eloquently integrated the work of other scientists also writing on death and dying topics, thereby bringing the science from other fields to nursing and facilitating research utilization in this nascent field.

Dr. Ida Martinson also noted the conspiracy of silence with both parents and health care providers not being aware that "many of the children did in fact know that they were dying" (I. M. Martinson, personal communication, December 8, 2013). Hinds et al. (2005) recently show that 18 of 20 children and adolescents 10 years of age and older were able to recall their treatment options and identified that death was a possible consequence of their decisions. This finding is striking and indicates that discussion of death awareness can combat the conspiracy of silence, even with those as young as 10 years.

Other nurses moved beyond talking about dying to helping individuals to plan in advance for the care one prefers at the end of life. Nurses raised awareness of the need for advance care planning among populations not commonly considered at end of life but clearly at risk for early death, such as in sickle cell disease, chronic kidney disease, and premature infants (Kavanaugh, Moro, Savage, Reyes, & Wydra, 2009). Dr. Virginia Tilden fostered advance care planning among nursing home residents who are more commonly viewed as near the end of life (Tilden, 2000; Tilden, Nelson, Dunn, Donius, & Tolle, 2000). Tilden, with her colleagues, also mounted statewide efforts to break the conspiracy of silence using a variety of approaches to educate the public, media, and professionals about advanced care planning, including starting the POLST (Physician Order of Life Sustaining Treatment) program in Oregon (Tolle & Tilden, 2002). Now a nationwide effort, POLST directs provision of the care patients prefer at the end of life.

Nurses also facilitated advance care planning for patients whose decisional capacity is uncertain or lacking. When decisional capacity is lacking, surrogates make decisions and need accurate information to assist them to accept or forego treatments, such as cardiopulmonary resuscitation (CPR), mechanical ventilation

(MV), or tube feeding (TF). One such intervention, Bonner's ActPlan is a group-based, 4-hour program delivered over 4 weeks and focused on educating African American caregivers about the dementia disease trajectory and risks and benefits of CPR, MV, and TF. This program encourages surrogate decision making in advance about whether to use these treatments in the future for the person with dementia (Bonner et al., 2014). Another intervention, Song's Patient-Centered Advance Care Planning program, is a 20- to 45-minute, individually focused, nurse-led discussion with an advance care planning decisional aid for patients in need of elective cardiac surgery and their surrogates (Song, Kirchhoff, Douglas, Ward, & Hammes, 2005). If future effectiveness trials also demonstrate that the interventions are effective, it would be appropriate to implement them widely to improve advance care planning, especially among vulnerable populations.

Efforts directed toward increasing awareness about death and dying have produced some important effects since Benoliel's pathfinding research was published. Unfortunately, much more work needs to be done to assure openness of communication about dying, given that the conspiracy of silence has not been eradicated.

MAKING MEANING: LIVING WITH THE CHRONICITY OF LIFE-THREATENING ILLNESSES

Living with life-threatening illness is an experience that occurs over variable time periods, some that represent the chronic nature of certain illnesses. Nurses have contributed to the understanding of the experiences, be they short or long, and helping children and adults make meaning of their feelings and the events associated with their illnesses. As profiled in the following sections, nurses developed and advocated for whole-person care, focused on the person and family living with the illness and not just the illness, and have been attentive to psychosocial and spiritual care for the dying and their families.

Developing and Advocating for Whole Person Care

Nursing as a discipline is well known for its focus on care of the whole person. It is not surprising that nurses developed care processes for persons living with life-threatening illnesses and advocated for systems of care that would implement care for the whole person. Often, nurse leaders' practice experiences stimulated research whose findings nurses then used to improve care. For example, Benoliel's clinical observation of the disfigurement following breast cancer prompted her study of women postmastectomy (Quint, 1963). The findings led to a meeting with Glaser and Strauss and her work on the dying patient (Benoliel, 1977, 2001, 2012). Her emphasis on the dying patient rather than the disease is exemplified by her work to create a social dependency scale, which was "a step toward creating a standardized instrument for assessing patients' requirements of assistance in performing activities or roles they normally can do for themselves" (Benoliel, McCorkle, & Young, 1980, p. 9). The scale measured activities such as bathing, feeding, dressing, toileting, walking, stair-climbing, transferring (from bed or chair), traveling, consciousness, role activity, social interaction, and social interest. Measuring the impact of illness on functional status was one way nurses documented the human experience of living with a life-threatening illness.

Lunney, Lynn, Foley, Lipson, and Guralnik (2003) addressed the importance of self- or proxy-reported function to predict dependency in activities of daily living before death. These investigators demonstrated that trajectories of functional decline differed for four illness trajectories—sudden death, cancer, organ failure, and frailty. Consideration of the trajectory of functional decline before death would be helpful to plan care needs for patients with these conditions. Examination of trajectories associated with other life-threatening illness could help to plan care for those groups, as well. The functional decline near death affects both the patient and the family.

Focusing on the Person and Family Living With Illness and Not Just the Illness

Benoliel was a forerunner in her concern for the family facing a death. In her holistic approach to care, she was concerned about services for children when there is a sudden death of a parent or a parent experiences a fatal illness (Benoliel, 1978). She also considered the challenges faced when the child was the person dying in the family and proposed the establishment of family-centered transition services. This family focus occurred a time when hospice programs were forming. It was also a time when Martinson was conducting her work with children dying at home, first in the United States and then in Hong Kong, China, Australia, and other countries (Davies et al., 1998). The early work with children dying at home focused on those with cancer, but now involves other fatal illnesses in addition to cancer.

Nurses working in oncology illustrated the nursing discipline's emphasis on the importance of family. McGuire (1979) examined what she termed "cancer prone families" an admittedly small percentage of all cancers. Nevertheless, she urges nurses to capture data on family and environmental risks as a contribution to a database that may provide clues as to both causes and potential cures. McGuire (1985) also discusses the needs of families with hereditary melanoma. Recently, McGuire examined the literature on the informal caregiver at the end of life and concluded that most of the studies were descriptive in nature with few intervention studies to guide practice (McGuire, Grant, & Park, 2012).

Consistent with McGuire's conclusion, the family experience as the person with a life-threatening illness receiving care in an intensive care unit (ICU) is a prime opportunity for nurses to facilitate communication and family understanding of the patient's condition and responses (Kirchhoff et al., 2002). When family members understand the patient's preferences for treatments at the end of life, it is easier for nurses to fulfill the roles that family members desire from ICU nurses. In the ICU, physical environment changes, end-of-life care education, "staff support, and better communication would improve care of dying patients and their families" (Kirchhoff et al., 2000, p. 36).

Tilden, Tolle, Nelson, and Fields (2001) also contributed to the focus on the family as the unit of care. Tilden's team studied barriers to optimal care from the perspective of family members and noted inadequate pain control and insufficient availability of physicians as problems (Tolle, Tilden, Rosenfeld, & Hickman, 2000). Stress associated with decisions to withdraw treatments was an important issue for family members, emphasizing the psychosocial impact of end-of-life care (Tilden et al., 2001).

Attending to Psychosocial and Spiritual Care for the Dying and Their Family

Dr. Betty Ferrell's explains that her palliative care research has focused on patients' and family caregivers' experiences in terminal illness and death at home. Over the past 30 years I have expanded that focus to include areas such as the experiences and roles of family caregivers, pain management at home, palliative surgery, and the integration of palliative care into routine cancer care. All of these studies have been based on our QOL [quality of life] model encompassing physical, psychological, social, and spiritual well-being (B. Ferrell, personal communication, December 9, 2013).

Ferrell and colleagues explicate the nature of suffering, the impact of caregiving on the family's QOL, and the burdens and challenges patients experience as they receive treatments for advanced stage non–small cell lung cancer (Koczywas et al., 2013).

Focusing on patients with cancer receiving hospice care, Dr. Susan McMillan identified strong support for psychophysiological, functional, and social/spiritual well-being components of quality of life (McMillan & Weitzner, 1998). Despite compromised functional abilities, patients receiving hospice care report social/spiritual well-being similar to healthy adults. McMillan's team also measured spiritual needs of caregivers of cancer patients in hospice and found their instrument was valid and reliable and that needs were of moderate magnitude and not associated with depression (Buck & McMillan, 2012). At the end of life, patients typically maintain their spiritual well-being, although there is great variability in unmet spiritual needs (Hampton, Hollis, Lloyd, Taylor, & McMillan, 2007). Using standardized measures, McMillan, Small, and Haley (2011) found excellence in hospice care in addressing psychosocial and spiritual needs, especially when there is sufficient attention to well-being domains by a team-based collaborative approach.

PROMOTING TEAM-BASED COLLABORATIVE APPROACHES TO CARE

Within the hospice and palliative care approaches to dying, there is a strong focus on the family as the unit of care and the patient and family as part of the team-based approach to care. Ida Martinson became interested in end-of-life care as a result of caring for her father-in-law so he could die at home, which was his wish (Martinson, 2001). Although interested in the timing of death, the focus of her research changed after an encounter with her next-door neighbor who was despondent that he would have to admit a child to the hospital to die. Martinson countered with the development of a research plan to study the feasibility of children dying at home, and she demonstrated subsequently that with support, 80% of the children in her study died at home (Martinson et al., 1986). Martinson (1993) reviews her prior research with children dying at home and examines the role of hospice care for dying children. She states,

> Focusing on the child living is also key and we encourage children to keep going to school or having schooling at home as well as taking the child out to get a Dairy Queen or go grocery shopping even if in a wheelchair. Team-based care was essential even when only a nurse was in the home. The nurse was in communication with the physicians and other team members as necessary. The family was the unit of care. To allow the option of the child dying at home, the family had to be involved. We followed the families up to two years post death; not too many teams had done that before. We demonstrated that involvement by families in care of a dying child in the vast majority of families was a worthwhile and very meaningful experience. (I. M. Martinson, personal communication, December 8, 2013)

Although there are differences, much of what Martinson described for children applies to any person who is dying.

Florence Wald, also an early pioneer in care of the dying, was influenced by a Cicely Saunders lecture that resonated with her interest in the needs of the dying and their families (Foster & Wald, 2001; Wald, 1994). She engaged in research with Dr. Morris Wessel and Rev. Ed Dobihal. That work led to the development of Hospice, Inc. and subsequently, the Connecticut Hospice, the first such program in the United States, for which she is known as the mother of hospice in America. Wald envisioned hospice care as an opportunity to change the care for the dying to emphasize the importance of managing symptoms with a particular focus on chronic pain; "the patient/family as the unit of care" and the importance of "support for the grieving" (Craven & Wald, 1975, pp. 1816–1822). Wald also developed the first in-patient facility designed to meet the needs of the terminally ill, which was also considered the most likely locus for research and innovation (Wald, Zoster, & Wald, 1980).

Dr. Inge Corless, another early leader of the hospice movement in the United States, developed an early hospice program and advocated for team-based care that was patient centered and family focused. She chronicled the development of the hospice movement, the legislation that set standards for hospice care, and the legacies of many hospice and palliative care leaders (Corless, 1985, 1987–1988, 2001, 2009).

McMillan applied a simple, research utilization-based intervention to improve teamwork in hospice. Using standardized measures in hospice care and sharing the results during the interdisciplinary team meeting, McMillan and colleagues found that depression improved in the experimental group over the control group, but other indicators of well-being improved in both groups (McMillan et al., 2011). They speculated that the interdisciplinary team was less accustomed to attending to depression than the other quality-of-life indicators, which were already a part of routine hospice care. This team-based approach to improving symptoms of patients with cancer and receiving hospice care is but one innovation nurses have made to enhance teamwork and thereby improve pain and symptom management.

MANAGING PAIN AND SYMPTOMS OF CHILDREN AND ADULTS

More than four decades ago, nurses focused on pain and symptom management at the end of life. Benoliel and Crowley (1974) wrote an early paper in which they not only examined the assessment of pain, but also suggested that the attitudes of nurses might interfere with effective pain management. Martinson also noted that pain was a subject of her investigations. "First many nurses and physicians did not believe the child had pain. Secondly the parents and child worried about addiction because of various drug education programs. Symptom management was very important for pain relief and helping both the child and parents sleep at night is critical" (I. M. Martinson, personal communication, December 8, 2013). Recognizing the importance of symptom control, McCorkle has focused her research on symptom management, the role of the advanced practice nurse in oncology, and interdisciplinary care, making major contributions to all of these fields (McCorkle, 2010; McCorkle et al., 2012). The impact of McCorkle's research is substantial, showing that interventions delivered by advanced practice oncology nurses are particularly effective in reducing depressive symptoms and result in a reduction in patients using emergency care services inappropriately.

The interest in symptom management was also manifested by researchers whose studies were in oncology and might not typically be included as a group in discussions of palliative care. For example, Dr. Marylin Dodd and her colleagues at the University of California, San Francisco (UCSF) developed a symptom management model that is used by many researchers to guide their studies (Dodd et al., 2001). Puntillo, one of Dodd's coauthors, has contributed important knowledge to symptom-measurement science for patients in intensive care settings and management of procedural pain to ensure comfort and favorable symptom outcomes (Puntillo et al., 2001). With the emergence of HIV/AIDS, it is not altogether surprising that another UCSF faculty member, Dr. William Holzemer, developed an International HIV/AIDS Nursing Research Network that engages in HIV research with a focus on symptoms, including fatigue, depression, neuropathy, and fear and anxiety, among other investigations, as well as an instrument to measure the signs and symptoms of HIV disease (Corless et al., 2008; Eller et al., 2010; Holzemer et al., 1999; Kemppainen et al., 2006; Nicholas et al., 2007). One of their research studies examined self-care management of symptoms and found that symptom frequency and intensity declined in the intervention group compared with the attention control group (Wantland et al., 2008).

Paice (2002), who has focused on pain and symptom management for many years, draws attention as well to the psychological aspects of care, including anxiety, depression, and delirium. Paice also made significant contributions to our understanding of pain and its treatment, including implementing system-level programs for quality improvement. Coyne et al. (2013), writing not only on pain, notes his contribution to be one of "constantly questioning interventions to improve pain and symptom management . . . and explored unique interventions to improve the quality of life of those with life-limiting diseases" (P. Coyne, personal communication, December 8, 2013). McGuire (1989) has made important contributions to the assessment and management of cancer pain, on managing mucositis, and more broadly on the topic of mucosal injury as a consequence of cancer therapy (McGuire, Rubenstein, & Peterson, 2004). Her work to develop and test a pain measure for patients who are not able to verbally communicate has the potential for great impact on palliative care.

Dr. Diana Wilkie has focused her research career on pain and symptom management for palliative care populations, including those near the end of life and those living with life-threatening illnesses. Wilkie contributed to pain measurement science considering pain as a multidimensional phenomenon with a novel focus on pain-control behaviors and facial expressions of pain (Wilkie, 1995; Wilkie, Keefe, Dodd, & Copp, 1992). She has studied a variety of successful interventions for pain and symptom management, including coaching patients to report their pain (Wilkie et al., 2010), massage therapy (Jane et al., 2011) and use of tailored computer-based multimedia education for patients and clinical decision support for providers (Huang et al., 2003). Her work originally focused on patients with cancer and more recently has extended to adults with sickle cell disease (SCD; Wilkie et al., 2010). From her initial observation that patients with SCD selected many descriptors of neurophathic pain, she and her colleagues have produced compelling evidence that for some patients with SCD, neuropathic pain is a part of their pain phenomenon and is likely contributing to their prolonged hospitalizations when pain is treated mostly as nociceptive pain. On the basis of those findings and using mechanism-driven approaches, old drug therapies may be repurposed for control of SCD pain (Molokie et al., 2014). Space precludes discussing all of the contributions of the talented nurse researchers and practitioners who have enhanced our understanding of pain and symptom management as part of palliative care.

INTEGRATING BEREAVEMENT WITHIN PATIENT-CENTERED AND FAMILY-FOCUSED DYING CARE

Benoliel (2001) encountered death in civilian hospitals and in the South Pacific during World War II as well as among family members. It was the latter that spurred her subsequent interest in thanatology. In a review of the origins of studies on loss and bereavement, Benoliel (1999) devoted a section of her paper to a consideration of loss from a nursing perspective (pp. 265–268), a forerunner of this chapter.

Other nurse researchers also have contributed to the understanding of bereavement. Legacy items prepared by a dying child are important for both the child to prepare for death and for the bereaved after the death (Foster et al., 2009). Improved symptom management for the dying person is associated with improved bereavement outcomes for the survivors (McCorkle, Robinson, Nuamah, Lev, & Benoliel, 1998). Evidence supports the need to monitor for depressive symptoms and complicated grief after a hospice death (Holtslander & McMillan, 2011). Interventions, such as bereavement debriefing sessions to assist bereavement work of health care providers after the death of a child, have been found to be useful (Keene, Hutton, Hall, & Rushton, 2010).

CONDUCTING RESEARCH WITH PEOPLE AT THE END OF LIFE

Nurse researchers have been exceptionally attentive to research issues as they have studied the dying person and their families as they face the end of life together. McMillan and Weitzer (2003) caution researchers about methodologic issues related to recruitment and retention that they should consider when conducting studies of patients with cancer near the end of life. Tilden, Drach, Tolle, Rosenfeld, and Hickman (2002) discuss case-finding techniques that facilitate community-based recruitment of survivors after the death of one dear to them. Wilkie and colleagues (2009) were some of the earliest researchers to use computer technologies for hospice patients and their family members to report their outcomes directly into tablet-based devices. Wilkie and colleagues (Gorman et al., 2008) showed that when the software was designed specifically for frail persons and those with few computer skills, not only was data collection feasible, but some patients, including minorities, also reported great satisfaction mastering a new skill near the end of their lives. Wilkie and colleagues (Huang, Ezenwa, Wilkie, & Judge, 2013) also developed technologies to assist with recruitment and retention of patients for end-of-life and palliative care studies and provided insights about collaboration with hospices. Trust building is important to successful collaborations. Researchers demonstrated feasibility for tape recording hospice nurses' interactions with patients to code communication (Ellington, Reblin, Clayton, Berry, & Mooney, 2012). The insights of these researchers are rich sources of experiential learning for investigators entering this field and others who would like to improve their research processes or outcomes.

EDUCATING NURSES TO IMPROVE CARE OF PEOPLE AT THE END OF LIFE

McCorkle and Benoliel co-developed the Transitions Services Program at the University of Washington in Seattle. This program was one of the first to focus on educating advanced practice nurses to provide care to the whole person and family with attention to treatments for psychosocial issues and symptoms experienced by patients with life-threatening illness.

Subsequently, two other educational programs (ELNEC, TNEEL) were developed and widely disseminated throughout the world to improve nursing education related to end-of-life and palliative care. Ferrell, Virani, Paice, Coyle, and Coyne (2010) developed ELNEC (End of Life Nurse Education Consortium), and since 2000, they have trained 17,500+ nurses in all 50 states and 78 countries. The program empowers nurses to improve key aspects of palliative care, including pain and symptom management, bereavement care, culturally respectful care, and addressing ethical concerns and care. Wilkie, Judge, Wells, and Berkley (2001) created and distributed the Tool Kit for Nurturing Excellence at the End of Life (TNEEL) to every nursing school in the United States and more than 8,000 U.S. clinical agencies and throughout Taiwan. This educational program is an interactive, engaging teaching tool for educators to use in teaching 27 topics related to end of life that was first distributed via CD-ROM, but now is available via Internet download (www.tneel.uic.edu) and as an Internet-based, self-study program offered by continuing education providers (www.tneel.uic.edu/tneel-ss). Inspired by TNEEL, the American Psychological Association now offers 10 online courses for end-of-life education for mental health workers. Universities, such as the University of Illinois at Chicago, also offer certificate programs focused on advancing palliative care nursing education. Within the past 15 years, the availability of palliative care education for nurses has increased substantially.

SUMMARY: IMPACT OF NURSES ON PALLIATIVE AND END-OF-LIFE CARE

Initiated by Benoliel in the 1960s, as we have noted, there has been an enormous impact from nurses' contributions to end-of-life and palliative care science and practice. Wald and Martinson were early leaders in the U.S. hospice care movement. In addition to Martinson, Hinds and Kavanaugh also conducted landmark studies focused on dying neonates and children. Tilden and Ferrell expanded knowledge about family caregivers. McCorkle, McMillan, McGuire, Ferrell, Paice, Coyne, Wilkie, Corless, and many others contributed in multiple ways to improving pain and symptom management, bereavement, and education of the next generation of nurse clinicians. Many nurses shared their insights about conducting research with the dying and their families. Although much has been accomplished, much is yet to be done to further improve palliative and end-of-life care.

Nurses will likely contribute to additional advances in many areas. There is a need to reduce the conspiracy of silence that still exists around death and dying topics, such as suicide and advance care planning. Interventions are needed to implement the science about pain and symptom management to improve comfort for the dying and thereby reduce the impact of poor symptom control on the bereaved. Translation of science from the research literature to the practice arena is needed for all areas of palliative and end-of-life care for all illnesses. Attention to populations across the life span in need of palliative care other than cancer is another area of need. Examples of such populations include persons with chronic conditions (dementia, neuromuscular disorders, heart failure, renal failure, pulmonary problems, and frailty), acute conditions (birth defects, genetic disorders, trauma, and multiorgan failure), and communicable diseases. Finally, there is a need for additional research related to psychosocial and spiritual care issues for the dying, their families, and their caregivers (lay and professional) before and after the death. In particular, the bereavement needs of health professionals require further attention. In many of these areas of need, it is important to build on existing research findings to more efficiently move the work forward, especially when the prior research has an intervention base. It is important to examine the early literature in the field to avoid missing important descriptive work that the early nurse leaders reported. Clearly, a literature review focused on the past 5 years is insufficient.

We were able to include only a small sample of the available literature by nurses who studied or advanced end-of-life and palliative care. Nurses have contributed significantly to both the science and practice of end-of-life and palliative care. Their holistic focus on both the dying person and the family contributed to the concepts of patient-centered and family-focused care across the life span that included a high priority on comfort during the dying process and bereavement care after the death. As well, nurses have provided insights about conducting rigorous research with the dying and their families. Nurses also have worked to increase education about palliative and end-of-life care. Over the years, nurses have addressed many of the issues Benoliel raised early in her career. Our roots are strong and nurses new to the field would learn much from exploring those roots to enrich their own research and practice.

REFERENCES

Benoliel, J. Q. (1970). Talking to patients about death. *Nursing Forum, 9*(3), 254–268.

Benoliel, J. Q. (1971). The dying patient: A nursing dilemma. *Washington State Journal of Nursing, 43*(1), 3–4.

Benoliel, J. Q. (1977). The interaction between theory and research. *Nursing Outlook, 25*(2), 108–113.

Benoliel, J. Q. (1978). A holistic approach to terminal illness. *Cancer Nursing, 1*(2), 143–149.

Benoliel, J. Q. (1999). Loss and bereavement: Perspectives, theories, challenges. *Canadian Journal of Nursing Research, 30*(4), 263–272.

Benoliel, J. Q. (2001). Thanatology and human rights. *Illness, Crisis and Loss, 9*(1), 8–14.

Benoliel, J. Q. (2012). The interaction between theory and research. *Nursing Outlook, 60*(5), 272–277.

Benoliel, J. Q., & Crowley, D. M. (1974). *The patient in pain: New concepts.* Atlanta, GA: American Cancer Society.

Benoliel, J. Q., McCorkle, R., & Young, K. (1980). Development of a social dependency scale. *Research in Nursing & Health, 3*(1), 3–10.

Bonner, G. J., Wang, E., Wilkie, D. J., Ferrans, C. E., Dancy, B., & Watkins, Y. J. (2014). Advance care treatment plan (ACT-Plan) for African American family caregivers: A pilot study. *Dementia, 13*(1), 79–95.

Buck, H. G., & McMillan, S. C. (2012). A psychometric analysis of the spiritual needs inventory in informal caregivers of patients with cancer in hospice home care. *Oncology Nursing Forum, 39*(4), E332–E339.

Corless, I. B. (1985). Implications of the new hospice legislation and the accompanying regulations. *Nursing Clinic of North America, 20*(2), 281–298.

Corless, I. B. (1987–1988). Settings for terminal care. *Omega, 18*(4), 329–340.

Corless, I. B. (2001). Women in thanatology illness. *Illness Crisis and Loss, 9*(1).

Corless, I. B. (2009). Florence Wald. *Illness Crisis and Loss, 17*(4), 281–398.

Corless, I. B., Voss, J. G., Nicholas, P. K., Bunch, E. H., Bain, C. A., Coleman, C., . . . Valencia, C. P. (2008). Fatigue in HIV/AIDS patients with comorbidities. *Applied Nursing Research, 21*(3), 116–122.

Coyne, P., Lyckholm, L., Bobb, B., Blaney-Brouse, D., Harrington, S., & Yanni, L. (2013). Managing pain with algorithms: An opportunity for improvement? Or: The development and utilization of algorithms to manage acute pain. *Pain Management Nursing, 14*(4), e185–e188.

Craven, J., & Wald, F. S. (1975). Hospice care for dying patients. *American Journal of Nursing, 75*(10), 1816–1822.

Davies, B., Deveau, E., deVeber, B., Howell, D., Martinson, I., Papadatou, D., . . . Stevens, M. (1998). Experiences of mothers in five countries whose child died of cancer. *Cancer Nursing, 21*(5), 301–311.

Dock, L. L., & Stewart, I. M. (1925). *A short history of nursing from the earliest times to the present day* (2nd ed.). New York, NY: G.P. Putnam's Sons.

Dodd, M., Janson, S., Facione, N., Faucett, J., Froelicher, E. S., Humphreys, J., . . . Taylor, D. (2001). Advancing the science of symptom management. *Journal of Advanced Nursing, 33*(5), 668–676.

Eller, L. S., Bunch, E. H., Wantland, D. J., Portillo, C. J., Reynolds, N. R., Nokes, K. M., . . . Tsai, Y. F. (2010). Prevalence, correlates, and self-management of HIV-related depressive symptoms. *AIDS Care, 22*(9), 1159–1170.

Ellington, L., Reblin, M., Clayton, M. F., Berry, P., & Mooney, K. (2012). Hospice nurse communication with patients with cancer and their family caregivers. *Journal of Palliative Medicine, 15*(3), 262–268.

Fee, E., & Bu, L. (2010). The origins of public health nursing: The Henry Street visiting nurse service. *American Journal of Public Health, 100*(7), 1206–1207.

Ferrell, B., Virani, R., Paice, J. A., Coyle, N., & Coyne, P. (2010). Evaluation of palliative care nursing education seminars. *European Journal of Oncology Nursing, 14*(1), 74–79.

Foster, T. L., Gilmer, M. J., Davies, B., Barrera, M., Fairclough, D., Vannatta, K., & Gerhardt, C. A. (2009). Bereaved parents' and siblings' reports of legacies created by children with cancer. *Journal of Pediatric Oncology Nursing, 26*(6), 369–376.

Foster, Z., & Wald, F. (2001). A crossroads. *Illness, Crisis, and Loss, 9*(1), 42–49.

Gorman, G., Forrest, J., Stapleton, S. J., Hoenig, N. A., Marschke, M., Durham, J., . . . Wilkie, D. J. (2008). Massage for cancer pain: A study with university and hospice collaboration. *Journal of Hospice and Palliative Nursing, 10*(4), 191–197.

Hampton, D. M., Hollis, D. E., Lloyd, D. A., Taylor, J., & McMillan, S. C. (2007). Spiritual needs of persons with advanced cancer. *American Journal of Hospice and Palliative Care, 24*(1), 42–48.

Hinds, P. S., Drew, D., Oakes, L. L., Fouladi, M., Spunt, S. L., Church, C., & Furman, W. L. (2005). End-of-life care preferences of pediatric patients with cancer. *Journal of Clinical Oncology, 23*(36), 9146–9154.

Holtslander, L. F., & McMillan, S. C. (2011). Depressive symptoms, grief, and complicated grief among family caregivers of patients with advanced cancer three months into bereavement. *Oncology Nursing Forum, 38*(1), 60–65.

Holzemer, W. L., Henry, S. B., Nokes, K. M., Corless, I. B., Brown, M. A., Powell-Cope, G. M., . . . Inouye, J. (1999). Validation of the sign and symptom check-list for persons with HIV disease (SSC-HIV). *Journal of Advanced Nursing, 30*(5), 1041–1049.

Huang, H. Y., Ezenwa, M. O., Wilkie, D. J., & Judge, M. K. (2013). Research tracking: Monitoring gender and ethnic minority recruitment and retention in cancer symptom studies. *Cancer Nursing, 36*(3), E1–E6.

Huang, H. Y., Wilkie, D. J., Zong, S. P., Berry, D., Hairabedian, D., Judge, M. K., . . . Chabal, C. (2003). Developing a computerized data collection and decision support system for cancer pain management. *Computers Informatics Nursing, 21*(4), 206–217.

Jane, S. W., Chen, S. L., Wilkie, D. J., Lin, Y. C., Foreman, S. W., Beaton, R. D., . . . Liao, M. N. (2011). Effects of massage on pain, mood status, relaxation, and sleep in Taiwanese patients with metastatic bone pain: A randomized clinical trial. *Pain, 152*(10), 2432–2442.

Kavanaugh, K., Moro, T. T., Savage, T. A., Reyes, M., & Wydra, M. (2009). Supporting parents' decision making surrounding the anticipated birth of an extremely premature infant. *Journal of Perinatal & Neonatal Nursing, 23*(2), 159–170.

Keene, E. A., Hutton, N., Hall, B., & Rushton, C. (2010). Bereavement debriefing sessions: An intervention to support health care professionals in managing their grief after the death of a patient. *Pediatric Nursing, 36*(4), 185–189; quiz 190.

Kemppainen, J. K., Eller, L. S., Bunch, E., Hamilton, M. J., Dole, P., Holzemer, W., . . . Tsai, Y. F. (2006). Strategies for self-management of HIV-related anxiety. *AIDS Care, 18*(6), 597–607.

Kirchhoff, K. T., Spuhler, V., Walker, L., Hutton, A., Cole, B. V., & Clemmer, T. (2000). Intensive care nurses' experiences with end-of-life care. *American Journal of Critical Care, 9*(1), 36–42.

Kirchhoff, K. T., Walker, L., Hutton, A., Spuhler, V., Cole, B. V., & Clemmer, T. (2002). The vortex: Families' experiences with death in the intensive care unit. *American Journal of Critical Care, 11*(3), 200–209.

Koczywas, M., Cristea, M., Thomas, J., McCarty, C., Borneman, T., Del Ferraro, C., . . . Ferrell, B. (2013). Interdisciplinary palliative care intervention in metastatic non-small-cell lung cancer. *Clinical Lung Cancer, 14*(6), 736–744.

Kübler-Ross, E. (1969). *On death and dying.* New York, NY: Scribner Book.

Lunney, J. R., Lynn, J., Foley, D. J., Lipson, S., & Guralnik, J. M. (2003). Patterns of functional decline at the end of life. *Journal of the American Medical Association, 289*(18), 2387–2392.

Martinson, I. M. (1993). Hospice care for children: Past, present, and future. *Journal of Pediatric Oncology Nursing, 10*(3), 93–98.

Martinson, I. M. (2001). Barriers and facilitators experienced during my career: From the perspective of being a woman in the field of thanatology. *Illness, Crisis and Loss, 9*(1), 63–69.

Martinson, I. M., Moldow, D. G., Armstrong, G. D., Henry, W. F., Nesbit, M. E., & Kersey, J. H. (1986). Home care for children dying of cancer. *Research in Nursing & Health, 9*(1), 11–16.

McCorkle, R. (2010). Interdisciplinary collaboration in the pursuit of science to improve psychosocial cancer care. *Psychooncology, 20*(5), 538–543.

McCorkle, R., Knob, M. T., Engelking, C., Lazenby, M., Davies, M., Sipples, R., . . . Lyons, C. (2012). Transition to a new cancer care delivery system: Opportunity for empowerment of the role of the advanced practice provider. *Journal of Advanced Practice Oncology, 3*, 34–42.

McCorkle, R., Robinson, L., Nuamah, I., Lev, E., & Benoliel, J. Q. (1998). The effects of home nursing care for patients during terminal illness on the bereaved's psychological distress. *Nursing Research, 47*(1), 2–10.

McGuire, D. B. (1979). Familial cancer and the role of the nurse. *Cancer Nursing, 2*(6), 443–452.

McGuire, D. B. (1985). Preventive health practices and educational needs in families with hereditary melanoma. *Cancer Nursing, 8*(1), 29–36.

McGuire, D. B. (1989). Cancer pain. Pathophysiology of pain in cancer. *Cancer Nursing, 12*(5), 310–315.

McGuire, D. B., Grant, M., & Park, J. (2012). Palliative care and end of life: The caregiver. *Nursing Outlook, 60*(6), 351–356, e320.

McGuire, D. B., Rubenstein, E. B., & Peterson, D. E. (2004). Evidence-based guidelines for managing mucositis. *Seminars in Oncology Nursing, 20*(1), 59–66.

McMillan, S. C., Small, B. J., & Haley, W. E. (2011). Improving hospice outcomes through systematic assessment: A clinical trial. *Cancer Nursing, 34*(2), 89–97.

McMillan, S. C., & Weitzner, M. (1998). Quality of life in cancer patients: Use of a revised hospice index. *Cancer Practice, 6*(5), 282–288.

McMillan, S. C., & Weitzner, M. A. (2003). Methodologic issues in collecting data from debilitated patients with cancer near the end of life. *Oncology Nursing Forum, 30*(1), 123–129.

Molokie, R. E., Wilkie, D. J., Wittert, H., Suarez, M. L., Yao, Y., Zhao, Z., . . . Wang, Z. J. (2014). Mechanism-driven phase I translational study of trifluoperazine in adults with sickle cell disease. *European Journal of Pharmacology, 723*, 419–424.

Nicholas, P. K., Kemppainen, J. K., Canaval, G. E., Corless, I. B., Sefcik, E. F., Nokes, K. M., . . . Gallagher, D. M. (2007). Symptom management and self-care for peripheral neuropathy in HIV/AIDS. *AIDS Care, 19*(2), 179–189.

Nightingale, F. (1860/1969). *Notes on nursing: What it is and what it is not.* New York, NY: Dover.

Paice, J. A. (2002). Managing psychological conditions in palliative care. *American Journal of Nursing, 102*(11), 36–42; quiz 43.

Puntillo, K. A., Benner, P., Drought, T., Drew, B., Stotts, N., Stannard, D., . . . White, C. (2001). End-of-life issues in intensive care units: A national random survey of nurses' knowledge and beliefs. *American Journal of Critical Care, 10*(4), 216–229.

Quint, J. C. (1963). The impact of mastectomy. *American Journal of Nursing, 63*, 88–92.

Quint, J. C., & Strauss, A. L. (1964). Nursing students, assignments, and dying patients. *Nursing Outlook, 12,* 24–27.

Song, M. K., Kirchhoff, K. T., Douglas, J., Ward, S., & Hammes, B. (2005). A randomized, controlled trial to improve advance care planning among patients undergoing cardiac surgery. *Medical Care, 43*(10), 1049–1053.

Tilden, V. P. (2000). Advance directives. *American Journal of Nursing, 100*(12), 49–51.

Tilden, V. P., Drach, L. L., Tolle, S. W., Rosenfeld, A. G., & Hickman, S. E. (2002). Sampling challenges in end-of-life research: Case-finding for family informants. *Nursing Research, 51*(1), 66–69.

Tilden, V. P., Nelson, C. A., Dunn, P. M., Donius, M., & Tolle, S. W. (2000). Nursing's perspective on improving communication about nursing home residents' preferences for medical treatments at end of life. *Nursing Outlook, 48*(3), 109–115.

Tolle, S. W., & Tilden, V. P. (2002). Changing end-of-life planning: The Oregon experience. *Journal of Palliative Medicine, 5*(2), 311–317.

Tolle, S. W., Tilden, V. P., Rosenfeld, A. G., & Hickman, S. E. (2000). Family reports of barriers to optimal care of the dying. *Nursing Research, 49*(6), 310–317.

Tilden, V. P., Tolle, S. W., Nelson, C. A., & Fields, J. (2001). Family decision-making to withdraw life-sustaining treatments from hospitalized patients. *Nursing Research, 50*(2), 105–115.

Wald, F. S. (1994). Finding a way to give hospice care. In I. B. Corless, B. G. Germino, & M. Pittman (Eds.), *Dying, death, and bereavement: Theoretical perspectives and other ways of knowing* (pp. 31–47). Boston, MA: Jones & Bartlett.

Wald, F. S., Zoster, Z., & Wald, H. J. (1980). The hospice movement as a health care reform. *Nursing Outlook, 28*(3), 173–178.

Wantland, D. J., Holzemer, W. L., Moezzi, S., Willard, S. S., Arudo, J., Kirksey, K. M., . . . Huang, E. (2008). A randomized controlled trial testing the efficacy of an HIV/AIDS symptom management manual. *Journal of Pain & Symptom Management, 36*(3), 235–246.

Wilkie, D., Berry, D., Cain, K., Huang, H. Y., Mekwa, J., Lewis, F., . . . Ko, N. Y. (2010). Effects of coaching patients with lung cancer to report cancer pain. *Western Journal of Nursing Research, 32*(1), 23–46.

Wilkie, D. J. (1995). Facial expressions of pain in lung cancer. *Analgesia, 1,* 91–99.

Wilkie, D. J., Judge, M. K. M., Wells, M. J., & Berkley, I. M. (2001). Excellence in teaching end-of-life care: A new multimedia toolkit for nurse educators. *Nursing and Health Care Perspectives, 22*(5), 226–230.

Wilkie, D. J., Keefe, F. J., Dodd, M. J., & Copp, L. A. (1992). Behavior of patients with lung cancer: Description and associations with oncologic and pain variables. *Pain, 51*(2), 231–240.

Wilkie, D. J., Kim, Y. O., Suarez, M. L., Dauw, C. M., Stapleton, S. J., Gorman, G., . . . Zhao, Z. (2009). Extending computer technology to hospice research: Interactive pentablet measurement of symptoms by hospice cancer patients in their homes. *Journal of Palliative Medicine, 12*(7), 599–602.

Wilkie, D. J., Molokie, R., Boyd-Seal, D., Suarez, M. L., Kim, Y. O., Zong, S., . . . Wang, Z. J. (2010). Patient-reported outcomes: Nociceptive and neuropathic pain and pain barriers in adult outpatients with sickle cell disease. *Journal of the National Medical Association, 102,* 18–27.

James L. Werth Jr.

5

LEGAL ISSUES IN END-OF-LIFE DECISION MAKING

The dying process and the time following death can and should be an intimate, personal process. Ideally, the person dies the way she or he wishes, perhaps at home, maybe surrounded by loved ones, and without drama. However, the reality is that conflict and controversy can become part of the end-of-life and after-death processes for many people because of the emotional nature of the events and the fact that the parties involved (both loved ones and professionals) can have very different perspectives and belief systems. Thus, instead of being a peaceful time of sharing and caring, family members/loved ones may be fighting with each other and/or with medical professionals, medical professionals may be making decisions with which the family members/loved ones disagree, and the dying person herself or himself may or may not be aware of or participating in the debates. As a result, there are many opportunities for disagreements to escalate to the point where lawsuits are threatened.

This chapter discusses many of the legal issues associated with dying and death. Entire books have been written on legal aspects of end-of-life decision making (e.g., Meisel & Cerminara, 2004), so in order to keep this chapter to a manageable length, the focus will be limited to a handful of precedent-setting cases and the repercussions of the rulings, a few state and federal laws, and related research. Because the developments described below build off each other, the most logical way of organizing the chapter is chronological order.

BACKGROUND

My involvement in end-of-life decision-making and interest in its legal aspects began in 1990 during my first year of graduate school when I went to a volunteer training to help me provide direct service to persons with HIV disease. The trainer, who was a social worker, talked about his clients who openly talked about considering suicide and struggling with his professional role and responsibilities in these situations. For my doctoral ethics course, I wrote a paper on "rational suicide and persons with AIDS" that examined the ethical and legal responsibilities that mental health professionals had when working with terminally ill clients who were considering suicide as an option. My first several articles and books were on the topic of rational suicide and the idea that some people could make a well-reasoned decision that death was the best option they had, given their circumstances (Werth, 1996, 2000; Werth & Rogers, 2005).

As I deepened and broadened my exploration of the issues surrounding dying, I noticed that it was artificial to separate out one type of end-of-life decision from others because, according to the research, the same things that may cause a person to consider suicide may also lead a person to request that life-sustaining treatment be withheld or withdrawn. Thus, I shifted my focus to end-of-life decision making more broadly. Because of my training in ethics, and later in law (I have a Master of Legal Studies degree), I continued to examine the legal and ethical aspects of life-and-death decisions. My most recent emphasis has been on the "duty to protect" when mental health professionals are working with clients who may be a danger to self and/or other people.

The focus of this chapter is on significant court cases, highly influential and relevant state and federal laws, and associated research. Each of the cases or laws reviewed has had a significant impact on the public's perception and understanding of end-of-life decision making, on legal developments that have implications for the options available to people who are dying and their loved ones, and/or have been the focus of significant and biased debate. In order to minimize the impact of my own views, I decided to use quotations from primary sources, such as the court decisions or the laws and regulations themselves.

1970s AND 1980s

Starting this timeline in the 1970s is a bit arbitrary because there certainly were important cases and laws before this period. However, if we look specifically at end-of-life-focused issues, it makes sense to begin with the case of Karen Ann Quinlan, which was decided in 1976.

In re Quinlan (New Jersey, 1976)

Karen Ann Quinlan was a 22-year-old single woman living in New Jersey when, "for reasons still unclear," she "ceased breathing for at least two 15-minute periods" (In re Quinlan, 1976, p. 23). She was diagnosed as being in a "chronic persistent vegetative state" (p. 24) but was not "brain dead" (p. 24). She was placed on a respirator because the physicians believed she could not breathe on her own, and she received artificial nutrition and hydration. Because she was not able to make decisions for herself, she was assigned a guardian *ad litem* who was given responsibility for "the person of" Ms. Quinlan. The court case revolved around her father's request for judicial authority to withdraw the life-sustaining mechanisms temporarily preserving his daughter's life, and his appointment as guardian of her person to that end. His request was opposed by her doctors, the hospital, the Morris County Prosecutor, the State of New Jersey, and her guardian *ad litem* (p. 22).

The court emphasized that Mr. Quinlan's decision came about only after conferring with his parish priest about "the moral rightness of the decision" (p. 30). The New Jersey Catholic Conference submitted an *amicus curiae* brief verifying that stopping the use of the treatment would be acceptable because it is considered "extraordinary treatment" (pp. 31–32).

The Court held that,

> Upon the concurrence of the guardian and family of Karen, should the responsible attending physicians conclude that there is no reasonable possibility of Karen's ever emerging from her present comatose condition to a cognitive, sapient state and that the life-support apparatus now being administered to Karen should be discontinued, they shall consult with the hospital "Ethics Committee" or like body of the institution in which Karen is then hospitalized. If that consultative body agrees that there is no

reasonable possibility of Karen's ever emerging from her present comatose condition to a cognitive, sapient state, the present life-support system may be withdrawn and said action shall be without any civil or criminal liability therefor on the part of any participant, whether guardian, physician, hospital or others. (p. 54)

Further, the Court stated, "By the above ruling we do not intend to be understood as implying that a proceeding for judicial declaratory relief is necessarily required for the implementation of comparable decisions in the field of medical practice" (p. 55).

This ruling was ground-breaking for several reasons. First, it established the legal right for a guardian of a person who is not legally competent to make her or his own decisions to decide that life-sustaining measures should be discontinued, even if death may result. Second, it emphasized the role of hospital ethics committees in end-of-life decision making. Third, it indicated that these types of decisions do not need to go before a court but instead could be handled by the parties involved.

In addition, it gave legal recognition to religious perspectives on end-of-life issues, especially the distinction between ordinary and extraordinary means and the principle of "double effect." Both of these concepts have been important parts of Catholic philosophy related to end-of-life decision-making. Beauchamp and Childress (1994) addressed both in their important text on biomedical ethics. These authors stated, "Ordinary has often been taken to mean 'usual' or 'customary,' whereas extraordinary has often been taken to mean 'unusual' or 'uncustomary'" (p. 200). The resultant conclusion is therefore that ordinary treatments must be given but extraordinary ones can be withheld or withdrawn. Beauchamp and Childress are critical of this distinction for a variety of reasons. One obvious problem is that it is context dependent because what may be customary in one situation will not be so in another, so this distinction is too broad to take into account the person's particular condition and what she or he wants done.

Similarly, Beauchamp and Childress (1994) are unpersuaded by the utility of the principle of double effect. This idea has four parts, each of which is necessary: (1) "the act must be good, or at least morally neutral"; (2) "the agent intends only the good effect" even if a "bad effect can be foreseen"; (3) "the bad effect must not be a means to the good effect"; and (4) "the good effect must outweigh the bad effect" (p. 207). To use the example of Ms. Quinlan, one analysis using the principle of double effect could proceed as follows: the removal of the ventilator is at least a morally neutral act in and of itself. The intent of removing the tube is to acquiesce to her wishes and to alleviate or prevent suffering, not to cause her to die. She does not need to die as a result of the removal of the ventilator to meet the goal of implementing her wishes. Not forcing her to continue to exist in a state undesired by her is better than her dying while unaware of doing so. Even though some do not view the principle of double effect to be persuasive, it has been important in allowing strongly religious individuals to allow people to die as opposed to maintaining life regardless of the circumstances.

After this case, courts across the country addressed various aspects of end-of-life decision making. Each of these had some import in individual states but none rose to the federal level until the case of Nancy Cruzan, which began when she was found unconscious in 1983. The final court case was decided in 1990 so it is discussed in the next section.

1990s

Cruzan v. Director, Missouri Department of Health
(U.S. Supreme Court, 1990)

In early 1983, Nancy Cruzan was a young woman living in Missouri when she had an automobile accident. She was found face down in a ditch and paramedics were able to restore her breathing and heartbeat at the site, but it was estimated that she was oxygen deprived for up to 14 minutes, leading to a coma and eventually a persistent vegetative state. Her husband consented to the placement of an artificial nutrition and hydration tube (Cruzan, 1990). After it was apparent that it was very unlikely that she would regain consciousness, "her parents asked hospital employees to terminate the artificial nutrition and hydration procedures. All agree[d] that such a removal would cause her death. The employees refused to honor the request without court approval" (pp. 267–268). Missouri had a living will law, and if Ms. Cruzan had such a document, which is used to specify the treatment a person does or does not want in certain circumstances (e.g., "I do not want to receive artificial nutrition and hydration if I am in a persistent vegetative state" or the converse), then her wishes as expressed in that document would have been followed, if they had applied to her medical condition. However, she did not have a living will and, given this, Missouri required a relatively high standard of proof ("clear and convincing evidence") regarding her wishes. When the case went to court, the Missouri Supreme Court had ruled that the statements Ms. Cruzan made to a housemate did not rise to the level of clear and convincing evidence, and, therefore, the Missouri Supreme Court denied the removal of Ms. Cruzan's tube.

The case was appealed to the U.S. Supreme Court, where the issue was "whether Cruzan has a right under the United States Constitution which would require the hospital to withdraw life-sustaining treatment from her under these circumstances" (p. 269). Later, the Court stated, "This is the first case in which we have been squarely presented with the issue of whether the United States Constitution grants what is in common parlance referred to as a 'right to die'" (p. 277).

The Court stated, "The principle that a competent person has a constitutionally protected liberty interest in refusing unwanted medical treatment may be inferred from our prior decisions" (p. 278). Further the Court said that "for purposes of this case, we assume that the United States Constitution would grant a competent person a constitutionally protected right to refuse lifesaving hydration and nutrition" (p. 279). Specifically, "It cannot be disputed that the Due Process Clause protects an interest in life as well as an interest in refusing life-sustaining medical treatment" (p. 281). Thus, the Court did enshrine withholding or withdrawing life-sustaining treatment as a Constitutional right. However, the Court then said,

> An incompetent person is not able to make an informed and voluntary choice to exercise a hypothetical right to refuse treatment or any other right. Such a "right" must be exercised for her, if at all, by some sort of surrogate. Here, Missouri has in effect recognized that, under certain circumstances, a surrogate may act for the patient in electing to have hydration and nutrition withdrawn in such a way as to cause death, but it has established a procedural safeguard to assure that the action of the surrogate conforms as best it may to the wishes expressed by the patient while competent. Missouri requires that evidence of the incompetent's wishes as to the withdrawal of treatment

be proved by clear and convincing evidence. The question, then, is whether the United States Constitution forbids the establishment of this procedural requirement by the State. We hold that it does not. (p. 280)

In other words, the U.S. Supreme Court ruled that Missouri "may apply a clear and convincing evidence standard in proceedings where a guardian seeks to discontinue nutrition and hydration of a person diagnosed to be in a persistent vegetative state" (p. 284). The majority then ruled that it could not say the Missouri Court committed a Constitutional error in stating that Ms. Cruzan's comments to her friend did not rise to the necessary level. Finally, the U.S. Supreme Court also held that Missouri was not obligated to accept the "substituted judgment" of family members who do not have proof rising to the appropriate level of evidence. Thus, the Court did not allow the removal of Ms. Cruzan's tube.

The Cruzan case was notable because it was the first time the U.S. Supreme Court examined the issue of end-of-life decision-making. Even though lower level courts had ruled on similar matters, the fact that the Court found a Constitutional right to the withholding or withdrawal of life-sustaining treatment was crucial for all the subsequent developments in this area. The attention given to the Missouri living will statute was important as well.

Patient Self-Determination Act (1990/1991)

The Patient Self-Determination Act (PSDA) was passed by Congress in 1990 and began implementation in 1991. The focus of the PSDA is on the use of advance directives. Advance directives typically refer to written instructions specified in two documents (or a single document combining these two pieces) about a person's preferences regarding health care treatment and decision makers if a person is unable to speak for herself or himself (Wilkinson, Wenger, & Shugarman, 2007). As noted above, a "living will" identifies what type of care is and is not wanted in different circumstances. A "durable power of attorney for health care" identifies one or more people who are authorized to make medical decisions for a person in the event that she or he is not competent to make her or his own choices. Wilkinson and colleagues (2007) noted that many experts believe that the power of attorney designation is more important than the living will because living wills often are not useful in particular situations, whereas the power of attorney can take the context into account and make decisions as situations evolve. However, a living will can provide important information for the holder of power of attorney to use when making decisions and can help loved ones cope if a decision is made to withhold or withdraw treatment, such as cardiopulmonary resuscitation, artificial nutrition and hydration, dialysis, or a ventilator, which then contributes to or leads to the death of the person.

The final regulations of the PSDA begin with a definition:

"Advance directive" means a written instruction, such as a living will or durable power of attorney for health care, recognized under state law (whether statutory or as recognized by the courts of the State), relating to the provision of health care when the individual is incapacitated. (Federal Patient Self-Determination Act Final Regulation, 1995, Section 489.100)

Because the PSDA does not apply to individual physicians, the "Requirements for providers" section is composed primarily of expectations of health care institutions. These organizations must have written policies and procedures about advance directives for adults receiving care at their facilities or by their providers. They are required to do the following:

1. Provide written information either before the person becomes a patient of the facility or at time of admission, depending on the type of institution, about
    a. a person's rights under State law "to make decisions concerning such medical care, including the right to accept or refuse medical or surgical treatment and the right to formulate, at the individual's option, advance directives. . . ."
    b. if relevant, "a clear and precise statement of limitation if the provider cannot implement an advance directive on the basis of conscience. . . ."
2. "Document in the individual's medical record whether or not the individual has executed an advance directive";
3. "Not condition the provision of care or otherwise discriminate against an individual based on whether or not the individual has executed an advance directive";
4. "Ensure compliance with requirements of State law . . . regarding advance directives. . . .";
5. "Provide education for staff concerning its policies and procedures on advance directives"; and
6. "Provide for community education regarding issues concerning advance directives. . . ." (Section 489.102)

The regulations also include a provision saying that

> If an adult individual is incapacitated—at the time of admission or at the start of care and is unable to receive information—(due to the incapacitating conditions or a mental disorder) or articulate whether or not he or she has executed an advance directive, then the provider may give advance directive information to the individual's family or surrogate in the same manner that it issues other material about policies and procedures to the family of the incapacitated individual or to a surrogate or other concerned persons in accordance with State law. The provider is not relieved of its obligation to provide this information to the individual once he or she is no longer incapacitated or unable to receive such information. Follow up procedures must be in place to provide the information to the individual directly at the appropriate time. (Section 489.102(e))

As is explicitly stated above, the PSDA focuses on adults. One of the continuing unsettled issues is the age at which adolescents and children can have a say in the medical decisions that may or may not extend or limit the length of their lives.

The obvious intent of the PSDA was to increase the use and usefulness of advance directives. However, these goals have not been realized. Wilkinson and colleagues (2007) reviewed the literature on advance directives for the U.S. Department of Health and Human Services. They found that only around 20% to 30% of people have an advance directive, with some groups more likely to have them than others, including people who are older, European Americans, and those of higher socioeconomic status. Honing in on people with the most need for advance directives and awareness of them, Wilkinson's team reported that fewer than 50% of patients considered severely or terminally ill had an advance directive in their record and approximately two thirds to three quarters of physicians did not know that their patients had advance directives.

The goal of advance directives is to increase the autonomy of patients and the likelihood that their wishes would be respected by providing direction for loved ones and medical teams. Unfortunately, even though all states have laws, there are federal laws, and all levels of courts have supported their use, fewer than half of people have completed an advance directive and, of those who have done so, it is likely that they have not had conversations with their physicians and loved ones about their wishes. There are other limitations to advance directives and the push for physician-assisted death was a way of addressing some of these issues.

Oregon Death with Dignity Act (1994/1997)

Although advance directives are helpful if a person is unable to make decisions for herself or himself, especially if there may be some medical interventions that are or could be used to keep the person alive, not everyone who is seriously ill is in this type of situation. For example, someone can have bone cancer and be in tremendous pain but be conscious. Further, some people find being in control to be very important and are anxious about uncertainty. Being diagnosed with a terminal illness can lead to great anxiety over what will happen. If someone is terminally ill but not on life-sustaining technology and is suffering and wants to die, the person can end her or his own life without involving anyone else (traditionally referred to as "suicide"), ask someone else for the means to end her or his own life but take the final action herself or himself (referred to by a variety of terms, including "physician-assisted suicide" or "physician-assisted dying" or "physician-assisted death"—opponents of this method refer to it as "physician-assisted suicide"), or ask someone else to take the final action ("voluntary active euthanasia"). Suicide is not illegal in any state, but it can be traumatic for loved ones, and there is the possibility of being worse off after attempting suicide but not dying. Euthanasia implicates another person and can lead to prosecution for murder or manslaughter, as was the case for Dr. Jack Kevorkian in Michigan. As a result, advocates for people who are terminally ill who wanted to create options that would allow these dying individuals to have more control over the manner and timing of death focused on legalizing physician-assisted death.

The first successful effort to pass a law allowing physicians to prescribe medication to a terminally ill person, knowing that the dying individual would use the medicine to end her or his own life, was the Oregon Death with Dignity Act (ODDA; ORS 127.800-996). The law has been very controversial, with much written by opponents and supporters. The material in this section is taken from the website maintained by the Oregon Public Health Division (OPHD, n.d.-a), which is required to gather data on the implementation of the law.

The ODDA was a citizen initiative that was originally passed in 1994. However, before it could be used, suits were filed, and the law was prevented from being implemented for several years. Following the U.S. Supreme Court decisions in *Washington v. Glucksberg* and *Vacco v. Quill*, described in the next section, the Oregon legislature returned the issue to the voters and in 1997 the public rejected an effort to repeal the law, which then allowed it to be used.

The ODDA requires that the person requesting medication be a resident of the state. According to the OPHD Frequently Asked Questions (OPHD, n.d.-b) page,

> The law states that, in order to participate, a patient must be: (1) 18 years of age or older, (2) a resident of Oregon, (3) capable of making and communicating

health care decisions for him/herself, and (4) diagnosed with a terminal illness that will lead to death within six (6) months. It is up to the attending physician to determine whether these criteria have been met. (Question/Answer 3)

The OPHD (n.d.-b) stated that, once these criteria have been met,

> The following steps must be fulfilled: (1) the patient must make two oral requests to the attending physician, separated by at least 15 days; (2) the patient must provide a written request to the attending physician, signed in the presence of two witnesses, at least one of whom is not related to the patient; (3) the attending physician and a consulting physician must confirm the patient's diagnosis and prognosis; (4) the attending physician and a consulting physician must determine whether the patient is capable of making and communicating health care decisions for him/herself; (5) if either physician believes the patient's judgment is impaired by a psychiatric or psychological disorder (such as depression), the patient must be referred for a psychological examination; (6) the attending physician must inform the patient of feasible alternatives to the Act including comfort care, hospice care, and pain control; (7) the attending physician must request, but may not require, the patient to notify their next-of-kin of the prescription request. A patient can rescind a request at any time and in any manner. The attending physician will also offer the patient an opportunity to rescind his/her request at the end of the 15-day waiting period following the initial request to participate. (Question/Answer 12)

Physicians are not required to participate in the ODDA, and some systems, such as those affiliated with the Catholic Church, have prohibited using the law at their sites.

Physicians are required to complete forms for the OPHD, so there have been yearly reports on the ODDA. According to the most recent report, since the law was implemented in 1997, 1,173 people had received prescriptions and 752 people had used the medication to die (OPHD, 2014). The number of people receiving prescriptions and using them has increased from 24 and 16, respectively, in 1998 to 116 and 85, respectively, in 2012 (the most recent year with complete data). In terms of demographics, most people who died as a result of taking the medication were older, European American, male, well educated, had cancer, died at home, were enrolled in hospice care, and had health insurance. Only two of the people who died in 2013 were referred for an evaluation by a psychiatrist or psychologist. "As in previous years, the three most frequently mentioned end-of-life concerns were: loss of autonomy (93.0%), decreasing ability to participate in activities that made life enjoyable (88.7%), and loss of dignity (73.2%)" (p. 3).

Other states were reluctant to implement a similar law until there was time to see the practical implications of the ODDA and determine whether any of the fears expressed about the ODDA had come to pass. Following 10 years of implementation without evidence of people being pressured to die or discriminatory actions by physicians, other states moved forward. In 2008, the state of Washington passed a citizen's initiative that mirrored the ODDA (see Washington State Department of Health, n.d.). In 2009, the Montana Supreme Court relied on the Montana Constitution to become the first state-level court to expressly allow physicians to prescribe medication to patients (see *Baxter et al. v. State of Montana and*

Steve Bullock, 2009). In 2013, the Vermont General Assembly became the first state legislature to pass a law allowing physician-assisted death (see Vermont Department of Health, 2014).

Washington v. Glucksberg (1997) and *Vacco v. Quill* (U.S. Supreme Court, 1997)

The U.S. Supreme Court was pulled into the debate over "physician-assisted suicide" (the Court's term) when it decided to hear two cases from opposite ends of the country. The issue to be addressed was whether state laws prohibiting "physician-assisted suicide" were Constitutional.

The first case in this section is *Washington v. Glucksberg* (1997).

> Petitioners in this case are the State of Washington and its Attorney General. Respondents Harold Glucksberg, M. D., Abigail Halperin, M. D., Thomas A. Preston, M. D., and Peter Shalit, M. D., are physicians who practice in Washington. These doctors occasionally treat terminally ill, suffering patients, and declare that they would assist these patients in ending their lives if not for Washington's assisted suicide ban. In January 1994, respondents, along with three gravely ill, pseudonymous plaintiffs who have since died and Compassion in Dying, a nonprofit organization that counsels people considering physician assisted suicide, sued in the United States District Court, seeking a declaration that Washington State's law that makes aiding another person to attempt suicide a felony is, on its face, unconstitutional. (pp. 707–708)

> Relying on the Cruzan decision along with other cases, the Ninth Circuit Court of Appeals used a liberty interest argument and ruled that "the State's assisted-suicide ban was unconstitutional 'as applied to terminally ill competent adults who wish to hasten their deaths with medication prescribed by their physicians'" (p. 709). Thus, when it was heard by the U.S. Supreme Court, the issue was framed and decided in this way: "The question presented in this case is whether Washington's prohibition against 'caus[ing]' or 'aid[ing]' a suicide offends the Fourteenth Amendment to the United States Constitution. We hold that it does not" (pp. 705–706). The Court concluded its analysis by stating, "Throughout the Nation, Americans are engaged in an earnest and profound debate about the morality, legality, and practicality of physician-assisted suicide. Our holding permits this debate to continue, as it should in a democratic society" (p. 735).

In the companion *Vacco v. Quill* (1997) case,

> Petitioners are various New York public officials. Respondents Timothy E. Quill, Samuel C. Klagsbrun, and Howard A. Grossman are physicians who practice in New York. They assert that although it would be "consistent with the standards of [their] medical practice[s]" to prescribe lethal medication for "mentally competent, terminally ill patients" who are suffering great pain and desire a doctor's help in taking their own lives, they are deterred from doing so by New York's ban on assisting suicide. Respondents, and three gravely ill patients who have since died, sued the State's attorney general in the United States District Court. They urged that because New York permits a competent person to refuse life-sustaining medical treatment, and because

the refusal of such treatment is "essentially the same thing" as physician-assisted suicide, New York's assisted-suicide ban violates the Equal Protection Clause. (pp. 797–798)

The Second Circuit Court of Appeals used an equal protection argument and stated that

"New York law does not treat equally all competent persons who are in the final stages of fatal illness and wish to hasten their deaths," because "those in the final stages of terminal illness who are on life-support systems are allowed to hasten their deaths by directing the removal of such systems; but those who are similarly situated, except for the previous attachment of life-sustaining equipment, are not allowed to hasten death by self-administering prescribed drugs." [citation omitted] In the court's view, "[t]he ending of life by [the withdrawal of life-support systems] is *nothing more nor less than assisted suicide.* [citation omitted] (emphasis added). The Court of Appeals then examined whether this supposed unequal treatment was rationally related to any legitimate state interests, and concluded that "to the extent that [New York's statutes] prohibit a physician from prescribing medications to be self-administered by a mentally competent, terminally-ill person in the final stages of his terminal illness, they are not rationally related to any legitimate state interest. We . . . now reverse. (pp. 798–799)

The practical significance of these rulings was that the U.S. Supreme Court left it to each state to decide how to proceed regarding whether to allow physicians to prescribe medications to terminally ill patients so the patient can use them to die as opposed to mandating that states allow physician-assisted death. The implications were that this opened the door to the implementation of the Oregon Death with Dignity Act, as noted above, and in other states, whether by citizen initiative, state court ruling, or legislative action.

2000s

The Case of Theresa Marie Schiavo (2000–2005)

The case of Theresa Marie ("Terri") Schiavo is long and complicated, involving state and federal law; the involvement of politicians and physicians and professors; and ultimately the involvement of the Pope, both houses of the Florida legislature, the Governor of Florida, both houses of the U.S. Congress, the President of the United States, and several appeals up to the U.S. Supreme Court. Descriptions of the events are available in a variety of places but it can be difficult to find non-biased descriptions of the events. The material from this section was summarized from the University of Miami Ethics Programs website developed by Cerminara and Goodman (2014a, 2014b). The events in this case are remarkable, so the interested reader is urged to review the website and the associated documents. The focus here is on the federal-level involvement in the case.

Mrs. Schiavo was 26 years old when, in February 1990, she had a cardiac arrest that led to brain damage as a result of oxygen deprivation. Because she could not eat or drink on her own, a tube was placed to provide her with artificial nutrition and hydration. Later that year, her husband, Michael, was appointed her guardian, without objection from her parents. In 1992, Michael was awarded medical malpractice awards that were to be used, in part, for his wife's medical expenses and to compensate him. In 1993, Michael and Mrs. Schiavo's parents disagreed over her care, and Mr. and Mrs. Schindler (her parents) went to court to have Michael removed as her guardian, but the court dismissed the suit. In 1994, a guardian *ad litem* submitted a report stating that Michael had been acting appropriately as Mrs. Schiavo's guardian.

In 1998, Michael petitioned to have the tube providing Mrs. Schiavo with artificial nutrition and hydration removed. Her parents opposed the request because they believed she would want to stay alive, so the court appointed a different guardian *ad litem*. This guardian *ad litem's* report stated that Mrs. Schiavo was in a persistent vegetative state with no chance of improvement, but it also said that Michael may be influenced by the possibility of inheriting the rest of the money from the malpractice settlements. In mid-February, 2000, the judge ruled that, based on the evidence before him, Mrs. Schiavo would have chosen to have the tube removed, so he ordered the tube be removed, but he later stayed the implementation of his order until 30 days after the exhaustion of all appeals by the Schindlers.

Following this initial ruling, there were 5 years of legal and political maneuvering. The Florida Supreme Court denied to hear any appeals of the trial court's decision until the state legislature passed a bill that was signed by then-Governor Jeb Bush. The bill was colloquially entitled "Terri's Law" and served the purpose of overruling court decisions that the tube should be removed. The Florida Supreme Court ruled that the law was unconstitutional. This ruling and several others were appealed to the U.S. Supreme Court, which denied hearing any of the cases. The Pope even became involved in the case by choosing to make a speech focused on people who were in persistent vegetative states.

The Florida legislature considered several more bills that would prevent the removal of artificial nutrition and hydration tubes from people in persistent vegetative states whose circumstances mirrored Mrs. Schiavo's, but none were passed by both houses. However, on March 16, 2005, the U.S. House of Representatives passed a bill that would allow certain cases, such as the current one, to be shifted to federal court. On March 17, the U.S. Senate passed a "private bill" applying specifically to Mrs. Schiavo's case but that differed from the U.S. House of Representatives bill. On March 18, the U.S. House Committee on Government Reform took several actions intended to prevent the removal of the tube, but it was still removed as scheduled following the latest round of court appeals. This was the third time that the tube had been removed. It was believed that Mrs. Schiavo would die within a few days unless the tube was reinserted again.

On March 19–20, the U.S. Senate and U.S. House worked to reach a compromise on their bills and on March 21 the bill was signed by then-President Bush (brother of Florida Governor Jeb Bush). On March 23, the Eleventh Circuit Court of Appeals denied the Schindler's appeal to have the tube reinstated and on March 24, the U.S. Supreme Court once again denied to hear the case. Several other appeals and efforts to force the tube to be reinstated were denied over the course of the next several days. On March 31, 2005, Mrs. Schiavo died. A subsequent poll indicated that the majority of respondents disagreed with how Governor Bush, President Bush, the Florida Legislature, and the U.S. Congress handed the case (PR Newswire, 2005). The autopsy report, released June 15, stated that Mrs. Schiavo's condition was "consistent" with what would be found in a person who was in a persistent vegetative state and that the "damage was irreversible."

The practical implications of the case were that what had previously been settled law following the cases of Karen Ann Quinlan and Nancy Cruzan remained settled. In addition, the roles of courts and legislatures remained in balance instead of privileging the decisions of state or federal legislators. On the other hand, the Pope's statements led to questions about allowable courses of action regarding the discontinuation of artificial nutrition and hydration because they were contrary to what had been considered settled doctrine following the Quinlan case described previously. Subsequently, clarification reestablished the earlier interpretation.

Gonzales v. Oregon (U.S. Supreme Court, 2006)

This was another U.S. Supreme Court case that related to the matter of whether physicians could prescribe medication to assist a person to die. In this particular case, the Court said, "The question before us is whether the Controlled Substances Act [CSA] allows the United States Attorney General to prohibit doctors from prescribing regulated drugs for use in physician-assisted suicide, notwithstanding a state law permitting the procedure" (p. 1). The state law at issue was the Oregon Death with Dignity Act, which was described earlier. The medications that physicians in Oregon prescribe to help people die are regulated by the CSA. In 2001, then-Attorney General Ashcroft issued an "Interpretive Rule" that said that "using controlled substances to assist suicide is not a legitimate medical practice and that dispensing or prescribing them for this purpose is unlawful under the CSA" (p. 2). Because physicians need a registration with the Drug Enforcement Administration in order to prescribe controlled substances, this Interpretive Rule would have rendered the Death with Dignity Act unusable. The Rule was challenged by the State of Oregon, a physician and a pharmacist, and a group of terminally ill patients. The Ninth Circuit ruled that the Interpretive Rule was invalid for two reasons: (1) it changed the balance between the state government and the federal government by transferring power that historically had been under a state's control to the federal government, and (2) the CSA was written to address drug abuse, not medical policy.

The Supreme Court considered several arguments by the attorney general as to why the Interpretive Rule was an acceptable use of his authority but decided, among other things, that the attorney general "is not authorized to make a rule declaring illegitimate a medical standard for care and treatment of patients that is specifically authorized under state law" (p. 11). Further, the Court said that Congress, through the CSA, "regulates medical practice insofar as it bars doctors from using their prescription-writing powers as a means to engage in illicit drug dealing and trafficking as conventionally understood" (p. 23), otherwise power is delegated to the states to regulate medical practice. Specifically to this point, the Court said that "Oregon's [Death with Dignity Act] is an example of the state regulation of medical practice that the CSA presupposes" (p. 24). For more information on the case, see the Physician-Assisted Dying webpage of the Oregon Department of Justice (n.d.).

The practical implication of this is that the Supreme Court's decision made it clear that the federal government had no role in regulating the use of medications that could be used to assist a patient to die, as long as the state where the prescribing occurred had a law specifically authorizing physicians to help people to die or permission was granted in other state laws or state governing documents. This decision meant that states were still allowed to implement physician-assisted death, consistent with the rulings in *Washington v. Glucksberg* and *Vacco v. Quill* described previously.

2010–PRESENT

Final Exit Network, Inc. et al. v. State of Georgia (2012)

Suicide is not illegal in Georgia; however, Georgia had a law related to "assisted suicide" and, in 2012, the Georgia Supreme Court ruled on a case related to the law.

> In 1994, the Georgia legislature enacted OCGA § 16-5-5 (b), which provides that any person "who publicly advertises, offers, or holds himself or herself out as offering that he or she will intentionally and actively assist another person in the commission of suicide and commits any overt act to further that purpose is guilty of a felony." Violation of the statute is punishable by imprisonment for not less than one nor more than five years. OCGA § 16-5-5 (b). The issue in this case is whether OCGA § 16-5-5 (b) is constitutional under the free speech clauses of the federal and state constitutions. (p. 1)

The case was appealed to the Georgia Supreme Court by the Final Exit Network and some of its members after they were indicted in 2010 for assisting a Georgia resident to die. In its analysis, the Court focused on the fact that

> not all assisted suicides [] are criminalized but only those which include a public advertisement or offer to assist. This distinction takes the statute out of the realm of content neutral regulations and renders it a selective restraint on speech with a particular content. (p. 3)

Because the issue under consideration was free speech, not the prohibition of physician-assisted death in and of itself, the State had to demonstrate a compelling interest and that the statute was limited to address that interest.

The Court stated that the law "does not ban assistance in all suicides, conduct which by itself is legal in Georgia. Many assisted suicides are either not prohibited or are expressly exempted from the [law]" (p. 4). The Court asserted,

> Had the State truly been interested in the preservation of human life, however, it could have imposed a ban on all assisted suicides with no restriction on protected speech whatsoever. Alternatively, the State could have sought to prohibit all offers to assist in suicide when accompanied by an overt act to accomplish that goal. The State here did neither. (pp. 4–5)

As a result, the Court stated, "We hold the State may not, consistent with the United States and Georgia Constitutions, make the public advertisement or offer to assist in a suicide a criminal offense" (p. 7).

The practical implications of this case were that, as a result of the ruling, the defendants were acquitted (Severson, 2012). In May 2012, the Georgia legislature passed a new law stating,

> Any person with actual knowledge that a person intends to commit suicide who knowingly and willfully assists such person in the commission of such person's suicide shall be guilty of a felony and, upon conviction thereof, shall be punished by imprisonment for not less than one nor more than ten years. (GA Code §16-5-5)

Beyond the effect on the law in Georgia, another significant implication of the case was the publicity given to the Final Exit Network and their advocacy for people who are dying and the use of helium as a means of helping people die (Severson, 2012).

CONCLUSION

Given the emotional nature of the dying process, it is not surprising that conflict and controversy will arise. State and federal laws and associated court cases have attempted to balance the competing interests involved while maximizing the control that the dying person has over the time she or he has remaining. This chapter highlighted some of the most important and well-known cases and laws in the end-of-life arena. As technology continues to advance and people live longer, we can envision that some areas that may lead to legal involvement could revolve around "rationing" of health care dollars, decision making when people have dementia and other progressive conditions that will affect decision-making abilities, and the extent to which ill individuals versus their medical teams make decisions about when treatment is "futile."

REFERENCES

Assisted suicide; notification of licensing board regarding violation, Georgia Code § 16-5-5 (2012).

Baxter et al. v. State of Montana and Steve Bullock. (2009). MT 449. Retrieved from http://applicationengine.mt.gov/getContent?vsId={88A87FE0-2501-438A-AC31-CCE62D37C894}&impersonate=true&objectStoreName=PROD%20OBJECT%20STORE&objectType=document

Beauchamp, T. L., & Childress, J. F. (1994). *Principles of biomedical ethics* (4th ed.). New York, NY: Oxford University Press.

Cerminara, K., & Goodman, K. (2014a). *Schiavo timeline, part 1.* Retrieved from http://www.miami.edu/index.php/ethics/projects/schiavo/schiavo_timeline/

Cerminara, K., & Goodman, K. (2014b). *Schiavo timeline, part 2.* Retrieved from http://www.miami.edu/index.php/ethics/projects/schiavo/schiavo_timline2/

Cruzan v. Director, Missouri Department of Health, 497 U.S. 261 (1990).

Federal Patient Self-Determination Act Final Regulation. (1995). *Federal Register, 60*(123), 33294–33295. Retrieved from http://som.unm.edu/ethics/_docs/patient-self-determination-act.pdf

Final Exit Network, Inc. et al. v. State of Georgia. 290 Ga. 508 (2012).

Gonzales v. Oregon, 546 U.S. 243 (2006).

In re Quinlan, 70 N.J. 10, 355 A.2d 647 (New Jersey, 1976).

Meisel, A., &Cerminara, K. L. (2004). *The right to die: The law of end-of-life decisionmaking* (3rd ed.). New York, NY: Aspen.

Oregon Death with Dignity Act, Oregon Revised Statute, 127.800-995 (1997).

Oregon Department of Justice. (n.d.). *Physician assisted dying.* Retrieved from http://www.doj.state.or.us/hot_topics/11072001.shtml

Oregon Public Health Division. (n.d.-a). *Death with Dignity Act.* Retrieved from http://public.health.oregon.gov/ProviderPartnerResources/EvaluationResearch/DeathwithDignityAct/Pages/index.aspx

Oregon Public Health Division. (n.d.-b). *Frequently asked questions.* Retrieved from http://public.health.oregon.gov/ProviderPartnerResources/EvaluationResearch/DeathwithDignityAct/Pages/faqs.aspx

Oregon Public Health Division. (2014). *Oregon's Death with Dignity Act – 2013.* Retrieved from http://public.health.oregon.gov/ProviderPartnerResources/EvaluationResearch/DeathwithDignityAct/Documents/year16.pdf

Patient Self Determination Act, Omnibus Reconciliation Act of 1990 (1990).

PR Newswire. (2005, April15). *The Terri Schiavo case.* Retrieved from http://www.the freelibrary.com/The+Terri+Schiavo+Case%3A+Paradoxically+Most+U.S.+Adults+ Approve+of+How...-a0131501504

Severson, K. (2012, February 6). Georgia court rejects law aimed at assisted suicide. *New York Times.* Retrieved from http://www.nytimes.com/2012/02/07/us/assisted-suicide-law-is-overturned-by-georgia-supreme-court.html

Vacco v. Quill, 521 U.S. 793 (1997).

Vermont Department of Health. (2014). *Patient choice and control at end of life.* Retrieved from http://healthvermont.gov/family/end_of_life_care/patient_choice.aspx

Washington v. Glucksberg, 521 U.S. 702 (1997).

Washington State Department of Health. (n.d.). *Death with Dignity Act.* Retrieved from http://www.doh.wa.gov/YouandYourFamily/IllnessandDisease/DeathwithDignity Act.aspx

Werth, J. L., Jr. (1996). *Rational suicide? Implications for mental health professionals.* Washington, DC: Taylor & Francis.

Werth, J. L., Jr. (2000). How do the mental health issues differ in the withholding/withdraw-ing of treatment versus assisted death? *Omega, 41,* 259–278.

Werth, J. L., Jr., & Rogers, J. R. (2005). Assessing for impaired judgment as a means of meet-ing the "Duty to Protect" when a client is a potential harm-to-self: Implications for clients making end-of-life decisions. *Mortality, 10,* 7–21.

Wilkinson, A., Wenger, N., & Shugarman, L. R. (2007, June). *Literature review on advance directives.* Washington, DC: U.S. Department of Health and Human Services. Retrieved from http://aspe.hhs.gov/daltcp/reports/2007/advdirlr.htm#note29

Thomas Attig 6

THE ETHICS OF CARING FOR THE DYING AND THE BEREAVED

This chapter explores the development of thinking about the ethics of care of the dying and the bereaved within the broader contexts of the history of thinking about the responsibilities of physicians and the emergence of medical/health care ethics in the last several decades. The chapter briefly describes how I became involved in this work within the death and dying field. It then discusses the history and substance of four fundamental principles recognized as central to a principle-based approach to health care ethics, introduces the idea of respect for persons as the basis for understanding end-of-life ethics as encompassing not only life and death decision making but all aspects of caregiving, and contrasts the principle-based approach with a narrative-based approach to an ethics of care at the end-of-life. The chapter describes the two core ideas of the narrative approach: (a) carefully attending to the details of personal stories of the terminally ill and bereaved to learn about their needs, vulnerabilities, suffering, and remaining potential for living meaningfully and (b) working in partnership with them to discern the right things to do in interactions with them and in supporting their living the next chapters of their lives as meaningfully as possible. The chapter concludes that these core ideas are the key reasons for thinking that narrative ethics is the best approach to discerning the right thing to do in respectful end-of-life care.

MY INVOLVEMENT IN END-OF-LIFE ETHICS

I joined the philosophy faculty at Bowling Green State University in the fall of 1972 and began teaching courses on ethics and on existential phenomenology. Many of my colleagues were exploring the applications of philosophy's critical thinking, conceptual, and normative disciplines in medicine, business, law, and the environment. Several had already developed or were preparing applied courses to serve the needs of students in the new College of Health and Human Services that added programs in gerontology, social work, child and family services, and criminal justice to an already established nursing program. In 1978, two of my colleagues and I published an introductory textbook on ethics and social philosophy that emphasized the applications of ethics to real-world problems (Facione, Scherer, & Attig, 1978). By 1981, our department had reshaped an undistinguished Masters in Philosophy program into the first Masters of Applied Philosophy program in the country. By 1987, while I was department chair, we established the world's first PhD in applied philosophy program.

I began teaching my course on the philosophy of death and dying in 1974 when there were relatively few university courses on death and dying, most in psychology or sociology. I believe that John Morgan at King's University College (the University of Western Ontario), Charles Corr at Southern Illinois University at Edwardsville, and I were the first in philosophy to offer university courses about death and dying.

I had originally proposed teaching a course on ethics and death, covering topics such as suicide, euthanasia, abortion, capital punishment, and killing in war, since I had taught several of them in the other applied ethics courses I had been teaching in the earliest years of my career. When the course was approved, I thought seriously about what students would need and came to doubt that focusing exclusively on ethical issues would be the best way to serve them. Instead, I sensed that they would be most concerned about not knowing what to do or say when interacting with the dying, their families, and the bereaved. And I already had serious doubts about any need to invoke ethical principles regularly in interactions with flesh-and-blood dying and grieving persons. (It hadn't yet occurred to me that these everyday interactions and my doubts about regularly invoking ethical principles were themselves ethical matters.) I read widely in psychology, sociology, history, and literature to find materials and became a kind of interdisciplinary one-man band. I scattered small bits by philosophers in parts of the course and included a couple of ethics topics in the syllabus, but I sensed I was leaving philosophy behind.

After 4 years of teaching the course, I wrote my first serious essay on the philosophy of death and dying, "Death, Respect, and Vulnerability" (1979). While writing it, I was surprised by how much philosophical thinking was coming out of me as a result of teaching the course and thinking about so many issues in a sustained way. I hadn't left my philosophical training or dispositions behind after all, and I was finding existential/phenomenological and ethical dimensions in so much of the core of the subject matter. It had become clear to me already that attending to the experiences of the dying and the bereaved as revealed through the stories they have to tell about them (the subject matter of existential-phenomenological reflection) was the most important thing in developing a well-grounded philosophy of death and dying and, in particular, thinking seriously about end-of-life ethics. My essay developed for the first time a full articulation of what respect for persons requires, including the dying, the bereaved, their families, and their caregivers. But I'm getting ahead of myself. Before discussing that core idea, it makes sense to say more about the emergence of medical/health care ethics.

THE HISTORY OF MEDICAL/HEALTH CARE ETHICS

Ethics is a philosophically disciplined reflective search for the best ways to determine *the right thing to do*. For more than 2 millennia, Western thinkers have wondered about ethics in general, the morality of aspects of practical life, including ways of living, decisions, actions, practices, and policies. They have rigorously analyzed and debated the best reasons for thinking that specific instances of these aspects of practical life are right, permissible, or wrong. They also have reflected and debated about the roles and relative merits of moral principles, responsibilities in relationships, and virtues as guides to doing the right thing. Space does not allow for a detailed review of this rich history. Instead, it makes sense to survey major historical themes that have held, and still hold, places in current thinking about the ethics of caring for the dying and the bereaved.

Traditional Medical Ethics

Nonmaleficence and beneficence
Ethics at the end of life was traditionally thought of as a part of medical ethics, and until recent decades, it was considered a matter of physicians' duties to

patients. Philosopher Albert Jonsen's *The New Medicine and the Old Ethics* (1990) traces this history. He begins by telling us that from the time of the ancient Greeks to the 1960s, the two duties of physicians were thought to be "Do no harm" (*the principle of nonmaleficence*) and "Promote the good of the patient" (*the principle of beneficence*).

Jonsen expands on three great strands of thinking that informed understanding of these two fundamental principles. First, the Hippocratic Oath for physicians is rooted in the Greek understanding of medicine as an art or craft (*techne*). Physicians are to work with patients in the same way builders or artists are to appreciate the limits of the materials with which they work, avoid damaging them, and bring out the best in those materials. The art of medicine on this understanding is confined to promoting the functioning of the body. Working beyond the limits of the craft is pride (*hubris*). This exclusive focus is hardly the full-blown concept of beneficence as we know it today.

Second, we get closer to a modern sense of beneficence when we think of St. Luke's story of the Good Samaritan (who, like Luke, may have been a physician). The Samaritan administers oil and wine in tending to the injured man's wounds. But he goes further at great inconvenience and at great risk of harm given hostility toward helping a stranger held in contempt by his culture. This generosity in helping one's neighbor in all circumstances is also part of the modern medical ideal of beneficence.

A third strand of tradition may be traced to the Order of Knights Hospitallers founded during the Crusades. Members, mostly from noble families, dedicated themselves to serving "our lords, the sick." This tradition of service was continued by religious orders and into the 18th century in the idea of the gentleman-physician and the ideal of *noblesse oblige* toward the sick. The idea was to minister to the sick in ways that "unite tenderness with steadiness and condescension with authority to inspire gratitude, respect, and confidence in patients." This ideal guided physicians in many parts of the world, was incorporated word-for-word into the Code of Ethics of the American Medical Association from 1847 until 1912, and lived on long afterward. Taken together, these three traditional strands of thinking about physicians' duties to patients—competent craftsmanship, helping no matter the circumstances, and noble service—defined the core of medical ethics from ancient times through the 1950s.

Challenges to Traditional Medical Ethics

Medical ethics becomes health care ethics

Jonsen goes on to describe how this traditional thinking was challenged profoundly beginning in the 1960s by three major changes in society. First, the rise of nursing to full professional status, the recognition that decision making in health care often requires technical competence from many disciplines, and growing appreciation that those decisions have broad implications for all aspects of patients' lives fed demand for a team approach to health care and decision making at the end of life. Such approaches are familiar and quite well developed in many hospice and palliative care settings. The narrow focus on physician duties to patients has given way, as has hierarchical and patriarchal thinking (at least to some considerable extent). It makes more sense to think of responsibilities of the health care team and all of its members to those they serve and to speak of *health care ethics* rather than *medical ethics*.

Patient Autonomy

A second, more radical, shift came with the patients' rights movement beginning in the 1960s. The movement took hold following revelations about abuses in medical research in which no informed consent had been secured. This led to the establishment of research ethics committees, first in the United States and then in the United Kingdom and Canada. Before long, the movement led to rethinking of the physician–patient relationship and a rejection of the traditional paternalism in medicine. Paternalism is the idea that it is the responsibility of the physician to decide and do what is, in his or her considered medical opinion, best for the patient. The movement insisted that persons (who may or may not become patients) are self-governing agents who know best their own preferences, interests, and values. It urged that physicians' professional expertise extends no further than medical matters of physical functioning, disease, and treatment alternatives. As an antidote to paternalism, the movement insisted on a *principle of respect for patient autonomy,* or the right of a person to decide what is best for himself or herself in the broadest possible terms, taking into account not only disease prognosis and the probabilities of success in treatment but also implications for the course and quality of their lives.

Codes of ethics from the 1970s onward have added respect for the patients' autonomy to the duties of nonmaleficence and beneficence. Nurses, social workers, and others have defined their roles, in part, as *advocates* for patients. The ideal of informed consent has held a central place in thinking in health care ethics since that time. It requires giving patients all relevant information in terms they can readily comprehend that will enable those who are able/competent to decide which, if any, proposed medical interventions or treatments they will accept. Advance directives, including living wills or giving others power of attorney to speak on behalf of patients when they cannot speak for themselves, are intended to ensure that patients' autonomous choices are respected. Surrogate decision-making procedures, used when patients have left no advanced directive or are not competent to consent, are intended to lead to decisions that reflect the deep character, values, or will of the patient. All of these procedures are designed to support respect for patient autonomy by all members of the health care team.

Justice

The third shift brought unprecedented attention to issues of justice in the delivery of health care. In earlier times, it was easy to think of medical or health care ethics as being confined to face-to-face interactions between caregivers and those in their care. Principles of nonmaleficence, beneficence, and eventually respect for autonomy could easily be thought to cover the territory of the variety of issues likely to arise. The means to meet the needs of the dying, such as they were, were for the most part readily available to all caregivers and could be offered to all who needed them. However, we do not live in those earlier times when end-of-life care options were far more limited. Spectacular life-extending technological advances in medicine and soaring health care costs have given rise to a host of ethical questions concerning the fair distribution of scarce resources. In circumstances in which we fall far short of meeting *all* vital needs for health care—worldwide and even within prosperous nations—rationing of health care resources is inevitable, priorities need to be set, and questions of justice come to the fore. These questions are by no means confined to matters of face-to-face interactions between caregivers and those in their care.

The core idea in the *principle of justice* is to "Treat people who are alike in their morally relevant respects alike and treat people who differ in morally relevant respects differently in proportion to those differences." In seeking fairness in distributing resources for end-of-life care, the morally relevant differences are defined in terms of *need*. At a global or societal level, justice requires (1) weighing the *general needs across a population* for end-of-life care as opposed to other vital needs for such things as food, clothing, shelter, relief from poverty, security, education, general health care, and preventive health care and (2) distributing resources proportionate to needs in these general areas. At the local or institutional level, justice requires weighing the *needs of individuals* for various forms of end-of-life care and allocating resources set aside for end-of-life care proportionate to their particular needs.

When the allocation of scarce resources is at issue, the demand for an accounting of the effectiveness of the diverse uses of the resources in meeting diverse needs increases. Cost–benefit analysis—or attempts to measure the benefits that derive from using resources for alternative purposes—is a standard tool for providing such an accounting. Measurement focuses on costs and benefits that can be quantified or counted. The material costs of various allocations are easily measured in terms of quantities of currency and material used. But some benefits are far more easily measured than others, and if there are no readily identifiable units of measurement for a range of benefits, those benefits tend to be discounted or thought unimportant. Quality, then, tends to reduce to quantity as such calculations are undertaken. And physical benefits tend to be more easily measured than psychological, emotional, social, or spiritual benefits. This raises serious issues in assessing the benefits of many of the efforts in palliative, end-of-life care, and consequently in doing justice to end-of-life care in the allocation of scarce resources.

Principle-Based Health Care Ethics

Taken together, the principles of nonmaleficence, beneficence, respect for personal autonomy, and justice comprise the core principles in the principle-based approach to ethics at the end of life that has emerged since the 1960s and still holds a dominant place in thinking and practice in the field. The most comprehensive and widely respected textbook in health care ethics, *Principles of Biomedical Ethics* (2012) by philosophers Thomas Beauchamp and James Childress, first appeared in 1985 and is now in its seventh edition. It summarizes the discussion and development of refined understanding of each of the four principles by the leading defenders of the principle-based approach to health care ethics and vividly illustrates application of the principles to cases. *The History and Theory of Informed Consent* (1986) by legal scholar Ruth R. Faden and philosopher Thomas Beauchamp is a definitive study of the subject at the heart of thinking about the principle of respect for autonomy and remains an important resource for physicians, philosophers, policy makers, religious ethicists, lawyers, and psychologists. *The Hastings Center Report* began publishing in 1971 and today features a popularly accessible range of articles that explore philosophical and ethical issues in medicine, health care, the environment, technology, and medical research: reports or reviews of empirical studies that raise philosophical and ethical questions; case studies with commentary, personal stories about receiving or providing health care; and brief commentary on events in the news. The establishment of ethical research review boards, mentioned above, was followed by the hiring of applied ethicists and/or development of ethics committees in hospitals intended to clarify the implications of the four principles for practice when questions arise, support effective communication between health care professionals and patients and families about ethical matters, and in some cases adjudicate disputes before disputants turn to courts for definitive relief.

RESPECT FOR PERSONS

What Respect Requires

In my earliest essay (Attig, 1979), I defended a distinctive understanding of what respect for persons requires. It makes sense to summarize that understanding here as we turn our attention toward criticisms of limitations of a principle-based understanding of ethics at the end of life and the emergence of an alternative, virtue-based, narrative approach to an ethics of care beginning in the early 1990s.

Think of aspects of your own experiences (real or imagined) of asking others to treat you with respect when you are ill with a life-threatening illness or condition, dying, or grieving. Think of how you would want your caregivers (professional, volunteer, or personal) to understand what matters most deeply to you in living: how much you value living on your own terms; what you devote your passion to; the activities, experiences, and relationships that you value most; what brings you joy, satisfaction, and fulfillment in life when you experience them. Think of how you would want them to be sensitive to how vulnerable you are to being compromised in (or even deprived of) thriving in these ways by illness, injury, loss, or other life events, or of how you would be vulnerable to their indifference, insensitivity, attempts to control, or other failings in interactions with you and responding to your suffering. Think of how, at the least, you would hope they wouldn't get in the way of your living and thriving in ways that matter to you, make things worse, or add to your suffering. Finally, think of how you would hope that they would help you in some constructive ways to continue to live, or return to living, in often seriously compromised life circumstances in ways that mean a great deal to you. Notice how you would want them to appreciate how, in your ways of thriving and your vulnerability to suffering, you not only are different from them but also are unique in your individuality.

The core idea of respect for persons in the preceding paragraph has four essential components. (1) Respect requires that we appreciate and understand a person's distinctive potentials for thriving, realizing value, or living well in ways that are meaningful for him or her. (Notice that living autonomously is but one among many possible ways of thriving, realizing value, or living meaningfully that are worthy of respect.) (2) Respect requires that we appreciate and understand how a person may be suffering now and is vulnerable to additional suffering. But although appreciating and understanding these things about a person are necessary if we are to respect the person, it is not sufficient. Respecting an individual is fundamentally a matter of responding to and interacting with the person in ways that reflect what we appreciate and understand about that person. (3) Respect requires that we avoid doing anything to hinder, compromise, interfere with, or even undermine the person's thriving, realizing value, or living meaningfully, or to compound the person's vulnerability, or add to the person's suffering. This requirement defines a minimal order of respect—the least we can do is to make sure that we don't make things worse. Lastly, (4) respect requires that we do what we can to promote or support the person's thriving, realizing value, or living meaningfully within the limitations imposed by illness, dying, or bereavement. This requirement defines a higher order of respect—doing what we can to contribute constructively. Everyday respect for one another in our families and communities requires that we at least avoid making things worse for others. When, however, we have accepted responsibilities to care for others, for example, in families or in service professions, respect for those we serve requires that we make positive contributions when we can. This fleshed-out idea of respect can be easily understood as defining an ethic of care or caregiving, or even an ethic of compassion that encompasses all aspects of end-of-life care, not just end-of-life decision making.

Against Thinking of Respect for Persons as an Ethical Principle

It is tempting to understand respect for persons as an ethical principle or as a framework for integrating the four ethical principles introduced earlier. We can easily find in it echoes of the principles of nonmaleficence, beneficence, and respect for autonomy. We can even find the principle of justice in the idea that all within the human community are equally entitled to respect—to not be harmed and to be given at least a fair share of positive support when resources are limited. Yet, I hesitate to think of respect for persons as an ethical principle because I have the following serious reservations about the usefulness of principles in guiding us to do the right thing in real-life circumstances:

- Principles are abstract and general, whereas real-life matters are concrete and specific.
- Principles are intended to be as clear and definitive as possible (like rigid rules or official protocols), whereas real-life circumstances are always unique, often exceptional, and permeated with ambiguity in ways that make it difficult to know how to apply principles.
- Principles can lead in contrary directions, and they do not in themselves tell us which is to take precedence when they conflict.
- Principles may tell us what our duties or obligations are or what is not permitted, but they say little about what might be ethically commendable "above and beyond the call of duty."
- We may sometimes hold to a principle as a way of evading responsibility for doing something we believe would actually be the right thing to do in particular circumstances—a kind of bad faith, as if the principle "made us do it."
- Although invoking principles may hold a prominent place in adversarial contexts where the point is to make a case or win an argument, for example, in a courtroom, university seminar, or legislature, interactions between caregivers and those in their care are rarely adversarial or argumentative in nature.

Respect for Persons as an Ethical Virtue

Some might wonder what ethics could be about if not about searching for the best principles to guide us toward doing the right thing. Ethical principles, such as the four we have been discussing, focus on *the character of actions themselves* or on *the consequences of actions* (what it is generally best to do). But the history of ethics also includes extensive reflection on another way of finding our way to doing the right thing more often than not. It holds that we should instead attend to *the character of persons* (how to be at one's best and how best to be together with others) and cultivate *virtues* such as humility, honesty, trust, reciprocity, sensitivity, compassion, generosity, gratitude, commitment, loyalty, cooperation, acceptance of responsibility, respect, care, love, integrity, and courage (Hursthouse, 2013).

Rather than thinking of respect for persons as an ethical principle, I think of it as an ethical virtue that should be cultivated if we want to do the right thing in interactions with others. As such, respect for persons disposes us to work very hard at appreciating the potential for thriving and finding meaning and the vulnerability of a particular person in his or her unique life circumstances and to act in accord with what that appreciation tells us. In contrast to principles as discussed above, respect functions as a virtue as:

- It attunes us to the concrete and specific in real-life circumstances.
- It appreciates the unique needs and vulnerabilities of individuals and the particularities of their life stories.
- It motivates the best that is in us to find the response that best reflects understanding of those unique vulnerabilities and needs.
- It moves us to consider more than the minimum that some principles require.
- It moves us to accept full responsibility for what we do.
- It invites us to focus on building relationships of mutual respect with those in our care when working toward consensus is a primary objective.

As an ethical virtue, respect is an aspect of character that we can strive to make our own so that it becomes part of who we are and enables us to express some of our deepest values as we draw on it to shape our interactions with others. It is one thing to try to work out the right thing to do *at an abstract distance* from real life through weighing principles. It is quite another to wonder how to be as respectful as possible by *turning inward* to find our disposition to respect those in our care and then *turning toward others* to learn what matters most to them as individuals, appreciate their particular vulnerabilities, and act accordingly.

THE TURN TO NARRATIVE ETHICS

Personal Stories as the Ethical "Heart of the Matter"

From the time I began teaching about death and dying nearly 40 years ago, I have held that in responding to the needs of the dying and the bereaved, their personal stories are "the heart of the matter" (Attig, 1995). Respect requires learning and appreciating the significance of the stories of this particular person's living with illness, dying, or loss. Only by attending carefully to the stories told by the terminally ill or dying, by those able to tell us about them when they cannot speak for themselves, and by the bereaved will we access the detailed understanding of what matters most to the storytellers and how they are vulnerable, as life-threatening or terminal illness or bereavement affect them not just physically, but emotionally, psychologically, behaviorally, socially, and spiritually and how such experiences change the shapes of their daily lives and the unfolding of their life stories. Without knowing the details of their stories, full respectful response to them as the unique individuals they are is impossible—on the one hand avoiding making things worse for them, and on the other hand supporting them in living meaningfully in their particular life circumstances.

Emergence of a New Movement in Health Care Ethics

Essential readings
Naturally, then, I have been heartened by the emergence in the last several decades of a new narrative ethics movement that centers on attending to, learning from,

and partnering with the tellers of such personal stories as the key to finding the right thing to do in health care, including at the end of life. The first landmark development in that movement was the appearance of psychiatrist and medical anthropologist Arthur Kleinman's *The Illness Narratives: Suffering, Healing, and the Human Condition* (1988). It set the tone for the movement by arguing that interpreting illness experience is an art tragically neglected by modern medical training, an art that could bridge the gap between patients and health care providers. Many others and I take sociologist Arthur Frank to be the key thinker in the development of narrative ethics. His three books, *At the Will of the Body: Reflections on Illness* (2002), *The Wounded Story-Teller: Body, Illness, and Ethics* (1997), and *The Renewal of Generosity: Illness, Medicine, and How to Live* (2004) offer groundbreaking insights into the experiences of embodiment and personal vulnerability and mortality of the ill and dying, the types of stories they have to tell, the relationship between the ill and dying and their caregivers, and the influences of institutional and broader cultural contexts in shaping these experiences and interactions. Most recently, physician and literary scholar Rita Charon, in *Narrative Medicine: Honoring the Stories of Illness* (2008), has deepened and enriched the movement by shedding light on the experiences and struggles of health care practitioners in listening to and witnessing the stories. She expands on the usefulness of literary interpretative techniques in developing narrative competence, plumbing the depths and singularities of the stories and the biographies of those living them, introducing the idea of parallel charting as a way for caregivers to explore the meanings of the stories told to them by those they serve and to write stories of their own experiences of caring for them, and articulating how narrative medicine can transform health care practice for the benefit of all involved in it and the broader community.

Arthur Frank on restitution, chaos, and quest stories

Because of space limitations, I will focus primarily on Arthur Frank's seminal contributions in explaining core features of narrative ethics. He writes of three types of stories, namely, restitution stories, chaos stories, and quest stories. *Restitution stories,* the paradigm stories of modern medicine, are stories in which "what ails you" gets fixed. Illness or debilitation presents itself as a problem to be overcome. Medical professionals know how to identify problems and select treatments that will solve them, leaving the one with the problem "as good as new." Typically, the physician or the treatment is the hero of the story. The sufferer cooperates with "what needs to be done," that is, he or she passively goes along for the ride and ends up fully recovered. Those who fail to go along are considered "noncompliant."

Chaos stories are told by those "living lives of overwhelming trouble and suffering." The taken-for-granted order and sense of purpose in their lives have broken down. The worlds of their experience are in disarray. Their daily routines are shattered. Their life stories have veered sharply off their expected courses. They suffer in all dimensions of their being at once. Their bodies are not working well, and they experience pain and other distressing symptoms. They are caught up in emotional turmoil. Their self-confidence, self-esteem, self-image, and sense of identity are undermined. They cannot do what they are accustomed to doing or enjoy the full range of experiences they find meaningful. There is tension and heartache in their ties with others. Their souls feel homesick for life as it was but can never be again. And their spirits are shaken by fear, discouragement, joylessness, despair, even doubt of their faith.

Quest stories are stories of the ill and dying as they move past the disruption within and beyond the suffering they are experiencing. They begin in awakening to the possibility that there is something to be gained (not at all clear from the beginning) from or through suffering. Like Joseph Campbell's classical treatment of the hero's journey (1949) they trace a course from *departure* (the call to make sense of or live meaningfully in response to what is happening), through *initiation* (on the road of trials), to the *return* (where the sufferer has learned new ways of experiencing within suffering). The distinctive heroism in these quest stories is not the heroism of a conqueror where something is defeated or brought under control, the heroism of the physician at the heart of restitution stories. In quest stories, the ill or dying person is the hero, who perseveres and has something to offer to listeners about what he or she is learning from unflinching engagement with the mysteries of human limitation, suffering, and mortality.

Mortality stories

Only rarely does Frank discuss stories that those who know they are dying have to tell; stories that I would call *mortality stories*. They are told by those living in circumstances that involve such things as irreversible physical decline, growing dependence on others, or withdrawal into permanent dementia. Chaos has over-matched their increasingly powerless egos. Ego-driven efforts of others to control the progress of disease are futile. The quest stories they tell go beyond teaching about living with illness and suffering to teaching about living with finiteness and mortality. Those who hear them can learn not only what physical health and well-being are but also a great deal about surrender and what really matters in living in all dimensions of being human.

Mortality stories are often told in contexts where difficult end-of-life decisions are made about such matters as declining or discontinuing curative treatments or procedures; requesting do-not-resuscitate (DNR) orders, terminal sedation, assisted suicide, or euthanasia; or interpreting and following living wills or other advanced directives when the dying become unable to speak for themselves. In many such situations, tension within the idea of what respect for persons requires, between respect for personal autonomy and respect for remaining potential for living meaningfully, have to be weighed carefully in individual cases. Adherents of the narrative approach to end-of-life ethics advocate making these decisions through respectful dialogue among the dying (where possible), their families, and their caregivers. Such dialogue is intended to foster appreciation of the unique needs and vulnerabilities of the dying and the particularities of their life stories; appeal to the virtue of respect in all parties to the discussion; and lead to consensus about the best thing to do, often under conditions of uncertainty. Betty Rollins' *Last Wish* (1985/1998) recounts a compelling example of such respectful dialogue in response to her mother's request for assistance in securing the means to kill herself. My own essay on rational suicide in terminal illness (Attig, 2005) offers more extensive discussion of the narrative ethics approach to addressing such decisions than can be included here.

Attig on stories of loss and grief

Frank's books do not include stories that those who are grieving have to tell. My own writings about loss and bereavement (Attig, 2000, 2004, 2011, 2012) have all centered on the *stories of loss and grief* that grieving persons tell and what respectful response to those who tell them requires. There are no parallels to restitution stories because loss and grief are not illnesses or pathologies, and there is no "fixing" of them by professionals. Stories of *grief reaction* are in many ways parallel to chaos stories told by the ill and dying. They are about what happens to us as brokenness and sorrow come over us when a loved one dies, including coming into crisis in all dimensions of our being. They are also about how loss transforms the world of our experience and taken-for-granted ways of living in it, shatters our illusions of control and invulnerability, unravels our daily life patterns, and disrupts the unfolding of our life stories. Stories of *grieving response* are parallel in many ways to quest stories. They are about how we actively engage with and seek meaningful ways of living in the shadows of what has happened to us in loss and grief reaction. They are about how we learn to carry the pain of missing those who died; relearn the worlds of our experience, including our physical surroundings, relationships with others, and aspects of ourselves; learn to continue loving the one who died in separation; and learn to live meaningfully with the mysteries that pervade life in the human condition.

When I first began thinking and teaching about loss and grief 40 years ago, the focus in grief counseling was on the affective dimension of our experiences. Emotions were not understood as reflections of our deep needs, but they were the heart of what grieving was thought to be. Being present with and comforting those in their thrall and as they dissipated over time was the be all and end all of caring response. There was some thinking about our active engagement with loss (grieving response), but it was overwhelmed by the emphasis on affect and grief reaction. There was little, if any, appreciation of the power of the mind to adapt to new realities. Some of my early teaching aimed at underscoring how valuable the mind is in helping us to understand and orient ourselves in reality, especially when loss changes it so profoundly. The power of reflection is surely one of the things that make sorrow-friendly practices, including counseling with another person, effective in helping the bereaved relearn how to live in the aftermath of loss.

Over time, I believe that the pendulum has swung too far in the other direction, as cognition now seems too heavily emphasized. It is heartening to see fuller appreciation of the cognitive dimension of grieving in a new emphasis on meaning-making and narrative therapy. But while the labors of grieving through relearning the world have a cognitive dimension, shifting our thinking, even revising the stories that we tell ourselves about our lives and the world around us, it is not the heart of grieving. Insights gained from telling our stories, attending to our grief reactions, and reflecting can, at their best, provide guidance in doing the multidimensional work of relearning the world. (See Chapter 1 for fuller discussion of grieving as relearning the world.)

The listener and storyteller as I–Thou

To understand the importance that Frank and other proponents of narrative ethics see in storytelling for both those who suffer and for those who care for them, it is helpful to follow philosopher Martin Buber (1923/2000) in distinguishing *I–It* and *I–Thou* relationships. In an *I–It* relationship, an experiencing subject or active agent (the *I*) engages with or uses an object (the *It*). Think of a driver at the wheel, a scientist with testing equipment, an artist with paint or clay, a musician with an instrument, a farmer with a plow. In an I–Thou relationship, one experiencing subject or active agent (the *I*) acknowledges and interacts with another experiencing subject or active agent (the *Thou*). (Note that in Old English "thou" is the familiar term of address and "you" the formal.)

It is easy to see the central aspect of restitution stories as stories in which medical personnel stand in I–It relationships with those in their care. Their focus on disease and efforts to control or overcome illness, or at least bring it into remission, is a focus on an It, a biochemical process, an object. There is no acknowledgment, or central role given, in restitution stories to the subjectivity of the ill person struggling to live with the disease and its consequences for the shape of his or her daily life or the course of his or her life story. The Thou (the experiencing subjectivity of "the patient") is at best a minor player in such stories. These stories are "modern" in their emphasis on medical "heroes" fixing things, controlling natural phenomena, struggling to change the bodies of others.

It is also easy to read the entirety of Frank's work as an insistent cry that the fundamental character of the caring relationship between caregiver and those in their care must be I–Thou, not I–It. Respectful care is care *for and about* the whole person who is living with the illness, not just the illness. Respectful care requires dialogue with the ill person to learn the extent to which he or she wants to be party to efforts toward restitution; clear communication about treatment alternatives and their likely impacts on their abilities to live their lives on their own terms; and respect for their values and rights to choose whether to "comply" with what seems medically best or not. Respectful care also requires checking in periodically on the person who is undergoing treatment to find out whether he or she really wants to continue.

Respectful care requires dialogue with the Thou in one's care when he or she is living an alternative story—living in chaos or on a quest to live meaningfully within or beyond chaos when restitution is no longer possible. It requires acknowledgment that care extends beyond efforts to fix physical *problems*. It requires recognition and comfort in response to the Thou who suffers while efforts to problem solve and fix are underway and when such efforts are seen to be futile. It requires support for the Thou who contends with life's *mysteries*, including suffering, limitation, vulnerability, and mortality. It requires dialogue with the Thou who struggles to change himself or herself in response to these unchangeable constants in the human condition.

Rather than *cultural competence*, or mastery of general information about a variety of cultures and the differences among them in beliefs and practices, respectful care requires *cultural sensitivity*, or attuning to how, if at all, the dying and bereaved, as unique individuals, identify with their cultures or experience them as supportive or unsupportive as they die or grieve (Hays, 2001). Culture may or may not shape or influence how the dying or the bereaved experience illness or accident, speak or think of sickness and death (e.g., whether they may be openly discussed), value an individual's life (or death), find meaning in suffering or express it, consent to or resist treatments, open to or refuse hospice and palliative care or grief counseling, approach decision making, trust authority or the health care system, give roles to healers and families in caregiving, value spiritual practices, choose to dispose of a body after death, express their grief, or engage in mourning practices.

Testimony and bearing witness

In writing about "testimony," Frank writes about the *teaching* and *learning* that derive from the ill telling their chaos and quest stories. In telling their stories, they bear witness to what they are experiencing in their bodies, in their suffering, and in their struggles to change their life courses in ways that are meaningful for them and those they care about and love. Bearing witness has moral significance as they take responsibility for how they live with their illness and for being *for* others in telling about it. They are learning themselves in the processes of telling and retelling their stories as they (a) emerge ever so gradually from nearly overwhelming chaos, (b) enter on a quest that is at first defined only by a resolve to "find something of value" in the experience, and (c) persevere and come eventually to realize just how the experience is changing them and how the new stories of their lives have unexpected meanings for them. Think of how we often discover things about ourselves as we repeat stories over and over again, changing the ways we tell them, noting new details, adopting new perspectives, seeing in a different light, highlighting different aspects, making new connections, and so on.

In bearing witness to their own experiences, they are appealing to others to be witness to (learn from) the stories they are living and what they can articulate of them, to reciprocate by being there *for* them in care, to empathize *with* them, to join them in I–Thou dialogue, to experience them as having something to offer in exchange for caring ministrations. They testify to truths about life that are generally unrecognized or even suppressed. They testify in contexts in which the modernist medical culture insists that restitution stories of ego successes in fixing things are the only ones worthy of attention. They testify about matters of the deep self—soul and spirit—learning to live with and change in response to mystery.

Frank elaborates on the nature of narrative ethics as calling the ill and those who care for them to distinctive commitments: the ill to living and telling their stories for their own sake and for others, their caregivers to responding appropriately to those stories, and both to resonating *with* one another in empathy and being *for* one another in dialogue. Narrative ethics calls the ill and their caregivers alike to *become* the best they can be in living their individual life stories and in living the story of their being with and for one another as life and caring continue in the shadows of illness and mortality.

Suffering and healing

Frank suggests that stories that grow out of and are about suffering have two sides—the one having to do with disintegration or the threat of it and the other with healing, or movement toward a new wholeness. He writes of how the embodied self can be unmade not only by illness itself but by external threats. Ill people feel genuinely vulnerable and threatened by the medical institutions designed to help them. They experience the anguish of surrendering their bodies to the medical world where treatments often compound suffering. Other people, in the name of attempting to achieve restitution, take charge of giving direction to the sufferers' lives. He also writes of movements toward a new wholeness that is possible despite the illness and through opening to others. He calls it a "half-opening" because the wounded storyteller can only go so far in telling of his or her suffering. In its chaotic aspects, it eludes articulation. Its depths cannot be fathomed. It always exceeds what can be said about it. Words fail in capturing it. It is, ultimately, a mystery. So, too, is the self of the sufferer, both to the sufferer and to those who witness their living and telling their stories.

Yet, in quest stories, sufferers can and do say something about their suffering and their embodied selves as they struggle to live new stories and find healing in them. They find healing, or new wholeness, in community with caregivers who are willing to care and listen. They take responsibility for living with their illnesses and telling what they can of what they experience. Though their bodies may yet be broken, their spirits are healed through the I–Thou connection of dialogue that overcomes the brokenness of loneliness and isolation. The healing takes place as the caregiver not only hears what is said but also values it and the teller. Tellers of quest stories (stories of reaching through and past chaos) attempt to change their own lives by affecting the lives of the caregivers who hear them.

LOOKING TO THE FUTURE

I anticipate that the principle-based approach to ethics at the end of life will have its adherents into the indefinite future. The best part of the approach is the reminder implicit in it of core values that almost all of us bring with us whenever there is serious discussion of ethical issues at the end of life—promoting the good, avoiding harm and suffering, honoring autonomy, and promoting justice. No doubt the approach will continue to have a place in adversarial contexts (legislatures, court rooms, and seminars) where there may be a point in trying to make a case or win an argument. But, sadly, there is considerable potential for use of the principle-based approach in ways that fail to witness, respect, and honor the personal stories that unique individuals have to tell about the singularities in their lives that are the heart of the matter in determining together with them the right thing to do as they live their last days and die. I worry when the approach is thought of and used as the equivalent of yet another set of protocols or recipes for caregiving that leaves caregivers at a distance from those in their care with a false sense of security about knowing the right thing to do with no need for discussion. I worry that the approach may still be abused in attempts by caregivers or ethics review boards to impose an arbitrary certainty in contexts at the end of life where uncertainty and ambiguity prevail. I worry that it will maintain a foothold in medical contexts where the primary responsibility is thought to be curing illness and treating physical symptoms or in grief-counseling contexts where it is thought to be avoiding or eliminating pathology, not respecting the whole persons of those who are ill, dying, or grieving.

I also anticipate that the current and growing momentum toward wider use of the narrative approach to ethics at the end of life will continue. The continuing spread of hospice and palliative care programs devoted to whole person care support that momentum, as do educational programs and growing public awareness of the need for whole person care and not merely respect for autonomy. I have also heard anecdotally that more and more applied ethicists and ethics committees in clinical settings are adopting narrative ethics approaches in their work. It may not always be possible to fully understand and honor the stories the dying and bereaved have to tell, but the narrative approach offers the best hope I see for achieving that result more often than not.

REFERENCES

Attig, T. (1979). Death, respect, and vulnerability. In A. de Vries & A. Carmi (Eds.), *The dying human* (pp. 3–15). Tel Aviv, Israel: Turtledove Press.
Attig, T. (1995). Can we talk? On the elusiveness of dialogue. *Death Studies, 19*(1), 1–19.
Attig, T. (2000). *The heart of grief: Death and the search for lasting love.* New York, NY: Oxford University Press.
Attig, T. (2004). Disenfranchised grief revisited: Discounting hope and love. *Omega, 49*(3), 197–216.
Attig, T. (2005). Rational suicide in terminal illness: The ethics of intervention and assistance. In K. Doka (Ed.), *Living with grief: Ethical dilemmas in end-of-life care* (pp. 175–197). Washington, DC: Hospice Foundation of America.
Attig, T. (2011). *How we grieve: Relearning the world* (rev. ed.) New York, NY: Oxford University Press.
Attig, T. (2012). *Catching your breath in grief . . . and grace will lead you home.* Victoria, British Columbia, Canada: Breath of Life Publishing.
Beauchamp, T., & Childress, J. (2012). *Principles of biomedical ethics* (7th ed.). New York, NY: Oxford University Press.
Buber, M. (2000). *I and thou.* New York, NY: Scribner. (Original work published in 1923, first translated into English in 1937)
Campbell, J. (1949). *The hero with a thousand faces.* New York, NY: Harper Collins.

Charon, R. (2008). *Narrative medicine: Honoring the stories of illness.* New York, NY: Oxford University Press.

Facione, P., Scherer, D., & Attig, T. (1978) *Values and society: An introduction to ethics and social philosophy.* Englewood, NJ: Prentice-Hall.

Faden, R., & Beauchamp, T. (1986). *A history and theory of informed consent.* New York, NY: Oxford University Press.

Frank, A. (1997). *The wounded story-teller: Body, illness, and ethics.* Chicago, IL: University of Chicago Press.

Frank, A. (2002). *At the will of the body: Reflections on illness* (rev. ed.) Boston, MA: Houghton Mifflin.

Frank, A. (2004). *The renewal of generosity: Illness, medicine, and how to live.* Chicago, IL: University of Chicago Press.

The Hastings Center. (1969–present). *The Hastings Center report.* Garrison, New York, NY: Author. Retrieved from www.thehastingscenter.org/Publications.

Hays, P. A. (2001). *Addressing cultural complexities in practice: A framework for clinicians and counselors.* Washington, DC: American Psychological Association.

Hursthouse, R. (2013). Virtue ethics. In E. N. Zalta (Ed.), *The Stanford encyclopedia of philosophy.* Retrieved from http://plato.stanford.edu/archives/fall2013/entries/ethics-virtue/

Jonsen, A. R. (1990). *The new medicine and the old ethics.* Cambridge, MA: Harvard University Press.

Kleinman, A. (1988). *The illness narratives: Suffering, healing, and the human condition.* New York, NY: Basic Books.

Rollins, B. (1985/1998). *Last wish.* New York, NY: Public Affairs.

J. William Worden   7

THEORETICAL PERSPECTIVES
ON LOSS AND GRIEF

SIGMUND FREUD

In this chapter, we will review the process of mourning and how thinking about people's adaptation to loss has developed over the past 100 years. Any survey of this type would obviously begin with Sigmund Freud, the father of psychiatry. Freud was visited by adult patients who showed various neuroses and neurotic behaviors. These neuroses stemmed primarily from repressed memories, often memories resulting from trauma. Freud tried to help patients recover repressed memories, first by putting pressure on the patient's head and then by using hypnosis. Later, he used free association, looking for hesitations and parapraxis in order to try and uncover repressed memories that would lead to insight and the freeing of neurotic conflicts.

Many of Freud's patients also showed grief symptoms that resembled symptoms of depression. To Freud, these two manifestations were similar but not the same, and out of his observations he wrote his classic book *Mourning and Melancholia* (1917), "mourning" referring to grief and "melancholia" referring to depression. In this book, he makes his classic distinction: "In Grief—the world looks empty to the person, and in Depression—the person experiences the self as empty."

Freud saw grief as necessary after losing a loved one to death. This process of mourning enabled the person to test the reality of the loss, not always an easy task. Mourning involved not only reality testing but also emotional withdrawal of one's attachment to the deceased (decathexis). Freud believed that a person's grief was resolved when decathexis from the lost loved one was complete and the grieving person's emotional energy could be reinvested in new relationships and activities. Freud termed these mourning activities "grief work."

Freud's theory of grief remained in vogue for the next 25 years, especially among his followers. He had his detractors, who created their own theories of mental health, but few, if any, focused on grief in the way Freud did.

ERICH LINDEMANN

The next theorist to make an impact on our thinking about the process of mourning was Erich Lindemann, who was then head of the Psychiatry Department at the Massachusetts General Hospital, the flagship teaching hospital for the Harvard Medical School.

Boston has two Catholic colleges that are great football rivals—Boston College and Holy Cross College. In the Fall of 1942, these two rivals met for their traditional game, and Holy Cross won the game. Afterward, a number of students and fans went to celebrate at the Coconut Grove nightclub in the Park Square area of

Boston. The club was packed, and during the evening one of the decorative light bulbs burned out. A busboy came to change the bulb. In order to see, he lit a match and accidentally set a decorative palm tree on fire. The fire spread rapidly, and in a short time 500 people were trampled, burned, and killed in that tragic event.

Lindemann decided to study the survivors from that disaster to further our understanding of grief and mourning. In addition to the families served by Mass General, he looked at families served by other hospitals in Boston and ended up with a sample of 101 grieving patients. Some of these had been in the fire and survived, whereas others were family members of those killed at the Coconut Grove.

He published his findings in a seminal paper titled, "Symptomatology and Management of Acute Grief" (1944). In this article, he makes the distinctions between normal grief and morbid grief. "Normal grief," described by the term "acute grief," occurs when the mourner confronts the loss and experiences the various emotional reactions stemming from it. Lindemann found the emotional reactions to be quite varied and much broader in scope than those described by Freud. "Morbid grief" is the term that he used to describe those who repressed their grief and avoided expressions of grief. Lindemann and his colleagues came up with a fairly simplistic treatment recommendation—"Express your grief and you will return to normal."

Although Lindemann's study advanced our thinking of grief and loss after a major disaster, there are at least two major limitations from his study. First, he did not focus on individual differences that caused mourners to have different expressions of grief and/or different outcomes. Second, he overlooked the issue of chronic grief. Some of these mourners moved rather quickly through their grieving experiences, while there was a subgroup of mourners for whom grief continued for a long period. It would have been helpful had this latter group been studied. Nevertheless, Lindemann must be credited for giving us this seminal study as we moved toward mid century.

JOHN BOWLBY

In the 1960s, John Bowlby began publishing groundbreaking work on attachment theory. His fruitful work continued for the next 25 years, and he was joined in collaboration by Colin Murry Parkes. Attachment theory has provided a key foundation for much of our thinking on bereavement, grief, and mourning, and continues today.

Parkes and Bowlby defined four phases of mourning that outline the trajectory of grief after the death of a loved one: The first phase is *shock and numbness*. This helps defend the person against the pain experienced by the death of a loved one. The second phase is *yearning and searching*. Searching for the lost loved one is very common after a death as one looks for the loved one to make sure that he or she is gone. Pining for the loved one is the affect most frequently associated with searching behavior. The third phase is *disorganization and despair*. Here the mourner struggles with questions such as "Who am I now without the dead loved one?" and "How can I go on without them?" Some of the most painful grief experiences come during this third phase. The fourth and final phase is *reorganization*. The goal of this phase is to mend the fabric of one's life and find a way to move on as a new person in a new reality (Bowlby & Parkes, 1970). Bowlby made the distinction between secure and insecure attachments, and Parkes focused much of his work on how attachment security plays a role in reactions to bereavement and in complications to the grieving process.

COLIN PARKES

Colin Parkes was not only a colleague of Bowlby, but one of the key bereavement theorists of the past 100 years. Parkes's interest in bereavement began in the 1950s, when his research focused on the impact of bereavement on both physical and mental health. His research asked the question whether bereavement can cause psychiatric morbidity and/or mortality (Parkes, 1964)? His research took place in three key venues. His first investigations took place while he was on the staff of the Tavistock Clinic in London. A second location was St. Christopher's Hospice in London where Parkes established, along with Cicely Saunders, the first hospice bereavement service and studied dying and bereavement there. A third research venue was the Harvard Medical School, where he was the principal researcher in the Harvard Bereavement Study. This study was based in the Laboratory of Community Psychiatry at the Massachusetts Mental Health Center (MMHC), where Gerald Kaplan did his pioneering work on crisis intervention. MMHC has played a pivotal role in the development of preventative psychiatry and community mental health. This Harvard study looked at the impact of bereavement on young widows and widowers in Boston under 45 years of age who were followed for 4 years after the death. This study enabled Parkes and colleagues to identify "risk factors" at the time of bereavement that predicted later adjustment. Early identification of persons predicted not to do well can help ensure that these "at-risk" people are singled out for early intervention in order to do preventative mental health work (Parkes, 1972; Parkes & Weiss, 1983).

Like Freud, Parkes sees grief work as necessary. This work involves helping the mourner deal with preoccupied thoughts of the loved one, helping him or her deal with painful repetitions of the loss experience, and helping the mourner to modify his or her assumptive world so as to make sense of the world without the deceased. Over the years, Parkes's research has strongly influenced the thinking of many other bereavement theorists, including Maddison, Raphael, Fleming, Silverman, Vachon, and Worden.

ELISABETH KÜBLER-ROSS

Elisabeth Kübler-Ross taught and practiced clinical medicine at the University of Chicago hospitals during the mid-1960s. It was there that she began to see a progression of stages in the lives of the dying patients that she treated. She used this information in her teaching and wrote the well-received book *On Death and Dying* (1969). In it she outlined her five stages of dying: denial, anger, bargaining, depression, and acceptance. There is hardly a health care provider trained in that period or since who has not heard of these five stages.

Along the way some who were seeking a quick and easy way to understand bereavement began applying these five stages to the bereavement process, though this was never her original intent (E. Kübler-Ross, personal communication, 1971). Whether this was her intent or not, Kübler-Ross's stage model has influenced the theories of grief over the past 40 years.

WILLIAM WORDEN

William Worden began his thinking and research on grief and loss in 1968 when he joined Harvard psychiatrist Avery Weisman at the Massachusetts General Hospital. Their 18-year collaboration, funded by grants from the National Institutes of Health, looked at various aspects of life-threatening illness and life-threatening behavior. A main focus of this research was people's participation in their own death, whether overtly by suicide or more subtly by giving up and losing the will to live. Out of this clinical and research focus on existential issues an interest in grief and bereavement naturally followed.

Worden was asked to put together a training course for health and mental health professionals, to educate them about grief and how to work with grieving individuals and families. To come up with a useful model, Worden borrowed the notion of developmental tasks from developmental psychology. There are certain tasks that the mourner must deal with as he or she adjusts to the death of a loved one. The idea of tasks seemed more fluid than that of stages. Tasks could be revisited and reworked over time. Not every task presented the same challenge to the mourner. The challenge depended on the attachment to the deceased, the circumstances of the death, prior loss experiences, changes and disruptions in daily life, and social support. This model gives the mourner a perspective on what she or he may be experiencing and gives the mental health professional a way to understand the patient/client, especially when the client presents for therapy feeling stuck in their grief. The task model was used in these training courses at Harvard and at the University of Chicago beginning in the early 1970s and culminated in the book *Grief Counseling & Grief Therapy: A Handbook for the Mental Health Professional* in 1982. Since then there have been three revised editions of this book (1991, 1998, and 2009).

There are four tasks of mourning that Worden believes apply to all mourners:

> *Task I—To accept the reality of the loss.* If one doesn't believe the loss is real, then one can't deal with the affect associated with the death. This task involves not only intellectual acceptance but emotional acceptance as well—the latter often taking some time to accomplish.
>
> *Task II—To process the pain of the loss.* Not every death is equally painful, but pain must be acknowledged and processed. To suppress or repress the pain before it is adequately processed can lead to a delayed grief reaction or to some type of somatic manifestation of the grief.
>
> *Task III—To adjust to an environment where the deceased is missing.* Under this task there are three types of adjustments that challenge the mourner: (1) External adjustments—What changes has the death brought that affects the functioning of daily life? (2) Internal adjustments—How has the death affected the person's self-definition? This includes how the death has challenged the person's sense of self-esteem and self-efficacy. (3) Spiritual adjustments—How has the death changed or shattered the person's basic assumptions about God and the world? How has it affected his or her core beliefs and values?
>
> *Task IV—To emotionally relocate and memorialize the dead person in a way that one can move on with life.* Unlike Freud's notion of decathexis, the mourner finds a healthy way to remember the dead person but in a way that can help the mourner move forward with life.

Although the tasks apply to all mourners, how they are worked through depends on individual differences. Worden outlined a series of six mediators that influence how a person handles the various tasks of mourning. These involve relationship and attachment issues, death factors, personality and social factors, as well as concurrent stressors. Worden's task model has been widely used around the world as a standard reference on grief counseling and grief therapy and has been translated into 14 languages.

THERESE RANDO

Therese Rando is a Rhode Island psychologist whose clinical practice and research have long focused on bereavement. Shortly after Worden's book appeared, Rando developed the Six "R" Model. She uses alliteration to help the clinician and the mourner remember what needs to be done. Although she doesn't use the term "tasks," she suggests six activities or processes that are important in adapting to a loss. These are: (1) Recognize the loss; (2) React to the separation; (3) Remember and re-experience; (4) Relinquish attachments and assumptions; (5) Readjust to a new world; and (6) Reinvest in new activities and new relationships. Many of these overlap with Worden's tasks of mourning, although with different wording and ordering (Rando, 1984, 1993).

SIMON RUBIN

Rubin and his colleagues (1981, 1999) in Israel have developed the Two Track Model for understanding the mourning process. This bifocal approach focuses on: (1) the biopsychosocial functioning of the individual who is grieving and (2) the ongoing emotional attachment and relationship of the mourner with the dead person. These two tracks are distinct axes that can intersect with each other. Both of these axes are important to mourning, but focusing on them separately can be useful to the clinician doing research and intervention with the bereaved.

The first track, *functioning*, focuses on several questions. What and how many emotional symptoms is the mourner experiencing (such as anxiety, depression, and somatization)? What is their family like, and how do they function in interpersonal interactions? Is the person able to work and to invest in life tasks? Has the death affected their self-esteem? What is the meaning of the death for their life?

The second track, *relationship*, on the other hand, looks at the mourner's closeness to and distance from the deceased, including his or her ability to accept the loss along with its ambivalences. How well is the person dealing with the emotional part of the loss—is there too much or too little? How is the death impacting on their self-perception? Is the person able to memorialize the lost loved one?

Personal functioning (Track 1) is only a part of a person's response to the loss. The ongoing relationship with the complexity of memories, thoughts, associations, and needs associated with the person who died is also important for a person's adaptation to the loss of a loved one (Track 2). Too often, clinicians have been overly focused on the former and have not paid sufficient attention to the latter. Rubin has developed an instrument to assess where a person is on these tracks, and this can be useful in clinical work and research (Rubin, 1999).

THOMAS ATTIG

Thomas Attig sees grieving as a process of *relearning the world* in the aftermath of loss (Attig, 1996/2011). However, his relearning is more than the cognitive process of *learning* that the world is different following loss. In his view, relearning the world is *learning how to live* meaningfully again as the whole persons we are in a world changed profoundly by loss. This involves learning how to carry the pain of missing the deceased; returning to and finding meaning (Attig, 2001) in engagement with familiar physical and social surroundings, activities, and experiences that remain viable; stretching into and making meaning in the inevitably new daily life and in an unanticipated future; learning to love in separation (Attig, 2000); and learning how to live in the shadows of mysteries that pervade life in the human condition, including finiteness, suffering, and death.

Attig is a philosopher whose training in existentialism and phenomenology has led him to respect the individuality of each grieving person and to insist that just as no two people *learn how to live* in exactly the same way, so no two people *relearn how to live* in exactly the same way. He urges the importance of appreciating each grieving person's unique life circumstances, personal history, and relationship with the deceased; the singularities of his or her experiences of loss and sorrow; and the particularities of the challenges he or she faces in learning how to live meaningfully again. In his view, understanding and attuning to the unique story that each grieving person has to tell is the *heart of the matter* in effective counseling or therapy.

STROEBE AND COLLEAGUES

In 1999, Margaret Stroebe and colleagues in the Netherlands introduced the Dual Process Model (DPM) to understand how mourners deal with death loss. The focus of this model is more on how people cope with a loss rather than it is on bereavement outcomes, although the assumption is that coping styles will affect adaptation to bereavement. This approach is based on two categories of stressors associated with bereavement: (1) those related to the *loss* and (2) those related to *restoration*. The mourner oscillates between coping with these two types of stressors, choosing at times to deal with one or the other but generally not both of them at the same time. Adaptive coping involves confronting these stressors while at other times avoiding them. Mourners oscillate between preoccupation with the grief itself and reengagement with a world transformed by their loss.

Oscillation is *key* to this theory, as it is the regulatory process that makes coping effective and makes this model unique from previous theories, such as phases or tasks. Oscillation suggests that the bereaved will confront aspects of loss and at other times avoid them. The same is true for aspects of restoration. According to the DPM model, coping with bereavement is a complex regulatory process of confrontation and avoidance, and such oscillation between the two types of stressors is necessary for adaptive coping.

The DPM has been widely received and has been studied in various research projects to further validate or modify it. Guidelines for using it in research have been offered by the authors (Stroebe & Schut, 1999, 2010).

CONTINUING BONDS

One of the most interesting changes in grief theory to come along in this past century is the notion of *continuing bonds*. You will recall that a key factor in Freud's thinking about the mourning process was that of decathexis. According to Freud, bereavement was not complete until the mourner was able to withdraw the emotional attachment to the deceased (*decathect*) and reinvest that emotional energy into a new relationship or, at least, back into life. This thinking was prevalent in grief theory into the 1980s.

In the mid-1980s Silverman and Worden studied a community-based sample of bereaved school-age children who had lost a parent to death. These children and their surviving parent were followed for a 2-year period after the death. What Silverman and Worden discovered was that a large number of these children stayed connected to their deceased parent rather than emotionally withdrawing and moving on. They stayed connected by making an effort to locate the deceased, through experiencing the deceased, by remembering the deceased, by reaching out for a connection, and attaching to the deceased through transitional objects. Through a process they called "constructing" the deceased, these children developed inner representations of the deceased that allowed them to maintain their relationships with the deceased, relationships that changed as the children matured and the intensity of grief lessened. Over time, the children relocate the dead persons in their lives and memorialize them in ways that allow their lives to move on (Silverman, Nickman, & Worden, 1992).

Concurrent with the Harvard Child Bereavement Study, Dennis Klass was working with bereaved parents in the Midwest. Klass found that many of these bereaved parents did not want to disengage from their deceased children but rather sought ways to keep a sense of their children's presence with them as they moved forward after their loss (Klass, 1988). Klass, who had an interest in cross-cultural adaptations to grief, has found that bereaved parents from other cultures also had a desire to remain bonded with their deceased children.

Based on Klass's studies and the findings from the Harvard Child Bereavement Study, a book was written titled *Continuing Bonds*—coining a new term—as well as a new way to look at the relationship between the mourner and the deceased (Klass, Silverman, & Nickman, 1996). The Harvard study found that not all children maintained bonds with their dead parent, but of those who did, continuous bonding was not detrimental but rather had a salutary effect on their overall adjustment after the loss (Worden, 1996).

Since the book *Continuing Bonds* was published, there have been some who have cautioned against overexcitement about bonds to the deceased. For some mourners, particularly those with "anxious–ambivalent attachments," excessive rumination can lead to chronic grief. For these mourners, maintaining bonds may not make for a healthy adaptation. They need to relinquish some of these overly close ties and learn how to manage their anxiety before they can move forward with their grief (Schut, Stroebe, & Boelen, 2006), (Stroebe & Schut 2005).

ROBERT NEIMEYER AND JANICE NADEAU

Another emphasis appeared in the late 1990s that influenced grief theory and involved meaning-making or meaning reconstruction. Although this notion was present in the thinking of earlier theorists, it received a new emphasis during this period. The death of a loved one can fill the mourner with a seemingly endless number of questions such as: "Why me?" "What will my life look like now?" "Who am I now that this death has occurred?" "How can I feel safe in this world?"

This emphasis on meaning-making was spearheaded by Robert Neimeyer and his colleagues at the University of Memphis. Neimeyer is a clinical psychologist who espouses a constructivist approach to psychotherapy, including grief therapy. According to Neimeyer, grieving is a process of reconstructing a world of meaning that has been challenged by loss. Although most people successfully navigate bereavement and retain or return to adequate functioning, a significant proportion struggle with prolonged grief, and are unable to find meaning in the wake of an unsought transition. For these individuals, constructivist therapy offers a number of strategies that foster meaning-making and help clients reestablish a coherent self-narrative that integrates the loss, while also permitting their life story to move forward along new lines.

Meaning reconstruction in response to a loss is the *central process* in mourning, according to Neimeyer. Meaning reconstruction involves at least two main tasks: (1) redefining the self and (2) redefining how one engages with the world. Achieving this will not necessarily return the mourner to pre loss functioning but rather help them develop a meaningful life without the deceased loved one (Neimeyer, 1999, 2001).

A second person to emphasize meaning reconstruction is family psychologist Janice Nadeau. Nadeau has emphasized the role of the family in meaning-making after a death. She believes that the way a family construes the loss will strongly affect the way that the family grieves. Because of this, family intervention is strongly encouraged for a bereaved family. Intervention that is geared to change a family's problematic meaning system can go a long way to affect the grief of individuals in the family as well as the grief trajectory for the entire family (Nadeau, 1998).

THE ELEPHANT NEEDS A PEDICURE: SIMILARITIES, DIFFERENCES, DIRECTIONS FOR THE FUTURE

Looking at the various theories of grief that have been proffered over the past 100 years is a bit like the fable of the blind men and the elephant. The description of what the elephant was like depended on what part of the elephant the various blind men were touching. Grief theory makes up the elephant—conceptions of the adaptation to the loss of a loved one with their various similarities and differences. However, the elephant needs a pedicure! Rather than recreating the elephant, we need to select and investigate specific parts of these theories (toes) and tweak them. I have selected eight areas that we need to look at and tweak—not sure how many toes an elephant has—but eight is a good round number. Here are my questions and suggestions:

1. *What is the place of attachment and separation in the bereavement process?* Freud (1917/1957) started us on our journey by suggesting that adaptation to death loss was made better by decathexis, or emotionally withdrawing from the deceased so that emotional energy could be reinvested in new relationships and activities. Bowlby and Parkes (1970) strongly suggest that attachment, be it secure or insecure, very much affects the outcome of bereavement. The idea of continuing bonds suggests that the mourner find ways to continue attachment to the deceased loved one. Worden (2009), in his Task IV, promotes the notion of finding an enduring connection with the deceased in the midst of embarking on a new life. Several questions need further investigation. For whom are continuing bonds a good thing, and for whom are they not a good thing? Do some bonds place an impediment on the mourning process? Also, we need to know which kind of bond makes for the best attachment (e.g., a memory or an object). And what happens to these bonds over time? A longitudinal study of these questions would be in order.

2. *What is the role of emotion, and when can feelings be detrimental?* Most of the theories outlined above acknowledge that emotions after a death are important and a natural part of grieving. Sadness is not the only emotion for the bereaved. Anger, guilt, shame, and loneliness are among the other feelings the bereaved grapple with. Worden (2009) focuses on dealing with affect as one of his tasks of mourning (II) and posits the mourner needs to acknowledge these feelings in order to make the best adaptation. There are others, such as Bonanno et al. (2002) and Wortman (1989), who suggest that the mourner can overfocus on feelings and that some who make the best adjustment to loss have few, if any, feelings.

Nolen-Hoeksema (2001) focuses on excessive rumination as a behavior that can get in the way of adjusting to a loss and push the mourner toward a prolonged and less productive pathway. We need further research into the role of affect and affect regulation and how these impact bereavement outcomes.

3. What is the role of "meaning finding" in adapting to a loss? Some like Neimeyer (2001) would say that it is the central process in mourning. Others like Parkes, Bowlby, Worden, and Stroebe would say it is important but is only one of a group of tasks or activities that need to be processed as one adapts to death loss. For many mourners, finding meaning after a death is not a big struggle. It is easily handled by seeing death as part of a life cycle, especially if the death is timely and occurs in season. For others, a sudden death or a death out of season becomes a big struggle for the mourner to make sense of and to integrate it into his or her life. This can take time and may need intervention. Further investigation of this is needed to see when intervention for meaning reconstruction is needed and for whom.

4. What is the importance of cross-cultural influences on grieving behavior? Some theorists have focused on this more than others. Rosenblatt says that "culture shapes grieving" (Rosenblatt, 2008), and others would agree. Parkes and colleagues (1997) have written *Death and Bereavement Across Cultures*, and Klass (1999) has written *Developing a Cross-Cultural Model of Grief*. Worden (2009) looks at culture as one of the important *mediators* of mourning that influences the tasks of mourning. There are wide variations across cultures as to how, and how much, people grieve, which challenges the universality of any theory of grief and grieving. Looking at death rituals of a particular society can give one some clue as to the meaning of death in that society (Rosenblatt, 1976). We need to recognize that much of bereavement research has been done by Europeans and Americans and is often written in English. As these societies become increasingly pluralistic, additional attention and research needs to focus on important cross-cultural differences that impact on how we see and work with mourning behavior.

5. What is the role of individual differences when one is grieving? There has been a tendency for those working with the bereaved and subscribing to a particular grief theory to assume that one size fits all. An extreme example of this would be applying Kübler-Ross's stages to every bereaved person and to expect them to pass through these stages in sequence. Similarly, one might do the same thing with the phases suggested by Parkes and Bowlby, though the author's dissuade this. Some have taken Worden's tasks of mourning and suggested that they are really stages rather than the dynamic and fluid tasks that the author described. Others do the same thing with the theories of Rando, Rubin, and Stroebe.

Psychologist Gordon Allport (1957) at Harvard was fond of saying, "Each person is like *all* other persons, each person is like *some* other persons, and each person is like *no* other person." This maxim would apply to the grief experience. Each person's grief is like all other people's grief; each person's grief is like some other people's grief; and each person's grief is unique and like no other person's grief. Any useful theory must account for individual differences. Worden (2009) did this by adding the *Mediators of Mourning* to his model. Although the tasks of mourning apply to any death loss, how difficult these tasks are and how the individual handles these tasks depend on these various mediators of mourning. Attig's theory of Relearning the World emphasizes the importance of individual differences and focuses on these as the counselor helps the mourner relearn the world. Not every mourner struggles in adjusting to the death of a loved one;

many do quite well, and many are what Bonnano calls "resilient" (Bonnano et al., 2002). The most useful theories will take into account the importance of individual differences and try to account for them.

6. Who should receive intervention, and who should not? It is clear that not every bereaved person needs intervention. Many, if not most, do very well in adapting to the death of a loved one without any special intervention. However, there are those who can profit by help with their grief. Who are these people? Schut (2010) and colleagues in the Netherlands, who do careful and seminal research, found that those who profited the most from intervention were those who sought it out rather than being enlisted in some type of research program. The mourner identified a need and sought help with this need. This makes a lot of sense. If on asking a person, "Are you having trouble dealing with the death?" and "Are you interested in seeing a grief counselor to help with that?" he or she answers "yes," there is a high probability that the individual will find grief counseling productive (Gamino, Sewell, Hogan, & Mason, 2009).

There is another way to approach intervention. This was first used by Parkes in the Harvard Bereavement Study and requires a longitudinal study (Parkes, 1972). Information is gathered on the bereaved close to the time of death, and these people are followed for several years to see how they do. Those not doing well several years later are identified with discriminating information from the earlier assessments. If these "at-risk" people can be identified early, then intervention can be done with them to prevent later negative sequelae. This preventative mental health approach can be quite useful rather than waiting until a person gets into difficulty and then seeks out help. Worden used this same approach with parentally bereaved children. He developed a screening instrument that could identify children 4 months after parental death who were going to be making a poor adaptation 2 years later, so early intervention could be offered to them (Worden, 1996). Some have been concerned that bereavement intervention can be harmful. There is little, if any, evidence to support this (Larson & Hoyt, 2007).

7. What is the relationship among trauma, grief, and traumatic grief? Stroebe, Schut, and Finkenauer (2001) offer a useful paradigm for thinking of this. Their distinctions are (1) grief without trauma, (2) trauma without grief, and (3) traumatic grief. In the latter, there is a loss that involves both grief and trauma. Traumatic stress interferes with grief over the loss, and grief interferes with trauma mastery (Rando, 1993). Traumatic grief raises the question as to which gets treated first, the trauma or the grief? There are some like Rando and Worden who believe that the trauma needs to be addressed first before the grieving can move forward. Stroebe would agree with this, but points out that there is considerable overlap between grief and trauma when doing intervention. We need more clarification on this in order to offer the most efficacious intervention.

There is a debate as to what causes traumatic bereavement. One camp focuses on the *event* itself. It is the type of death that significantly impacts the level of trauma following a loss. It is the event and not the person's reaction to it (Stroebe et al., 2001). An alternate view focuses on *the mourner and his or her relationship to the deceased* rather than on the event. This focuses on the relational and interpersonal impact on bereavement rather than the objective nature of the death (Rubin, Malkinson, & Witztum, 2003). To try and further clarify this, Worden followed 70 conjugally bereaved widow/ers for 2 years following the death of their spouses. Multivariate analysis showed that a violent death was the strongest predictor of trauma 2 years after the death. This was followed by the coping style of the mourner (passive coping, and the inability to redefine events). In the end, research will probably show that both points of view are important. In addition to the event itself, we need to see what an individual brings to a traumatic event as well as what he or she experiences afterward.

8. Is grief work necessary? The answer to this question depends on what you mean by "grief work." Freud coined this term early in his study of grieving behavior, and it continued in vogue for much of the twentieth century. He coined that term on the assumption that grief is psychological work that one neglects at one's peril. His grief work focused on reality testing the loss and the expression of painful emotions (Freud, 1917/1957).

Grief work in general refers to what one goes through when adapting to the death of a loved one. Most of the theorists considered in this chapter would endorse this term in one form or another. Lindemann, Bolwby, Parkes, Worden, Rando, Rubin, and Stroebe each outline behaviors that will help a person move through his or her grief and make an adequate adaptation. There is a general assumption by most of these that being able to do something active is preferable to being passive. This idea of being active is certainly central to Worden's tasks of mourning model (Worden, 2009).

Wortman and Silver (1989) began to criticize the notion of grief work in their classic paper, "The Myths of Coping with Loss." One point they challenged was that great distress should be experienced after every loss and that the failure of this was problematic. They report a lack of empirical evidence for this, which in their thinking makes grief work a myth. However, they overlook individual difference, which makes some losses intensely devastating for the mourner and other losses much less so. Any experienced clinician knows this is so.

Another myth that they identify is that of "working through" the loss. They posit that those who work through do not ultimately cope better than those who do not. The problem here is with the definition of "working through." Various research studies approach this concept in different ways. More research is needed to discern what types of confrontation and what types of avoidance are important and for whom. A clearer definition of "working through" is needed along with intervention programs and activities that can help establish the efficacy and validity of this notion.

There have been others who have criticized the notion of "grief work" in favor of a different way to look at grief and grieving. George Bonnano has been a leader in this area. Others like Folkman (2001), Janoff-Bultman (1992), and Rosenblatt (1983) come to mind. Even with these criticisms, Stroebe and colleagues point out that the grief work concept remains a powerful analytic tool for understanding the way people adapt to bereavement. It captures at least part of the essence of coming to terms with loss, at least in our own culture. It must also be noted that although the major theorists did consider grief work to be fundamental to adaptive grieving, their writing reflects an awareness of greater complexity (Stroebe, 2001). It is this complexity on which our research needs to focus.

It is the author's opinion that we need to establish common agreements in bereavement theory and research. This consensus makes up most of the elephant. Then we need to tackle the toes that are the questions suggested above and focus our empirical research on these and other relevant questions. This will increase our knowledge of how the whole is greater than the sum of its parts. We do not need an orthogonal shift in our paradigm as much as we need to modify what we think we know through better research.

REFERENCES

Allport, G. (1957). Class lecture notes.

Attig, T. (2000). *The heart of grief: Death and the search for lasting love.* New York, NY: Oxford University Press.

Attig, T. (2001). Relearning the world: Making and finding meanings. In R. A. Neimeyer (Ed.), *Meaning reconstruction & the experience of loss* (pp. 33–53). Washington, DC: American Psychological Association.

Attig, T. (2011). *How we grieve: Relearning the world* (rev. ed.). New York, NY: Oxford University Press. (Original work published 1996)

Bonanno, G. A., Wortman, C. B., Lehman, D. R., Tweed, R. G., Haring, M., Sonnega, J., . . . Nesse, R. M. (2002). Resilience to loss and chronic grief: A prospective study from preloss to 18-months postloss. *Journal of Personality & Social Psychology, 83,* 1150–1164.

Bowlby, J., & Parkes, C.M. (1970). Seperation and loss within the family. In E.J. Anthony & C.M. Koupernik (Eds.), The child in his family (pp. 197–216). New York: Willey.

Folkman, S. (2001). Revised coping theory and the process of bereavement. In M. Stroebe, R. O. Hansson, W. Stroebe, & H. Schutt (Eds.), *Handbook of bereavement: Consequences, coping, and care* (pp. 563–584). Washington, DC: American Psychological Association.

Freud, S. (1957). Mourning and melancholia. In J. Strachey (Ed. & Trans.), *Standard edition of the complete works of Sigmund Freud* (Vol. 14, pp. 237–260). New York, NY: Basic Books. (Original work published 1917)

Gamino, L. A., Sewell, K. W., Hogan, N. S., & Mason, S. L. (2009). Who needs grief counseling? A report from the Scott & White Grief Study. *Omega, 60,* 199–223.

Janoff-Bultman, R. (1992). *Shattered assumptions: Toward a new psychology of trauma.* New York, NY: Free Press.

Klass, D. (1988). *Parental grief: Solace and resolution.* New York, NY: Springer Publishing Company.

Klass, D. (1999). Developing a cross-cultural model of grief: The state of the field. *Omega, 39,* 153–178.

Klass, D., Silverman, P., & Nickman, S. (Eds.). (1996). *Continuing bonds: New understandings of grief.* Washington, DC: Taylor & Francis.

Kübler-Ross, E. (1969). *On death and dying.* New York, NY: Macmillan.

Larson, D., & Hoyt, W. (2007). What has become of grief counseling: An evaluation of the empirical foundations of the new pessimism. *Professional Psychology: Research and Practice, 38,* 347–355.

Lindemann, E. (1944). Symptomatology and management of acute grief. *American Journal of Psychiatry, 151*(6 Suppl.), 155–160.

Nadeau, J. W. (1998). *Families making sense of death.* Thousand Oaks, CA: Sage.

Neimeyer, R. (1999). Narrative strategies in grief therapy. *Journal of Constructivist Psychology, 12,* 65–85.

Neimeyer, R. (Ed.). (2001). *Meaning reconstruction and the experience of loss.* Washington, DC: American Psychological Association.

Nolen-Hoekskema, S. (2001). Ruminative coping and adjustment to bereavement. In M. S. Stroebe, R. O. Hansson, H. Schut, & W. Stroebe (Eds.), *Handbook of bereavement research: Consequences, coping, and care* (pp. 545–562). Washington, DC: American Psychological Association.

Parkes, C. M. (1972). *Bereavement: Studies of grief in adult life.* New York, NY: International Universities Press.

Parkes, C. M., Laungani, P. & Young, B. (1997). Death and bereavement across cultures, London: Routledge.

Parkes, C. M., & Weiss, R. S. (1983). *Recovery from bereavement.* New York, NY: Basic Books.

Rando, T. A. (1984). *Grief, dying, and death.* Champaign, IL: Research Press.

Rando, T. A. (1993). *Treatment of complicated mourning.* Champaign, IL: Research Press.

Rosenblatt, P. (2008). Grief across cultures: A review and research agenda. In M. S. Stroebe, R. O. Hansson, H. Schut, & W. Stroebe (Eds.), *Handbook of bereavement research and* practice: *Advances in theory and intervention* (pp. 207–222). Washington, DC: American Psychological Association.

Rosenblatt, P. C., Walsh, R. P., & Jackson, D. A. (1976). Grief and mourning in cross-cultural perspective. New Haven, CT: Human Relations Area Files Press.

Rubin, S. S. (1981). A two-track model of bereavement: Theory and application in research. *American Journal of Orthopsychiatry, 5,* 101–109.

Rubin, S. S. (1999). The Two-Track Model of Breavement: Overview, retrospect, and prospect. Death Studies, 23, 681–714.

Rubin, S. S., Malkinson, R., & Witztum, E. (2003). Trauma and bereavement: Conceptual and clinical issues revolving around relationships. Death Studies, 27, 667–690.

Schut, H. (2010). Grief counseling efficacy: Have we learned enough? *Bereavement Care, 29,* 8–9.

Schut, H. A., Stroebe, M. S., & Boelen, P. A. (2006). Continuing relationships with the deceased: Disentangling bonds and grief. Death Studies, 30, 757–766.

Silverman, P. R., Nickman, S., & Worden, J. W. (1992). Detachment revisited: The child's reconstruction of a dead parent. *American Journal of Orthopsychiatry, 62,* 454–503.

Stroebe, M., & Schut, H. (1999). The dual process model of coping with bereavement: Rationale and description. *Death Studies, 23,* 197–224.

Stroebe, M. (2001). Bereavement research and theory: Retrospective and prospective. American Behavioral Scientist, 44, 854–865.

Stroebe, M., & Schut, H. (2005). To continue or relinquish bonds: A review of consequences for the bereaved, *Death Studies, 29,* 477–494.

Stroebe, M., & Schut, H. (2010). The dual process model of coping with bereavement: A decade on. *Omega, 61,* 273–289.

Stroebe, M., Schut, H., & Boerner, K. (2010). Continuing bonds in adaptation to bereavement: Toward theoretical integration. *Clinical Psychology Review, 30,* 259–268.

Stroebe, M., Schut, H., & Finkenauer, C. (2001). The traumatization of grief: A conceptual framework for understanding the trauma-bereavement interface. *Israel Journal of Psychiatry & Related Sciences, 38,* 185–201.

Wortman, C. B., & Silver, R. C. (1989). The myths of coping with loss. *Journal of Consulting and Clinical Psychology, 57,* 349–357.

Worden, J. W. (1996). *Children and grief: When a parent dies.* New York, NY: Guilford.

Worden, J. W. (2009). *Grief counseling & grief therapy* (4th ed.). New York, NY: Springer Publishing Company.

Leeat Granek

8

THE PSYCHOLOGIZATION OF GRIEF AND ITS DEPICTIONS WITHIN MAINSTREAM NORTH AMERICAN MEDIA

For much of my academic career, I have been thinking and writing about the medicalizing and psychologization of grief (Granek, 2008, 2010, 2013a, 2013b). I became interested in this topic by accident. Like most academics who study grief, I came to the subject out of my own personal experiences of loss. I was halfway through my doctoral degree in the History and Theory of Psychology Program at York University in Toronto, Canada, when my mother, who had been ill for a long time, and to whom I was very close, died from breast cancer. Her death was followed by a succession of other losses that year that made it difficult to think about, or focus on, anything else but my intense feelings of grief. In line with my habit as a lifelong reader, I began to consume everything I could get my hands on that had to do with loss—both in the academic literature and in popular texts, such as memoirs and books on the topic. I wanted to understand my experience; to have some kind of frame around it so that I could control what was happening to me. I read self-help books. I read memoirs. I read novels. I read poems. I read pop psychology articles. I watched Oprah. I read the Bible. I read article after article that I printed from Psyc-Info, and nothing satisfied me. I couldn't find myself or my experiences in any of the texts, especially in the academic ones that came out of my own field of psychology.

In these explorations of grief, I noticed that one common theme in everything I was reading (expect in my beloved novels) was the sense that there was a danger that grief could go terribly wrong and become pathological if it went on for too long or too intensely. As a mourner, I could not understand this thread that seemed to cut across the academic and popular literatures on grief. My own experience of grieving seemed to be pointing to a long journey in which the intensity and duration of these feelings were par for the course. Intuitively, it seemed to me that if you loved someone intensely, you also grieved for them with the same passion with which you cherished them when he or she was still alive.

In my dissertation, I wrote that my grief felt like a spiraling mandala of darkness and sorrow, and in the beginning, I felt like I was being swirled in its currents. Eventually, I took a step back from this chaos, and at some point, I was far enough from my experience of grief to recognize that the mandala had a definite pattern that was peculiar to my North American culture, but close enough to feel the heat from the spinning motion. In other words, I was close enough to the pain for it to be embodied, but far enough away from it to take a meta-view over what had happened. In retrospect, I believe that this was the perfect starting place to begin researching the topic of grief. It was at this point—the point between chaos and emotional neutrality—that my thinking about grief began to profoundly change and take on a more critical view.

GRIEF AS A PSYCHOLOGICAL OBJECT OF STUDY IN A MODERNIST CONTEXT

Medicalizing or psychologizing grief means turning what was once considered a normal, human reaction to the loss of a loved one or, in some cases, grief caused by other losses into a mental or medical disorder necessitating psychological or medical intervention. Because I have written extensively about the pathologization of grief elsewhere, I refer readers to these publications for a thorough historical, cultural, and social account of the ways in which grief has become increasingly pathologized in the last century (Granek, 2008, 2010, 2013a, 2013b). What is important to delineate is that today, in North American societies, grief is considered to be a psychological process that has a starting point, a middle point, and an end point. The task of the griever is to do "grief work" and get back to the job of living full, productive lives as soon as possible. If the griever is not able to "move on" fast enough or "well enough," it is their responsibility to seek professional help, which often takes the shape of a therapist or a prescription for medication.

The emergence of grief, then, as a psychological, scientific object of study is an early 20th-century invention (Granek, 2008, 2010). The psychologization and pathologization of grief is situated within several other cultural and historical movements that have been part of the shifting understanding of mourning as a medical entity. These contexts include the rise of modernism and the focus on the psychological self as a site of meaning and the subsequent fear of death and grief (Becker, 1973; Kellehear, 2007; Seale, 1998); the proliferating role of therapeutic experts in managing everyday life (Illouz, 2008); and an adherence to a progress narrative that emphasizes happiness, innovation, and a forward-moving mentality while denying sadness and mourning (Cable, 1998; Gorer, 1967). Modernism emphasizes science, reason, progress, and an emphasis on the individual self. The focus is on functionality, rationality, and efficiency in all areas of living (Gergen, 1991, 1992). As such, modernism developed in tandem with a decline in religion and a belief in science instead of God (Bauman, 1992; Gorer, 1967). Whereas it used to be the case that religion and traditional societies offered social processes around mourning that ascribed rituals and practices to deal with death, and subsequently grief, the modernist focus on the self has left people bereft of meaning, community, and structure with which to manage grief. When applied to grief, this modernist paradigm assumes that:

> People need to recover from their state of intense emotionality and return to normal functioning and effectiveness as quickly and efficiently as possible. Modernist theories of grief and related therapeutic interventions encourage people who have experienced loss to respond in just this way. Grieving, a debilitating emotional response, is seen as a troublesome interference with daily routines, and should be "worked through." Such grief work typically consists of a number of tasks that have to be confronted and systematically attended to before normality is reinstated. Reducing attention to the loss is critical, and good adjustment is often viewed as breaking of ties between the bereaved and the dead. (Stroebe, Gergen, Gergen, & Stroebe, 1992, p. 1206)

THE PATHOLOGIZATION/PSYCHOLOGIZATION OF GRIEF

As already noted, grief within the psychologized frame is constructed as a potentially pathological condition that necessitates psychological intervention in order for people to heal as quickly as possible (Granek, 2010). This view is so widely held that a form of grief was recently considered for inclusion in the *Diagnostic and Statistical Manual of Mental Disorders* (*DSM-5;* American Psychiatric Association, 2013). Moreover, the American Psychiatric Association has now removed the bereavement exclusion from the major depressive episode diagnosis; this means that anyone showing sufficient symptoms of clinical depression after a major loss can be diagnosed with clinical depression even if these symptoms are caused by bereavement-related losses (Granek, 2013a). By virtue of its inclusion as a psychological object of study, what was once considered to be a natural reaction to death has fallen under the purview of the psy-disciplines (e.g., psychology, psychiatry, social work, and other mental health professions), and has therefore become monitored, understood, and experienced in a way that previous generations could not have conceptualized (Granek, 2010). As with other psychological diagnoses in recent years (e.g., social anxiety disorder; Lane, 2007), *the specific criteria of what constitutes pathology are less important than the notion that one can evaluate one's grief on a continuum of normality/abnormality at all*. Regardless of *how* grief has become pathologized within the disciplines, the very inclusion of it as a psychological/psychiatric subject has had a drastic effect on the way people understand their experience of bereavement (Granek, 2008, 2010; Granek & O'Rourke, 2011).

In this frame where all grief is considered *potentially* pathological, some grief is described as "excessive," a "disease," "out of the norm," and a "mental disorder" (Forstmeier & Maercker, 2007; Horowitz, 2005–2006; Prigerson & Jacobs, 2001; Prigerson et al., 2009; Shear & Frank, 2006; Shear et al., 2011). The extreme end of pathologizing grief is the diagnosis of complicated grief (CG), sometimes referred to as traumatic grief, prolonged grief, or pathological grief (Stroebe & Schut, 2005–2006). CG is a proposed diagnostic category for the *DSM* (Forstmeier & Maercker, 2007; Prigerson et al., 1995, 1997a, 1997b; Shear et al., 2011). Although CG is currently *not* an official diagnosis, it is widely used by researchers and clinicians and is often diagnosed in patients and clients alike.

The determination of frequencies of CG depends on the definition, for which there is currently no consensus. The leading proponents of including CG in the *DSM* are Prigerson and her colleagues (Prigerson et al., 1995, 1997a, 1997b; Prigerson & Jacobs, 2001), Horowitz and colleagues (1997), and Shear and colleagues (2011). Table 8.1 outlines the specified criteria for each of these schools of thought on what constitutes complicated or prolonged grief disorder.

The main difference between Horowitz et al. (1997) and Prigerson and Maciejewski (2005–2006) is the criteria for duration and the number of symptoms necessary for diagnosis. Although Prigerson stipulated that a diagnosis can be made 6 months postloss, she also indicated that all four criteria categories must be met. Horowitz, on the other hand, proposed that diagnosis should be made 14 months after loss; he also has a smaller number of criteria to be met in order to be diagnosed. As with Prigerson, Shear suggests that there is little difference between the symptoms of acute grief and complicated grief but it is the duration and intensity of the symptoms that distinguish pathology. She noted that grief becomes complicated when the symptoms of acute grief last for longer than 6 months and, therefore, become persistent.

TABLE 8.1 Proposed Criteria for Complicated or Prolonged Grief Disorder

PATHOLOGICAL GRIEF PROPONENTS	CRITERIA	CUTOFF FROM TIME OF BEREAVEMENT
Prigerson and colleagues (2009)	*a.* Event: Bereavement (loss of a significant person)	6 months
	b. "Chronic yearning, pining and longing for the deceased"; physical or emotional suffering as a result of the desired, but unfulfilled, reunion with the deceased) daily or to a disabling degree	
	c. Five or more out of nine symptoms, such as: "confusion in one's role in life," "difficulty accepting the loss," "avoidance of reminders of the reality of the loss," "inability to trust others," "bitterness or anger about the loss," "difficulty about moving on," "numbness," "feeling that life is unfulfilling," and "feeling dazed or shocked about the loss"	
	d. Diagnosis should not be made until at least 6 months have elapsed since time of death	
	e. The disturbance causes clinically significant impairment in social, occupational, or other important areas of functioning	
	f. The disturbance is not better accounted for by major depressive disorder, generalized anxiety disorder, or posttraumatic death disorder	
Horowitz and colleagues (1997)	*a.* Bereavement	14 months postloss
	b. In the last month, any three of the following seven symptoms with a severity that interferes with daily functioning: **Intrusive symptoms:**	
	1. Unbidden memories or intrusive fantasies related to the lost relationship	
	2. Strong spells or pangs of severe emotion related to the lost relationship	
	3. Distressingly strong yearnings or wishes that the deceased was there	
	Signs of avoidance and failure to adapt:	
	4. Feelings of being alone too much or personally empty	
	5. Excessively staying away from people, places, or activities that remind the subject of the deceased	
	6. Unusual levels of sleep interference	
	7. Loss of interest in work, social, caretaking, or recreational activities to a maladaptive degree	
Shear and colleagues (2011)	*a.* Person has been bereaved	6 months postloss
	b. At least one of the following symptoms of persistent intense acute grief has been present for a period longer than is expected by others in the person's social or cultural environment	
	1. Persistent intense yearning or longing for the person who has died	

(continued)

TABLE 8.1 Proposed Criteria for Complicated or Prolonged Grief Disorder (*continued*)

PATHOLOGICAL GRIEF PROPONENTS	CRITERIA	CUTOFF FROM TIME OF BEREAVEMENT
	2. Frequent intense feelings of loneliness or like life is empty or meaningless without the person who has died	
	3. Recurrent thoughts that it is unfair, meaningless, or unbearable to have lived when the loved one has died, or a recurrent urge to die in order to find or join the deceased	
	4. Frequent preoccupying thoughts about the person who has died, e.g., thoughts or images of the person intrude on usual activities or interfere with functioning	
	c. At least two of the following symptoms are present for at least a month:	
	1. Frequent troubling rumination about circumstances or consequences of the death, e.g., concerns about how or why the person died, or about not being able to manage without the loved one, thoughts of having let the deceased person down, etc.	
	2. Recurrent feeling of disbelief or inability to accept the death, like the person can't believe or accept that the loved one is really gone	
	3. Persistent feeling of being shocked, stunned, dazed, or emotionally numb since the death	
	4. Recurrent feelings of anger or bitterness related to the death	
	5. Persistent difficulty trusting or caring about other people or feeling intensely envious of others who haven't experienced a similar loss	
	6. Frequently experiencing pain or other symptoms that the deceased person had, or hearing the voice or seeing the deceased person	
	7. Experiencing intense emotional or physiological reactivity to memories of the person who died or to reminders of the loss	
	8. Change in behavior due to excessive avoidance or the opposite, excessive proximity seeking, e.g., refraining from going places, doing things, or having contact with things that are reminders of the loss, or feeling drawn to reminders of the person, such as wanting to see, touch, hear or smell things to feel close to the person who has died	
	d. The duration of symptoms and impairment is at least 1 month	
	e. The symptoms cause clinically significant distress or impairment in social, occupational, or other important areas of functioning, where impairment is not better explained as a culturally appropriate response	

The theme in all of these understandings of CG is the trend toward inclusiveness. Most proponents of CG as a disease category concede that there is an ambiguous line between normal grief and pathological grief, but argue that this is not significant in making a diagnosis of CG. Researchers in the field claim that although normal grief and pathological grief *look* the same, it is a matter of *duration and intensity* that marks the distinction between them.

DEPICTIONS OF PATHOLOGICAL/PSYCHOLOGICAL GRIEF IN MAINSTREAM MEDIA

Before discussing the impact of the pathologization of grief, it's necessary to understand how these messages about pathologized grief get circulated in the public domain. How do these psychological depictions of grief influence the public's experiences of mourning? In this next part of the chapter, I illustrate how the scientific notions of pathological grief described in the first half of this chapter get represented in the mainstream media, and in the process influence how the public understands and subsequently experiences its own grief. I focus on the most popular mainstream media sources that affected millions of people daily up until the mid-2000s to examine how psychological notions of grief get circulated in mainstream culture. Hacking (1995) describes this process as "looping," a trajectory by which psychological ideas get circulated in mainstream culture and subsequently picked up and taken on by the lay public.

The looping of grief begins with the psy-disciplines' construction of it as an individualized, psychologized, and private event, as described in the introduction to this chapter (Granek 2013a, 2013b). This construction then gets relayed to the public through various representations in mainstream media, including film, television, and newspapers. The relaying of psychological messages about grief in these media illustrates two interlocking features of the looping process. First, the representation of psychological constructions of grief in the media is reflective of how these classifications became interpreted and changed by agents in the public who themselves are immersed in and responsive to culture. In other words, people who direct films, write newspaper articles, and produce television are in and of themselves immersed in the culture, and are thus excellent examples of how the psychological classification of grief is understood, interpreted, and experienced by the public. Second, these media examples illustrate how psy-classifications become further looped to the lay public by serving as disseminators of psychological messages about grief that have been mediated by the aforementioned North American cultural agents. As will be shortly illustrated, grief is an excellent example of this looping phenomenon. As it became known in the public over the last 30 years, it began to take on a life of its own, and people who may never have had any knowledge of psychology or psychiatry began to understand their own and other people's experiences of grief through a psychological lens.

Representations of Grief in Film

In contemporary North American culture, television and film are mediators in which people get introduced, immersed, and identify with narratives and themes of their culture (Bell, Haas, & Sells, 1995). Indeed, one of the primary ways in which the psychological construct of grief got introduced into public consciousness is through the medium of film (Sedney, 2002). In the following section, I analyze two films, *Ordinary People* and *Reign Over Me*, for their depiction of grief as a psychological phenomenon. I chose these films both because they were viewed by millions of people at the time they were released and because they are representative of the two decades preceding the contemporary debates about grief as a pathological disorder. Although several years have passed since they were released, they continue to capture the collective imagination and appear to retain their cultural currency as the films people most remember in relationship to grief. To understand the current cultural conceptions of pathological grief, it is necessary to understand the historical trajectory of the media messages circulated in mainstream culture.

One of the most well-known films dealing with grief in North America is Robert Redford's *Ordinary People,* released in 1980. This film was so popular with audiences that it won four Oscars, five Golden Globes, and several other prestigious film awards. The film depicts the Jarrett family, who are trying to return to normal life after the attempted suicide of their teenage son, Conrad, who had recently come home from a long stay in a psychiatric hospital, where he received electric shock therapy and psychoanalysis. Alienated from his friends and family, Conrad's parents push him to seek help from a psychiatrist, Dr. Berger, who coaxes out of him that he had been involved in a sailing accident that killed his older brother, Buck. Calvin Jarrett, the father, awkwardly struggles to connect with his surviving son, who is depicted as clinically depressed and suffering from what Dr. Berger calls "survivor guilt" and "posttraumatic stress disorder." Beth Jarrett, the matriarch of the family, struggles to maintain a sense of normalcy and has become obsessed with maintaining the appearance of perfection in the family.

This film depicted the psy-disciplines' construction of psychological grief and introduced the public to the relationship between grieving and psychology and psychiatry. Conrad's attempted suicide as a reaction to his brother's death necessitates psychiatric intervention, including shock therapy and regular sessions with a therapist. As Conrad successfully works with his psychiatrist and learns to express his feelings, he has major, dramatic breakthroughs in therapy that help him do his "grief work," including the recognition that he shouldn't feel guilty for surviving and that it is okay to be angry.

Calvin, Conrad's father, begins to go to therapy, too, and finds ways to connect with his son and, in the process, feel the pain of his own grief. Although Calvin is an essential figure in the movie, the true hero of the film is Dr. Berger. He is patient, compassionate, emotionally and physically available, and always perceptive and analytic in his interpretations of what is happening with Conrad and Calvin as they struggle through their grief work. He is the catalyst and the container in which the men work through their grief.

If Dr. Berger is the hero, then Beth, the mother, is portrayed as the villain. In reaction to one son's death and the other's attempted suicide, she shuts off emotionally. She wants to go back to normal as fast as possible and throughout the film expresses her desire to "keep grief a private matter" to be solved within the family. Beth is depicted as being in denial about her pain and refuses to talk about Buck's death, or show any emotion or vulnerability to her family members. Out of all the characters, Beth is depicted as the least likeable and appears to be stubborn, and heartless, for withholding her feelings and refusing to go to therapy to work it out with her husband and son. Indeed, the end of the film has Beth abandoning her family to fulfill what her husband calls her "selfish desires."

Although the primary goal of the film may have been to portray an ordinary family going through extraordinary stress, there is implicit messaging about grief and grieving that is revealing in terms of what it tells us about the psychological construction of grief at this time and how it was woven into popular representations.

The audience learned that the grief of ordinary people can lead to suicide, hospitalization, and shock therapy; can go on too long (Conrad suffers from chronic mourning accompanied by numbing); can lead to major psychiatric problems (Conrad suffers from "survivor guilt," "clinical depression," and "posttraumatic stress disorder"); and can break up families and tear people apart. The film further suggested that grief *must* be treated to avoid these problems. Not only is therapy for grieving, therefore, "necessary," as Conrad's father tells his son in the first 5 minutes of the film, but one wonders whether without it, one will end up like Beth: a selfish, cold, and self-absorbed person.

Another example is *Reign Over Me*, which was released in late 2007. The main character in *Reign Over Me* is so far removed from reality that he is in a state beyond denial. In his grief, he has regressed into adolescence, where he travels around Manhattan on a scooter and retreats into a world of video games, compulsive late-night kitchen renovations, and classic rock, which he listens to on oversized headphones. His grief at losing his three daughters and his wife in the 9/11 terrorist attack in New York City is so incapacitating and so extreme it appears that he is suffering from some kind of psychotic disorder. Any mention of his dead family sends him into extreme rages where he throws and breaks furniture.

Although such grief reactions are extremely rare, these two popular films give the impression that grief is a dangerous and out-of-control condition that necessitates therapy. One of the main plot lines in *Reign Over Me* (2007) is the urgent need of the bereaved man's friend to get him into therapy to deal with his loss. The message in these films is that grief needs to be treated and resolved, or else one is at risk of being in denial about the death of loved ones, or going on violent rampages to avoid talking about them.

Representations of Grief on Television

Although grief is often depicted as pathological and requiring therapy in the movies, television programs also use psychological constructs in their portrayal of grief. One of the most successful talk shows ever produced was the *Oprah Winfrey Show*, which ran for 25 years on television. The show was hosted by Oprah Winfrey and was aired in 135 countries worldwide, and close to 9 million viewers tuned in to her show daily. Her influence on the American public was so profound that any endorsement from her (whether a recommendation of a new book, a product, or a political candidate) was met with overwhelming enthusiasm. Two of her most popular guests were Dr. Phil McGraw and Dr. Robin Smith, two psychologists who started out as guest experts and eventually expanded to have their own spin-off shows that teach "life skills" and coach people on "relationship issues" worldwide. Because Oprah was so popular, and because her influence was so pervasive in North America, she is a particularly good source to use to examine as an example of how mainstream media depicts psychological understandings of grief.

A general search on Oprah's popular website targets all of Oprah's media outlets, including her magazine, her show, and the radio programs hosted by Oprah, Dr. Phil, and Dr. Robin. The keyword search "grieving" yielded 140 hits that had to do with grief caused by the death of a loved one. Although it is impossible to describe all of these sources, a look at a few key examples will provide an illustration of the way grief is conceptualized on these shows. A common theme in these sources is the psy-disciplines' construction of grief as a psychological disorder and as a condition that needs to be treated with professional help. The first show, entitled "9/11 Widow Stuck in Her Grief," aired in October 2005 (Winfrey, 2007a). On this show, Dr. Phil outlined four stages of grief and gave several suggestions on how people can move on with their lives after a death. In Dr. Phil's view, the four stages of grief include shock, denial, anger, and resolution, and in order to reach closure and resolution, one must "define success differently, change the form of your relationship with the deceased, ask for help, set up a support system, and work actively on your grief process" (Winfrey, 2007b). Dr. Phil goes on to give several more suggestions in a time of crisis that include "giving oneself permission to grieve," "voicing of one's feelings," "maintaining a normal routine," and avoiding "being in denial" (Winfrey, 2007b).

Several messages about grief are evident in this show that was so popular it was aired several times and eventually expanded to include a series on grieving and loss of loved ones. The title of the show *"9-11 Widow Stuck in Her Grief"* conveyed the premise of the program. Although the show was about "helping" widows "heal from their grief," a large part of the program was about differentiating what is normal from what is pathological when it comes to grieving (i.e., who is still "stuck" and who has "moved on"; Winfrey, 2007a). On this show, both the grieving widows and the 9 million Americans (as well as the many others who watched the repeats or read about it on the website) learned that there is a "right" and a "wrong" way to grieve.

The resolution of grief, according to Dr. Phil, is to take action in a number of ways. One of the main things Dr. Phil advocates is asking for help when doing one's grief work. Dr. Phil is quoted on the website as saying, "You must be willing to ask for help" and "time heals nothing. It's not the passage of time; it's what you do with that time. One day of doing the right thing can replace a year of doing the wrong thing. Don't let yourself spend days and weeks in denial and withdrawal" (Winfrey, 2007c).

The "right" thing, according to Dr. Phil, means seeking therapy and the "wrong" thing means being in denial, withdrawing, and not doing one's "grief work." Other suggestions include "giving yourself permission to heal." Dr. Phil said, "Don't fight your emotions; work through them. If you don't, you will have unfinished emotional business" (Winfrey, 2007c). Much like the messages transmitted in *Ordinary People* (1980), and *Reign Over Me* (2007), the implicit message is that one must do one's grief work or else there may be "unfinished emotional business" that could make one go insane. The message to the bereaved here is not a suggestion that doing one's "grief work" may help, but rather a very threatening warning that one *must*, one is *obligated* to seek help, or else there will be consequences.

Perplexingly, while one is expected to do all of this grief work, Dr. Phil also suggests that one should continue to "maintain a normal routine." "Take each day at a time. Even if you don't feel like doing your regular activities, do so anyways. Behave your way to recovery" (Winfrey, 2007c). Here the message seems to be that while one should do grief work in the privacy of a therapeutic relationship, the individual should also continue to put on a happy face and go back to normal as quickly as possible. The pathologization of grief in a therapeutic culture leads naturally to privatization; when one is "stuck in grief," or is suffering from pathological grieving, the onus of responsibility is on the bereaved to seek help for his or her sadness rather than inflicting it on others. The job of the mourner is to go back to normal and "go back to regular activities" even if he or she doesn't feel like it. Finally, although the undercurrent of all this advice is to turn one's sadness into something positive, Dr. Phil explicitly says this only at the end:

Releasing negative energy will allow you to feel better. Channel this energy into positive situations. Become active in your community, be a role model for your children or voice your opinion to representatives in Washington—just do something positive with this negative energy. (Winfrey, 2007c)

In summary, the message for people who are grieving is that they should seek help for their sadness; they should move on with their lives and go back to normal as soon as possible; they must do their grief work to avoid pathology; they should avoid being "in denial" or "withdrawing from life"; and finally, and perhaps most important, they should stop wallowing in their sadness and do something positive with their negative energy. The inability of most people to follow through with these multiple injunctions and demands is inevitable. The majority of those who are bereaved do not become heroes by doing something positive with their sadness. Indeed, the majority feel sad for a very long time. The disparity between what people experience and what they are told they *should* experience or do with their grief is likely what leads many people to seek professional help for their sadness.

Representation of Grief in Newspapers

Popular magazines and newspapers are other media outlets through which the psy-disciplines' construction of grief is transmitted and interpreted by the public. Baugher (2001) noted that no matter how tragic a story is, how many people have died, or how many are grieving, the message in mainstream American media outlets is that grief will soon be over. In a 2-year study looking at how newspaper outlets portray grief, Baugher (2001) found that many articles have headlines about how long grief should last and convey the implicit message that one should move on. For example, he noted that many headlines include the world "still" in their titles implying that one is "still stuck" grieving losses several years later (i.e., "Father Still Mourns Loss of His Son, 16, Ten Years After the Attack" or "Still Mourning Her Son's Death after Eighteen Years"). Another point Baugher (2001) made in sync with Dr. Phil's philosophy, is that in newspapers, grief is often written about when people turn it into something positive in the form of activism or personal growth. The message is that grief should be productive and enlightening rather than sad and depressing. Walter, Littlewood, and Pickering (1995) have similarly argued that news coverage after disasters in which many deaths have occurred tends to affirm the value of human attempts at rational control. People who are expressively grieving are often displayed as heroes brave enough to speak about their sadness in the news. Walter et al. (1995) suggested that these displays of grief enforce the psy-conception of expressive grieving as the normal and right way to cope with loss, and to reach a good and healthy resolution.

Like movies and television, newspapers also have a profound influence on people's ideas and understanding of modern grief. *The New York Times* is a daily newspaper published in New York City and distributed internationally. Founded in 1851, the newspaper is known as the authoritative reference for modern events and is one of the most well-read papers in North America and the world today. In 2007, the paper reported a circulation of roughly 1,120,420 copies on weekdays and 1,627,062 copies on Sundays. *The New York Times* also has an extensive website that is accessed by 18 million people per month. The combination of their daily and weekend newspapers and their website makes *The Times* a particularly relevant media source to examine for its impact on people's understandings of grief.

In the 1980s, Daniel Goleman, a psychologist, wrote several articles about grief for *The Times*. In an article entitled *Mourning: New Studies Affirm Its Benefits* (1985), Goleman introduced the public to the research of psychologists doing work on bereavement and grieving. Although the title is misleading in that it suggests the piece would be about the benefits of mourning, the majority of the article was about how grieving can go wrong. As with the messages transmitted on Oprah, and in many newspaper articles, Goleman (1985) reiterated the point that although people's responses to grief differ widely, and most people don't follow a set of stages when grieving, there are nonetheless typical patterns and the possibility of pathology. He wrote:

> *Mourning, when successful* removes one from the stream of life to ponder one's own place in the world and one's relationship with the dead person, and finally to return to that stream having *adjusted to living with the loss. . . . When mourning goes awry*, the rest of the life suffers. Over a protracted period, perhaps years, the mourner is so overwhelmed and obsessed that *the grief is debilitating and distorts many aspects of life.* (Goleman, 1985, p. C1) (Italics added)

The idea that mourning can be successful implies that mourning can also be unsuccessful, and, indeed, Goleman discussed the possibility of debilitating and obsessive pathological grief toward the end of the paragraph. Goleman also reiterated the idea that grieving is a process, and that there is work to be done that goes in successive stages in order for one to "adjust to the loss" and "move on" (Goleman, 1985). The psy-construction of grief is also evident through Goleman's interview with Mardi Horowitz, a contemporary advocate for the inclusion of complicated grief in the *DSM*. "For some people," said Horowitz, "mourning the loss involves a process so unbearably painful, protracted or tenaciously blocked that it can be described as pathological grief" (Goleman, 1985, p. C1).

In 1988, Goleman wrote another article for *The Times* entitled the *Study of Normal Mourning Process Illuminated Grief Gone Awry*. Although the last article was about grieving in general with an introduction to pathological grief, this article dealt specifically with complicated grief. Again, Goleman (1988) interviewed Dr. Horowitz at length, but also included a short quote by Dr. Volkan, another researcher advocating for complicated grief's inclusion in the *DSM*. Goleman (1988) quoted Horowitz, who stated, "the death of a loved one is the prototypical psychological catastrophe, a blow to the unconscious sense of personal inviolability that most of us carry." Goleman (1988) wrote:

> Mourning a loved one is always painful, but some people find the process more difficult than others, either *becoming too distraught or holding too much emotion in. . . .* The research is also spawning new *psychological treatments for those who have trouble grieving.* Most of the treatments focus on *helping mourners follow the normal path.* (Goleman, 1988, p. C1) (Italics added)

It is worth noting that death in itself, and grieving for a loved one, is not an unusual trauma or a catastrophe in the way that is implied. Death is constant and expected. Although it is emotionally straining to cope with loss, it is not out of the ordinary to grieve. The idea that grief is a "psychological catastrophe" is part of the psy-disciplines' construction of grieving. If the loss of a loved one can be considered a psychological problem, it can also be treated as one. Indeed, as Goleman's (1988) statement implied, grieving can go awry by either the person becoming too distraught, or not distraught enough. The role of the psychologist, therefore, is to aid the mourner to "follow the normal path" of the grieving process with new treatments.

Following the terrorist attacks on September 11, 2001, a series of articles about grieving were published in *The Times*. Robert Klitzman (2002), a psychiatrist, wrote about using antidepressants to deal with his grief over his dead sister and suggested that this might be a good solution for others, too. Another article written by Erica Goode (2001) was entitled *A Nation Challenged: Psychological Trauma: Stress Will Chase Some into Depths of their Minds*. The piece was about grieving after 9/11 and the development of treatment for survivors who suffered from posttraumatic stress disorder and pathological grieving (Goode, 2001). Similarly, in 2006, Anthony DePalma wrote about grief assistance available to those who lost a relative in the World Trade Center attacks. He noted:

> The American Red Cross shows that for many of those directly affected by the Sept 11 attacks, grief remains a constant companion nearly five years later. The report shows that two-thirds of the responders, survivors, and victim's relatives who sought help from the Red Cross to deal with their emotions in the aftermath of 9/11 believe that grief still interferes to a large or moderate extent with their lives. Overall, just over 40% of the 1,500 adults surveyed said that they still needed additional services to help them recover. Foremost among the services needed, according to the survey, were mental heath treatments. (p. B3)

Although each of these articles differs in content and purpose, they all share the same underlying message for the public. Whether it be grief resulting from a personal loss or grief resulting from a national one such as 9/11, all conclude that grief has a normal path that can go awry, and that help is not only available but necessary, either in the form of psychological therapy or medication. The representation of the psy-classification of grief is evident in the reporting on these issues. Interestingly, none of the newspaper reporters questioned the validity of pathological grief, which is likely an indication of its widespread acceptance in the culture. Further, as is evident from reports like DePalma's (2006), where the majority sought psychological help for their grief, and almost half reported still needing psychological or psychiatric intervention 5 years after the attacks, the public clearly experiences their grief as abnormal and in need of help. Moreover, both the reporter and the people being written about seem surprised that grief should remain present nearly 5 years after 9/11. The evaluation of how long grief should last, the very idea that grief should be "over and done with," can also be interpreted as the incorporation of the psy-classification of grief into people's understanding of their experiences.

DISCUSSION

In this chapter, I have suggested that the pathologization/psychologization of grief within the psy-disciplines has had an impact on the way in which mourning is understood and managed in day-to-day life. Moreover, I have shown *how* these pathological depictions of grief were represented in mainstream media in the last few decades, and how, in turn, these depictions have influenced the public's understanding of their own grief. These media messages include the obligation to be "normal" in one's expression of grief; the evaluation of oneself in psychological terms of what normal versus pathological grief looks like; the pressure to turn one's grief into a celebratory experience for personal growth; the pressure to do one's grief work; and the obligation to seek professional, psychological help if one cannot do this on one's own. The result for the grieving person is profoundly felt on an individual level, as is evidenced by all of the things grieving people *need* and *should* do, but is also felt by the society in which the grieving person lives.

One of the primary outcomes of the psy-construction of grief is the creation of a culture in which these kinds of expectations and scripts around grief become the norm regardless of whether they are viable for those who are grieving. As I have indicated, many of these expectations around grief may be untenable and place enormous demands on the mourner. As a result, people who believe they *should* meet these grieving milestones feel they need professional help to achieve these goals. The psychological imperative of accepting and resolving one's grief is a good example of this pressure. Many people will never accept or resolve their sadness over losing someone they have loved. The pressure on them to do so, however, not only makes them self-conscious about whether they are doing their grief work properly, but also infuses them with a sense of guilt and failure over being unable to meet these demands (Gilbert, 2006). The outcome for mourners is a sense of shame and embarrassment over both their sadness and their inability to overcome it.

Moreover, to conceptualize grief as a potential pathology that can be cured with therapy or medication is to individualize and privatize what used to be a communal responsibility of grieving the dead (Mellor & Shilling, 1993). Indeed, the vocabulary of grief has been thoroughly psychologized and in the process has become individualized. Terms such as "coping," "recovery," "healing," "denial," and "grief work" or "grief process" are all constructions of the psy-professions, and today psychotherapy and medication are common ways in which grieving is dealt with (Granek, 2008). The psychological construction of grief has enforced the idea that grief can be pathological, and that the best way to avoid this, or to cope with grief that has gone awry, is to turn to a professional who has the tools and the knowledge to help one overcome sadness and return to normal as quickly and efficiently as possible. There is thus a closed circle whereby the psy-disciplines both problematize grief and then offer a solution to the problem. Finally, the questionable act of turning grief into a disorder has reduced the diminishing range of what is considered acceptable human emotion by the psy-disciplines. To pathologize grief is to claim that the widespread response to feeling sadness over a loss is a disorder that needs to be treated. The outcome is that people are afforded less compassion, less time, and less space to grieve their losses.

LOOKING AHEAD

In a previous paper, I have suggested that the field of psychology is suffering from a kind of disciplinary wound, where as a field, we have become disassociated from our historical roots when it comes to the study of grief and loss (Granek, 2013a). The focus in the grief-and-loss field today is almost always on its dysfunctional nature, and this laser-like focus on pathology has come at the expense of other questions we might be asking about grief.

The psychoanalyst and philosopher Robert Stolorlow noted, "Pain is not pathology" (Stolorow, 2011, p. 7). The field of thanatology would do well to remember this simple but profound fact that is worth repeating again. *The pain of grief is not pathological.* The study of grief and loss in the last century has lost sight of this very important distinction. Certainly, this does not mean that grief and loss should not be studied. Indeed, I myself am a researcher in this field, and subscribe to the idea that grief can, and indeed should, be examined in a variety of ways, including empirically. There is unequivocally room for research on grief and its accompanying processes. However, looking at grief solely as an object to be studied, manipulated, predicted, diagnosed, and treated, and only within a pathological frame, is limited in scope, imagination, and integrity.

The field of thanatology has the potential to change the frame entirely. Instead of focusing on the one question of whether or not grief is a pathology—a question that has dominated the field for the last several decades, and most certainly dominated the media lately, we can ask a whole new set of questions about grief—questions that include: What don't we know about grief? Why don't we know it? Why are we looking at grief in these particular ways? What are different ways we can study and think about grief? How do our limited scientific tools curb what we can know about grief? And most important, how might we go about finding new ways of generating research, collaboration, and partnerships to gain a more complex picture of what this necessary and powerful human experience of grief is all about?

REFERENCES

American Psychiatric Association. (2013). *Diagnostic and statistical manual of mental disorders* (5th ed.). Arlington, VA: American Psychiatric Publishing.

Baugher, R. (2001). How long (according to the media) should grief last? *Columbia Journalism Review, 39*(6), 58.

Bauman, Z. (1992). *Mortality, immortality and other life strategies.* Cambridge, UK: Polity Press.

Becker, E. (1973). *The denial of death.* New York, NY: Free Press.

Bell, E., Haas, L., & Sells, L. (1995). *From mouse to mermaid: The politics of film, gender, and culture.* Bloomington, IN: Indiana University Press.

Cable, D. C. (1998). Grief in American culture. In K. J. Doka & J. C. Davidson. (Eds.), *Living with grief: Who we are, how we grieve* (pp. 61–70). Washington, DC: Hospice Foundation of America, Brunner/Mazel.

DePalma, A. (2006, May). Survey finds that grief is a constant companion for those at the scene of the 9.11 attacks. *New York Times,* p. B3. http://www.nytimes.com/2006/05/26/nyregion/26survivor.html

Forstmeier, S., & Maercker, A. (2007). Comparison of two diagnostic systems for complicated grief. *Journal of Affective Disorders, 99*(1–3), 203–211.

Gergen, K. J. (1991). *The saturated self: Dilemmas of identity in contemporary life.* New York, NY: Basic Books.

Gergen, K. J. (1992). *The social constructionist movement in modern psychology.* Washington, DC: American Psychological Association.

Gilbert, S. (2006). *Death's door: Modern dying and the ways we grieve.* New York, NY: W.W. Norton.

Goleman, B. D. (1985, February 5). Mourning: New studies affirm its benefits. *New York Times,* p. C1. http://www.nytimes.com/1985/02/05/science/mourning-new-studies-affirm-its-benefits.html

Goleman, B. D. (1988, March 29). Study of normal mourning process illuminates grief gone awry. *New York Times,* p. C1. http://www.nytimes.com/1988/03/29/science/study-of-normal-mourning-process-illuminates-grief-gone-awry.html

Goode, E. (2001, September 18). Stress from attacks will chase some into the depths of their minds. *New York Times,* p. B1. http://www.nytimes.com/2001/09/18/health/psychology/18PSYC.html

Gorer, G. (1967). *Death, grief, and mourning* (1st ed.). Garden City, NY: Doubleday.

Granek, L. (2008). *Bottled tears: The pathologization, psychologization, and privatization of grief* (Unpublished doctoral dissertation) York University, Toronto, Canada.

Granek, L. (2010). Grief as pathology: The evolution of grief theory in psychology from Freud to the present. *History of Psychology, 13*, 46–73.

Granek, L. (2013a). The complications of grief: The battle to define modern mourning. In E. Miller (Ed.), *Complicated grief: A critical anthology*. Washington, DC: NASW Press.

Granek, L. (2013b). Disciplinary wounds: Has grief become the identified patient for a field gone awry? *Journal of Loss and Trauma, 18*(3), 275–288.

Granek, L., & O'Rourke M. (2011, Spring). *What is grief actually like: Results of the slate survey on grief*. Retrieved from http://www.slate.com/id/2292126/

Hacking, I. (1995). The looping effects of human kinds. In D. Sperber (Ed.), *Causal cognition: An interdisciplinary approach* (pp. 351–183). Oxford, UK: Oxford University Press.

Horowitz, M. (2005–2006). Meditating on complicated grief disorder as a diagnosis. *Omega: Journal of Death and Dying, 52*(1), 87–89.

Horowitz, M. J., Siegel, B., Holen, A., Bonanno, G., Milbrath, C., & Stinson, C. H. (1997). Diagnostic criteria for complicated grief disorder. *American Journal of Psychiatry, 154*, 904–910.

Illouz, E. (2008). *Saving the modern soul: Therapy, emotions, and the culture of self-help*. Berkeley, CA: University of California Press.

Kellehear, A. (2007). The end of death in late modernity: An emerging public health challenge. *Critical Public Health, 17*(1), 71–79.

Klitzman, R. (2002, September 10). Cases. *New York Times*, p. F5. http://www.nytimes.com/2002/09/10/health/cases-when-grief-takes-hold-of-the-body.html?module=Search&mabReward=relbias%3Ar%2C{%221%22%3A%22RI%3A6%22}

Lane, C. (2007). *Shyness: How normal behavior became a sickness*. New Haven, CT: Yale University Press.

Mellor, P. A., & Shilling, C. (1993). Modernity, self-identity and the sequestration of death. *Sociology, 27*, 411–431.

Prigerson, H. G., Horwitz, M. J., Jacobs, S. C., Parkes, C. M., Aslan, M., Goodkin, K., . . . Maciejewski, P. K. (2009). Prolonged grief disorder: Validation criteria proposed for DSM-V and ICD-11. *PLoS Med, 6*(8), e10000121.

Prigerson, H. G., & Jacobs, S. C. (2001). *Traumatic grief as a distinct disorder: A rationale, consensus criteria, and a preliminary empirical test*. Washington, DC: American Psychological Association.

Prigerson, H. G., Maciejewski, P. K., Reynolds, C. F., Bierhals, A. J., Newsom, J. T., Fasiczka, A., . . . Miller, M. (1995). Inventory of complicated grief: A scale to measure maladaptive symptoms of loss. *Psychiatry Research, 59*(1–2), 65–79.

Prigerson, H. G., Shear, M. K., Bierhals, A. J., Pilkonis, P. A., Wolfson, L., Hall, M., . . . Reynolds, C. F. (1997a). Case histories of traumatic grief. *Omega: Journal of Death and Dying, 35*(1), 9–24.

Prigerson, H. G., Shear, M. K., Frank, E., & Beery, L. C. (1997b). Traumatic grief: A case of loss-induced trauma. *American Journal of Psychiatry, 154*(7), 1003–1009.

Seale, C. (1998). *Constructing death: The sociology of dying and bereavement*. Cambridge, UK: Cambridge University press.

Sedney, M. A. (2002). Maintaining connections in children's grief narratives in popular film. *American Journal of Orthopsychiatry, 72*(2), 279–288.

Shear, K., & Frank, E. (2006). *Treatment of complicated grief: Integrating cognitive-behavioral methods with other treatment approaches*. New York, NY: Guilford.

Shear, M. K., Simon, N., Wall, M., Zisook, S., Neimeyer, R., Duan, N., . . . Keshaviah, A. (2011). Complicated grief and related bereavement issues for *DSM-5*. *Depression and Anxiety, 28*, 103–117.

Stolorow, R. (2011). From mind to world, from drive to affectivity: A phenomenological contextualist psychoanalytic perspective. *Attachment: New Directions in Psychotherapy and Relational Psychoanalysis, 5*, 1–14.

Stroebe, M., Gergen, M. M., Gergen, K. J., & Stroebe, W. (1992). Broken hearts or broken bonds: Love and death in historical perspective. *American Psychologist, 47*, 1205–1212.

Stroebe, M., & Schut, H. (2005–2006). Complicated grief: A conceptual analysis of the field. *Omega: Journal of Death and Dying, 52*(1), 53–70.

Walter, T., Littlewood, J., & Pickering, M. (1995). Death in the news: The public invigilation of private emotion. *Sociology, 29,* 579–596.

Winfery, O. (2007a). *9/11 Widow stuck in her grief.* Retrieved from http://www.oprah.com/showinfo/911-Widow-Stuck-in-Her-Grief

Winfrey, O. (2007b). *Dr. Phil helps grieving wives.* Retrieved from http://www.oprah.com/tows/pastshows/tows_past_20011002_c.jhtml

Winfrey, O. (2007c). *Coping with the emotional aftermath.* Retrieved from http://www.oprah.com/tows/pastshows/tows_past_20010919_b.jhtml

9

DEVELOPMENTAL PERSPECTIVES ON DEATH AND DYING, AND MATURATIONAL LOSSES

OUR STORIES

Judith's Story

All career choices are influenced by professional opportunities and personal histories, and mine were no exception. I was born to parents whose "first child" was a miscarriage, and their loss made me aware of how losses are often hidden, even if powerfully felt. In college, my best friend was killed by a drunk driver, and I felt alone and unvalidated in my grief. Later, I worked as a social worker with oncological and perinatal populations and frequently saw bereaved individuals whose grief was not validated. I felt compelled to validate their right to grieve losses that are less recognized.

I encouraged bereaved people to "hold" their grief, and I was delighted when *Continuing Bonds* (Klass, Silverman, & Nickman, 1996) was published as it provided support for the interventions I was using with bereaved parents. I tended to dissuade them from the notion that "acceptance" and "closure" were the goals (Kübler-Ross was in vogue at the time). I recognized their need to mourn the attachments that had grown; they needed permission to stay connected to the children they had birthed in their minds and bodies.

Entering doctoral work, I expected to be the first to examine what I called "Unvalidated Grief." Imagine my sense of loss (and validation!) on discovering Doka's *Disenfranchised Grief* (1989). Someone had finally named the experience I felt, and saw so often in others. His next book (2002) explicitly identified how social norms are tied to disenfranchised loss, and, further, how coping with loss is predicated on the availability of support. These premises, combined with the power of attachment, are foundational to how I understand loss and grieving.

My doctoral research focused on women with desired pregnancies who had to make decisions about whether to end a pregnancy affected by fetal anomaly, and deal with the stigma of choosing to end it. Doka's work, combined with Arlie Hochschild's concept of "feeling rules" (1979), led me to consider how social structures and expectations frame the experience of loss and grief. I was fascinated by how technology changed experiences of grief and loss. The attachments heightened by visualization of the fetus made decisions terribly difficult when a fetal anomaly was diagnosed. Women's experience of stigma while grieving made the disenfranchised aspects of the loss all the more poignant.

I was also interested in how understandings of loss change over the course of a lifetime. Neimeyer's (2001) focus on meaning-making, together with the idea that all losses entail "re-learning the world" (Attig, 2001) in a way that may inspire growth, remain major themes in my work. It is clear to me that grief and loss

121

evolve within social contexts; people may grow from loss when supported and given opportunities for meaning-making and help with relearning their world. Likewise, growth can inspire loss. Carolyn and I write about how maturational growth entails loss of the way one was, loss that is disenfranchised. I remain intrigued that growth can inspire a sense of loss, just as loss can inspire growth.

Carolyn's Story

My first brush with death occurred at 16, when my father died. This propelled me into a major in psychology in order to help others. In the late 1960s, I enrolled in a masters in social work (MSW) program where my only exposure to ideas about death and grief were John Bowlby (1951) and Kübler-Ross (1969). In doctoral work in the late 1970s, I was introduced to Bertha Simos's (1979) seminal work, *A Time to Grieve: Loss as a Universal Human Experience*. Reflecting back, I realize that Simos's work helped me grasp basic concepts about loss: it cannot be escaped and is an ongoing and essential part of the human condition; it affects all people at all phases of the life cycle. These ideas have powerfully influenced three of my books (Oktay & Walter, 1991; Walter, 2003; Walter & McCoyd, 2009).

My interest in death work began after the death of my first husband when I was 47. My understanding of the subject was fundamentally changed by an Association for Death Education and Counseling (ADEC) conference presentation in 1996 by Klass, Silverman, and Nickman on how "continuing bonds" with the deceased could promote the healing process. Previously, I had learned that there is closure to the process of mourning and that you need to put the deceased behind you before entering a new relationship. This did not mesh with what I experienced as a young widow. I mourned my beloved husband while resuming life as a single woman. I devoured *Continuing Bonds*, and ideas began to percolate for a book (Walter, 2003) that included stories from widowed adults and domestic, gay, and lesbian partners across the life span.

The narratives for the book revealed similarities in the grief process, but also differences related to the developmental phase and societal support for the relationship. Doka's (1989) notion of disenfranchised grief helped me understand the painful stories related by gay men and women. The theme of "continuing bonds" appeared in the story of nearly every interviewee. Almost universally, the bereaved respondents shared stories of how they made meaning from their losses. Neimeyer's (2001) concept of meaning-making/reconstruction of identity and Attig's (2001) idea that those who suffer give meaning to their experiences were vividly apparent.

I completed this book in 2003. Subsequent research for a new MSW course, "Grief and Loss Across the Life Cycle," brought me to the dual-process model (Stroebe & Schut, 1999). This describes the "cycling" common to bereavement as one moves from the deep emotions of grief to rebuilding life. The dual-process model has also informed Judie's work and thus our work together. *Grief and Loss Across the Lifespan* (Walter & McCoyd, 2009) reflects our understanding of how life-cycle tasks influence the experience of loss and the understanding of death.

OUR DEVELOPMENTAL PERSPECTIVE

We adhere to the developmental perspective grounded in the assumption that individuals continually change over the life course as a result of physical growth, new experiences, cognitive development, and evolving relationships. We also believe that experience with death is shaped by developmental tasks, issues, and challenges specific to each life-cycle phase. Although we focus on developmental aspects of grief, we also observe the irony that though grief can debilitate some, it stimulates growth in others. In this chapter, we discuss how the individual's life-stage development affects the response to death loss, and note the circumstances under which grief may best provoke growth.

Developmental biology as well as psychological and social contexts impact death understandings. The experience of loss and death at different times in childhood means understandings vary as a result of the physical and cognitive developments that have occurred. These combine with the child's attachments to the lost entity to create experiences that impact a child's experience of death. When a young adult faces the loss of a parent or friend, the loss experience is shaped by his or her struggle to establish intimacy with a partner, or to find his or her place in the adult world. Although this early development is the easiest to understand, older adults also have new experiences that affect the way they cope with and understand death. To understand how individuals encounter death, one must understand biopsychosocial development over the life course.

Certain types of death losses tend to be encountered for the first time at particular ages. Although there are many "off-time losses" that are challenging because they are not part of a cohort experience, we focus here on losses typical to each age. For instance, children often experience death for the first time when a grandparent or pet dies. Many young adults face the loss of a grandparent, and some the death of a friend. For midlife adults, the loss of a parent is common. Older adults commonly experience the death of a spouse or life partner. Earlier "off-time" partner death is more challenging precisely because it is not a common experience.

Age and development also affect the way one is perceived to grieve. These perceptions constitute a form of disenfranchised grief that we refer to as disenfranchised developmental aspects of grief, such as when children are not included in funerals. Life stages frame grieving for older adults too as when they get little support after a death because they are believed to be inured to such loss by their age and experience.

Finally, we also address a form of loss that may not be conceived as loss, much less a form of death. We believe that maturational growth may involve a "mini death" that requires some mourning and/or recognition. As one develops, parts of the self and earlier behaviors and ways of being have to die. The adorable toddler with food in his hair will be told to quit playing with his food and grow up. The teenager will get a job, but will also be held accountable for paying more expenses. The older adult will retire from paid work, but will also lose the status afforded by professional identity. The individual is "growing," yet also experiencing the death of a part of self. These maturational losses become the context for coping with death.

PERINATAL PERIOD AND INFANCY

The beginning of a pregnancy is supposed to be a joyous occasion, yet about 70% of all pregnancies end in the first trimester, most before recognition of the pregnancy. Another 5% to 10% end in stillbirth or the death of a neonate (in the first 28 days of life; Freidenfelds, 2013). We do not understand what the fetus/neonate experiences and cannot consider a fetus' experience of death. We do know that the mother/parent/s have begun an attachment process and that they experience significant loss and grief when a pregnancy ends or a baby is born and dies. Women who experience such loss often try to protect themselves by attempting to avoid attachment in subsequent pregnancies until they believe the pregnancy will be successful

(Cote-Arsenault & Donato, 2011). This type of death has unique qualities in that others are not available to share the grief as virtually no one has gotten to "know" the fetus in utero, whereas the mother has likely endowed the "baby" with an identity and set of hopes and dreams that become a major part of the loss. Further, as is true in childhood generally, parents are expected to keep children safe, so when children die, most parents are not only bereft but feel they failed in their duty. This is particularly true of mothers who believe that their bodies should provide a safe environment for growth and feel that their bodies have betrayed them when a miscarriage or stillbirth occurs (Bennett, Litz, Sarnoff Lee, & Maguen, 2005).

The experience of an infant following the death of a loved one is difficult to know, but it is clear that the death of a caregiver will have an impact on the infant, particularly after about 6 months of age (Coates & Gaensbauer, 2009). Prior to that, infants cope as long as someone provides consistent, attuned caregiving and a routine for them. It is not just the physical necessities of care that are required, but also attunement to the infant's emotional states and help with affect regulation. Some of what is known has been derived from separations infants and toddlers experience when they have parents in the military. These separations can become permanent as a result of death, or may be temporary, but infants' lack of time sense and the verbal ability to process past and future mean that they are at particular risk during their parent's deployments (Paley, Lester, & Mogil, 2013).

Infants tend to respond to the death of close family and relatives by disturbance in sleep cycles and more difficulty self-soothing (Markese, 2011). Consistent, caring guidance and maintenance of a predictable routine will help the infant readjust to a world without that person. The "September 11, 2001, Mothers, Infants and Young Children Project" studies families whose father died on 9/11. This research illuminates how the mother's stress impacts fetuses in utero (via her cortisol and other hormonal impacts) and challenges the mother's ability to remain attuned to the infant during her own grief (Markese, 2011). The degree of distress and the coping ability of the surviving parent were shown to mediate infants' and toddlers' grief responses, but much of the literature indicates negative impacts on the security of the attachment with higher likelihood of parent–child conflict, behavioral problems, and externalizing behaviors as infants grow (Markese, 2011). The most important intervention is to assist the primary caregiver to remain attuned and responsive to the infant after the death of any caregiver.

TODDLERHOOD THROUGH PRESCHOOL-AGED CHILDREN

Toddlerhood (2 years of age) through the beginning of elementary school is a time of rapid development; bodies grow, and children move from total dependence on an adult to a growing ability to provide self-care and form attachments of their own. Most critically, toddlers develop the ability to speak and communicate their thoughts to caregivers (and researchers). They do not yet have the cognitive ability to understand death fully, something Speece and Brent (1984) assert requires understanding irreversibility (once dead, the entity remains dead), nonfunctionality (the dead cannot function), and the universality of death (all living beings will die eventually). They found that most children develop the ability to understand each of these notions by around age 7, with irreversibility and nonfunctionality understood as early as 2 or 3 years old by some. Dual process seems to function more quickly as young children cycle between tears and running off to play, seemingly a normative coping style for youngsters.

Most research indicates that when surviving parents or caregivers respond in consistent, empathic ways to young children, they are not as likely to show depression or externalizing behaviors later in childhood (Markese, 2011). Preschoolers are still new to the use of language as a way of interacting and symbolizing affect, and they are often most able to communicate their thoughts and feelings via play. Euphemism-free explanations, assurances of safety, and consistent routines have all been shown to assist bereaved young children. Notably, therapeutic interventions aimed at young children have *not* been shown to be highly effective (Currier, Holland, & Neimeyer, 2007). It seems that children need routines and attuned caregiving that allows them to talk about a death more than they need therapeutic groups or therapy.

Recent research indicates that children whose parents talk directly about death and who share the sadness, allowing children to express their own sadness while not dwelling on it, avoided the most negative outcomes over time (Markese, 2011). Nearly all clinicians have stories from their practices that recount how young children were given euphemistic explanations that became problematic in and of themselves. (In Judie's practice, a 3½-year-old, told that his beloved dog was "put to sleep," developed sleep disturbances and ultimately told his parent that he did not want to die and go to heaven with the dog if he went to sleep in his room.) Direct communication is best.

Magical thinking is typical at this stage, and children may believe their angry thoughts caused the death of the deceased. Seeing the body of the deceased and explaining the concrete nature of death (irreversibility and nonfunctionality, particularly) is generally advised. Attendance at funerals may assist younger children to cope with the death; one should help the child build accurate expectations for the service and/or burial, answer the child's questions, and provide for the child to be with a trusted adult who is not herself severely affected by the death. Older toddlers and preschoolers will benefit from explanations such as "Grandpa's body got very old and worn out and he died, which means his body doesn't work anymore. We will bury his body, but we will always remember Grandpa." Small rituals like leaving a stone on a tombstone when visiting or letting a balloon "go up to heaven for Grandpa" are useful in maintaining a continuing bond with the deceased.

The death of a young child often provokes parents to feel guilty for failing to protect her. Additionally, fewer people outside the family know the child because she or he is not yet integrated into society. This means that mourners have fewer social supports who actually knew the child, and so although sympathy may be extended, it does not come with the same shared experience of loss.

Maturational losses occur in conjunction with rapid growth during this time. Typical toddler behavior that brought positive attention is now reprimanded. The child goes off to preschool and finds that she or he must adhere to rules about when to talk and what to do. A piece of the child has "died" in that he or she is no longer granted approval unconditionally. This must be experienced as a loss of self, one that children may lack the ability to process.

ELEMENTARY SCHOOL-AGED CHILDREN

By elementary school, children industriously learn and produce; they engage in creative, athletic, and other endeavors. The ability to produce promotes a sense of mastery; in contrast, the child who is unable to meet this level of industry often feels inadequate or inferior (Erikson, 1959/1980). The brain is growing and becoming more complex. Children attribute human characteristics to inanimate objects, and magical thinking (a belief that their thoughts can influence events) is strong. Clearly, if a death occurs, a child is at risk if he or she believes that his or her thoughts may have caused the death.

We will limit discussion of elementary school-aged children's responses in deference to Linda Goldman's fine chapter on work with children. We do note that many of the observations of preschool children and their responses to death parallel those of the younger children in elementary school, just as the information about tweens and teens (below) can apply to older children. The first experiences of loss are common at this age as children have their first pets die, or experience the death of their grandparents. Many have had their first exposures to death via fairy tales, Disney movies, and other children's literature in which the death of a character's parent often precedes the drama of that "child's" story (e.g., Bambi, Simba, Cinderella, and many others). These gradual exposures can allow the child to learn the experience of loss, grieving, and healing without having experienced a direct death.

Maturational losses are common for elementary school-aged children. They experience the loss of being the fully cared for child and grow into an academic setting where they are expected to achieve and perform for recognition and approval. Although school can be a haven for children who have not had the unconditional love of parents (because they can finally earn praise in the academic setting), others lose the sense of being loved purely for who they are, not just what they can produce. Children can now see that one child excels at spelling, another at kickball, and these comparisons mean the child must grapple with an egocentric loss—a "death" of the fully approved of and loved part of self. These maturational losses can make them particularly vulnerable to the loss of a parent because the safety of home no longer compensates for losses experienced at school.

TWEENS AND TEENS

Tweens to teens encompasses ages 12 to at least 19, though some assert that this adolescent period of identity consolidation and relationship formation extends into the late 20s or early 30s. Neuroscientists report that the adolescent brain changes rapidly as prefrontal cortex integration is accomplished (Siegel, 2014), a physiological phase said to last until about age 25. Theories about adolescence now integrate Erikson's identity versus identity diffusion task with the young-adult task of intimacy versus isolation. Adolescence covers a range of development as tweens differentiate themselves from their families and no longer view themselves as children, a loss of identity, albeit desired. The changing nature of their attachments and self-perceptions may give insight into the intensity of adolescent experiences of death and loss.

Christ, Siegel, and Christ (2002) note that the typical egocentricity of early adolescence gives way to more empathy and awareness of others' perspectives; younger adolescents tend to feel uniquely afflicted with grief, whereas older adolescents understand others' grief as well as their own. They assert that the adolescent task of moving away from the family of origin means that they are more susceptible to ambivalence if a family member dies. Until adolescence, most bereaved children cycle (Stroebe & Schut, 1999) quickly between restoration (a focus away from grief) and grief orientation (mourning) phases, with more time spent in restoration. Adults tend to spend more time in grief orientation, especially right after loss. Teens' Dual Process may seem unpredictable as they shift from childlike to adult patterns.

Adolescents also experience what Oltjenbruns (1996) calls "double jeopardy," a tendency to avoid emotional expression because it seems childish to the teen to be emotional at a time he or she is trying to identify with the less expressive adult role. Yet teens who stifle emotion and disclosure when they are most in need of comfort risk being cut off from vital support. Grief interventions for adolescents cannot be "prescribed" by adults, but only offered to adolescents in ways that respect self-determination and budding adulthood. Interventions that allow them to process their grief while focused on other activities tend to be most successful. Such interventions include creative expression (developing or discussing lyrics to music, working on a craft, etc.) or physical activities more acceptable to teens than play therapy or face-to-face talk therapy.

Wilkinson, Croudace, and Goodyer (2013) note that adolescents who have a tendency toward rumination are more likely to experience depression and other psychopathology. They also found that problem solving and distraction were associated with more resilient outcomes and less depressive symptoms. These associations suggest that interventions with adolescents should help them to avoid isolated rumination and promote distractions (while still assuring that dual process is observed and the teen is spending time in both grief and restoration phases).

When death losses occur, they are most often those of childhood (grandparents, pets), yet this is also a time when peers may be exposing themselves to higher risks and suicide, making homicide and accidental death more common. These sudden, unpredicted deaths often spur spiritual and existential questions for teens (Balk, 1999). Although Rask, Kaunonen, and Paunon-Ilomonen (2002) found that teens reported little or no offers of support when a friend died, it is unclear whether teens have difficulty experiencing proffered support as enacted support. The maturational losses of changing teen identities may be part of what makes adolescence so vulnerable a time to experience another's death.

YOUNG ADULTS

Social scientists are reconsidering the span of early adulthood (Furstenberg, Kennedy, McLoyd, Rumbaut, & Settersen, 2004) because the markers for this transition (choosing a career, marriage, and parenthood) are now delayed for many until well into the 20s or 30s. The restructuring of identity for young adults is prolonged and easily disrupted by any death, such as loss of a parent. Bagnoli (2003) suggests that the reconstruction of the deceased ("imagining the lost other") in order to define one's self is much more challenging when a parent dies and can no longer validate the young adult's quest for identity. Moreover, the family is altered just as the young adult is working to reduce physical and emotional dependence on parents in favor of an adult-to-adult relationship.

Young adults must develop intimate relationships without losing themselves in the process. This can be inhibited by the self-absorption required by grieving, and yet the death of a parent is "off time" for a young adult and is particularly traumatic because wholly unexpected. Most young adults are unfamiliar with death and cannot offer informed support, so that a bereaved peer is often disenfranchised from support.

Young adults try to find a place in the adult world through meaningful work. They tend to be goal-oriented and their sense of time is projected forward with an attitude that everything is possible and that life is just. Stein et al. (2009) suggest that a death can thwart progress or be a motivator; but a death that is anticipated (grandparent) is typically less distressing than an off-time death because it is less likely to disrupt belief that the world is just.

Practitioners must validate the losses of young adults, which often go unrecognized by family and friends. As Bagnoli (2003, p. 206) observes, most are determined "to carry on with life as usual, regardless of the pain," needing to demonstrate to the world and to themselves that they can make it on their own.

Practitioners should help them recognize the pain and anger that may undergird this determination.

Neimeyer, Baldwin, and Gillies (2006) found that bereaved young adults who used continuing bonds in conjunction with their meaning-making experienced fewer symptoms of complicated grief, and those who found a "silver lining" to their loss and/or experienced transformative personal/spiritual outcomes did best. To this end, practitioners should urge young adults to tell and retell the story of their loss.

One of the first maturational losses faced by young adults is emotional and physical separation from their parents. This loss often goes unrecognized by the young adult and others in his or her life because everyone is focused on the ability of the young adult to live independently. Disenfranchised loss is particularly poignant around the loss of a romantic relationship that is often not validated by others who see the young adult as having many more opportunities to invest in other relationships. The young adult is left to grieve in silence, as those around her or him do not understand the depth of his or her sadness. These maturational separations may make the separation of death all the more painful at this stage.

MIDDLE ADULTHOOD

With increased longevity and the prolongation of early adulthood, middle adulthood extends from 50 to 70 years old or more. Midlife adults take stock of their lives and confront mortality. With a heightened sense of mortality, they focus on generativity, which involves making contributions that transcend death, to society and particular people. The need to be generative colors all losses during this phase. When a midlife adult loses an adult child, the sense of generativity can be negatively impacted because they see this child and potential grandchildren as their major contribution to future generations. Midlife adults, like others who experience the death of loved ones, may have their sense of generativity heightened as they make meaning from their loss, or inhibited as the grief process depletes them.

When deaths occur, the midlife adult may experience heightened mortality concerns. Enduring a death at this phase differs from bereavement in early adulthood because midlife adults have usually experienced a death by this life stage; it is not experienced as "off time." Adults in midlife can expect more support from family and friends because they too have experienced the deaths of loved ones.

The loss of a parent, although more expected at this phase, still remains somewhat disenfranchised because society does not define this death as a major disruptive loss. Umberson's (2003) research likens the intensity of this loss of a parent to that of losing an adult child. Marks, Jun, and Song (2007) found that parent loss in midlife is associated with a significant decrease in both psychological and physical well-being. Not surprisingly, ambivalent prior relationships with parents predict difficulty with grieving. Adult children may demand more of their marriage following the death of a parent, which may contribute to marital discord (Abeles, Victor, & Delano-Wood, 2004).

Marshall (2004) found that the loss of both parents is a "two staged transition" because following the loss of the first parent, the bereaved adult focuses more on the surviving parent's grief. The loss of the second parent triggers reflection about the death of the first parent, so that the adult child grieves for her or himself more fully then. Dare (2011) found that the impact of aging and the death of parents place extra demands on women, who often are responsible for care of the remaining parent. Because midlife adults are involved in reassessing their lives and identities, the death of a parent may hasten such redefinition.

Professionals should work with bereaved midlife adults to identify their strengths and weaknesses and to recognize their accomplishments (often denied during this process of loss/change). Bereaved clients should be helped to connect and reconstruct continuing bonds and memories of the deceased while maintaining meaningful ties with the living. Practitioners should validate disenfranchised grief, help bereaved adults express their emotions and find meaning in the loss, especially in relation to shifts in identity. Practitioners should be alert to decreasing partner support and suggest marital therapy to strengthen interpersonal communications. A bereavement-group option where adults can verbalize their experiences with others who have lost parents may be an excellent alternative or addition to individual and marital/family intervention (Abeles et al., 2004).

RETIREMENT/REINVENTION

Although transition and change generally breed uncertainty, retirement is unsettling because change happens on many fronts. Leaving a job or career requires reevaluation of a work identity. This transition, although reminiscent of the adolescent need to create a new identity, can be frustrating because adults in this phase of life *expect* to know who they are. The death of a professional or work identity can also jeopardize the sense of mattering to society or to oneself. Schlossberg (2013) claims that regardless of gender or socioeconomic status, retirees need to feel important, appreciated, and noticed. In a word, to matter.

Retirees regulate this loss and redefine themselves while losing the routines on which they have depended. The yearning and searching so typical after other losses also marks this phase of life. The search for a path through this transition marks the "work" of this phase. Balancing part-time work (paid or volunteer), leisure activities, relationships, and time for self is paramount.

The loss of work identity is often accompanied by a loss of financial resources and security, the loss of relationships tied to the workplace, and changes in friendships and family. Retirees may need new friends and may need to let go of other cherished relationships (particularly difficult for women), perhaps even a marital partner. The search for an "encore self" takes precedence.

In work with retirees, it is helpful to recognize how long it takes to complete this transition. As with any loss or death, retirees and relevant others expect this transition to be settled sooner rather than later. But it proceeds fitfully, with false starts and dissatisfactions. This is often surprising and frustrating to adults who have handled other life changes more straightforwardly.

If during this transition retirees are also faced with a death or loss of health, the disorientation can make finding a sense of balance (the main task of this phase) even more difficult. Addressing the death of a family member or intimate friend can truncate the search for identity and hinder the search for how to matter—to make a difference to others and themselves. However, the search for meaning that often follows the death of family and friends can facilitate the formation of a new identity.

Redefining the self is less difficult when regrets are reframed as lessons and we have permission to change at our own pace, especially when this process is shared with others. Some believe that the solution for uncertainty is planning and preparation (Life Planning Network [LPN], 2013); others that planning is quite difficult because the journey moves erratically. Ibarra (2003) believes that trying out new activities and "selves," taking action and experimenting with new options helps retirees to discover themselves at this phase of life. Schlossberg (2013) believes that new activities and "selves" can be combined and recommends constructing a personal narrative to identify passions, and what matters, and to modify ambition and practice resilience.

OLDER ADULTS

Adults in their mid-70s and older face the major challenge of accepting life so as to achieve a sense of integrity. Older adults need to take pride in achievements while examining personal goals they have not met. This emotional work prepares older adults to develop a perspective on death, a major task of this life phase. Azaiza, Ron, Shoham, and Tinsky-Roimi (2011) found that although there is no relationship between an older adult's religiosity and death anxiety, belief in an afterlife is associated with less death anxiety. Rappaport et al. (1993) reported that older adults with a developed purpose in life are open to new meanings or possibilities and do not focus solely on mortality. The Positive Aging movement (Life Planning Network, 2013) urges seniors to use their wisdom, experience, and passion to reinvent themselves beyond midlife. *New Senior Woman* (Fleisher & Reese, 2013) provides vignettes of senior women who are redefining this stage of life. Fleisher and Reese's blog, *Elder Chicks*, provides space each week for older women to share their accomplishments, thoughts, and worries.

Major health challenges shape how older adults manage losses. Further, seniors may endure multiple losses and, as it is hard to process more than one loss at a time, mourning becomes complicated. However, these losses can also provide opportunity for growth in self-reflection and reinvention.

The loss of a spouse is one of the most frequent losses of older adulthood and it, too, creates a need to reexamine one's identity. Naef, Ward, Mahrer-Imhof, and Grande (2013) suggest that identity transformation in the midst of changed daily life characterizes this bereavement experience. Older bereaved adults must reorient themselves in their social world and assume new roles and learn new skills in order to experience growth. Although older adults can sometimes weather loss more easily than those in other life phases, older partners may also have more long-practiced roles that must change (Hansson & Stroebe, 2007). In a highly mobile society, and as personal networks shrink with the illness and death of friends, spousal relationships among the elderly assume increasing importance because fewer intimates can provide support.

Our cultural tendency to dismiss the impact of loss on the elderly because they have experienced more deaths and losses than others trivializes their experience with loss. This can lead to self-disenfranchisement. Hansson and Stroebe (2007) caution that when examining the reactions of older adults to death and loss, one needs to remember that their cohort exhibits more intragroup differences than cohorts in other life phases. Resilience among the elderly has been documented by Lieberman (2011) and many others. Liberation from some of life's stress helps older adults cultivate themselves and their relationships (Lieberman, 2011). Sexual desire persists among the elderly, and brain development continues among those who take on new experiences, tasks, and relationships. Essential to resilience is the capacity to rely on helpful social connections, but as noted above, personal networks typically are narrowed by death and illness. Thus, it is important that older adults consciously work to maintain robust social relations.

In the last phase of life, many changes and losses assault the self. It is helpful for older adults to reminisce about past accomplishments and ways they might suggest possibilities for the present. Practitioners should bear witness to past emotional insults and help older adults mourn their losses. Both older (Caserta & Lund, 2007) and newer studies (John & Lang, 2012) demonstrate how restoration-oriented coping (dual process's time of adaptation and response) helps widows and widowers. Reorientation and rebuilding networks after the loss of a spouse were associated with affective well-being. However, Naef et al. (2013) found that problem-focused/restoration-oriented coping was more important during the later stages of bereavement, whereas immediately after the loss, widows needed to come to terms with the more emotional aspects of the death. Naef et al. (2013) found that widows were comforted by continuing a relationship with their lost partner via conversations, sensing of presence, memories, dreams, and taking on an activity of the deceased. Holland, Thompson, Rozalski, and Lichtenthal (2013) found that widowed older adults periodically reassessed bereavement-related regrets and other aspects of the continued relationship with the deceased. Kim, Kjervik, Belyea, and Choi (2011) found that meaning-making was a central factor in recovery from spousal loss.

NEW DIRECTIONS AND DEVELOPMENTS

Research increasingly accounts for the life stage of the bereaved. In the past, our societal silence about death meant that we seldom explored younger individuals' experiences of loss and death. Now, studies of pregnant women and their offspring after September 11, 2001, may generate new findings about the impact of grief on the fetuses and young children of bereaved women. Death's impact on infants is better understood as we develop new techniques to observe and measure infant–caregiver interactions rather than rely solely on caregiver reports (Markese, 2011). Instead of being too fragile to hear about death, we find that young children are surprisingly resilient when provided a consistent, attuned caregiver in conjunction with opportunities to process their feelings and questions directly (Currier et al., 2007). Additionally, new research aims to differentiate traumatic and complicated grief in children (McLatchey, Vonk, Lee, & Bride, 2014) and explore the best ways to identify and intervene with struggling children.

Research continues on young adults' loss of a child, but there is little new research on young adults' experiences of parental death. As adults live longer, we need more research on midlife as a time of cumulative loss (deaths of parents, spouses, siblings, and friends). More research is needed on widowers, an oft-neglected group. The dual-process model has been used productively in recent research with adults (Coifman & Bonanno, 2010) and to guide practitioners in work with adults in all life phases. We will benefit from continued research on DPM and its nuances. These new directions for research, combined with more focus on meaning-making and normative trajectories of grief, will allow us to help grievers in more tailored and informed ways.

REFERENCES

Abeles, N., Victor, T. L., & Delano-Wood, L. (2004). The impact of an older adult's death on the family. *Professional Psychology: Research and Practice, 35*(1), 234–239.

Attig, T. (2001). Relearning the world: Making and finding meaning. In R. Neimeyer (Ed.), *Meaning construction and the experience of loss* (pp. 33–53). Washington, DC: American Psychological Association.

Azaiza, F., Ron, P., Shoham, M., & Tinsky-Roimi, T. (2011). Death and dying anxiety among bereaved and nonbereaved elderly parents. *Death Studies, 35*, 610–624.

Bagnoli, A. (2003). Imagining the lost other: The experience of loss and the process of identity construction in young people. *Journal of Youth Studies, 6*(2), 203–217.

Balk, D. E. (1999). Bereavement and spiritual change. *Death Studies, 23*, 485–493.

Bennett, S. M., Litz, B. T., Sarnoff Lee, B., & Maguen, S. (2005). The scope and impact of perinatal loss: Current status and future directions. *Professional Psychology: Research and Practice, 36*(2), 180–187.

Caserta, M. S., & Lund, D. A. (2007). Toward the development of an inventory of daily widowed life: Guided by the Dual Process Model of coping with bereavement. *Death Studies, 31*, 505–535.

Christ, G. H., Siegel, K., & Christ, A. E. (2002). Adolescent grief: "It never really hit me . . . until it actually happened." *Journal of the American Medical Association, 288*, 1269–1279.

Coates, S., & Gaensbauer, T. J. (2009). Event trauma in early childhood: Symptoms, assessment, intervention. *Child and Adolescent Psychiatry Clinics of North America, 18*(3), 611–626.

Coifman, K. G., & Bonanno, G. A. (2010). When distress does not become depression: Emotion context sensitivity and adjustment to bereavement. *Journal of Abnormal Psychology, 119*(3), 476–490.

Cote-Arsenault, D., & Donato, K. (2011). Emotional cushioning in pregnancy after perinatal loss. *Journal of Reproductive & Infant Psychology, 29*(1), 81–92.

Currier, J. M., Holland, J. M., & Neimeyer, R. A. (2007). The effectiveness of bereavement interventions with children: A meta-analytic review of controlled outcome research. *Journal of Clinical Child and Adolescent Psychology, 36*, 253–259.

Dare, J. S. (2011). Transitions in midlife women's lives: Contemporary experiences. *Health Care for Women International, 32*, 111–133.

Doka, K. J. (1989). *Disenfranchised grief: Recognizing hidden sorrow*. New York, NY: Lexington Books.

Doka, K. J. (Ed.). (2002). *Disenfranchised grief: New directions, challenges and strategies for practice*. Champaign, IL: Research Press.

Erikson, E. H. (1980). *Identity and the life cycle*. New York, NY: W.W. Norton. (Original work published 1959)

Fleisher, B., & Reese, T. (2013). *The new senior woman*. Lanham, MD: Rowman and Littlefield.

Freidenfelds, L. (2013). Pro-Choice, Pro-Life, and the History of Miscarriage. Symposium on "Maternal Bodies, Fetal Bodies." October 2013, Rutgers University, New Brunswick, NJ.

Furstenberg, F. F., Kennedy, S., McLoyd, V. C., Rumbaut, R. G., & Settersen, R. A. (2004). Growing up is harder to do. *American Sociological Association, 3*(3), 33–41.

Hansson, R. O., & Stroebe, M. S. (2007). Coping with bereavement. *Generations, 31*(3), 63–65.

Hochschild, A. R. (1979). Emotion work, feeling rules, and social structure. *American Journal of Sociology, 85*(3), 551–575.

Holland, J. M., Thompson, K. L., Rozalski, V., & Lichtenthal, W. G. (2013). Bereavement-related regret targets among widowed older adults. *Journal of Gerontological Behavioral Science and Social Science, 10*, 1093–1120.

Ibarra, H. (2003). *Working identity*. Boston, MA: Harvard Business School Press.

John, D., & Lang, F. R. (2012). Adapting to unavoidable loss during adulthood. *Gerontological Psychology, 25*(2), 73–82.

Kim, S., Kjervik, D., Belyea, M., & Choi, E. (2011). Personal strength and finding meaning in conjugally bereaved older adults: A four-year prospective analysis. *Death Studies, 35*, 197–218.

Klass, D., Silverman, P. R., & Nickman, S. L. (1996). *Continuing bonds: New understandings of grief*. Washington, DC: Taylor and Francis.

Kübler-Ross, E. (1969). *On death and dying: What the dying have to their doctors, nurses, clergy and their own families*. New York, NY: Macmillan.

Lieberman, S. (2011). *Getting old is a full time job: Moving on from a full time job*. Houston, TX: Susan Lieberman.

Life Planning Network. (2013). *Live smart after 50: The expert's guide to life planning for uncertain times*. Boston, MA: Author.

Markese, S. (2011). Dyadic trauma in infancy and early childhood: A review of the literature. *Journal of Infant, Child, and Adolescent Psychotherapy, 10*(2–3), 341–378.

Marks, N. F., Jun, H., & Song, J. (2007). Death of parents and adult psychological and physical well-being: A prospective U.S. National Study. *Journal of Family Issues, 28*(12), 1611–1638.

Marshall, H. (2004). Midlife loss of parents: The transition from adult child to orphan. *Ageing International, 29*(4), 351–367.

McClatchey, I., Vonk, M., Lee, J., & Bride, B. (2014). Traumatic and complicated grief among children: One or two constructs? *Death Studies, 38*(2), 69–79.

Naef, R., Ward, R., Mahrer-Imhof, R., & Grande, G. (2013). Characteristics of the bereavement experience of older persons after spousal loss: An integrative review. *International Journal of Nursing Studies, 50*, 1108–1121.

Neimeyer, R. A. (2001). *Meaning construction and the meaning of loss.* Washington, DC: American Psychological Association.

Neimeyer, R. A., Baldwin, S. A., & Gillies, J. (2006). Continuing bonds and reconstructing meaning: Mitigating complications in bereavement. *Death Studies, 30*, 715–738.

Oltjenbruns, K. A. (1996). Death of a friend during adolescence: Issues and impact. In C. A. Corr & D. E. Balk (Eds.), *Handbook of adolescent death and bereavement* (pp. 196–215). New York, NY: Springer Publishing Company.

Oktay, J. S., & Walter, C. A. (1991). *Breast cancer in the life course: Women's experiences.* New York, NY: Springer Publishing Company.

Paley, B., Lester, P., & Mogil, C. (2013). Family systems and ecological perspectives on the impact of deployment on military families. *Clinical Child & Family Psychology Review, 16*(3), 245–265.

Rappaport, H., Fossler, R. J., Bross, L. S. and Gilden, D. (1993). Future time, death anxiety, and life purpose among older adults. *Death Studies, 17*, 369–379.

Rask, K., Kaunonen, M., & Paunon-Ilomonen, M. (2002). Adolescent coping with grief after the death of a loved one. *International Journal of Nursing Practice, 8*, 137–142.

Schlossberg, N. (2013). *Revitalizing retirement: Reshaping your identity, relationships and purpose.* Washington, DC: American Psychological Association.

Siegel, D. J. (2014). *Brainstorm: The power and purpose of the teenage brain.* Los Angeles, CA: Tarcher.

Simos, B. G. (1979). *A time to grieve: Loss as a universal experience.* New York, NY: Family Service Association of America.

Speece, J. W., & Brent, S. B. (1984). Children's understanding of death: A review of three components of death concept. *Child Development, 55*, 1671–1686.

Stein, C. H., Abraham, K. M., Bonar, E. E., McAuliffe, C. E., Fogo, W. R., Faigin, D. A., . . . Potokar, D. (2009). Meaning making from personal loss: Religious, benefit finding and goal-oriented attributions. *Journal of Loss and Trauma, 14*, 83–100.

Stroebe, M., & Schut, H. (1999). The dual process model of coping with bereavement: Rationale and description. *Death Studies, 23*, 197–224.

Umberson, D. (2003). *Transition to a new adult identity.* New York, NY: Cambridge University Press.

Walter, C. A. (2003). *The loss of a life partner: Narratives of the bereaved.* New York, NY: Colombia University Press.

Walter, C. A., & McCoyd, J. L. M. (2009). *Grief and loss across the lifespan: A biopsychosocial perspective.* New York, NY: Springer Publishing Company.

Wilkinson, P. O., Croudace, T. J., & Goodyer, I. M. (2013). Rumination, anxiety, depressive symptoms and subsequent depression in adolescents at risk for psychopathology: A longitudinal cohort study. *BMC Psychiatry, 13*, 250–267.

Part II: Institutional Developments

David Clark   **10**

HOSPICE CARE OF THE DYING

ATTRACTIONS OF HOSPICE

Cicely Saunders once said to me, "Hospice is like fly paper. Once you're stuck on it, you can't get off." She was right. I began researching actively into hospice developments in 1989, and a quarter century later find myself still more and more engaged in these and related issues, seeking to make sense of the patterns of growth, the paths taken and not taken, the strengths, the weaknesses, the challenges that remain. I am not alone. Hospice ideals and hospice organizations have proved attractive to multiple constituencies. They appeal to the activist, to the practitioner, to the scholar and researcher, as well as to the philanthropist, the politician, the person of faith, the communitarian, the citizen, the volunteer, and ultimately to the beneficiaries of the care that hospices provide—dying people and those close to them. Perhaps most notable about this attraction is the sense in which hospice creates spaces for thinking and acting differently when it comes to caring for people at the end of life. Hospice is both a service and a set of ideals; a way of doing and a way of thinking.

When the modern hospice movement got underway in the 1960s, it drew on older associations of care and solicitude and kindled a desire to connect with deeper traditions of hospitality, of pilgrimage, and of shelter along a journey. At the same time it appealed to those concerned about the increasingly problematic relationship between medicine and death, whether that emanated from medicine's neglect of the dying or from its overinvolvement in the face of life's ending. Some of its appeal was in the grammar: Are we dealing here with a noun or an adjective? The question was put in a paper by some notable early activists in the United States (Butterfield-Picard & Magno, 1982). Using the noun refers to the formal organizational structures in which hospice care is delivered—the setting or building, the mode of delivery. Using the adjective describes the conceptual framework of care—the premise that when the quantity of life is limited, the quality of life must be optimal. I am drawn to this distinction—but also the connections between the two approaches. For all care has some element of place in which it occurs, and hospices have done remarkable things to create "healing spaces" even for those who are close to death (Worpole, 2009). But of course places of care without the right philosophy are really empty vessels. Much of the modern history of hospices has been about balancing these tensions of noun and adjective—and we see this woven through pathways of hospice development in many contexts. For reasons of space here I have concentrated on American and British experiences, but the remarkable thing about hospices and hospice has been an ability to pour into many different cultural molds and settings, sometimes to improbable effect—and so I also allude briefly to some of this where I can.

FOUNDATIONAL STRANDS OF EARLY DEVELOPMENT

Idealism and Skepticism

Hospice care has deep historical roots, with associations going back at least to European medieval traditions of prehospital care. But in the 20th century it came to signify something quite specific—a reaching out to those in the terminal phase of illness, often in a manner influenced by religious or wider personal and social commitments and with a goal of engaging with the fundamentals of human mortality—making the departure from life dignified, meaningful, and free from suffering. This modern version of hospice care also had wider goals. Yes, it was about services and systems of care. But it also spoke to a specific social agenda—the recognition of death as a part of the fabric of life; the need for medicine and health care to reconnect with the care of dying and bereaved persons; and the notion that hospice could provide a new approach to care at the end of life, one that might find root and take hold elsewhere in the health care system, if perhaps slightly altered in the process.

Nevertheless, and despite the enthusiasm of its protagonists, there were detractors and doubters. Hospice could appear prescriptive, even preachy. It was perhaps too caught up in an idealism that would be difficult to apply beyond a limited number of services and initiatives run by committed activists. Viewed from the perspective of the public health system it could be seen as a limited approach, focused mainly on malignant and end-stage disease and therefore unlikely to be capable of meeting needs at the population level. To survive and thrive, hospice would need to speak the language of the modern medical establishment—and in the world of medical modernization that was gathering pace in the 1960s and 1970s that would include fluency in assessing outcomes, modeling interventions against best evidence, and some acumen in assessing the costs and benefits of particular approaches. Although "hospice" often captured public interest and attention, it played less well with medical culture, could be seen as overly attached to charitable or religious perspectives, or to social activism, and ran the risk of being dismissed or marginalized as the preserve of an enthusiastic but ultimately slightly anachronistic few. As one British detractor declaimed, it appeared "too good to be true and too small to be useful" (Douglas, 1992). In America, there was also the concern about "death groupies" attracted to hospice who were "full of good intentions and slightly crazy ideas" (Butterfield-Picard & Magno, 1982). Not all physicians were doubters, however, and the history of modern hospice includes many examples of medical doctors who have stepped off their professional tramlines to engage in a field in which alternative approaches might be possible and where working alliances could go beyond the obvious professional networks of the medical system. Interviews with a wide array of such individuals from many different countries have shown that their motivations and subsequent path were often shaped directly by a personal contact or meeting with Cicely Saunders herself (Wright & Clark, 2012).

Here is just one example: As interest in hospice care gathered momentum in Australia, David Allbrook, an English doctor working in Perth, invited Cicely Saunders to visit the city and give a lecture. Rosalie Shaw was an intern in 1977 and took a week off work to travel from Victoria to Perth to hear her speak. She found it an inspirational experience. Rosalie Shaw recalls:

> I sat in awe of Cicely Saunders as many people do, and she did so well. She just told stories to an audience that was normally very intellectual and

erudite, and I remember being fascinated. Then at the end of it—maybe I imagined this, but this is how I remember it—instead of the normal clapping there was a sort of hushed silence, as though everyone in the audience thought that something very special was happening here. (Rosalie Shaw, Hospice History Project interview, January 23, 2007)

"Hospice" and "Palliative" Care

Some of those influenced in this way by Cicely Saunders quickly sought to adapt her thinking to other contexts. For example, in the early 1970s the Canadian surgeon Balfour Mount had become impressed with the work of hospice, but sought a way to translate its ideas and practices into mainstream health care delivery. He coined the term "palliative care" to this end, and it not only became widely used in the coming decades, but over time it came to denote a related but different approach to that of hospice. Indeed, palliative care, once defined, soon developed an uneasy relationship to hospice. The new field had a formalized "model" of care; it sought to transcend diagnostic groups and to engage earlier in the trajectory of illness. It seemed to have the potential for wider impact at the system level and became associated with attempts at "mainstreaming" beyond specialist services. Palliative care in this guise espoused holistic and multidisciplinary principles. Over time, it came to adopt the perspectives of public health as a driver for its development, but often it ran into difficulties in implementing them "at scale."

In particular, from the late 1980s, palliative medicine emerged as a recognized specialty in some countries and highlighted the need for a close relationship to the profession of medicine and the importance of a scientific basis for interventions, particularly those focused on pain and symptom management. The specialist field was, if anything, more ambivalent to hospice. Although some physicians who trained in this new area of medicine did go on to work in hospice services, many preferred to seek wider impact by operating within acute hospital settings, and some sought entry to the work of academic medicine and the teaching programs of medical schools and colleges. By such means, a cultural divide opened up between the two areas, and the interactions, tensions, and differences between the two continue to occupy much debate and reflection.

Yet the two approaches—of "hospice" and "palliative" care—have now been adopted and adapted in various ways around the world, and in some countries they exist in quite explicit juxtaposition. Although the former enjoys fairly high public recognition in some societies, the latter remains poorly understood beyond those who practice it. In a sense, one remains a social movement, whereas the other is a health care specialty. The overlap between them can be complementary but can also create a certain tension. If hospice is death embracing, palliative care emphasizes quality of life; whereas hospice frequently draws on a social model, for palliative care the model is increasingly medical; if hospice promotes community engagement, palliative care supports professional development. These have become salient distinctions over time, but they tend to get glossed over and are sometimes difficult to discuss in public. Interestingly, when specialty recognition was obtained in the United States in 2006, the name adopted was Hospice and Palliative Medicine, but the membership does appear to comprise two rather distinct groups with differing goals and orientations, the former toward community-based and home care services (Gazelle, 2007) and the latter toward an acute, early intervention hospital-based model (Ravi et al., 2013).

Cicely Saunders and St Christopher's Hospice

We can trace these linked but separate dimensions right back to the approach being developed by Cicely Saunders in London from the late 1950s and that led to the opening of the world's first modern hospice—St Christopher's—in 1967. Saunders trained in social work, nursing, and then medicine at a major London teaching hospital. She was influenced by that which had preceded her in the late 19th and early decades of the 20th century. So she studied and learned from the hospices and homes for the dying that had appeared in small numbers across Europe and the United States during that period. These institutions had three sets of concerns: religious, philanthropic, and moral. They placed a strong emphasis on the cure of the soul, even when the life of the body was diminishing. They drew on charitable endeavors, and were often concerned to give succor to the poor and disadvantaged. They were not, however, places in which the medical or nursing care of the dying was of any real sophistication (Humphreys, 2001). They were nonetheless critical in influencing the thinking of Cicely Saunders, as she developed her ideas in the 1950s.

St Christopher's Hospice can rightly be called the first "modern" hospice. It sought to combine three key principles: excellent clinical care, education, and research. It therefore differed significantly from the other homes for the dying that had preceded it and aspired to establish itself as a center of excellence in a new field of care. Its success was phenomenal, and it soon became the stimulus for an expansive phase of hospice and palliative care development, not only in Britain, but also around the world. Under Saunder's leadership and subsequently, St Christopher's seemed to be extremely successful in bridging the paradigms of hospice and palliative care.

Sharing a passion for innovation and inspiration, Cicely Saunders was particularly attracted to America in her search for new ideas about the care of the dying (Clark, 2001). During the 1950s, she had read Alfred Worcester's *The Care of the Aged, the Dying and the Dead* (Worcester, 1935). Worcester's purpose was to educate the next generation of practitioners, based on his long experience and in the absence of effective formal training for doctors in care of the dying. He set out a detailed manual for medical care at the end of life, beginning by outlining the signs and symptoms of dying, moving on to specific areas, such as mouth care, posture, alleviation of restlessness, the need for fresh air, the avoidance of "whispering," and so on. Worcester was both pragmatic and principled about telling patients and family members the truth about their prognosis, and equally emphatic about the proper use of morphine: "large and frequent doses may be needed. There is no limit to the amount that may properly be given" (Worcester, 1935, p. 45). Inspired by this work, Saunders had also followed up other leads in the American literature: a study in Boston of terminal cancer care among 200 patients (Abrams, Jameson, Poehlman, & Snyder, 1945) and a paper on social casework with cancer patients (Abrams, 1951). By casting her net in this way to include North America, she was able to introduce herself and a British audience to a wider range of potential influences. She made three crucial visits to the United States in 1963, 1965, and 1966.

On reaching the United States for the first of these, Saunders discovered that a cornucopia of links and connections opened up for her. In New York at the House of Calvary (which traced back a direct line to Jeanne Garnier's *Les Dames du Calvaire*, founded in France in 1842), at Rosary Hill Home, St. Rose's Home, and at St. Vincent's Hospital she found echoes of the Catholic ambience of St. Joseph's Hospice, in which she had learned her craft in London. In contrast to the traditionalism of these places, she also came face to face with the modernist regime of the American medical system: the emphasis on aggressive, curative approaches; the denial of death; and the ambivalence about truth telling. But there were also doctors and nurses disillusioned by this approach with whom she found a common and shared concern and with whom she established contact. Perhaps more than anything, however, it was the opportunities that America afforded for access to a range of disciplines and perspectives that was so important. Here she could meet chaplains, such as Carleton Sweetser, struggling with the care of the dying in a modern hospital setting, and also social workers like Theodate Soule, at the United Hospital Fund of New York. In addition, there were some psychologists, sociologists, and anthropologists who, unlike most of their contemporaries in Britain, were also contributing to developments in this area. There was also a new cadre of pain specialists, such as Stanley Wallenstein and Ray Houde, at Memorial Hospital, New York, and Henry Beecher at Massachusetts General Hospital, from whom she received encouragement and inspiration in her own studies. It was indeed a rich mixture of influences and skills, and one that was later to become such an important aspect of the modern multidisciplinary specialty of hospice and palliative care.

Reaction to American Health Care and Cancer Treatment

But there were significant contextual challenges within American health care at this time as well as within the emergent cultural orientation to dying and death—and not least in the public disposition toward cancer. After World War II, there had been unprecedented optimism about what medicine could achieve. By the early 1950s, there was hope of "a penicillin for cancer." There even began to be more openness about the disease, which might no longer be the death sentence of the past. New chemotherapeutic agents were thought to have the potential to eradicate even metastatic disease. The sick role theory of illness behavior, promulgated by Talcott Parsons from the early 1950s, was entirely predicated on the power of medicine to restore health in short order to the suitably compliant patient—even with cancer. The mood was one of hubris.

Meanwhile, death, when it occurred, was increasingly likely to take place in hospital. Hospital care expanded from the late 1940s, and by 1960, 50% of all American deaths were taking place there. Emily Abel, in her book on the history of care for the dying in 19th and 20th century America (Abel, 2013), maintains that many of these patients were subjected to invasive medical and surgical treatments of an experimental nature, which they readily endured in the belief that death could be kept at bay and avoided, almost indefinitely. It was social scientists and researchers, rather than clinicians, who first articulated a concern about the direction of travel and the growing denial of death within medical culture and practice. Herman Feifel's (1959) edited volume, *The Meaning of Death*, broke new ground. The work of Glaser and Strauss (1965), Quint (1966), and Sudnow (1967)—all based on field studies in American hospitals in the early to mid-1960s—generated a new critique of the culture of dying. At the same time, social workers and health services researchers began to uncover details of the inadequacies of care for the terminally ill—particularly those with cancer. Late diagnosis or disclosure was a common occurrence. Reports from Chicago and Boston showed the disastrous consequences of sending home poor and disadvantaged terminally ill patients without adequate support. But the alternatives seemed no better. As Abel puts it: "In most instances, enrolling relatives in terminal care facilities meant sending them away to die alone" (Abel, 2013, p. 135).

For Abel, this deeply ingrained marginalization of, and aversion to, the care of the dying within the American medical system explains why it is that the late 20th century entry of hospice and palliative care thinking and practice has proved so challenging and why progress has been slow and difficult. Hospice proliferated in the United States as a reaction against the wrong sort of involvement of medicine with the dying. Hospice reintroduced the idea of the family as the unit of care and placed a strong emphasis on care in the home. Hospice reacted against the excesses of hospital care at the end of life and offered a new model of holistic care that combined the physical and social needs of patients with their psychological concerns and spiritual preoccupations. But as we have been seeing, although many rallied to its support, it also met with resistance, with alternative models, and sometimes with outright hostility.

Yet there is a sense during these years that for Cicely Saunders, America was offering encouragement, even when her spirit flagged in the face of the enormity of getting St Christopher's started. A special relationship was forged between Cicely Saunders and her American friends and colleagues during the middle years of the 1960s. The relationship turned out to be part of an extraordinary groundswell of interest in the care of the dying and the bereaved, out of which new social movements and professional specialties were quickly to emerge, not only in Britain and the United States, but worldwide.

American Support for Hospice Through Medicare

In this America made very significant early progress. It was quick to establish legislative support and financial reimbursement for hospice, though it was much slower to move forward the formal recognition of palliative medicine as a specialty, which was not to come for another almost quarter century. Within a few years of the first state-certified hospice commencing operations in 1974, Senator Edward Kennedy was giving massive support to a phenomenon that he saw as having wide-ranging importance: "Hospice is many things. Hospice is home care with inpatient back-up facilities . . . pain control . . . skilled nursing . . . a doctor and a clergyman coming to your home. . . . But most of all, hospice is the humanization of our health care system" (Buck, 2014, p. 13). This was in 1978; 4 years later, in 1982, hospice became an entitlement under the Medicare program. Part of the driver was that in the mid-1970s the Robert Wood Johnson Foundation joined forces with the newly formed Health Care Finance Administration and the John A. Hartford Foundation to fund a comprehensive study of the cost and efficacy of hospice care—the National Hospice Study. This large-scale project broke new ground and set out to evaluate the impact of hospice care on terminally ill patients and their families. It was a key element in establishing the value of hospice—and the case for reimbursement (Marx, Blendon, & Aiken, 1978).

Joy Buck explores in detail this early history of American hospice and its relationship to Medicare (Buck, 2007). The issue had found high-level political interest, of a kind rarely seen elsewhere in other countries. But even as Hospice Medicare came into being, Ronald Regan was sounding warning bells about the wider system that he viewed as wasteful, fraudulent, and uncontrollable. Buck notes that translating the hospice ideal into a reimbursable model of care, without changing its nature was a major—and is still to some extent an unresolved—challenge. Over time, it drew criticism from the emergent medical subspecialty of palliative care, which lacked a reimbursement stream to support it. American hospice seems throughout its brief history to have been embroiled in funding, legal, and policy issues. In 1978, a small group of hospice entrepreneurs and activists formed the National Hospice Organization and the National Hospice Education Project. Their mission, according to Buck, was to both create and corner the market for hospice at the national level, and in this context standardization of hospice was a critical element in achieving success. Three basic models of hospice organization now prevailed. First, hospital-based hospice programs; second, home hospice programs affiliated with urban/suburban Visiting Nurses Associations; third, independent hospices, which evolved from community-based volunteer efforts to reform care of the dying.

The Global Spread and Adaptation of the Hospice Ideal

Modern hospice developments occurred first in affluent countries, but in time they also took hold in poorer settings, often supported by mentoring and partnership arrangements with more established hospices in the West. In the United Kingdom there was an initial emphasis on voluntary inpatient hospices, many of which had Christian origins. Echoes of this model can also been seen elsewhere, but almost always nuanced to the local context and conditions. For example, in Germany the influences of religion and civil society were strong, and the early hospice services were more likely to be community based with limited medical involvement. In India, some hospices were opened but seemed ill suited to local conditions, where huge population need required a different, more public health-oriented approach—such as that subsequently developed by the Neighbourhood Networks in Palliative Care, in Kerala. In Romania, the first hospice had many of the attributes of its British equivalents, but was adapted to a culture in which voluntary engagement was relatively unfamiliar and where religious traditions had been suppressed under a communist dictatorship. Hospice Africa Uganda developed as a model organization for sub-Saharan Africa. Starting in 1993 with the aim of supporting affordable, suitable, and accessible palliative care, it went on to influence national health policy, to gain access to sustainable supplies of cheap oral morphine, and to develop training and outreach programs both in-country and further afield.

In many settings, hospice developments were closely allied to civil society, to notions of service, social reform, and even political change. In Eastern Europe, hospices quickly emerged after the collapse of communist systems and as part of a new enthusiasm for social action and public engagement; indeed, in Poland, hospice activists were among those who were instrumental in bringing about the collapse of the old regime through the Solidarity movement. UK developments built on a tradition of local involvement in delivering services with voluntary input. This was not always a model that translated easily to other contexts. France and Spain, for example, are good examples in which the focus of *palliative care* development was in the public health system rather than the field of social activism. Indeed, in these countries the word "hospice" itself had problematic associations—with poverty, disadvantage, and even those in need of institutional containment.

Becoming Institutionalized, but at a Price?

By the early 1990s, however, new services were appearing in many countries, and in some, such as the United Kingdom and the United States, hospices were becoming an established part of a mixed economy of care. Significantly, the idea of hospice—with its emphasis on holistic approaches that included physical, spiritual, psychological, and social care—and with its attention to the needs of patient and family, was attracting growing interest, well beyond a core circle of activists and enthusiasts. Teaching programs emerged in colleges and universities, tentative steps were taken toward establishing research-based evidence in support of further development, specialist journals as well as journalistic and more popular writings found a growing readership, and policy makers started to factor in "hospice" to their thinking and planning.

But these gains and successes also brought their problems. As early as 1986, Emily Abel sounded a warning bell. In her important paper on institutionalizing innovation in the hospice movement (Abel, 1986), she argued that the early leaders of the hospice movement shared a number of attitudes with the founders of the alternative institutions of the 1960s and early 1970s: nostalgia for simple, old-fashioned ways, dissatisfaction with bureaucratic and authoritarian institutions, faith in the power of nature, a determination to avoid domination by experts, and a desire to improve the quality of personal relationships. However, as hospices became better established, they were gradually incorporated into the dominant health care system and lost their uniqueness. Some affiliated with hospitals or home health agencies. Even autonomous organizations became subject to pressures for accommodation because of a reliance on the established order—for resources, personnel, and political acceptance. Organizations receiving payment under the new Medicare benefit had to adhere to a set of regulations that might distort the movement and were at risk from a government that saw them primarily as a vehicle to save money. Paradoxically, Abel argued, as hospices grew in popularity, the critical force of the movement was being blunted.

The theme was taken up a few years later when two British sociologists, Nicky James and David Field, adopted the perspective of Max Weber to trace a narrative of "routinization" and "bureaucratization" within the hospice movement (James & Field, 1992). These authors suggest that a process of diversification and legitimation meant that hospices in the United Kingdom became increasingly subject to mainstream influence. Using Weber's concept of charisma, they suggest there are a number of factors leading to the routinization of hospice care, including the ways in which it was sponsored and developed at the local level, and pressures toward bureaucratization and professionalization. They conclude by asking whether it is possible for the hospice movement to sustain its founding ideals as these processes advance. These papers remain relevant and stimulating. Do they betray a somewhat romantic nostalgia on the part of historians and sociologists remote from the daily realities of delivering hospice services? Or should we take from them a bold willingness to grasp the nettle of an issue likely to prove problematic for both "hospice" and "hospices" if ignored?

HOSPICE CARE TODAY: EVALUATION AND CONTROVERSY

Systematic Evaluations

In 2004, Joan Teno and others established good evidence of the quality of hospice care in the United States (Teno et al., 2004). This was the first attempt in the country to examine the adequacy or quality of end-of-life care in institutional settings compared with deaths at home. It used Teno's favored "mortality follow-back" method to survey family members or other knowledgeable informants representing 1,578 people who had died in the year 2000. Informants were asked over the telephone about the patient's experience at the last place of care at which the patient spent more than 48 hours. Family members of patients receiving hospice services were more satisfied with overall quality of care—70.7% rated care as "excellent," compared with fewer than 50% of those dying in an institutional setting or with home health services. The study concluded that many people dying in institutions have unmet needs for symptom amelioration, physician communication, emotional support, and being treated with respect; and that family members of those who received care at home with hospice services were more likely to report a favorable dying experience.

This was complemented in 2007 by a publication that for the first time provided solid evidence of the cost-reduction benefits of hospice care. The authors point out that since their inclusion in Medicare, hospices have been expected to reduce health care costs, but the literature on their ability to do so has been mixed. The 2007 study focused on the length of hospice use that maximizes reductions in medical expenditures near death. The authors used a retrospective case-control study of Medicare decedents (1993–2003) to compare 1,819 hospice decedents with 3,638 controls, matched through their predicted likelihood of dying while using a hospice. The study showed that hospice use reduced Medicare program expenditures during the last year of life by an average of $2,309 per hospice user: $7,318 in expenditures for hospice users compared with $9,627 for controls. On average, hospice use reduced these Medicare costs during all but two of the hospice users' last 72 days of life; about $10 on the 72nd day prior to death; and with savings increasing to more than $750 on the day of death. Maximum cumulative expenditure reductions differed by primary condition. The maximum reduction in Medicare expenditures for each user was about $7,000, which occurred when a decedent had a primary condition of cancer and used a hospice for their last 58 to 103 days of life. For other primary conditions, the maximum savings of around $3,500 occurred when hospice was used for the last 50 to 108 days of life. Given the relatively short length of hospice use observed in the Medicare program, the authors argued that increasing the length of hospice use for 7 in 10 Medicare hospice users would increase savings to the program (Taylor, Ostermann, Van Houtven, Tulsky, & Steinhauser, 2007).

Financial Challenges in American Hospice Care

A global report on the quality of death in 40 countries published in 2010 placed the United States in ninth position in terms of the quality of its end-of-life care provision (Economist Intelligence Unit, 2010). The report highlighted the high overall cost of health care in the United States, where expenditure had risen sharply in recent years, now accounting for one dollar in every six spent. In particular, it pointed to the financial burden to patients at the end of life, driven up by the low availability of public funding and social security spending on health care.

Financial considerations remain central to thinking about the provision of hospice and palliative care in the United States. Medicare reimburses hospice providers at a flat daily rate, based on four levels of home and inpatient care, assuming patients have a terminal illness and an estimated 6 months or fewer to live. The Medicare Payment Advisory Commission (MedPAC) recommended amendments to the system, starting in 2013, to give relatively lower payments the longer the treatment lasts. In a 2009 report to Congress, the agency suggested that the present system provides incentives for hospice providers to admit long-stay patients and claimed this may have led to inappropriate use of the benefit among some hospices (MedPac, 2009).

Seen this way, the question arises as to whether Medicare's per diem payment structure may create financial incentives to select patients who require less resource-intensive care and have longer hospice stays. For-profit and nonprofit hospices may respond differently to such financial incentives. A study published in 2011 in the *Journal of the American Medical Association* set out to compare patient diagnosis and location of care between for-profit and nonprofit hospices and to examine whether the number of visits per day and the length of stay vary by diagnosis and profit status (Wachterman, Marcantonio, Davis, & McCarthy, 2011). The results proved to be of major import and showed that for-profit hospices had a lower proportion of patients with cancer and a higher proportion of patients with dementia and other noncancer diagnoses. After adjustment for demographic, clinical, and agency characteristics, there was no significant difference in location of care by profit status. However, for-profit hospices compared with nonprofit hospices had a significantly longer length of stay and were more likely to have patients with stays longer than 365 days, and less likely to have patients with stays of fewer than 7 days. Compared with cancer patients, those with dementia or other diagnoses had fewer visits per day from nurses and social workers. The study concluded that compared with nonprofit hospice agencies, for-profit hospice agencies had a higher percentage of patients with diagnoses associated with lower skilled needs and longer lengths of stay. Commenting on these results, Charles von Gunten captured the thoughts of many working in the field, noting that: "The for-profit agencies whose shares are traded publicly on the stock exchanges and report large profits do, in fact, "cherry pick" less expensive patients who live longer" (Von Gunten, 2011).

Since those remarks, the position has become murkier. The hospice in which von Gunten was working at the time of this comment was closed on bankruptcy grounds 2 years later. The case of the San Diego Hospice closure has yet to be subject to detailed academic analysis, though it has fostered much commentary through social media and the Internet. Key to the discussion has been how Medicare regulations requiring that those entering hospice programs have a prognosis of 6 months or less appear to be interfering with clinical judgments of need and are creating barriers to allowing the sickest of patients from accessing the most appropriate care in the most suitable setting. As Suzana Makowski has observed:

> While the intention of these regulations is to avoid abuse and thus avoid cost, it actually is adding to the cost of care, by preventing patients from having the needed supports at home and often giving them little choice but to go to hospital. Hospice care should not have such rigid entry requirements. Entry should not be based on criteria that are not evidence based and that have not evolved with the science over the last 30+ years. (Makowski, 2013)

San Diego Hospice was established in 1977 and had grown into one of the largest academic hospice programs in the United States, caring for over 1,000 patients per day and engaged in a wide range of fellowship and training programs, including international activities focused on the development of leadership skills for palliative care workers across the world. It was subject to extended audit by Medicare during the 2 years leading up to closure in 2013 on the grounds that it was caring for patients who were not eligible for specialized care or, if they were, may not have had their prognoses properly documented. Setting alight underlying concerns across the sector, the closure at San Diego rocked the U.S. hospice community.

It was followed by much wider debate about the implications of Medicare hospice funding for meeting the needs of frail and vulnerable patients who might not be likely to die in 6 months—and in particular of the role of for-profit hospices within this. Newspaper headlines made claims such as "Hospice firms draining billions from Medicare" and asserted that Medicare rules had created a boom-ing business in hospice care for people who are not dying. There were assertions that the "nondeath discharge" figures for hospice were increasing dramatically and that the hospice industry was resistant to change in a system that served its interests rather well. The *Washington Post* stated, "This vast growth took place as the hospice 'movement,' once led by religious and community organizations, was evolving into a $17 billion industry dominated by for-profit companies. Much of that is paid for by the U.S. government—roughly $15 billion of industry revenue came from Medicare last year" (Whoriskey & Keating, 2013).

Robust rebuttals soon appeared from elsewhere in the press and from within the hospice and palliative care community. Howard Gleckman, writing in *Forbes*, observed "the *Post* article misses a bigger question: Why are growing numbers of people willing to enroll in hospice—and often forego traditional medical treatment—long before they are dying?" (Gleckman, 2014). The article noted that for the vast majority of hospice patients, care is provided where they live (at home or in a nurs-ing facility) rather than in a hospital. Skilled nurses, social workers, chaplains, and volunteers—attuned to the needs of their frail, mostly elderly patients—provide the kind of holistic care that is increasingly valued by older people. The paradox for the health care system is that the patient must be dying in order to get it. Nev-ertheless, it is clear there are perverse incentives. Medicare pays hospice a fixed daily rate (a capitated payment). Although this remains fairly constant, costs of care for any one patient can be quite variable—high on admission and in the final days of life, but lower in the intervening period. The opportunities for financial gain are clear to see.

But if some patients are enrolled for too long on hospice, others (about a third) receive its services for less than 1 week—arguably far too short a period for patients and families to derive optimal benefit. Gleckman therefore concluded: "So let's fix the payment system. But more importantly, let's step back and think about what hospice does and how to replicate it elsewhere in the health system" (Gleckman, 2014). Bruce Scott, a hospice-trained physician, elaborated on these points and concluded:

> Despite having grossly exaggerated the cost to Medicare, falsely suggested that discharged patients weren't actually dying, and deceptively used statis-tics to advance their narrative, the [*Washington Post*] authors did raise some important points as well. They described some fairly unpleasant recruitment tactics. I consider some of these tactics to be unethical. I would not want to be involved with a hospice that used them. . . . They are not, however, against the current rules, nor are they illegal. And they are the same sorts of things that happen at businesses around the country. I want hospices to be better than businesses around the country. My gut feeling is that hospices ARE in general better than businesses around the country. . . . But we can't expect all hospice firms to be better than other corporations just because it's the nice thing to do. (Scott, 2014)

This is doubtless an issue that will continue to run. It demonstrates how con-sequential the achievement of a Medicare hospice benefit has been, and how a set of unanticipated and unintended consequences has resulted since the scheme was introduced in 1982. The United States seems to be significantly alone, however, when compared internationally, in generating a hospice "industry" with such a substantial for-profit component.

Reframing From Hospice and End-of-Life Care to Palliative Care?

A second quite specific issue has also come to dominate debate about hospice in the United States—and it is a view that has had a certain hearing elsewhere also. This concerns the so-called "reframing" from hospice and end-of-life care to *palliative* care. It is promulgated by focusing on the concern of patients and families that physicians will abandon them if hospice care is recommended. Thus it is observed:

> The notion of a "good death," which hospice effectively enables for many people, has greatest salience *after* a loved one has died. From this perspective, it is argued, most people and families facing a serious illness do not want a "good death"; they want a cure. The special feature of the frame of palliative care, therefore, is to allow patients, families and physicians to accept care and amelioration of pain while they pursue active treatment. (Patrizi & Spector, 2011, p. 29)

Palliative care, seen in this way, is not something that commences when all else has failed, but is rather an integrated component of mainstream medical practice, to be pursued legitimately alongside other clinical goals. Such an approach has in turn led to a new definition of palliative care, which, strikingly, makes no reference to dying, death, or bereavement (Center to Advance Palliative Care, 2011).

This explicitly consumerist orientation to the delivery of palliative care is based on the assertion that the model of care must follow the demands and orientations of the patients and users. It argues that delivering palliative care has achieved better symptom control, improved communication and greater alignment with patient and family wishes as its primary goals, and that only once these are achieved is it appropriate to engage with questions of meaning, mortality, and the reality of death. This seems a departure from Cicely Saunder's model, which has been widely adopted by hospices and in which a central focus is on finding personal and/or religious closure at the end of life and where a wider social goal is also being pursued, in addition to the specific task of providing care to patients and families—that of making society better.

Inspired by charismatic leadership, hospice was a movement that condemned the neglect of the dying in society; called for high-quality pain and symptom management for all who needed it; sought to reconstruct death as a natural phenomenon, rather than a clinical failure; and marshaled practical and moral argument to oppose those in favor of euthanasia. Indeed, for Cicely Saunders and her followers, such work served as a measure of the very worth of our culture: "A society which shuns the dying must have an incomplete philosophy" (Saunders, 1962, p. 1046). These views are still much shared among hospice activists and protagonists who refuse to reduce "hospice" to a set of services shaped by "evidence" and delivered through specific reimbursement models.

Nevertheless, it is impossible for hospice to entirely resist these factors, and to seek to perpetuate hospice ideals while disregarding movements and trends within the wider health care system would be extremely unwise. This has been well recognized in the United Kingdom, which in 2013 saw the publication—after 2 years of inquiry—of the finding of a *Commission into the Future of Hospice Care*, published by the national charity Help the Hospices (Commission into the Future of Hospice Care, 2013). Designed to provide strategic direction for UK hospices, the report calls on hospices to adapt their practices to meet the rising demand for services, and to work more closely with other care services, commissioners, and providers in the sector.

The Commission imagines a future in which hospices work in partnership so that high-quality palliative and end-of-life care can be provided to all, across many different settings. It is committed to a future in which hospice care is dynamic, innovative, and responsive and is adapting constantly to meet the needs of people with life-shortening illness as well as their relatives and family carers. It identifies a future in which hospice care helps people cope with the reality of dying, death, and bereavement, and does this with confident expertise. It is a future in which hospice care is shaped by systematic knowledge of need and supported by robust evidence of effectiveness and one in which hospice care dovetails with the National Health Service, local authorities, and care homes; as well as being shaped by the communities that each hospice seeks to serve.

The report illustrates how the demand for palliative and end-of-life care will rise in the coming decades. It highlights the growing vulnerability and frailty of those who will need care, as well as the increasing complexity of their needs. This requires a responsibility to assess future needs for palliative and end-of-life care on a population basis, and to be active and outward looking in developing new partnerships and understandings that can enable these needs to be met. Hospices should seek to reach more people both through their care and their influence—for example, working as partners, campaigners, and educators across local health and care systems to achieve greater leverage. Hospices should also commit to innovate and evaluate new approaches that have the potential to extend the practice and ethos of their care. Hospices should make their care more accessible, around the clock and throughout the week, as well as doing more to reach out to those who have not traditionally used their services.

The Commission identifies five key steps that hospices might take to ensure they are fit for purpose, able to achieve maximum impact, and well placed to deliver the best outcomes for those with palliative and end-of-life care needs—now and in the future:

- Prepare for significant change in the context of palliative and end-of-life care
- Strengthen understanding of the contribution of hospice care
- Establish hospice care as a solution to future challenges in palliative and end-of-life care
- Strengthen the connection between hospices and their local health and social care systems and their local communities
- Strengthen the leadership of hospice care

Appearing at around the same time as the controversial coverage of hospice issues in the United States, this report from the United Kingdom reflects a shared but divergent history. Although American hospices have a clear and mandated source of reimbursement for their work, in the United Kingdom the hospice sector receives only about one third of its running costs from the National Health Service. The United Kingdom has seen no "for profit" hospice development and holds close to the value of local, independent charitable organizations that deliver hospice services in ways that are closely attuned to the needs and sentiments of their local communities. At the same time, these hospices are sometimes seen as isolationist, lacking engagement with the wider health and social care system, and to an extent as unattractive workplaces for specialist palliative care physicians. It is clear that on both sides of the Atlantic, hospice faces some significant challenges. Nevertheless, the strength of its mission and the importance of its service role point to a continuing relevance, albeit one that will need to be tempered by appropriate methods of organization and funding.

CHALLENGES AND HOPES FOR THE FUTURE
OF HOSPICE CARE FOR THE DYING

This chapter has sketched out the brief but rich history of modern "hospice" and "hospices," concentrating on developments in the United States and the United Kingdom, but highlighting the spread of influence and the adaptation of ideas in other cultures and jurisdictions. "Hospice" appears to be a far better recognized and understood "brand" than "palliative care," though, as we have seen, the two have developed together along parallel and sometimes divergent tracks. Whether separate or combined, it is clear that the need for the services provided by hospice and palliative care is set to grow. Around 58 million deaths occur in the world every year, and the number may rise to 90 to 100 million by midcentury and beyond. Population aging and changing patterns of mortality and morbidity mean that care for people in the final stages of life has become a pressing humanitarian issue with global dimensions.

This is leading to a strengthening field of hospice, palliative care, and end-of-life provision that is taking various forms across different resource contexts and cultures. It has raised significant questions for wider health services and policy, clinical practice, ethics, law and public perceptions, preferences and behaviors. Hospice has a key role to play in current debates about care at the end of life. To do so effectively, it must rise above some of its financial, cultural, and organizational limitations. Connor (2007–2008) described hospice care as a "small rebellion" when it first got underway. Clearly, it has become much more than that. The question now is whether it has the capacity and the confidence to deal with the challenges and the opportunities that lie ahead.

REFERENCES

Abel, E. K. (1986). The hospice movement: Institutionalising innovation. *International Journal of Health Services, 16*(1), 71–85.

Abel, E. K. (2013). *The inevitable hour: A history of caring for patients in America*. Baltimore, MD: The Johns Hopkins University Press.

Abrams, R., Jameson, G., Poehlman, M., & Snyder, S. (1945). Terminal care in cancer. *New England Journal of Medicine, 232*, 719–724.

Abrams, R. D. (1951, December). Social casework with cancer patients. *Social Casework,* pp. 425–431.

Buck, J. (2007). Netting the hospice butterfly: Politics, policy, and translation of an ideal. *Home Healthcare Nurse, 25*(9), 566–571.

Buck, J. (2014). Ideals, politics, and the evolution of the American hospice movement. In B. Jennings & T. W. Kirk (Eds.), *Hospice ethics.* pp. 113–14, New York, NY: Oxford University Press.

Butterfield-Picard, H., & Magno, J. B. (1982). Hospice the adjective, not the noun: The future of a national priority. *American Psychologist, 37*(11), 1254–1259.

Center to Advance Palliative Care. (2011). *Response to misleading WaPo hospice*. Retrieved from http://www.pallimed.org/2014/01/response-to-misleading-wapo-hospice_9.html

Clark, D. (2001). A special relationship: Cicely Saunders, the United States, and the early foundations of the modern hospice movement. *Illness, Crisis and Loss, 9*(1), 15–30.

Commission into the Future of Hospice Care. (2013). Retrieved from http://www.helpthehospices.org.uk/our-services/publications/http-wwwhelpthehospicesorguk-our-services-commission-/

Connor, S. (2007–2008). Hospice and palliative care in the United States. *Omega, 56*(1), 89–99.

Douglas, C. (1992). For all the saints. *British Medical Journal, 304*(6826), 479.

Economist Intelligence Unit. (2010).

The Quality of Death: Ranking End of Life Care across the World. (2010.) *A report from the Economist Intelligence Unit commissioned by the Lien Foundation* (p. 36). Retrieved from http://www.slideshare.net/economistintelligenceunit/the-quality-of-death-ranking-endoflife-care-across-the-world?related=1. Accessed September 5, 2014.

Feifel, H. (1959). *The meaning of death.* New York, NY: McGraw Hill.

Gazelle, G. (2007). Understanding hospice—An underutilized option for life's final chapter. *New England Journal of Medicine, 357,* 321–324.

Glaser, B., & Strauss, A. (1965). *Awareness of dying.* Chicago, IL: Aldine.

Gleckman, H. (2014). *The real story behind the latest hospice controversy.* Retrieved from http://www.forbes.com/sites/howardgleckman/2014/01/03/the-real-story-behind-the-latest-hospice-controversy/

Humphreys, C. (2001). "Waiting for the last summons": The establishment of the first hospices in England 1878–1914. *Mortality, 6*(2), 146–166.

James, N., & Field, D. (1992). The routinisation of hospice: Charisma and bureaucratisation, *Social Science and Medicine, 34*(12), 1363–1375.

Makowski, S. (2013). *Prognosis: Weeks to months—On the end of an era at San Diego hospice.* Retrieved from http://www.pallimed.org/2013/02/prognosis-weeks-to-months-on-end-of-era.html

Marx, M., Blendon, R., & Aiken, L. (1978). Study of the cost and efficacy of hospice care. In *Linda H. Aikens Papers* (Box 1, Folder 39, pp. 652–657). Philadelphia, PA: Center for the Study of the History of Nursing, University of Pennsylvania.

MedPac. (2009, March 17). *Report to the congress: Medicare payment policy.* Washington, DC: Author. Retrieved from http://www.medpac.gov/documents/Mar09_EntireReport.pdf

Patrizi, P., Thompson, E., & Spector, A. (2011). *Improving care at the end of life: How the Robert Wood Johnson Foundation and its grantees built the field.* Princeton, NJ: Robert Wood Johnson Foundation.

Quint, J. (1966). Obstacles to helping the dying. *American Journal of Nursing, 66*(7), 1463–1678.

Ravi, B., Parikh, R. B., Kirch, R. A., Thomas, J. D., Smith, J., & Temel, J. S. (2013). Early specialty palliative care—Translating data in oncology into practice. *New England Journal of Medicine, 369,* 2347–2351.

Saunders, C. (1962, August 17). And from sudden death . . . *Nursing Times,* pp. 1045–1046.

Scott, B. (2014). *Response to misleading WaPo hospice article: Part the third.* Retrieved from http://www.pallimed.org/2014/01/response-to-misleading-wapo-hospice_9.html

Sudnow, D. (1967). *Passing on: The social organisation of dying.* Englewood Cliffs, NJ: Prentice-Hall.

Taylor, D. H., Ostermann, J., Van Houtven C. H., Tulsky J. A., & Steinhauser, K. (2007). What length of hospice use maximizes reduction in medical expenditures near death in the US Medicare program? *Social Science and Medicine, 65*(7), 1466–1478.

Teno, J. M., Clarridge, B. R., Casey, V., Welch, L. C., Wetle, T., Shield, R., & Mor, V. (2004). Family perspectives on end-of-life care at the last place of care. *Journal of American Medical Association, 291*(1), 88–93.

Von Gunten, C. (2011). Did you ever? *Journal of Palliative Medicine, 14*(5), 534–535.

Wachterman, M. W., Marcantonio, E. R., Davis, R. B., & McCarthy, E. P. (2011). Association of hospice agency profit status with patient diagnosis, location of care, and length of stay. *Journal of the American Medical Association, 305*(5), 472–479.

Whoriskey, P., & Keating, D. (2014). *Hospice firms draining billions from Medicare.* Retrieved from http://www.washingtonpost.com/business/economy/medicare-rules-create-a-booming-business-in-hospice-care-for-people-who-arent-dying/2013/12/26/4ff75bbe-68c9-11e3-ae56-22de072140a2_story.html

Worcester, A. (1935). *The care of the aged, the dying and the dead.* Springfield, IL: Charles C Thomas.

Worpole, K. (2009). *Modern hospice design: The architecture of palliative care.* London, UK: Routledge.

Wright, M., & Clark, D. (2012). Cicely Saunders and the development of hospice palliative care. In H. Coward & K. I. Stajduhar (Eds.), *Religious understandings of a good death in hospice palliative care* (pp. 11–28). Albany, NY: State University of New York Press.Economist Intelligence Unit. (2011). *Quality of Death,* 13.

Bernard J. Lapointe and Dawn Allen

11

HOSPITAL-BASED PALLIATIVE CARE

While the home is generally reported to be the preferred setting to receive end-of-life care, and despite it being the wish of a majority of patients to die at home, hospitals are the place where most people die. As shown by a recent comparison of institutional deaths across 45 countries, "for half of countries more than 54% of deaths occur in the hospital" (Robinson, Gott, & Ingleton, 2014, p. 18). Furthermore, despite a global trend toward more patients dying at home, the trend in the so-called developed world is expected to move in the opposite direction. Owing to changing demographics, advances in health technology, and improvements in health care, people in resource-rich countries are living longer and dying more often from one or more complex chronic illnesses. As a result of this more complex and less predictable health profile, combined with social realities such as social isolation of the elderly, we will see a significant increase over the next two decades in the number of people dying in hospital rather than at home. In fact, predictions in the United Kingdom estimate that only 1 in 10 people will die at home by 2030, which will require a significant injection of resources into an already stretched health care system (Al-Qurainy, Collis, & Feuer, 2009).

In addition to the demographic factors and the impact of medical advances, diagnoses of critical or terminal illness are most often made during an acute-care episode in a hospital. This reality explains why at any one time 13% to 36% of all hospital patients meet the criteria for palliative care, though not all will receive it (Gott, Sam, Ahmedzai, & Wood, 2001). However, only a minority of eligible patients access palliative care. This, in addition to the large number of people in need of episodic care for serious chronic terminal illness, highlights the critical need for palliative care and the role it should play in the acute-care hospital context.

However, since the early 19th century, hospitals have generally been viewed as being neglectful of the needs of dying patients—focusing instead on a curative model of care.

> Hospital use by patients with chronic, incurable, or terminal conditions was discouraged; individuals seeking shelter or comfort during their last hours were refused admission. Physicians not only perceived care of the dying as being outside the scope of medical work, they viewed death as a threat to their professional advancement. (Siebolt, 1992, p. 19)

Since the 19th century, rapid progression of modern scientific medicine—brought about by the development of antimicrobial strategies, the advancement of surgery, and the development of technologies such as the x-ray—has significantly contributed to a focus in medical culture on analyzing illness from the perspective of the

Pastorian paradigm (disease, diagnosis, treatment). This culture too often led to patients dying in the hospital, abandoned by professionals, and left to struggle physically, psychologically, and spiritually during the last days of their lives.

Despite today's perception that the hospital setting is inadequate for terminally ill patients, its appropriateness needs to be considered in light of factors such as the availability (or not) of a family caregiver, the intensity of the symptoms involved, and the availability of competent home care.

> The finding that on some occasions the acute hospital setting can be perceived as a safe haven at the end of life, a place where a dying person can go to in times of need or because no other option is available suggests that it is, and probably continues to be, an essential end-of-life care setting in certain situations. (Reyniers, Houttekier, Cohen, Pasman, & Deliens, 2014, p. 81)

Thus there is an urgent need for drastic change in the way we care for and allow people to live until they die, particularly if they are hospitalized.

In the 1960s, hospitals' curative focus and its dismal impact on the care that dying patients were receiving became the source of indignation for many. One of the first to act on this indignation was Dame Cecily Saunders, the founder of the modern hospice. Her philosophy is best captured in the famous phrase "You matter because you are you, and you matter to the end of your life." St Christopher's Hospice, founded by Saunders in 1967, emphasized a holistic approach to care that included careful pain and symptom relief as well as attention to the spiritual, psychological, and social needs of patients and their families. Her vision also always combined teaching and clinical research. Another powerful advocate, Elisabeth Kübler-Ross, actively denounced what became commonly known as the "plight of the dying":

> Dying nowadays is more gruesome in many ways, namely, lonelier, mechanical, and dehumanized [...] our concentration on equipment, on blood pressure, our desperate attempt to deny the impending death which is so frightening and discomforting to us that we displace all our knowledge onto machines, since they are less close to us than the suffering face of another human being which would remind us once more of our lack of omnipotence, our limits and failures, and last but not least perhaps our own mortality. (Kübler-Ross, 1969, p. 9)

Not surprisingly, independent hospice facilities were, initially, the preferred model because they were a departure from the traditional medical model and because of their commitment to nonaggressive, supportive care with a focus on quality of life in the final days.

Although in many countries the hospice palliative care movement was developed at the margins of the traditional health care system, in Canada the first formal palliative care programs were developed within tertiary care hospitals, both within the first months of 1975. Dr. Paul Henteleff developed a palliative care ward at St. Boniface General Hospital in Winnipeg. In Montreal, Dr. Balfour Mount, who coined the term *palliative care*, established the first service to have a full complement of services (dedicated unit, consult team, home care, bereavement support) at the Royal Victoria Hospital. Both initiatives were driven by the belief that hospital care and modern medicine could be transformed to provide comfort—a humanist approach to the care of the dying. These two programs were the first in the world to attempt to integrate the philosophy and the practice of palliative care within a modern teaching hospital rather than a stand-alone hospice.

My own interest and involvement in hospital-based palliative care came when I was a young physician in the mid-1980s working in a sexually transmitted disease (STD) clinic in downtown Montreal at the moment the HIV-AIDS epidemic exploded. In this work, I witnessed many very difficult deaths due to a lack of end-of-life homecare services. This, combined with the stigma of the disease and the resulting denial of access to care, heightened my awareness of the lack of compassion for the dying inherent in both society and the medical system. Many of the patients whose suffering I witnessed were close friends who were denied institutional palliative care on the pretext that palliative care was only for cancer patients.

My personal response to this reality was one of profound anger and disillusionment, not unlike Kübler-Ross' response to the abysmal quality of care for dying cancer patients during the first decades of the modern hospice movement. Again, modern medicine revealed itself as lacking in compassion and competence, especially for end-of-life care. At that moment, I understood the grave and urgent need to train health professionals (including myself) in basic end-of-life care; I also recognized the need for systemic change within the health care system.

In my search for solutions, I decided to join the Royal Victoria Hospital program, which under Mount's leadership was already accepting AIDS patients and treating people, not just disease. The inclusion of patients with progressive neuro-degenerative diseases and other forms of end-stage chronic illnesses was clearly defined from the onset of the program, a radical departure from many hospice programs admitting only patients with advanced malignant disease, a choice coherent with a long tradition of holistic medicine at McGill, illustrated in this quote by William Osler: "Ask not what disease the person has, but rather what person the disease has."

Similar to Dr. Mount, I truly believed that I could play an integral role in improving access to quality end-of-life care for my patients, specifically those suffering from HIV-AIDS. We needed to refocus care from cure to comfort, ensuring that both patients and their families were prepared for the end. This change needed to happen from within the hospital system, not only because hospitals are where ill people seek help, but also because they are where health professionals receive training and where cross-pollination among various disciplines occurs.

To effect deep and lasting change that would dramatically alter the way in which physicians cared for the dying while improving the way hospitals responded to patients with chronic life-limiting illnesses, I believed that a "Trojan horse" approach was best. We needed to inspire change from within the system.

WHERE WE BEGAN AND HOW WE HAVE CHANGED—A BRIEF HISTORY OF HOSPITAL-BASED PALLIATIVE CARE

The Beginnings

A chain of events triggered by a panel discussion on death and dying in February 1973 at a local church led to Dr. Mount's development of a palliative care service pilot project at the Royal Victoria Hospital, a McGill University–affiliated institution. At a time when more than two thirds of Canadians were dying in hospitals, Mount and colleagues were inspired by the radical departures from traditional mediocrity in terminal care that characterized Dr. Cicely Saunders's movement and St Christopher's Hospice. "Could her significant achievements be duplicated in a general hospital?" asked Ajemian and Mount in one of their early reports (Ajemian & Mount, 1980, preface). In this pilot project at the Royal Victoria Hospital (RVH), Mount and his team showed that the care of the dying and their families could be greatly improved by a palliative care program built around four axes: an inpatient palliative care unit (PCU), a palliative consultation team to follow inpatients in the hospital, home palliative care service, and bereavement service. The true originality and visionary quality of this model is its integration of these four axes in a seamless care delivery service that recognized the need to adapt the way we care in order to address the needs of patients and families "right now," wherever the patient is located. Hospice came to be understood not as a setting, but as a way to care.

The creation of a PCU, not unlike the model of the free-standing hospice developed by Saunders, allowed for the geographic regrouping of patients and families facing terminal illness when they could not be cared for at home. The PCU, instead of a busy, noisy acute-care ward, became a homelike environment where the traditional, hierarchical, physician-driven model was put aside in favor of a true interdisciplinary team approach that emphasizes total care by all members of the team, including volunteers. This alone was quite revolutionary in a modern teaching hospital. The creation of a PCU also allowed for a team approach to further the development of concepts in terminal care; for the training through clinical immersion of a wide spectrum of professionals who were able to replicate the model in their clinical environment; and for the development of a training environment for future professionals, in particular, medical or surgical residents and nursing students. The provision of home care by the same palliative care service professionals, in collaboration with specific home care agencies, allowed for a better coordination of the care, a better control of symptoms, and a better sense of personal identity. The same nurse or physician who had been in contact with the patient during the hospitalization remained involved with home care ensuring continuity of care and presence. Too often, we have seen the development of a PCU within a hospital but without any real link to the other wards, a kind of PCU on stilts. For Mount, ensuring communication with other treating teams and promoting early access to palliative care were essential. The consultation team rapidly became a resource within the hospital, providing clinical support and advice on how best to care for terminally ill patients hospitalized on other wards, thus enabling a large number of clinicians to learn and integrate the palliative approach within their daily care. Finally, Mount and colleagues strongly believed that competent support during the bereavement period would help prevent the morbidity linked with a difficult grieving process.

The leadership demonstrated by Mount was quickly recognized by medical leaders such as *Canadian Medical Association Journal* editor David Shephard, who wrote in July 1976:

> Whether a patient were in the PCU [palliative care unit] or at home (where he would be cared for by the PCU's domiciliary service), the back-up facilities of the parent hospital would always be available—but in addition the presence of the PCU within the hospital, would mean that its resources in terms of personnel and expertise would be available to the hospital, so that the PCU staff would assist staff in other wards in developing their skills in terminal care. Thus the presence of a PCU would foster use of consultant and counseling services and aid in-hospital education on terminal care. And likewise, a two-way relationship between the staff of the PCU and physicians elsewhere

would foster education not only of these physicians in care of the terminally ill but also of PCU staff by visiting physicians. (Shephard, 1976, p. 98)

Again this idea of cross-pollination had taken root, demonstrating that palliative care was an essential service for all patients no matter where they moved within the health care system.

Furthermore, Mount and colleagues, like Saunders, held firmly to the fundamental belief that it was not enough to simply deliver palliative care; it needed to be rigorously studied, carefully taught, and thoughtfully practiced in order to improve the quality of palliative interventions. Since its very beginnings, one of the central aims of the palliative care service at the RVH has been for colleagues to collectively reflect on all aspects of palliative care in order to develop new concepts in terminal care, and to do this regularly.

The International Congress on Palliative Care

In 1976, shortly after the doors opened for the Royal Victoria Hospital Palliative Care Service in Montreal, Dr. Mount and his colleagues hosted the first International Congress on Palliative Care, then known as "the International Seminar on Terminal Care." Among the 317 delegates at that Congress were Dame Cicely Saunders (from the United Kingdom), who gave a talk on "the philosophy of total care of the terminally ill" and Elisabeth Kübler-Ross (from Germany) whose two presentations focused on "the psychological needs of the patient and family" and on "grief work." The second Congress, held in 1978, almost tripled in size. With an unexpected 828 delegates, the organizers had to arrange for an overflow room with closed-circuit TV (B. Mount, personal communication, February 4, 2014). With each new Congress, attendance grew and included people from all corners of the world. Most recently, the Congress has hosted over 1,600 delegates from over 65 countries around the globe. A backward glance over the International Congress since its inception reveals growth not only in the breadth of its reach (i.e., the number of people from around the world who have developed clinical and academic programs in palliative care), but increasing depth and maturity of the field of palliative care as a whole. A perusal of the Congress programs shows us the development of palliative care education across the professions; research (qualitative and quantitative) across many disciplines, in both the arts and sciences of palliative care; high quality, standardized volunteer training programs; and the birth and rapid growth of pediatric palliative care, to name just a few.

Perhaps even more indicative of the growth of palliative care, however, is the number of palliative care congresses held annually around the world: the European Association of Palliative Care, the Latin America Palliative Care Congress, the Asia Pacific Palliative Care Congress, and there are many more. Together, these congresses represent the vibrant conversation of an active, international community committed to the best possible palliative care for all people with life-limiting illness, and their families.

The conclusions of the 1975–1976 pilot project of the Royal Victoria Palliative Care Service were clear: the medical, emotional and spiritual needs of the terminally ill and their families were generally neglected in the delivery of health care. These needs could be met by a trained interdisciplinary team of professional caregivers and volunteers. Moreover, a palliative care service for the terminally ill could be effectively integrated into a general hospital, and act as a monument not to the incurability of some diseases but to the dignity of man in his final days (Ajemian & Mount, 1980).

Models and Funding for Hospital-Based Palliative Care

Understanding the recent history of health care policy and funding is essential to understanding how models of palliative care delivery have emerged and developed. Beyond the motivation of being able to effect change from within, the decision to integrate palliative care services within a tertiary academic hospital arose from a consideration of the society's capacity to support such an innovation. Because of the particular sociopolitical context in Canada in 1974, hospital-based palliative care services (as opposed to free-standing hospices) were the path of least resistance, considering the difficulty in securing funding for new structures. The Canadian Medical Health Act of 1966 ensured government-funded universal health care and initially meant adequate funding of palliative care hospital beds either scattered throughout the hospital or within a specific palliative care ward. It is interesting to note that contrary to the lack of beds in modern-day hospitals, hospital occupancy rates were relatively low in the 1970s, often lower than 70%. Beds could therefore be easily made available by health care administrators.

Similarly, although hospice was the preferred model of care in the United States, funding was hard to obtain. Therefore, although hospice advocates feared integration into hospitals where their services would be less valued and more easily cut, such integration was often the only way to go. "In fact, during the late 1970s hospital-based programs were the most popular model; by 1980, 46% of all hospice programs were affiliated with hospitals" (Siebolt, 1992, p. 13).

Around the world, hospital-based palliative care programs are now delivered in a combination of organizational models, including some or all of the following:

- inpatient PCUs (dedicated beds)
- scattered dedicated beds in acute or chronic care units
- specialist palliative consultative or advisory teams that follow patients between settings of care as required
- day-therapy hospice
- ambulatory palliative care consultative teams available early in the disease trajectory
- bereavement services

Many models have been developed over the past 40 years to meet the needs of hospitalized palliative care patients. But is a model that has a consultation team alone sufficient? According to the Institute of Medicine: "inpatient consultation teams have been shown to improve patient symptoms, enhance family satisfaction and wellbeing, while significantly reducing hospital costs by aligning medical treatments to patient goals and reducing misutilization" (Morrison 2013, p. 204). It has often been argued that patients can be managed adequately on an acute-care service, with the support of a consultation team. However, for patients with symptoms that are difficult to control, other medical needs that require specialized attention, or for distressed families, optimal care is difficult to achieve on a busy acute-care service.

A recent literature review of general nurses' experiences of end-of-life care in an acute-care hospital identifies a number of substantial barriers to providing excellent care:

- improper education and knowledge
- lack of time to spend with patients

- mitigating the hospital-setting conflict of curative care versus comfort care (including the inappropriate use of active treatment)
- inadequate communication with team members and patients
- issues with pain and symptom management

Nurses participating in this study also emphasized personal issues that arose throughout treatment. These included a sense of inadequacy in the provision of care, stress, lack of access to professional support, and feelings of incompetence (McCourt, Power, & Glackin, 2013, pp. 510–516). Another study suggested that death anxiety is likely to be amplified in nurses who are providing care that is not accepting of the patient's impending death, and may result in behaviors like the observed reluctance to interact with the family and patient, and a focus on care tasks as a way of avoiding such interaction. "What, when superficially observed, appeared as frantic activity in the hours or minutes before a patient's death is more likely a representation of death anxiety, denial and withdrawal, where nurses focus on care tasks and disengage as a way of coping" (Bloomer, Endacott, O'Connor, & Cross, 2013, p. 762).

In many countries, including the United States, the development of hospital-based palliative care services has been largely influenced by the fee-for-service system, a system that very often fails to provide support for the interdisciplinary team beyond physician reimbursement. This very often leaves the directors of the in-hospital palliative care service to rely on charitable contributions to provide the care of an extended palliative care team, and this despite the fact that palliative care makes economic sense. A recent literature review of the economic impact of palliative care found that: "Palliative care is most frequently found to be less costly relative to comparator groups, and in most cases, the difference in cost is statistically significant" (Smith, Brick, O'Hara, & Normand, 2014, p. 148).

In fact, palliative care teams in both the United States and Canada have demonstrated significant cost savings to the health care system and, thereby, provide a strong business and economic case for further funding. Owing to this reality, "the number of hospital palliative care teams has grown rapidly and as of 2011, 63% of all US hospitals reported a palliative care team and over 85% of hospitals with over 300 beds" (Morrison, 2013, p. 204). Moreover, "high volume inpatient palliative care units have also been shown to be highly cost effective for hospitals. In one study a dedicated palliative care unit reduced daily hospital costs by 66% as compared with usual care patients" (Smith et al., 2003, p. 699).

The model fostered by the early pioneers of in-hospital palliative care was and is unique in the sense that it was developed within acute care and guided by a vision that challenged the traditional model of hospitals' medical care delivery. These early pioneers helped to develop a vision of the integration of palliative care that remains foundational to all modern models. The fundamental elements of these palliative care models represent a shift in the focus of care, the nature of the care team, and the values that drive care practices.

CORNERSTONES AND FOUNDATIONS OF HOSPITAL-BASED PALLIATIVE CARE

The focus of palliative care is on practices that improve any and all dimensions of patients' quality of life. Because living with advanced, life-limiting illness affects all aspects of one's life, an interdisciplinary team of care professionals and volunteers is essential for care of the whole person. Not only do the various members of the team offer complementary expertise to address the existential, psychological, social, and physical needs of the dying patient, but they work collaboratively toward a shared care goal established with the patient and his/her family.

The staffing of palliative care teams in hospitals varies according to characteristics of the hospital and the population it serves, funding resources, and national health care policies. In hospital-based PCUs, the complexity of patients' needs requires a high staff-to-patient ratio. Ideally, a full palliative care team includes the patient, the patient's family, volunteers, social work, physical therapy, occupational therapy, psychology, and chaplaincy, in addition to a team of specialized nurses and a team of palliative medicine physicians. If staff doesn't also include music and art therapists, links to palliative care expertise in these professions should be established resources. "While the number of professionals involved in each case may vary, the great advantage of the staff team is to have all professions available in the same physical area, with possibilities for daily meetings and interactions" (Hanks et al., 2010, p. 171).

Central to the concept of the "team" in the palliative care context is that all who are involved in the therapeutic triad—the patient, the family, and the professional caregiver—are recognized as being at risk for significant stress, each requiring clearly defined support mechanisms. This implies the need for team development and team support. Given the focus on quality of life (not just quality of health), an interdisciplinary team—which includes trained volunteers as well as the patient and his or her loved ones—serves as the core care team. The quality and success of this team depend on the careful and selective recruitment of all team members, as well as sufficient time for training and debriefing in areas such as conflict resolution and bereavement. The extent to which volunteers are embedded in the care team is unique to palliative care. Their presence provides comfort to patients, respite to families, and a unique perspective on the patients' well-being for the clinical staff. The inclusion and treatment of volunteers in the care team is also indicative of the ways in which the palliative care model bucks the physician-dominated hierarchy so common in health care teams and so inappropriate in end-of-life care. Similarly, another central element of palliative care is the team's ongoing commitment to compassionate, attentive care and unconditional respect for patients while resisting the tendency to revert to the disease–diagnosis–treatment paradigm so common in modern medicine. The team's ability to swim against the stream of traditional medical care is nourished through research and education that focus on the interface of the sciences and humanities.

Another cornerstone of hospital-based palliative care is what is referred to in French as *l'accompagnement*, a concept inadequately captured in the English translation "accompaniment." In English, accompaniment is best thought of as what Dr. Mount refers to as "radical presence," that is, being fully present to one's own and another's humanity (Mount, 2014). The name of France's palliative care association, *La société française d'accompagnement et de soins palliatifs*, is indicative of the centrality of humanity and person-to-person care in palliative care. In the hospital context, true accompaniment is possible only if all professionals are able to transcend technical care and build supportive, more personalized relationships with patients and their families, and provide respite and bereavement care.

As early as 1976, palliative care providers recognized the benefits of offering early integrated palliative care services along with standard oncology care for patients with advanced malignant disease.

Patients still receiving chemotherapy or other forms of therapy aimed at modifying the disease trajectory may be followed by the consultation team, on the home care program, and in the palliative care clinic […] palliative care services team involvement in this phase of the disease is beneficial as it allows the formation of supportive relationships with the palliative care team that facilitate a smooth continuum of care when the patient's condition deteriorates. (Ajemian & Mount, 1980, p. 271)

Because the transfer from active treatment to palliative care can sometimes cause conflict and fear, the early involvement of the palliative care team can also reduce the difficulty associated with this shift in goals of care by introducing quality-of-life interventions in conjunction with disease-specific interventions. Today, the early implementation of palliative care is commonly accepted as beneficial to the quality of life for patients with advanced cancer and their families. Recent studies (e.g., Temel et al, 2010; Greer et al, 2013) have shown that early intervention:

- decreases symptom burden
- helps patients develop tangible goals of care around prognosis and treatment, through, in part, frequent discussions of advance care directives
- optimizes health care resource use and treatment expenditures
- facilitates access to medical technology or interventions only available in hospital, such as stabilization of a malignant fracture, radiotherapy, or installation of a venting gastrostomy

> Introducing palliative care services soon after diagnosis for patients with advanced cancer helps to enhance quality of life, reduce depression, improve the quality of care at the end of life, and possibly improve survival (i.e., in the case of those with metastatic non-small cell carcinoma). (Greer, Jackson, Meier, & Temel, 2013, p. 360)

The fundamental elements of palliative care described in this section emerged in response to a number of problems with the hospital-based treatment of dying patients. Although progress has been made on many fronts for hospital-based palliative care, many challenges still remain.

CURRENT CHALLENGES IN HOSPITAL-BASED PALLIATIVE CARE

The most obvious and perhaps the most urgent challenge we face in hospital-based palliative care in developed countries is our rapidly aging population. In the United Kingdom, "the percentage of annual deaths is projected to rise by 17% from 2012 to 2030; the percentage of deaths amongst those aged 85 years or more is expected to rise to 44% by 2030" (Wee, 2013, p. 195).

Furthermore, nononcological terminal diseases are increasingly prevalent and require the embracing of palliative approaches to care in disciplines such as cardiology, neurology, nephrology, and HIV-AIDS.

These new demands also come at a time of a fiscally strained health care system. Although free-standing hospices are often dependent on charitable funding, they tend to have more autonomy and control over their palliative care programs. Publicly funded palliative care services may benefit from longitudinal funding of staff (particularly nursing and physicians), but are often controlled from a distance by hospital administrators who have variable levels of understanding and commitment to the practice of palliative care. In this context, the overriding challenge for hospital-based palliative care is to resist the culture (practices and values) of the acute-care-focused hospitals in which the programs reside. Institutional integration necessarily means sacrificing some autonomy, but the assimilative tendencies of large institutions have had a substantial impact on the fundamental elements of palliative care. These include reduced staffing; loss of control over staff recruitment; reduced time for team-based training, debriefing, and problem-solving; and reduced time to be fully dedicated to the supportive care of patients and families. Furthermore, the physical design of acute-care settings favors functionality over aesthetics, highlighting the value of curative care over comfort care. In so doing, hospitals can rarely offer patients privacy, aesthetic comfort, or respect—all of which play a central role in quality of life.

The assimilative power of the efficiency-oriented culture of acute-care hospitals can be seen in staff recruitment that is driven by a system of seniority rather than best fit according to interest and skills, and in team members being held to institutional standards of productivity. Treadmill palliative care services can emerge in response to hospital standards for bed use and length-of-stay estimates that drive the admitting and even discharging of patients. In an ideal world, the quality of home-based palliative care would be so good that limited access to the PCU would make sense, but this is not the reality.

In contrast to the inclusion of patients as core members of palliative care teams, in many parts of today's hospitals, patients are viewed as clients. Similarly, as palliative care becomes more immersed in the acute-care culture of hospitals, we are witnessing the insidious transformation of physicians from palliative care specialists into symptomologists working within the disease–cause–treatment paradigm that palliative care has long sought to change.

This transformation toward symptomology and the biomedical approach to end-of-life care is further encouraged by the values and demands of academia in university-affiliated teaching hospitals. The notion of the "expert" that shapes so much of academic culture sanctifies a knowledge that often excludes the patient experience and directly contradicts the person-to-person interaction at the heart of palliative care philosophy. Furthermore, by embracing official academia, which demands productivity as evidenced in primarily biomedical research, palliative care risks compromising its role in leading the resistance against the trend to elevate scientific knowledge over knowledge based in the humanities.

The accreditation of our educational programs by professional bodies has been key to the rapid progression of the clinical discipline of palliative medicine. However, this accreditation carries with it the demands to conform to particular ways of knowing and doing, rather than encouraging creative approaches to developing this discipline and valuing its role in questioning the assumptions and values of the contemporary biomedical approach. Also, many aspects of palliative care that don't fit within the biomedical model (e.g., bereavement and spiritual care) are frequently disinvested, underfunded, or nonexistent.

In addition to the assimilative powers of mainstream medicine (including its academic arm), another powerful challenge to hospital-based palliative care (and palliative care generally) is the superficial understanding and appropriation of its principles, which leads to underresourced services, undertrained staff, and inappropriate research methodologies. As a Trojan horse, palliative care finds itself in the difficult position of needing to achieve recognition within the medical community without compromising its resistance to the biomedical paradigm (e.g., epistemologies, research methodologies, and care practices). The development of palliative care specialty and subspecialty programs embodies this tension between hospital-based palliative care's need for recognition and its commitment to resistance.

Many agree that palliative medicine needs to be internationally recognized as a specialty to ensure that physicians who are developing palliative care competence are able to provide high-quality care in keeping with the constant developments in clinical knowledge and evidence. Palliative medicine is now a recognized discipline in many countries, including the United Kingdom, France, Australia, Hong Kong, Taiwan, New Zealand, the United States, and soon in Canada. (For an analysis of international certification, see *The Mapping of Medical Training and Physician Certification in Palliative Medicine in Europe*, a project of the European Association of Palliative Care, n.d.) Although I strongly agree with this trend toward the development of palliative medicine as a recognized specialty, I also feel that particular vigilance is needed to protect the core principles and elements of palliative care as we move forward.

LOOKING AHEAD: PROTECTING THE FUTURE OF HOSPITAL-BASED PALLIATIVE CARE

Attention to the Medicalization of Dying

In what is often referred to as our death-denying society, there is a potential for hospital-based palliative care to give a false sense of comfort to the larger society that death and dying are taken care of in hospitals; that they are a medical matter and therefore not the responsibility of the community. The tendency toward medicalized dying is one that hospital-based palliative care must continuously resist. We need to question how this particular provision of palliative care may insidiously contribute to a view of death as a medical phenomenon. Protecting the distinctive features of palliative care in the hospital context is likely the best way to manage this tension.

Protecting the Care Environment

Since its inception, hospital-based palliative care has emphasized the physical environment as a key component for good end-of-life care. With time, however, the rules and regulations of the larger institution have begun to chip away at efforts to create a more homelike environment for patients and families. Increased demands for more space from the many busy acute-care divisions threaten the preservation of quiet, private spaces for patients and their families. Additionally, the importance of including family (and pets) as part of the circle of care is challenged by rules that restrict visitors to specific hours and may exclude pets entirely. For the most part, PCUs have been successful in bending such rules to meet the needs of their patients and families. But one can never assume that this institutional flexibility is a given; it requires vigilant protection.

Protecting the Palliative Care Team and Service

As funding in hospitals specifically and health care more broadly become more and more constrained, it is increasingly difficult for hospital-based palliative care services to maintain the multidisciplinary team that ensures the supportive accompanying presence that is so central to palliative care. In times of fiscal constraint, it is always difficult to protect those aspects of care that fall outside the biomedical model of most care institutions. Spiritual care and bereavement follow-up are just two such aspects of palliative care that require protection if we are to maintain our commitment to caring for patients (and families) as whole persons.

Volunteers are another feature of the care team that is under threat of being lost in the current fiscal environment of technology and biomedically focused health care. Little progress (and perhaps even loss) has occurred since the inception of palliative care volunteer programs. As a care discipline, we are at risk of losing the powerful contribution of these caregivers who are often uniquely positioned to witness the more subtle signs of a patient's changing state of well-being (e.g., agitation, overmedication, depression) as well as gaps between care plans and reality.

For palliative care to maintain its integrity within the hospital context, we need to be able to offer a full range of services that do not become muddled in the technology-oriented culture of modern hospitals. It is not enough to simply deliver care; rather, we need to continue to insist on the importance of embodying the ethos of care. As Mount once stated: palliative care is "a model that recognizes medical technology as a means to an end rather than an end in itself" (Mount, 1980, p. 381).

Protecting and Promoting Innovative Approaches to Research and Education

As palliative care becomes more and more integrated into mainstream medicine, there is a tendency to adopt biomedical norms for research. Palliative care must never forget that its originality stems from its multidisciplinary structure and its ability to live at the intersection of the humanities and the sciences, where patients are not objects of study but participants in and inspiration for both our research and training programs.

Palliative care health professionals consistently benefit from interactions with hospital-based colleagues in a variety of disciplines. We can always grow personally and professionally when learning to see the world through another's eyes. Similarly, we can gain a much more nuanced understanding of disciplinary differences (and thus a more holistic picture of care) when witnessing the challenges that colleagues in those disciplines must face.

In conclusion, within the hospital setting, palliative care needs to continue to embrace new solidarities and welcome the disenfranchised. We need to continue to be the safe haven for all patients as they face their final journey. The very presence of palliative care in hospitals reflects a recognition by our society that care of the dying is the responsibility of the collective, and that the care we provide is a reflection of the practice of hospice palliative care as a whole, which recognizes that "hospitality is not to change people, but to offer them space where change can take place" (Nouwen, 1986, pp. 70–71).

REFERENCES

Ajemian, I., & Mount, B. (Eds.). (1980). *The R.V.H. manual on palliative/hospice care: A resource book*. Salem, NH: The Ayer.

Al-Qurainy, A., Collis, E., & Feuer, D. (2009). Dying in an acute hospital setting: The challenges and solutions. *International Journal of Clinical Practice, 63*(3), 508.

Bloomer, M. J., Endacott, R., O'Connor, M., & Cross, W. (2013). The "dis-ease" of dying: Challenges in nursing care of the dying in the acute hospital setting: A qualitative observational study. *Palliative Medicine, 27,* 757, 762.

European Association of Palliative Medicine. (n.d.). *The mapping of medical training and physician certification in palliative medicine in Europe.* Retrieved from http://www.eapcnet.eu/Themes/Education/Physicians/MappingofMedicalEducation.aspx

Gott, C., Sam, H., Ahmedzai, S. H., & Wood, C. (2001). How many inpatients at an acute hospital have palliative care needs? Comparing the perspectives of medical and nursing staff. *Palliative Medicine, 15*(6), 451–460.

Greer, J., Jackson, A., Meier, D., & Temel, J. (2013). Early integration of palliative care services with standard oncology care for patients with advanced cancer. *CA: A Cancer Journal for Clinicians, 63*, 349–362.

Hanks, G., Cherny, N., Christakis, N., Fallon, M., Kaasa, S., & Portnoy, R. (Eds.). (2010). Section 4.1: The specialist palliative care unit. In *Oxford textbook of palliative medicine* (eBook ed.). New York, NY: Oxford University Press.

Kübler-Ross, E. (1969). *On death and dying*. New York, NY: Macmillan.

McCourt, R., Power, J. J., & Glackin, M. (2013). General nurses' experiences of end-of-life care in the acute hospital setting: A literature review. *International Journal of Palliative Nursing, 19*(10), 510–516.

Morrison, R. S. (2013). Models of palliative care delivery in the United States. *Current Opinion in Supportive and Palliative Care, 7*(2), 201–206.

Mount, B. (1980). Looking to the future. In I. Ajemian & B. Mount (Eds.), *The R.V.H. manual on palliative/hospice care: A resource book*. Salem, NH: The Ayer.

Mount, B. (2014, February 18). *Radical presence*. Paper presented at Montreal General Hospital, Montreal, Quebec, Canada.

Nouwen, H. (1986). *Reaching out: The three movements of the spiritual life*. New York, NY: Doubleday.Page 70–71

Reyniers, T., Houttekier, D., Cohen, J., Pasman, H., & Deliens, L. (2014). The acute hospital setting as a place of death and final care: A qualitative study on perspectives of family physicians, nurses and family carers. *Health & Place, 27*, 77–83.

Robinson, J., Gott, M., & Ingleton, C. (2014). Patient and family experiences of palliative care in hospital: What do we know? An integrative review. *Palliative Medicine, 28*(1), 18–33.

Shephard, D. (1976). Terminal care: Towards an ideal. *Canadian Medical Association Journal, 115*(2), 97–98.

Siebolt, C. (1992). *The hospice movement, easing death's pains*. New York, NY: Twayne.

Smith, S., Brick, A., O'Hara, S., & Normand, C. (2014). Evidence on the cost and cost-effectiveness of palliative care: A literature review. *Palliative Medicine, 28*(130), 130–150.

Smith, T. J., Coyne, P., Cassel, B., Penberthy, L., Hopson, A., & Hager, M. (2003). A high-volume specialist palliative care unit and team may reduce in-hospital end-of-life care costs. *Journal of Palliative Medicine, 6*(5), 699–705.

Temel, J. S., Greer, J. A., Muzikansky, A., Gallagher, E. R., Admane, S., Jackson, V. A., . . . Lynch, T. J. (2010). Early palliative care for patients with metastatic non–small-cell lung cancer. *New England Journal of Medicine, 363*(8), 733–742.

Wee, B. (2013). Models of delivering palliative and end-of-life care in the UK. *Current Opinion in Supportive and Palliative Care, 7*, 195–200.

Betty Davies

12

PALLIATIVE CARE FOR CHILDREN

In this chapter, I describe the development of pediatric palliative care (PPC) based on a journey through 45 years as a nursing student, clinician, educator, and researcher. I describe what inspired my involvement in this field, reflect on significant markers in the early development of PPC, and define PPC. I then identify significant current work in the field, selected challenges, and a hope for the future. I do not in any way intend this chapter to be comprehensive. Instead, it offers a personal reflection on the most important developments in caring for children who live in the shadow of death.

MY ENTRY INTO THE FIELD

As a nursing student in the late 1960s, I was taught that nursing had three goals: to keep people healthy and prevent illness, to care for those who are sick, and to help those who cannot recover to die with dignity. But we were taught very little about dying, death, and bereavement. So as a second-year student, I had little knowledge to guide my first encounter with a patient who died. Breathless, and with knees shaking, I reported to the charge nurse that Mrs. Jones had died. While still engaged in a phone conversation about a medication order, the nurse pointed to the resource books and whispered, "The procedure book is over there." This translated to "Look up the procedure for caring for a body after death and follow it." Carrying out the procedure was traumatic, but it was also the start of my interest in caring for the dying.

At that time, there were few resources to explore. In the 1960s, the fact that death was not an issue for open discussion in Western society was clearly evident in my university-affiliated school of nursing. I do not remember ever talking about death, other than with one exceptional nursing instructor who worked side by side with me to care for a badly burned child. It was the way things were at the time. Death was not a topic of instruction nor a topic of conversation between physicians and patients with serious diagnoses; it was seldom a topic between patients and their families. In an early study of what happens for patients dying in hospital, in the majority of cases the physician and family members chose not to tell the patient of his or her prognosis (Duff & Hollingshead, 1968). At about the same time, Glaser and Strauss (1966) documented that seriously ill people knew they were dying and described various patterns of communicating with seriously ill adults about their awareness of death. This work gently lifted a corner of the blanket of silence that allowed clinicians to begin to change their views.

However, as a young student, I was unaware of this work and of the fact that others shared similar concerns. I had no idea that one could study "death." So, I continued to learn from my patients. My clinical instructors seemed to think that my caring for Mrs. Jones' body after her death had given me "experience" with death, so my subsequent patient assignments frequently included those for whom death was a clear possibility. I came to learn that this likely saved considerable discomfort for my instructors, who themselves did not know how to help students care for dying patients.

Always aiming to be a pediatric nurse, I was excited to begin this rotation; I did not expect to learn about death from children, but the lessons continued. Susie, age 4, had leukemia. Her favorite stuffed toy was a small green frog with red spots. As I bathed Susie's little body, the characteristic bruises and red spots of leukemia were evident. Holding up "Froggy" with both hands and pointing to his spots, she said matter-of-factly, "Froggy has spots because his blood is sick, very sick. He has more spots every day. His spots will never go away." I continued to gently dry her, responding only a quiet "umhmm." She sighed, and affirmed, "I have spots just like Froggy's." I was in awe of Susie's simple but accurate description; this child knew more about her condition and her prognosis than anyone realized.

EARLY WORK IN THE FIELD

The earliest work in the field that has come to be known as *pediatric palliative care* centered on the care of children who were dying—children with leukemia like Susie. This focus evolved over time. In her descriptions of the history of childhood, Schorsch (1979) notes that death among children was once so frequent that it was a matter of course. During the 16th to 19th centuries, children in Early Modern England (1500–1800) were subject to many diseases and physical hardships. Death frequently occurred during the first year of life; surviving children were at risk from the great epidemic diseases of bubonic plague and smallpox and from the more common illnesses of dysentery, scarlet fever, measles, whooping cough, and unidentifiable illnesses that killed perhaps 30% of England's children before the age of 15. Besides disease, accidents were common sources of children's sickness, disability, and death. As the specialty of pediatrics (from the Greek *paidi* for child and *iatriki* for medicine) had yet to emerge, children were treated as small adults in hospitals and were cared for as much as conditions would allow, which often left them in dangerous, dirty situations conducive to illness and death. Still, the distressing grief of mothers and fathers whose children died is apparent in diaries and letters of that period, kept in the same wards as adults. Any charitable institutions tended to be more for children who were abandoned by their parents or orphaned than for sick youngsters. Most of the population, particularly the poor, struggled for existence.

Only in the 20th century did the health of children begin to improve significantly. Moreover, the horrors of the Second World War motivated a desire to prevent such pain and suffering from ever occurring again, especially among children. Pioneering new developments in medicine, science, and public health contributed to a healthier world for children in the developed countries. The discovery of penicillin, other antibiotics, and vaccines saved children's lives from the ravages of the diseases that had killed them before. Acute lymphocytic leukemia, discovered in the early 1960s, and other childhood cancers took over as the most frequent cause of death by disease in children. The focus turned to how children like Susie and their families coped (e.g., Binger et al., 1969) and how health care professionals might help these families (e.g., Ablin et al., 1971). Development of chemotherapy and radiation therapies came to mean that death from leukemia and many other cancers was no longer inevitable. When I cared for Susie, most children with leukemia died; now 90% of children with acute lymphoblastic leukemia survive. She and other children were cared for on general pediatric units; only in 1975 were the first specialty units for children with cancer created.

There was also a growing interest in the psychosocial realm of experience and the effects of early childhood experiences. The Second World War had reinforced a generalized coping strategy of silence by shutting down conversation about death, but it also inspired the first ever accounts of children's understanding of death. The assassination of President Kennedy in 1963 had a notable effect on children, and adults struggled with the question of how best to help these grieving children. Researchers interested in studying children and death turned to Piaget's theory of cognitive development as a framework. His work with healthy children about the development of a concept of death indicated that a mature concept of death is not formed in children until after the age of 9 years. Thus, it was assumed that ill children under the age of 10 years were not aware of their diagnosis or prognosis and had little or no anxiety about their bodies or future. Therefore, professionals working with children with cancer or any life-threatening illness assumed that the findings with healthy children also applied to their patients and reasoned that if adults did not discuss the seriousness of their illness with them, the children would not experience anxiety. But my experience with Susie and other children like her taught me that this was not the case. Thus, I was ecstatic to eventually read Waechter's (1971) work.

Waechter, a pediatric nurse, conducted the first systematically controlled research directly with ill children to determine their awareness of a life-threatening condition. Her findings showed that children were indeed aware of their own serious illness and their impending death, and as a result, they were anxious about dying or death. Similar to Glaser and Strauss, Waechter lifted a corner of the blanket of silence about death among hospitalized children with serious illness. Subsequently, the replication by Spinetta, Rigler, and Karon (1973) of her findings, and Bluebond-Langner (1978) made a strong case for children's awareness of their own illness and dying, and argued for parents and health care professionals to not care for them in silence.

THE 1970s AND 1980s

Significant developments in PPC during the 1970s and 1980s focused on the location of care for children with cancer and subsequently other life-threatening conditions (LTC). Martinson's work at the University of Minnesota, funded by the U.S. National Cancer Institute from 1976 to 1978, was groundbreaking. Traditionally, children with cancer, including those in the terminal stage of their illness, received treatment and care in hospitals, but Martinson demonstrated that a child's care could be provided as effectively by the parents and by nurses at home, thus introducing the option of home care for families who desired it (Martinson et al., 1986; Moldow & Martinson, 1980). Subsequent studies reported on improved outcomes for the siblings and parents of home care compared with hospital care for children with cancer (Lauer, Mulhern, Bohne, & Camitta, 1985; Lauer, Mulhern, Wallskog, & Camitta, 1983).

In 1985, Ann Goldman, at Great Ormond Street Hospital in London, developed the first program for children dying from malignant diseases in hospital oncology units. She, along with two clinical nurse specialists, was involved with children from the time of diagnosis and throughout the disease trajectory to manage symptoms and to work with local care providers to facilitate home care and hospital care as needed. In Canada, the first hospital-based PPC program was in the Toronto Hospital of Sick Children in 1986; the second at Montreal Children's Hospital.

The development of hospices for children created another venue of care for children and their families. From the start, children's hospice focused on children with LTC in addition to children with cancer. During my early clinical years, most babies with conditions broadly referred to as "congenital" died during the perinatal period, but the development of neonatology and technological innovations in caring for premature babies of younger and younger gestational age meant they now survived. Consequently, a steadily increasing number of children were living with chronic, complex LTC. Such a child and her mother, desperate for help in meeting her child's needs for total care, motivated Sister Frances Dominica, a nurse and Anglican Sister, to create Helen House in 1982 with the mission of providing respite as well as end-of-life care and bereavement follow-up for families of children with LTC (Burne, Dominica, & Baum, 1984). Situated in Oxford, England, Helen House was the world's first free-standing children's hospice and has served as the model for other hospices in the United Kingdom and throughout the world.

Four other events during these two decades were of significance to the development of PPC. First, in the United States in 1983, Ann Armstrong-Dailey created Children's Hospice International (CHI), a nonprofit organization with the objective of providing education, legislation, and support for families of children with terminal illness (http://www.chionline.org/). Second, Corr and Corr edited a book, *Hospice Approaches to Pediatric Care* (1985), with the worthy goal of bringing together those within the hospice movement and members of the pediatric health care community so they could learn from each other. Third, in 1989, the first International Conference on Children and Death was hosted in Athens, Greece, under the auspices of the University of Athens by Dr. Danai Papadatou, a clinical psychologist, and her pediatrician father, Professor Costas Papadatou. This conference, the first to bring together practitioners, educators, and researchers to converse about their work, resulted in a compilation of their cross-discipline endeavors (Papadatou & Papadatou, 1991).

The fourth development pertained to grief and bereavement, an important aspect of PPC. When death was the expected outcome for children with cancer, those who worked with dying children were concerned about the impact of a child's death on parents, siblings, and the family (e.g., Fischoff & O'Brien, 1976; Tietz, McSherry, & Britt, 1977). Well aware of this impact and the lack of attention to children's grief, a pediatric oncology nurse, Beverly Chappell, founded the Dougy Center for Grieving Children in Portland, Oregon, in 1982 (Chappell, 2007). This program was the first of its kind and has served as the model for over 165 other such programs throughout North America, Asia, and elsewhere. I can personally attest to the rapid growth in children's bereavement services: While preparing the needs assessment for a children's hospice in Vancouver, Canada, in the late 1980s and early 1990s, the search for bereavement services to which a survey could be sent yielded a very small number; today, on maps designating the location of such services in the United States and Canada, there are too many to count accurately.

The field of neonatal palliative care also started during this time with attention to the bereavement needs of families. In 1981, Rana Limbo, a nurse working with Bereavement Services in the Gundersen Health System located in La Crosse, Wisconsin, developed a comprehensive approach to caring for families whose babies died during pregnancy or shortly after birth. The program, known as Resolve Through Sharing (RTS), was unique in health care at the time and is now known and used worldwide (http://www.bereavementservices.org/resolve-through-sharing).

THE 1990s

During the 1990s, PPC grew substantially. In 1991, the Association for Children with Life Threatening or Terminal Conditions and their Families (ACT), now known as Together for Short Lives, was formed in the United Kingdom, the first such organization to focus on working to achieve better quality of life and care for all life-limited children and their families, accomplished in part by the publication of numerous resource documents, such as three editions of *A Guide to the Development of Children's Palliative Care Services* (2009). In 1993, the first *Oxford Textbook for Palliative Medicine* (*OTPM*) included an edited section on PPC (Davies, 1993) that affirmed that PPC was indeed a legitimate field of study related to, but different from, adult palliative care. The *OTPM* included a PPC section until the first *Oxford Textbook on Palliative Care for Children* was published in 2005, now in its second edition (Goldman, Hain, & Liben, 2012). Also in 1993, the International Work Group on Death, Dying and Bereavement (IWG), one of the first professional organizations in this field, published a *Statement on Pediatric Palliative Care*, putting forward basic principles of PPC (IWG, 1993). Not until the end of the decade did the American Academy of Pediatrics publish a position statement on PPC (American Academy of Pediatrics Committee on Bioethics and Committee on Hospital Care, 2000) clearly indicating that PPC was of interest to pediatric medicine.

Starting in 1995, during annual conferences of the Canadian Hospice and Palliative Care Association, the Pediatric Palliative Care Interest Group brought together individuals from across Canada to advocate for PPC. In 1998, in the United States, the National Hospice and Palliative Care Organization (NHPCO) supported ChiPPS (Children's Project on Palliative/Hospice Services), initiated by an international, multidisciplinary group of PPC professionals to foster development of PPC. The work of ChiPPS resulted in a Compendium of PPC as well as a training curriculum for PPC (the basis for the NHPCO PPC Online Training Series), recommendations for how to improve the care of children living with LTC, as well as published articles and an e-newsletter that continues today as a widely used e-Journal, all of which can be found at the NHPCO website (http://www.nhpco.org/resources/pediatric-hospice-and-palliative).

Clinically, the 1990s also brought the development of several additional hospital-based PPC programs in the United Kingdom, the United States, Australia, and New Zealand, each following the pattern of beginning in pediatric oncology. In the United States, for example, the Pediatric Advanced Care Team (PACT) began as a demonstration project at Dana-Farber Cancer Institute in 1997, and in 2001 expanded to include all children with life-threatening illnesses at Boston Children's Hospital. As hospital-based Pain and Symptom Teams, Comfort Care Teams, or PPC Teams formed, they functioned primarily on a consultative basis providing support and advice to the primary care team in addition to the child and family.

Furthermore, professionals and parents began to discuss the need for targeted palliative care programs in neonatal and perinatal populations.

Children's hospices continued to expand in the United Kingdom (where they now number 44). In Vancouver, Canada, Canuck Place Children's Hospice, the first free-standing children's hospice in North America, opened in 1995. There are now six children's hospices in Canada, with two additional hospices under construction, one of which is a second Canuck Place facility in another geographic area of the province. Children's hospices also developed in some European nations, such as Belarus, and in Africa. Bereavement programs for children continued to grow, primarily in Western nations, and not necessarily associated with PPC.

DEFINITION OF PEDIATRIC PALLIATIVE CARE

Arising from the activity of the 1990s were increasingly clear and comprehensive definitions of PPC (ACT, 2009; World Health Organization, 2006) that serve as the basis for the definition provided here. PPC is both a philosophy and a type of care; it is not synonymous with end-of-life care. Palliative care for children represents a special field, albeit closely related to adult palliative care.

Palliative care for children is an active and total approach to care of a child's body, mind, and spirit as well as supporting the family. It begins at the time of recognition or diagnosis of disease, even if prior to birth, continues throughout the illness, which may last for many years and regardless of whether or not a child receives treatment directed at the disease, to the time of death and beyond for family members. Ideally, palliative care complements medical care that focuses on cure and the prolongation of life.

PPC requires a broad multidisciplinary approach in providing compassionate and nonjudgmental care that addresses physical, emotional, social, and spiritual and existential elements, enhancement of quality of life, and relief of suffering of the child and family. PPC includes management of symptoms, provision of respite, coordination of services, including transition services where needed, end-of-life care, and bereavement support. PPC can be provided in tertiary care facilities, community health centers, hospices, and children's homes. Optimally, PPC should create a seamless continuum of care for families among providers, across settings and over time.

Life-Threatening Conditions

PPC focuses on children from 0 to 19 years but may also include those whose diagnosis is made in childhood and who unexpectedly live beyond this age into young adulthood. PPC also applies when LTC are diagnosed prior to or at birth. Life-limiting (or life-shortening) conditions are those for which there is a high likelihood of death before adulthood; there is no hope of cure. LTC are those for which curative treatment may be feasible but can fail. Because all complex chronic conditions in childhood are fraught with uncertainty, some prefer the term "life-threatening" rather than "life-limiting," the former term implying an element of hope (Liben, Papadatou, & Wolfe, 2008). LTC are multisystem, often progressive over time, affect cognitive and physical development, and are physiologically diverse. They may be rare and variable, and often there is lack of disease-specific research. Prognosis may change over time as treatment options become available, but in the meantime, the parents of children with LTC are integral to the care these children receive at home and in health care settings. ACT (2009) has delineated four categories or quadrants of LTC (Table 12.1).

TABLE 12.1 Categories of Life-Threatening Conditions in PPC

Quadrant 1 (Q1)	Quadrant 2 (Q2)
Life-threatening conditions for which curative treatment may be feasible but can fail, e.g., cancer, irreversible organ failures	Premature death is inevitable, but long periods of intensive treatment prolong life and allow participation in normal activities, e.g., cystic fibrosis
Quadrant 3 (Q3)	**Quadrant 4 (Q4)**
Progressive conditions without cure; treatment is exclusively symptomatic and may extend over years, e.g., neurodegenerative, metabolic disease	Irreversible nonprogressive conditions with severe disability susceptible to health complications and premature death, e.g., severe cerebral palsy, anoxic brain injury

Source: Adapted from ACT (2009).

In Western nations, children in need of PPC today are increasingly those with Q3 conditions. ACT (2009) estimates that almost half of nontraumatic pediatric deaths are from these conditions. With no curative treatments, these children face an unknown life span and endure unstable and painful symptoms. They and their families experience emotional and spiritual challenges as the condition progresses along an uncertain trajectory toward death. Until cures are found, clinicians are obligated to maximize comfort and quality of life. Children with LTC suffer many physical problems that are currently managed inadequately (Malcolm, Forbat, Anderson, Gibson, & Hain, 2011), and their families struggle with health, psychological, social, and spiritual challenges (Steele & Davies, 2006). However, there is little research in this group compared with children who have other conditions, such as cancer. In the face of noncurable conditions, or when a potential cure has failed, children and their families seek comfort and quality of life.

PPC/Children's Hospice

PPC is primarily associated with care given to children in hospital with LTC for whom death is likely. Hospice for children refers to prototypical palliative care in which symptoms are managed and respite is provided throughout the course of the illness; end-of-life care is given during the final days or hours of life; and bereavement support or grief counseling is offered *before* death as children and their families experience numerous losses due to the diagnosis, the treatment and its ramifications, and the impending death of a child, and to families at the time of and following death. Often, children's hospice care is associated with a specialized, free-standing facility in the community that may or may not be directly affiliated with a hospital. In some places, it may refer to care provided for children in a section of an adult hospice (e.g., Hospice of the Sun Coast in Florida) or a home hospice care program offered by a children's hospital (e.g., the Karuna program within Children's Hospitals and Clinics of Minnesota) or by community organizations (e.g., the Diana Community Nursing Services in the United Kingdom). Regardless of location, however, the principles of PPC remain the same and guide the care that is given.

PPC Contrasted With Adult Palliative Care

Although based on similar philosophies of care, PPC differs from adult palliative care in several ways: (1) The number of children requiring palliative care is small relative to adults, but the death of a child is never seen as a normal or natural event and impacts greatly on parents, siblings, extended family, peers, communities, and health professionals, and needs are often more extensive. (2) Conditions in childhood are extremely rare with diagnoses specific to childhood (though some children survive into young adulthood); irregular disease trajectories mean that uncertainty about medical prognostication and day-to-day life is inherent in the situation. (3) The duration of children's illnesses varies widely, lasting from a few days to months or many years, often leading to long-term relationships between the children and their families with their pediatric care team. (4) Many of the illnesses are familial, so a family may have more than one child with the illness. (5) Care embraces the whole family—parents and siblings are particularly vulnerable—and parents bear a heavy responsibility for personal and nursing care as children are dependent on them. (6) Continuing childhood physical, emotional, and cognitive development require health care providers to be aware of and adapt to each child's changing levels of communication and ability to understand their illness, treatments, and prognosis. (7) Provision of education, play, and social interaction is essential and adds to the complexity of care provision and to the range of professionals involved.

However, because both adult and PPC share the same philosophical perspective, they can learn from each other. For example, as the palliative needs of adults change in response to increasing long-term chronic conditions, many aspects of PPC, such as working closely with and making decisions in partnership with family caregivers, dealing with pervasive uncertainty, and being creative to meet the developmental needs of children, may have much relevance for adult palliative care (Meier & Beresford, 2007).

CURRENT DEVELOPMENTS IN PPC (2000–THE PRESENT)

International Organization

Established in 2005 and situated in South Africa, the International Children's Palliative Care Network (ICPCN) works with national and regional associations to achieve the best quality of life for children and young people, their families, and carers worldwide. For example, in 2010, the U.K. Department of International Development (DFID) funded a proposal submitted by Help the Hospices to work with ICPCN to improve access to palliative care for children with HIV/AIDS in Malawi and the Maharashtra state of India, over a 5-year period. As well, ICPCN is spearheading a global campaign in 2015 to increase worldwide awareness of PPC and to explore what the developed world can to do help those in the developing world. ICPCN represents the voice of children in the Worldwide Palliative Care Association (WPCA), which promotes universal access to affordable quality care through the support of regional and national hospice and palliative care organizations.

Other international growth is evident in the expansion of PPC organizations and conferences. The First Middle Eastern Conference on PPC was held in Kuwait in 2005; the European Congress on Paediatric Palliative Care held its first two conferences in Rome in 2012 and 2014. ICPCN sponsored the First International Children's Palliative Care Conference in Mumbai, India, in February 2014. In Canada, the International Congress on Palliative Care, the longest-standing and largest palliative care conference worldwide, has gone from a scattering of PPC presentations, to a full 2-day preconference on PPC along with additional PPC presentations throughout the 5-day event.

Standards and Principles of Care, Charter of Rights

Standards documents have been designed to promote a standard, consistent approach to PPC regardless of whether that care is delivered at home, in a hospital, in a long-term care facility, or in a hospice. Standards for sustainable, consistent, and equitable provision of PPC have been proposed by the United Kingdom's Together for Short Lives (2013); The Canadian Network of Palliative Care for Children, under the auspices of the Canadian Hospice and Palliative Care Association (2006); the Task Force on Palliative Care for Children of the European Association of Palliative Care (EPAC; 2007); and CHiPPS as part of NHPCO in the United States (2009). In addition, the ICPCN (2008) published a Charter of Rights for children with LTC with the goal of having the Charter accepted and ratified by governments and health departments throughout the world. These documents address common key principles and values pertaining to the child and family as the unit of care, quality of life, location of care, whole person approach, attention to child and family culture and religions, goals of care, respite and bereavement, and involvement of an interprofessional team.

Educational Programs and Specialization

These standards must now be met by all those, both professionals and volunteers, who work in PPC. Thus, instruction about PPC should be included in basic professional education. Also needed is continuing education for practicing professionals who did not have this specialized training. This aspect has been well developed in the United States during the past decade. The End of Life Nursing Education Consortium (ELNEC), a national initiative to improve palliative care administered by the American Association of Colleges of Nursing, adapted its core curriculum for pediatrics in 2003 and updated it to include enhanced perinatal and neonatal content in 2009. The ELNEC Pediatric Curriculum Modules are also available as online training through the Hospice Education Network (www.hospiceonline.com). Similarly, EPEC (Education in Palliative and End-of-Life Care), established to provide education for physicians (www.epec.net), inaugurated its EPEC–Pediatrics program in 2012. Both ELNEC and EPEC programs are based on a "train the trainer" concept, and both have expanded internationally. Despite the increasing development of PPC programs in Europe, survey results showed that 33% of 43 European countries had no known PPC activity in 2011 (Knapp et al., 2011). Thus, appropriate and ongoing education and training are particularly important. Particularly useful for making PPC training accessible and affordable to all who need it is the ICPCN-developed free e-learning program (www.elearnicpcn.org/).

Specialization is growing within PPC. Pediatric palliative medicine is now recognized as a subspecialty in the United Kingdom, the United States, and Canada. Certification for hospice and palliative pediatric nurses in the United States is now offered by the National Board for Certification of Hospice and Palliative Nurses. Increasingly, specialization is also possible for other disciplines, such as social work. Also during this current decade, perinatal palliative care as a specialty has burgeoned, for example, with the creation of the Pregnancy Loss and Infant Death Alliance and the publication of a neonatal end-of-life protocol that was subsequently circulated worldwide (Catlin & Carter, 2002). Nurse leaders subsequently created care paths that applied palliative care principles to clinical practice (Gale & Brooks, 2006; Sumner, 2001). In 2004, Carter, Levetown, and Friebert published a groundbreaking *Practical Handbook*, now in its second edition (Carter, Levetown, & Friebert, 2011). Education continues through Resolve through Sharing and ELNEC, and considerable research is being conducted in the field. The National Association of Neonatal Nurses (NANN) recommends that neonatal nurses be trained and participate in offering services entailed in providing palliative and end-of-life care.

Provision of Services

During the past decade, PPC international development has grown dramatically, with new PPC programs in several European nations, such as Russia, South Africa (such as Soweto/Johannesburg), Costa Rica, and Mexico. In Greece, the nationwide bereavement program of Merimna was expanded to include the first PPC home care service in that country (www.merimna.org.gr). As well, the first free-standing children's hospice in the United States, George Mark Children's House, opened in 2004 in San Leandro, California. Another facility for children, partnered with an established hospice, opened in Arizona in 2010. As for why there are only two children's hospices in such a large nation, it is likely because there is very little to no direct reimbursement for palliative care services for children in the United States, and it is perceived that finding a way to sustain an organization/facility is difficult because philanthropy alone is so variable. It seems, however, that larger cultural differences, perhaps the same ones that sustain the U.S. health care system as it is, may play a role as children's hospices in the United Kingdom, Canada, and Europe operate mostly on donated funds. In the past decade, the Children's Hospice International Children's Program of All-Inclusive Coordinated Care (ChiPACC) initiative provided essential pilot studies to foster continued advocacy and initiatives at the state and national levels. Florida, one of the ChiPACC pilot states, was able to implement a Home and Community-Based Waiver to provide PPC services to medically fragile children. Now Colorado, California, and North Dakota have approved active waivers. Also, Concurrent Care, a provision of the Affordable Care Act implemented in 2010, allows for Medicaid-eligible children to receive both hospice and curative care at the same time—something that was a significant barrier for families that could benefit from the services provided by hospice. Currently, NHPCO is hosting a networking teleconference call every other month for state leaders in PPC to help them learn from each other, to provide support for the states trying to get waivers in place, and to ensure that concurrent care implementation is supported.

Research in PPC

The Institute of Medicine (IOM) published three reports, including one that shone a spotlight on the plight of dying children and their families in the United States (Field & Behrman, 2003) and called for national attention to address, build, and sustain a robust research agenda in end-of-life/palliative care. In 2010, the evaluative report that reviewed the research in palliative care between 1997 and 2010 indicated that fewer than 10% of all research publications focused on PPC. There is still a long way to go to provide research evidence on which to base PPC. However, considerable progress has occurred in the past 15 years in many areas, including symptom management in children with cancer, particularly pain, suffering, and fatigue; the experience of families of children with degenerative neuromuscular disorders; the epidemiology of deaths in children who require PPC; the responses of professionals who provide care to children who die; parental caregiving and the possibility of posttraumatic growth; the experiences of fathers and of siblings; the needs of culturally diverse families; and the impact of childhood death on parental bereavement. More research is needed on the evaluation of PPC services and the development of appropriate tools for such assessments.

Despite steadily increasing numbers of research projects, challenges derive from the relatively small population of children and the relatively few PPC professionals. I believe that one path to success is through infrastructure funding that makes it possible for research to occur. For example, the Canadian Institute of Health Research (CIHR) funded nine specialty research groups as Palliative Care New Emerging Teams in 2004. PedPalNET, an interdisciplinary (Medicine, Nursing, Social Work) core of five researchers, was the only PPC team funded in the competition (Straatman, Cadell, Davies, Siden, & Steele, 2008). The seed money from CIHR enabled the members of the PedPalNET group to secure additional funding totaling nearly $3.6 million (excluding all investigators' salaries that are not covered by research funding in Canada) to support a wide range of multidisciplinary projects across biomedical/clinical questions, psychosocial issues, and health services inquiries. The group worked with 48 collaborators and engaged with 14 partner organizations in Canada, the United States, the United Kingdom, and Australia and, through a second CIHR funding competition, received funding to expand and continue work as PedPalASCNet (A Network for Accessible, Sustainable, Collaborative Research in Pediatric Palliative Care) with PPC clinicians across the country—all made possible by the CIHR infrastructure support.

Another successful form of infrastructure support is available through the creation of research positions that allow individuals the freedom to conduct and lead research programs, encourage and foster the development of excellence in children's palliative care, and seek to influence national and international services and policy. I am aware of three such examples: The United Kingdom's True Colours Chair in Palliative Care for Children and Young People at the University College, London, Institute of Child Health and Great Ormond Street Hospital in 2010; in the United States, the Director of Research position with Children's Hospital of Philadelphia's Pediatric Palliative Care Program; and in Sweden at the Erstra Skondal University College, the newly established Galo Foundation's Professorship in Palliative Care with a Focus on Children and Youths. Such examples may help to convince administrators and funders, in a climate of diminishing resources, of the value of creating infrastructure to support the research and evaluation that is required to provide the basis on which optimal care can be provided.

CHALLENGES

Despite the advancement of the field of PPC, a range of barriers and associated challenges have been articulated (Davies et al., 2008; Liben, Papadatou, & Wolff, 2008), some of which are highlighted here along with others I see as pertinent.

Uncertainty of Prognosis

Uncertain prognosis and unpredictable disease trajectory are characteristic of children in PPC, particularly those with LTC. This uncertainty and unpredictability may hamper clinicians' ability to predict treatment responses or overall chances of a child's survival, affect decision making by both clinicians and parents, discourage the coexistence of "cure versus palliative" thinking, and undermine credibility and trust. They delay referrals to palliative care, hindering conversations in anticipation of when, where, and how next steps might occur. Earlier rather than later discussions allow more time for both clinicians and families to hear, to question, to reflect, and to understand. Indeed, "uncertainty is not something to be avoided, but rather is an inherent dimension of PPC. An uncertain prognosis should serve as a signal to initiate palliative care, rather than to avoid it" (Davies et al., 2008, p. 6).

Efficiency Model of Health Care Institutions

The efficiency model that currently guides the operation of most health care institutions jeopardizes the operationalization of person-centered or family-centered care despite formal statements proclaiming these concepts as guiding values. As a result, the flexibility of time and effort that is required to attend to the cultural and spiritual needs of children and families is not supported. For example, the optimal delivery of information to Chinese and Mexican families involves giving information, discussing the implications of the information for both the parents and the health care providers, and then assessing and addressing parents' responses to the information (Davies, Contro, Larson, & Widger, 2010), a process that may take more time and effort on the part of clinicians. Similarly, guidelines for spiritual assessment also depend on talking with children and parents to learn about and then address their spiritual concerns (Davies, Brenner, Orloff, Sumner, & Worden, 2002). These are examples of skills integral to offering optimal PPC that are seldom considered an efficient use of limited time in the current modus operandi of acute care settings.

Dominance of the Medical Model

The increasing focus on the dominance of the medical model, rather than a truly team-based interdisciplinary approach, presents an additional challenge. Of course, the adoption of pediatric palliative medicine is indeed a necessary and integral aspect of furthering the field of PPC, particularly in relation to exploring and developing the underlying mechanisms of the many rare and unusual diagnoses that now fit within PPC and in developing and testing treatments that may eventually ease the suffering of the children with these diagnoses and of their families. But along with the medical approach comes resolute adherence to the scientific model of controlled clinical trials as the gold standard, the quantification of symptoms and interventions. Indeed, these approaches have their rightful place. But optimal PPC exists at the crossroads of the traditional scientific approach and the experience of human beings at what is often the most critical time of their lives. PPC needs to be based on both science and art where practical and meaningful insights are gained from the biomedical or psychological approach as well as from the broader humanistic approaches of sociology, history, philosophy, and the person-centered and family-centered foundations of nursing, social work, and theology. On a personal level, I have found there is a camaraderie among PPC team members that seems rare in other fields; we all share a common philosophy that has person/family-centered care at the core. But the pressures of disciplinary, as well as academic and institutional, norms are profound, greatly compounding the personal and professional stress of many who struggle every day to provide optimal PPC—which is, in fact, an additional challenge.

Consequences for Seamless Continuity of Care

Taken together, the foregoing challenges impede the seamless continuity of care across the various dimensions of PPC—particularly respite, transitional, and bereavement care. Where respite care is offered on a regular basis so parents have a break, parents cope better with the demands of caring for their sick child. Respite care is a central aspect of pediatric hospice facilities or home hospice programs, but most parents do not have access to a children's hospice. Periodic admissions to hospital for acute episodes only compound parental responsibilities and worries; having a child in hospital is not respite. The need for respite services has been documented (ACT, 2009). Thus, designating even a few respite beds in acute care settings and developing enhanced home hospice/respite service would facilitate clinicians working across settings to foster the best possible care for families.

Improvements in medical and nursing therapies mean many children with LTC are surviving longer; this trend will continue as medical science advances. Thus, managing the transition of young people from pediatric to adult services must be well coordinated, include the young person and the family in long-range planning, and take into account the young person's developmental and individual needs. One of the few hospices to provide respite for young people is Helen House, now expanded to Helen and Douglas House in Oxford, which opened in 2004. Being able to stay longer in this facility decreases a need for extensive transition services.

Support for grief resulting from the numerous losses that accompany PPC should begin at the time of diagnosis and continue for as long as needed post-death (CHPCA, 2006; EAPC, 2007; NHPCO, 2009). Children's hospices typically offer active grief counseling to families as they encounter the numerous losses that occur along the trajectory of the child's illness. Upon the child's death, the bereavement needs of families are met through support groups and other gatherings that families find helpful. Palliative care programs in hospitals seem to pay less attention to the grief of the families in their care, though some hospitals have bereavement follow-up programs whereby sympathy cards are sent to families of children who died, or annual memorial services are held for the families that wish to attend. Social workers or chaplains often do their best to attend to grieving families, but must typically focus on the needs of other children in their care and cannot attend to grieving family needs in this regard, particularly after they leave the hospital program. Moreover, little attention is directed to the grief responses of the professionals whose daily work involves repeatedly dealing with issues of loss, with support remaining solely informal among team members. Grief takes time, effort, and patience for those grieving and for helpers, and the current system limits the perception of such activities as efficient use of limited resources.

Societal Views

The final challenge exists within the broader society where the certainty of mortality is dealt with through the pervasive presence of violence and death in the news and entertainment media, but where conversation about life's uncertainties surrounding illness, loss, disability, death, and grief is seldom heard and where conversation about children's dying and death is inaudible. Yet within the field of PPC, such conversations are a reality. My hope is that those who are committed to the field of PPC, both emotionally and intellectually, will continue to find the satisfaction in their work that will enable them to forge onward, consistently striving for the vision that guides them, and that as they keep improving the worlds of the families in their care, they will also change the world in which we all live.

REFERENCES

Ablin, A. R., Binger C. M., Stein, R. C., Kushner, J. H., Zoger, S., & Mikkelson C. (1971). A conference with the family of a leukemic child. *American Journal of Diseases of Childhood, 122*(4), 362–364.

American Academy of Pediatrics Committee on Bioethics and Committee on Hospital Care. (2000). Palliative care for children. *Pediatrics, 106*(2), 351–357.

Association for Children with Life-Threatening or Terminal Conditions and Their Families (ACT), Royal College of Paediatrics and Child Health. (2009). *A guide to the development of children's palliative care services* (3rd ed.). Bristol, CT: Author.

Binger, C. M., Ablin, A. R., Feuerstein, R. C., Kushner, J. H., Zoger, S., & Mikkelsen, C. (1969). Childhood leukemia: Emotional impact on the child and family. *New England Journal of Medicine, 280*(8), 414–418.

Bluebond-Langer, M. (1978). *The private worlds of dying children*. Princeton, NJ: Princeton University Press.

Burne, S. R., Dominica, F., & Baum, J. D. (1984). Helen House—A hospice for children: Analysis of the first year. *British Medical Journal Clinical Research Education, 289*, 1165–1168.

Canadian Hospice Palliative Care Association. (2006). *Pediatric hospice palliative care: Guiding principles and norms of practice*. Ottawa, Ontario, Canada: Author. Retrieved from http://www.chpca.net/media/7841/Pediatric_Norms_of_Practice_March_31_2006_English.pdf

Carter, B. S., Levetown, M., & Friebert, S. E. (2011). *Palliative care for infants, children and adolescents: A practical handbook* (2nd ed.). Baltimore, MD: Johns Hopkins University Press.

Catlin, A., & Carter, B. (2002). Creation of a neonatal end of life palliative protocol. *Journal of Perinatology, 22*(3), 184–195.

Chappell, B. (2007). *Children helping children with grief: My path to founding the Dougy Center for grieving children & their families*. Troutdale, OR: New Sage Press.

Corr, C. A., & Corr, D. M. (Eds.). (1985). *Hospice approaches to pediatric care*. New York, NY: Springer Publishing Company.

Davies, B. (1993). Section editor: Paediatric palliative care. In D. Doyle, G. Hanks, & N. MacDonald (Eds.), *Oxford textbook of palliative medicine* (1st ed., pp. 679–733). Oxford, UK: Oxford University Press.

Davies, B., Brenner, P., Orloff, S., Sumner, L., & Worden, W. (2002). Addressing spirituality in pediatric hospice and palliative care. *Journal of Palliative Care, 18*(1), 59–67.

Davies, B., Contro, N., Larson, J., & Widger, K. (2010). Culturally-sensitive information-sharing in pediatric palliative care. *Pediatrics, 125*(4), e859–e865.

Davies, B., Sehring, S., Partridge, J. C., Cooper, B., Hughes, A., Phip, J., . . . Kramer, R. (2008). Barriers to palliative care in children: Perceptions of health care providers. *Pediatrics, 121*, 282–288.

Duff, R. S., & Hollingshead, A. B. (1968). *Sickness and society*. New York, NY: Harper and Row.

End-of-Life Nursing Education Consortium—Pediatric Palliative Care (ELNEC-PPC). (2009). *ELNEC-Pediatric palliative care*. Washington, DC: American Association of Colleges of Nursing. Retrieved from http://www.aacn.nche.edu/elnec/about/pediatric-palliative-care

European Association for Palliative Care; Steering Committee of the EAPC Task Force on Palliative Care for Children and Adolescents. (2007). IMPaCCT: Standards for paediatric palliative care in Europe. *European Journal of Palliative Care, 14*(3), 109–114.

Field, M. J., & Behrman, R. E. (Eds.). (2003). *When children die: Improving palliative and end-of-life care for children and their families*. Washington, DC: National Academies Press.

Fischoff, J., & O'Brien, N. (1976). After the child dies. *Journal of Pediatrics, 88*, 140–146.

Gale, G., & Brooks, A. (2006). Implementing a palliative care program in a newborn intensive care unit. *Advances in Neonatal Care, 6*(1), 37–53.

Glaser, B., & Strauss, A. L. (1966). *Awareness of dying*. Chicago, IL: Aldine.

Goldman, A., Hain, R., & Liben, S. (2012). *Oxford textbook of palliative care for children* (2nd ed.). Oxford, UK: Oxford University Press.

International Children's Palliative Care Network. (2008). *The ICPCN charter of rights for life limited and life threatened children.* Assagay, South Africa: Author. Retrieved from http://www.icpcn.org/icpcn-charter/

International Work Group on Death, Dying and Bereavement. (1993). Palliative care for children. *Death Studies, 17,* 277–280.

Knapp, C., Woodworth, L., Wright, M., Downing, J., Drake, R., Fowler-Kerry, S., . . . Marston, J. (2011). Pediatric palliative care provision around the world: A systematic review. *Pediatric Blood Cancer, 56*(7). doi:10.1002/pbc.23100

Lauer, M. E., Mulhern, R. K., Bohne, J. B., & Camitta, B. M. (1985). Children's perceptions of their sibling's death at home or in hospital: The precursors of differential adjustment. *Cancer Nursing, 8,* 21–27.

Lauer, M. E., Mulhern, R. K., Wallskog, J. M., & Camitta, B. M. (1983). A comparison study of parental adaptation following a child's death at home or in the hospital. *Pediatrics, 71,* 107–112.

Liben, S., Papadatou, D., & Wolfe, J. (2008). Paediatric palliative care: Challenges and emerging ideas. *Lancet, 371,* 852–864.

Malcolm, C., Forbat, L., Anderson, G., Gibson, F., & Hain, R. (2011). Challenging symptom profiles of life-limiting conditions in children: A survey of care professionals and families. *Palliative Medicine, 25*(4), 357–364.

Martinson, I. M., Moldow, D. G., Armstrong, G. D. Henry, W. F. Nesbit, M. E., & Kersey J. H. (1986). Home care for children dying of cancer. *Research in Nursing and Health, 9,* 11–16.

Meier, D. E., & Beresford, L. (2007). Pediatric palliative care offers opportunities for collaboration. *Journal of Palliative Medicine, 10*(2), 284–289.

Moldow, D. G., & Martinson, I. M. (1980). From research to reality—Home care for the dying child. *American Journal of Maternal Child Nursing, 5*(3), 159–166.

National Hospice and Palliative Care Organization. (2009). *Standards of practice for pediatric palliative care and hospice.* Alexandria, VA: Author. Retrieved from http://www.nhpco.org/quality/nhpco's-standards-pediatrics-care

Papadatou, D., & Papadatou, C. (Eds.). (1991). *Children and death.* New York, NY: Hemisphere.

Schorsch, A. (1979). *Images of childhood: An illustrated social history.* New York, NY: Mayflower Books.

Spinetta, J. J., Rigler, D., & Karon, M. (1973). Anxiety in the dying child. *Pediatrics, 52,* 841–845.

Steele, R., & Davies, B. (2006). Impact on parents when a child has a progressive, life-threatening illness. *International Journal of Palliative Nursing, 12*(12), 576–585.

Straatman, L., Cadell, S., Davies, B., Siden, H., & Steele, R. (2008). Paediatric palliative care research in Canada: Development and progress of a new emerging team. *Paediatric Child Health, 13,* 591–594.

Sumner, L. H. (2001). Pediatric care: The hospice perspective. In B. R. Ferrell & N. Coyle (Eds.), *Textbook of palliative nursing* (pp. 556–559). New York, NY: Oxford University Press.

Tietz, W., McSherry, L., & Britt, B. (1977). Family sequelae after a child dies due to cancer. *American Journal of Psychotherapy, 31,* 417–425.

Together for Short Lives. (2013). *Standards framework for children's palliative care* (2nd ed.). Bristol, UK: Author. Retrieved from http://www.togetherforshortlives.org.uk/assets/0000/5003/Standards_framework_update_2013.pdf

Waechter, E. H. (1971). Children's awareness of fatal illness. *American Journal of Nursing, 71,* 1168–1172.

World Health Organization. (2006). *WHO definition of palliative care.* Geneva, Switzerland: Author. Retrieved from http://www.who.int/cancer/palliative/definition/en/

Stephen Connor

13

THE GLOBAL SPREAD OF HOSPICE AND PALLIATIVE CARE

Modern hospice and palliative care is approaching a significant anniversary: In 2017 it will be 50 years since the founding of St Christopher's Hospice. The hospice movement grew very slowly in its early decades, wherease during the last 20 years it has gained acceptance and is now viewed as an essential part of any complete health care system. The National Hospice Organization listed 138 hospice providers in the United States in 1980. By 2012, the number of providers had grown to more than 5,500 (National Hospice and Palliative Care Organization [NHPCO], 2013).

A similar pattern of growth in hospice palliative care occurred in Western Europe and Australia and is now spreading to the rest of the world. Slowly, palliative care is becoming available in low- and middle-income (LMI) countries where the need is greatest. Eighty percent of the need for palliative care is in LMI countries (Connor & Sepulveda, 2014).

In 2011, more than 54 million people died on our planet, over a million a week. That number will grow considerably in the decades ahead as the postwar population dies and population globally increases. According to the World Health Organization (WHO), a bare minimum of 20 million of those will need specialized palliative care, and when considering those who will need palliative care before the year of their death that number will at least double to 40 million (Connor & Sepulveda, 2014).

Most will be old (69%) and some very young (6%). The most common need for palliative care is cardiovascular diseases followed by cancer, respiratory disease, and a long list of other noncommunicable diseases. More than 6% will die from either HIV or tuberculosis (TB) or both. The biggest need for children's palliative care is for congenital disorders and neonatal conditions, followed by a host of complex chronic conditions. A significant number of children die from preventable conditions like protein energy malnutrition. Clearly the need for hospice and palliative care is enormous and now a necessary part of every health care system.

This chapter focuses on the global need for hospice and palliative care and the growing efforts to address the economic, political, and cultural challenges of bringing effective end-of-life care to the millions in need around the world.

PERSONAL REFLECTION

Like many drawn to work in hospice and palliative care, I was drawn to the spiritual and philosophical dimension of care of the dying. I had an epiphany in 1974 while attending the first conference of the Naropa Institute in Boulder, Colorado. During a lecture by Richard Alpert (Ram Das) on the yogis of the *Bhagavad Gita*, a light bulb went off in my head. Ram Das was doing a lecture on death showing pictures of monks meditating in front of corpses and California Highway Patrol footage of mangled bodies in auto accidents and was asking the question, "Why do we have so much difficulty accepting who death is a part of life everywhere?"

I had spent the previous 2 years working in heroin addiction treatment and was becoming cynical about counseling addicts who were sent to treatment under duress. Suddenly I said to myself, "I should be working with cancer patients not drug addicts." When one considers how to use one's time while alive, according to many religions and philosophies, reducing suffering can be considered action that is of the most value. So I returned home to Monterey, California, and eventually helped found the Hospice of the Monterey Peninsula in 1976. From that point I have continued to work in hospice and palliative care without interruption as a psychologist, researcher, executive, consultant, author, educator, and advocate.

FOUNDATIONAL WORK ON THE GLOBAL DEVELOPMENT OF PALLIATIVE CARE

St Christopher's Hospice

It is generally acknowledged that the founding of St Christopher's Hospice outside London in 1967 by Dame Cicely Saunders was the beginning of the worldwide hospice movement. In this chapter, we will refer to both hospice and palliative care as palliative care, even though Dr. Balfour Mount did not coin the term *palliative* until 1975. The word *hospice* in French Canada was related to a house for the poor. I once asked Cicely what her view was on whether we should use the words "hospice" or "palliative care" and she said, "I don't care what you call it, what's important is doing it."

It was obligatory in the early days to make a pilgrimage to St Christopher's to learn about palliative care. I made mine in 1977 and was quite inspired. From its founding, St Christopher's vision was not just to be a place to care for the dying but to be a beacon, a model center for research and education where others could come to learn and be inspired to return home to develop their own forms of palliative care. Cicely Saunders also said, "Go around and see what is being done and then see how your own circumstances can produce another version; there is need for diversity in this field." People from all over the world have continued to come to St Christopher's for knowledge and inspiration and have returned home to build palliative care in their own settings.

Elisabeth Kübler-Ross

Along with Cicely Saunders, Elisabeth Kübler-Ross stands as a key figure in the development of international palliative care. Her book *On Death and Dying* (1969) became an international best seller and opened a door in society to begin to openly talk about issues of death, dying, and bereavement. Although her career was controversial, there is no doubt that her influence on the social conversation was immense. She opened doors for many who were trying to promote a dialogue about death and dying and laid the groundwork for the hospice movement to grow and gain acceptance.

The hospice movement was part of a growing consumer movement in the 1970s that attempted to take back control over critical elements of living, whether it was teaching Lamaze for childbirth, creating purchasing cooperatives and food networks, treating alcoholism, or supporting cancer patients and those facing life-threatening illness. Support groups of every type sprang up for every social concern. From birth to death people wanted to take control back from institutions and, in the case of hospice, it was to help terminally ill patients to be able to stay at home, cared for by their families rather than being in hospitals and health care facilities.

Elisabeth (as she preferred to be called) also created a network of Elisabeth Kübler-Ross centers around the world on the basis of a model program that was started in Southern California called Shanti Nilaya (home of peace). These centers still operate today in Austria, Belgium, France, Germany, Japan, Mexico, Netherlands, and Switzerland.

International Work Group on Death, Dying, and Bereavement

Both Elisabeth Kübler-Ross and Cicely Saunders were founding members of the International Work Group on Death, Dying, and Bereavement (IWG), which was formed in November 1974 out of an international convocation of workers in the field of death, dying, and bereavement in Columbia, Maryland (www.iwgddb.org). The convocation was organized and funded by Ars Moriendi, an organization devoted to the study of the professional response to death, dying, and bereavement.

The IWG built on the work of Cicely Saunders's development of the hospice movement; Herman Feifel's work reported on in *The Meaning of Death*; in 1958; Elisabeth Kübler-Ross's work; John Hinton's book *Dying* in 1966; Colin Murray Parkes's work with London widows and publication of his book *Bereavement* in 1972; a meeting of Kübler-Ross, Saunders, and Parkes in 1965; and conferences organized by Robert Fulton in Minnesota in 1967 and Robert Kastenbaum in Detroit in 1969.

The initial goals and purposes of the IWG were to (1) conduct meetings of workers active in the field of death, dying, and bereavement, whose level is sufficiently high that the atmosphere is one of shared collegiality and in which there is no audience; (2) stay in the forefront of the field of death, dying, and bereavement; (3) promote *Wissenchaft* (sharing and studying what we know); (4) be international in scope, taking into account local and national issues but transcending them; and (5) be catalytic.

The mission statement of the IWG says it is "a nonprofit organization that supports leaders in the field of death, dying and bereavement in their efforts to stimulate and enhance innovative ideas, research, and practice." Its vision is "a world where dying, death, and bereavement are an open part of all cultures." IWG's "defining value without which nobody can qualify for membership of the IWG is a capacity for leadership in some aspect of the field of Death, Dying & Bereavement. This may reflect leadership in the ideas and theories that guide us, leadership in the research that provides justification for these ideas and the practices that follow, innovation reflecting the application of these ideas, communication of the ideas to others, and/or organisation of services based upon them."

Today the IWG consists of 171 leaders in death, dying, and bereavement from nations throughout the world. The group meets approximately every 18 months to form workgroups that push the boundaries of thought and understanding of the human encounter with death. IWG is a kind of incubator for leaders in this field.

International Association of Hospice and Palliative Care

Dr. Josefina Magno founded the International Association of Hospice and Palliative Care (IAHPC) in 1980, initially as the International Hospice Institute, later the American Academy of Hospice and Palliative Medicine and the International Hospice Institute and College (IHIC; www.hospicecare.com). In 1996, Derek Doyle was elected the first president of the College of the IHIC. Dr. Doyle brought an international perspective by stressing that IHIC's objective was not to promote a unique palliative care model but to encourage and enable each country, according to its resources and conditions, to develop its own model of palliative care provision. Thus, the IAHPC was formed in 1997 to support this goal.

Today the IAHPC is a leading international organization advocating for the development of palliative care globally. They have a number of ongoing programs to support palliative professionals globally, including support for traveling palliative care scholars to do palliative care training and for professionals from LMI countries to attend international conferences. They have worked with the World Health Organization (WHO) to improve the model list of essential medicines, have developed an international directory of providers and educational programs, contribute to improved access to opioids through the United Nations (UN) Commission on Narcotic Drugs, have developed a palliative care encyclopedia, and have made many other contributions to the field.

National Hospice and Palliative Care Organization

The National Hospice and Palliative Care Organization (formerly the National Hospice Organization [NHO]) is the largest membership organization for hospice and palliative care providers in the United States. NHO was founded in 1978 to improve the care of the terminally ill in the country. The NHPCO was one of the first national organizations formed to promote the development of hospice through support for state associations and individual providers. Currently all U.S. state associations and most hospice providers are members of NHPCO.

The first hospice standards for providers were developed by NHO in 1979, and NHPCO has continued to provide leadership to hospice providers throughout the United States and has contributed significantly to international palliative care development. In 2004, the Foundation for Hospices in Sub-Saharan Africa (FHSSA) affiliated with the NHPCO. FHSSA is unique in that it initiates, maintains, and sustains active relationships between frontline organizations in Africa and the United States. This partnering program now has almost 100 members.

Montreal conference
The International Congress on Palliative Care was first held in 1974. This conference has continued to be held in Montreal every other year since and has attracted thousands of health care professionals to the field of palliative care. Primarily a clinical conference, attending this conference has been another right of passage for those interested in the care of the dying. Many of those attending became instant converts to the field. Dr. Balfour Mount, one of the founders of palliative care, was the leader of this conference until his recent retirement.

End-of-Life Nursing Education Consortium and Education for
Physicians on End-of-Life Care
These training programs are standardized basic palliative care education programs for physicians and nurses. These curricula cover the basics of pain assessment and treatment, management of other symptoms, including respiratory distress, nausea and vomiting, bowel obstruction, skin and bowel care, determining prognosis, breaking bad news, cultural and spiritual considerations, last days of life, grief and bereavement, and other subjects.

The important thing about Education for Physicians on End-of-Life Care (EPEC) and End-of-Life Nursing Education Consortium (ELNEC) is that they have provided consistent educational content to ensure that basic skills are conveyed. In addition to didactic material, there are many case studies, film vignettes, and exercises to engage the participants. Though originally developed to teach in the United States, these programs have been translated into several languages and have been very useful in helping to spread palliative care throughout the world.

Association for Death Education and Counseling

In 1976, a group of interested educators and clinicians organized the Forum for Death Education and Counseling. Over the years, the organization grew to become the Association for Death Education and Counseling (ADEC; www.adec .org). ADEC is the oldest interdisciplinary organization in the field of dying, death, and bereavement. ADEC's primary goal is to enhance the ability of professionals and laypeople to meet the needs of those with whom they work in death education and grief counseling. ADEC holds an annual conference, conducts webinars, and promotes research and practice.

The mission of ADEC is to be an international, professional organization dedicated to promoting excellence and recognizing diversity in death education, care of the dying, grief counseling, and research in thanatology. Based on quality research, theory, and practice, the association provides information, support, and resources to its international, multicultural, multidisciplinary membership and to the public.

CURRENT WORK ON DEVELOPMENT OF PALLIATIVE CARE

Regional Hospice Palliative Care Associations

The spread of hospice palliative care globally has been assisted greatly through the development of national, especially regional, associations. The first regional association was the European Association for Palliative Care (www.eapcnet.eu), formed in 1988 to "bring together many voices to forge a vision of excellence in palliative care that meets the needs of patients and families." The EAPC consists of 55 associations in 32 countries.

The Asia Pacific Hospice Palliative Care Network (APHN; www.aphn.org) evolved over a series of meetings from March 1995 until May 2001. The mission of the APHN is to promote access to quality hospice and palliative care for all in the Asia Pacific region. The APHN consists of 193 organizations and 1,220 individuals from 33 countries.

The Latin American Association for Palliative Care (Asociación Latino Americana de Cuidado Paliativo [ALCP]) was established in Buenos Aires, Argentina, in April 2001 by six palliative care professionals from the region. The mission of the Association is to promote the development of palliative care in Latin America and the Caribbean by bringing together health professionals interested in improving the quality of life of patients with incurable progressive diseases, as well as their families.

The African Palliative Care Association was formed in 2004 in Arusha, Tanzania, and has its headquarters in Kampala, Uganda. The African Palliative Care Association's (APCA) mission is to ensure palliative care is widely understood, integrated into health systems at all levels, and underpinned by evidence in order to reduce pain and suffering across Africa, with the vision of promoting access to palliative care for all in Africa.

The regional associations have been responsible for helping to establish and strengthen the more than 70 national associations worldwide. The growing palliative care movement globally was strengthened through the formation of all these provider groups and other professional associations. Each association speaks for palliative care in its country or region, but what is lacking is a strong voice to speak for palliative care in the international arena.

Worldwide Hospice Palliative Care Alliance

The Worldwide Hospice Palliative Care Alliance (WHPCA; originally the World-wide Palliative Care Alliance) was formed to be this voice in the international arena. When major policy was undertaken at the United Nations and its many bodies, including the General Assembly, the Economic and Social Council, the WHO, the United Nations Children's Fund (UNICEF), Commission on Narcotic Drugs, UN Office on Drugs and Crime, World Bank Group, and so forth, no one representing palliative care in an organized way participated.

The WHPCA (www.thewpca.org) is an alliance of the regional and national hospice and palliative care associations worldwide. The principal purpose of the WHPCA is to advocate for hospice and palliative care. To bring policy issues before the international palliative care leadership and to ensure that palliative care is included in policies, such as those now focusing on noncommunicable diseases, HIV, drug-resistant TB care, care and support programs for adults and children, social protection, access to opioids, universal health coverage, health system strengthening, and many more significant policy issues.

In addition, WHPCA is home to World Hospice and Palliative Care Day (WHPCD; www.worldday.org) and the international news service "ehospice" (www.ehospice.com). Each year on the second Saturday in October, events are held worldwide to promote hospice awareness for WHPCD according to an agreed theme.

Mapping and Report Cards

A number of influential reports have been developed to track the development of palliative care globally. One of the earliest of these was a report from the International Observatory on End of Life Care at Lancaster University in the United Kingdom. This report, commissioned by the WPCA, divided all countries in the world into four categories:

- Those countries with no palliative care services and no champions interested in its development
- Those countries with palliative care champions that had not yet begun to provide palliative care services
- Those countries that are currently providing palliative care that is outside the mainstream health care system
- Those countries where palliative care is provided and has begun to be integrated into the health care system

At the time of the publication of this report (Wright, Wood, Lynch, & Clarke, 2008), 50% of countries were yet to provide any palliative care.

Another influential report was published in 2010 by the Economist Intelligence Unit on the quality of dying in 40 countries (OECD [Organisation for Economic Co-operation and Development] and BRICS [Brazil, Russia, India, China, and South Africa] countries). This report took in all factors associated with dying in a particular country, including palliative care. Not surprisingly the United Kingdom ranked first in this quality-of-death index. The most influential report on palliative care development is the new Global Atlas of Palliative Care at the End of Life, which includes an update to the global mapping exercise done in 2006.

The Global Atlas of Palliative Care at the End of Life

The Global Atlas of Palliative Care at the End of Life (Connor & Sepulveda, 2014) is a newly published book that paints a picture of palliative care worldwide. The *Atlas* addresses nine key issues for global palliative care:

1. What is palliative care?
   Current WHO definitions of palliative care are very broad and not operational. There is a need to clarify that palliative care is not just for the dying but for patients with chronic as well as life-threatening illness, there is no time or prognostic limit on the delivery of palliative care, palliative care is needed at all levels of care, and that palliative care is needed in all settings.
2. Why is palliative care a human rights issue?
   The basis for palliative care as a human right is found in the International Human Right to Health from the International Covenant on Economic, Social and Cultural Rights (ICESCR) calling for the "right of everyone to the enjoyment of the highest attainable standard of physical and mental health" (Office of the High Commissioner for Human Rights, 1996, Article 12.1).
3. What are the main diseases requiring palliative care?
   Prior to publication of the *Atlas*, WHO had only published on the need for palliative care for cancer and HIV. Now the full listing of diseases requiring palliative care is given, including cardiovascular diseases, chronic obstructive pulmonary disease, diabetes, dementias, kidney disease, liver disease, motor neuron disease, and drug-resistant TB. For children, congenital anomalies are a major cause of need for palliative care as are neonatal conditions, cancer, endocrine disorders, protein energy malnutrition, and so forth.
4. What is the need for palliative care?
   According to the WHO, a bare minimum of 20 million people need palliative care at the end of life, which increases to at least 40 million when considering those needing palliative care before the end of life.
5. What are the barriers to palliative care?
   The WHO public health model is used to understand the barriers to palliative care.
6. Where is palliative care currently available?
   A mapping exercise was done to describe the development of palliative care for each country in the world. In 2006, only 50% of countries were delivering some palliative care. By 2011, that number had increased to 58%.
7. What are the models of palliative care worldwide?
   The *Atlas* describes seven model palliative care programs in all regions of the world.
8. What resources are devoted to palliative care?
   A listing of financial resources devoted to palliative care is given along with philanthropic and bilateral support, research support, and education resources.
9. What is the way forward?
   The *Atlas* offers an advocacy agenda for advancing the field of palliative care.

   The WHO and the WHPCA jointly published the *Atlas* as an advocacy document that sets a benchmark for palliative care globally. The *Atlas* provides a baseline from which to measure progress in palliative care development worldwide. Major findings include that 80% of the need for palliative care is in LMI countries whereas 80% of the existing palliative care is provided in only 20 of the most developed countries. A minimum of 40 million patients need palliative care annually, including 20 million at the end of life; fewer than 10% of these patients are receiving any form of specialized palliative care.

There are many barriers to palliative care development, and they include lack of access to essential medicines, particularly oral morphine; lack of education for professionals and the public in palliative care; lack of resources to implement palliative care; and lack of policies that support inclusion of palliative care in health care systems. The lack of access to morphine is an especially difficult issue. According to a recent study (Seya, Gelders, Achara, Milani, & Scholten, 2011), only 7% of countries have adequate access to opioids. In 83% of countries, there is low to nonexistent access, 4% have moderate access, and 6% have insufficient data to know. Morphine-equivalent opioid use per capita is used to measure consumption using data from the International Narcotics Control Board. The average consumption of morphine per capita globally is only about 6 mg, whereas in the United States average consumption is almost 74 mg.

According to the *Atlas*, at present there are an estimated 16,000 hospice or palliative care teams worldwide serving about 3 million patients and their families annually. If we compare that to the estimated need of 40 million patients, then only about 7% of the need is being met, certainly less than 10%. These programs are concentrated in North America, Western Europe, and Australia, whereas the greatest need for palliative care is in the LMI countries. Clearly, the *Atlas* tells us that a huge amount of work is needed to close this gap.

The *Atlas* can be downloaded at http://www.thewpca.org/resources/global-atlas-of-palliative-care/

World Health Organization

The WHO is the directing and coordinating authority for health within the United Nations system. It is responsible for providing leadership on global health matters, shaping the health research agenda, setting norms and standards, articulating evidence-based policy options, providing technical support to countries, and monitoring and assessing health trends.

Recently the WHO Executive Board passed a resolution to provide guidance to member states on the inclusion of palliative care in health systems. Key recommendations from this resolution included the following:

- Develop policies to integrate palliative care into health system across all levels
- Ensure adequate domestic funding and allocation of human resources
- Integrate training into curricula for health workers at basic, intermediate, and specialist levels and provide continuing education on palliative care
- Assess domestic palliative care needs
- Review and revise drug control legislation as needed
- Include pain and palliative care sections into national essential medicines lists.

Further, the resolution calls on WHO to undertake the following activities and to report back to the World Health Assembly in 2016:

- Ensure palliative care is integrated into all relevant global disease control and health system plans
- Include palliative care into country and regional cooperation plans

- Update or develop guidelines on palliation, with specific mention of guidelines on treatment of pain
- Develop and strengthen guidelines on integration of palliative care into health system
- Support member states in reviewing and improving drug legislation
- Work with INCB to support accurate estimates for opioid analgesics
- Collaborate with UNICEF to promote pediatric palliative care
- Monitor global situation of palliative care
- Work with member states to encourage adequate funding and improved cooperation for palliative care programs and research
- Encourage research on palliative care models
- Report back in 2016 on implementation of resolution

These actions and activities will guide the future development of palliative care worldwide and one hopes will be more than words but will become actions that can be monitored and evaluated.

CHALLENGES AND HOPES FOR THE FUTURE

There are many challenges that remain for global palliative care development yet there is reason for optimism in that finally substantial progress will be made. If all people have the possibility of a good-enough death, then it can be said that we've succeeded; however, that hope is still many years away.

WHO Public Health Model

The WHO public health model is the roadmap for developing palliative care globally (Figure 13.1). These four major ingredients are time and again the real goals for achieving on-the-ground palliative care development in each country. It is essential that palliative care is included in policy, that essential palliative care medications are available, and that competent education is available at all levels. These ingredients are needed so that palliative care providers can then implement services to those who need them.

Policy
The kinds of policy support that are needed to establish palliative care in a country include the following:

- Assessment of the need for palliative care in the country
- Development of standards for palliative care programs
- Development of clinical guidelines and protocols
- A national strategy for implementing palliative care
- Modification of laws and regulations to allow for palliative care to be delivered and to eliminate barriers to accessing medicines and care
- Recognition of palliative care as a specialization in health care
- Inclusion of palliative care in national health plans, including those for cancer, noncommunicable diseases, HIV, TB, and so forth.

Doing this work and influencing those in national leadership positions requires a long-term commitment to building palliative care. It requires palliative care leaders and champions who are willing to make sacrifices, and it requires a lot of patience. Fortunately, international bodies like the WHO are finally calling on countries to do exactly what is necessary.

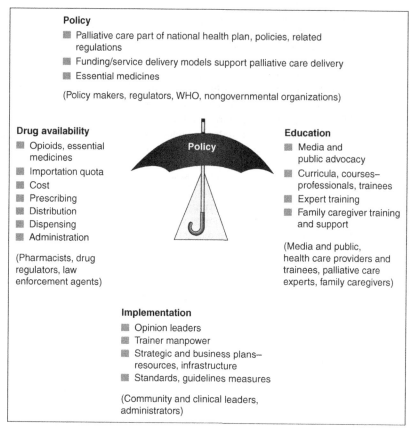

Policy
■ Palliative care part of national health plan, policies, related regulations
■ Funding/service delivery models support palliative care delivery
■ Essential medicines

(Policy makers, regulators, WHO, nongovernmental organizations)

Drug availability
■ Opioids, essential medicines
■ Importation quota
■ Cost
■ Prescribing
■ Distribution
■ Dispensing
■ Administration

(Pharmacists, drug regulators, law enforcement agents)

Education
■ Media and public advocacy
■ Curricula, courses– professionals, trainees
■ Expert training
■ Family caregiver training and support

(Media and public, health care providers and trainees, palliative care experts, family caregivers)

Implementation
■ Opinion leaders
■ Trainer manpower
■ Strategic and business plans– resources, infrastructure
■ Standards, guidelines measures

(Community and clinical leaders, administrators)

FIGURE 13.1 The Public Health Model for Palliative Care.
Source: Stjernsward et al. (2007). Used with permission.

Medicine availability

According to the international human right to health, expressed in the UN International Covenant on Economic, Social, and Cultural Rights, everyone should have access to the medications he or she needs. The disparities in access to opioids stem from misinterpretation of the 1961 Single Convention on Narcotic Drugs. Although the Single Convention called for a balance between prevention of illicit use of these medicines and access for medical and scientific purposes, almost all of the emphasis within countries has gone to restricting access to prevent illicit use with very little attention to the need for medical use. This has caused a huge problem globally as already noted.

What is needed is to restore this balance so that access for medical use is restored to its equal place with actions to prevent misuse. This will require countries to change laws and regulations that, for instance, say that only oncologists can prescribe opioids, or that prescriptions must be countersigned by the head of the hospital or health care institution to be valid, or that patients can only receive limited amounts per day or per prescription.

Education

In many respects, we don't need to create palliative care as a new and separate care delivery system as we need to educate existing health care providers to provide basic palliative care services. The percentage of patients who need specialized palliative care services has been estimated to be approximately 35%. That means that primary health care workers could probably care for two thirds of the palliative care patients if they had the skills to do so. To achieve this, it will be necessary for every nurse, physician, social worker, psychologist, and other therapists to receive at least basic palliative care training in school.

In addition to professional training, there are large numbers of professionals who are practicing or are in postgraduate status who need palliative care education. Palliative care needs to be added to ongoing continuing education and for those who wish to become a specialist or subspecialist. In LMI countries, qualifying clinicians to practice and to teach palliative care is a special problem that will require training abroad as well as ongoing mentoring.

Professionals need training that must be done in parallel with community education and engagement. If a physician doesn't have access to morphine or isn't trained to prescribe it, it is likely the patient will suffer. Likewise, if a physician is able and willing to prescribe but the patient refuses to take the medication, the patient will suffer. Over and over in different countries, it has been shown that we need to teach the public that they have a right to relief from pain and that they should demand that their physicians should give them relief, which should be readily available. The UN Special Rapporteur on torture has said that denying access to pain relief can amount to inhuman and degrading treatment.

Implementation

When all the ingredients for palliative care, namely, policy, medicines, and education, are available, we still need to be able to have quality palliative care services to deliver the care. This can take many years. In the United States, after almost 40 years, about 45% of all people who die of all causes receive at least 1 day of hospice care and many more receive some palliative care outside hospice in hospitals and from palliative care-trained clinicians. Still there are many patients who do not receive hospice or palliative care who need it and for those who do, it is often so near death that we call it brink-of-death care.

The median length of service in hospice in the United States is only 18 days. About one third of all admitted hospice patients receive 7 days or less of care (NHPCO, 2013). There are many social, psychological, cultural, and financial barriers to delivering palliative care to those who need care.

In closing, we believe that access to palliative care is a human right. Painful dying is not inevitable and the means are at hand to relieve most suffering. What is required is the willingness to face what is most difficult for humans. To acknowledge death as part of living and to bring the now considerable palliative care knowledge and skills to bear to help our patients and families to live as well as they can in the shadow of death.

REFERENCES

Connor, S., & Sepulveda, C. (Eds.). (2014). *Global atlas of palliative care at the end of life*. London, UK: World Health Organization/Worldwide Palliative Care Alliance.

Economist Intelligence Unit. (2010). *The quality of death: Ranking end of life care across the world*. London, UK: Author.

Feifel, H. (Ed). (1958). *The meaning of death*. New York, NY: McGraw-Hill.

Hinton, J. (1966). *Dying*. Baltimore, MD: Penguin Books.

Kübler-Ross, E. (1969). *On death and dying*. New York, NY: Macmillan.

National Hospice and Palliative Care Organization. (2013). *NHPCO's facts and figures: Hospice care in America (2013 ed.)* Alexandria, VA: Author.

Office of the High Commissioner for Human Rights. (1996). *International Covenant on Economic, Social and Cultural Rights*. Retrieved form http://www.ohchr.org/EN/ProfessionalInterest/Pages/CESCR.aspx

Parkes, C. M. (1972). *Bereavement: Studies of grief in adult life*. New York, NY: International Universities Press.

Seya, M. J., Gelders, S. F., Achara, O. U., Milani, B., & Scholten, W. (2011). A first comparison between the consumption of and the need for opioid analgesics at country, regional, and global levels. *Journal of Pain and Palliative Care Pharmacotherapy, 25*(1), 6–18.

Stjernsward, J., Foley, K., & Ferris, F. (2007). The public health strategy for palliative care. *Journal of Pain and Symptom Management, 33*(5), 486–493.

Wright, M., Wood, J., Lynch, T., & Clarke, D. (2008). Mapping levels of palliative care development: A global view. *Journal of Pain and Symptom Management, 35*(5), 469–485.

Vanderlyn R. Pine **14**

DEATH AND FUNERAL SERVICE

Growing up in the 1940s, I used to watch funerals on an almost weekly basis. They seemed completely normal and very important. My dad and grandfather were funeral directors, and their funeral home was in my backyard. Lots of people came to funerals back then in my small hometown, and my dad and grandfather knew almost all of them. It was obvious to me that their work was of great significance because, among other things, all of the clergymen would greet them fondly when they came to conduct a funeral, and they often would comment to me what fine men they were.

My dad and grandfather were held in special esteem by everybody in town. It seemed strange to me that when there was *not* an actual or imminent death, people joked about the "undertaker" and teased me about death and funerals. Other kids were the worst, but I heard it from adults as well. As I grew older, I learned to smile but not to enjoy nicknames like "Digger" or "Pine Box." I heard many death-themed jokes more times than I can or wish to count. As a teenager, I planned never to be a funeral director, and often said so. I do not recall having an aversion to death, but I definitely did not want to be a funeral director with the constant teasing that had become so familiar.

Although my family had been relatively free of deaths, my grandfather Pine died in December 1952, my grandmother Pine in December 1954, and in January 1957, my dad died suddenly and unexpectedly. Actually, while he was directing a funeral, he fell dead just before the ceremony was about to begin. My death-free life had changed dramatically in a roughly 4-year period, and I now did not have a paternal side of my family.

After my dad's death, I withdrew from Dartmouth College and went home to operate the funeral business with my mom. Never had I spoken to my father or mother about the operation of the funeral home nor had we discussed their attitudes toward death, funerals, loss, or grief. I went to funeral school, became a licensed funeral director, and worked for several years in the family business.

Throughout the early 1960s, I took courses at a local college in English literature and creative writing, always hoping that someday I would be able to finish college as an English major. As time passed, however, I came to realize that it was possible to study death and society. As I delved into the subject, I discovered that a book edited by Herman Feifel (1959), with essays written in the mid-1950s had set the social science ball rolling.

In 1963, a special edition of *The American Behavioral Scientist* published a collection of essays about death, further paving the way for interested scholars. Year 1965 was a watershed year for death studies with publication of books by Fulton (1965), Glaser and Strauss (1965), and Gorer (1965). These sources became critical underpinnings of my own emerging interest in dying and death. In 1966, I was able to return to Dartmouth as a full-time student. I changed my major and became totally absorbed in sociology. My interest became more sharply focused on death-related issues. That fall semester, I was asked to teach a course called "Death" in the Dartmouth Experimental College. I gave lectures on death and funeral behavior and prepared working papers on dying and death. I received an AB degree from Dartmouth in 1967.

After a year of graduate study at New York University (NYU), I returned to Dartmouth as a special graduate student in 1968 and became a research and teaching assistant for James A. Davis. That fall, a tragic event exposed me to a different kind of social research. There was an airplane crash near Dartmouth, killing 32 people. The local funeral director was challenged by the immensity of the tragedy, and he asked if I would help him. I worked with him as a funeral director and was able to investigate aspects of multiple death disasters on the scene that would have been inaccessible to other researchers. The experience was reported in my master's thesis and later as a research report and then a published paper (Pine, 1974b).

In 1968, I received a National Institute of Health, Public Health Service Pre-Doctoral Research Fellowship and returned to NYU to complete my doctorate. In 1969, my first published article appeared on cross-cultural funeral customs. Without knowing it at the time, I fortuitously was becoming a member of the emerging "death studies" field. I had become a friend of Herman Feifel, Bob Fulton, Edgar Jackson, Howard Raether, and others who were studying and writing about dying, death, grief, and bereavement. I received a PhD degree from NYU in 1971.

In 1970, I was appointed as an assistant professor of sociology at SUNY, New Paltz. Soon, I submitted a detailed, well-documented proposal to introduce a new course to be called "Death in American Society." Most of the faculty concurred with my logical presentation about the value of such a course, the overall rationale, the curriculum of what I hoped to cover, and the extensive reading list I had prepared. A few faculty members were skeptical of such a taboo topic as a college course. One even made the same kind of nasty teasing comments that had so turned me off about funeral directors when I was a child.

After in-depth talks with Feifel, Fulton, Bob Kastenbaum, Gene Knott, and Dan Leviton, by then good friends and conversational colleagues, I designed a lecture course that I hoped would attract a fair number of students. In the inaugural fall semester of 1973, the class opened with 237 students enrolled. The course Death in American Society became a popular staple of the sociology department for the next 25 years until my retirement. By then, I had taught more than 3,700 college students about dying, death, grief, and bereavement.

HISTORICAL ANTECEDENTS TO POST–WORLD WAR II FUNERAL DIRECTING

The earliest American death workers had been members of other trades or occupational groups, and "undertaking" was largely a part-time job. In colonial America, most of the activities following a death were carried out by family members or friends. A coffin was purchased from a local cabinetmaker or carpenter, a horse-drawn wagon or hearse rented from a local livery stable, and the grave dug in a small church or community cemetery by family and/or friends. Depending on the ethnic, religious, and/or family customs that prevailed for the bereaved, there were mourning activities that followed community mores.

In the 19th century, death care became more specialized, and it became increasingly common for items of merchandise and transportation to be provided by a person who was willing to "undertake" the provision of funeral activities.

These so-called "undertakers" often combined the death activities with a cabinet-making business that made coffins or a livery stable business that provided horse-drawn hearses.

During the Civil War, the practice of battlefield embalming of dead soldiers enabled the return home of their bodies. As a result, American families, especially in the North, became aware of the possibility of temporarily preserving the dead by embalming. This new funerary practice became more widely known following the assassination of President Abraham Lincoln, who had been embalmed and whose body was viewed by hundreds of thousands of citizens as he was transported by train from Washington, DC to his burial place in Springfield, Illinois. The train stopped at cities and railroad stops on the way, with public viewing of his body on the train at every stop.

Funeral customs in the early years of the 20th century were tinged with Victorian era and post–Civil War practices. Infant, child, adolescent, and younger adult mortality was common and especially powerful influences on the emerging practices of that era. Specifically, in 1900, 53.4% of all the deaths were of children between 0 and 14 years of age, 17.4% of the deaths were of adolescents and young adults ages 15 through 44, and about 12.7% of the deaths were of middle-age adults ages 45 through 64. Only about 16.5% of all deaths were of people 65 years and older. Put differently, more than 70% of all deaths were of children, adolescents, and younger adults (U.S. Bureau of the Census, 1900).

As a result, many of the funeral customs of this era were intended to note the deaths of these younger folks. Such deaths were sad and mournful occurrences, certainly not viewed as celebratory. It was an era in which it was common for parents to bury their children. In the post–World War II era, the age of those who died inexorably became older, and children became increasingly likely to handle the deaths of their parents. Honoring the dead evolved to reflect the demographics of decedents being older, and it became more acceptable to celebrate a life well-lived of an elderly person. By midcentury in 1950, the proportions of deaths for each age group had shifted dramatically. The proportion of deaths in the age category from 0 to 14 was down to about 9.4%, those aged from 15 to 44 years was also down to about 10.2%, about 27.8% of all deaths were of adults from age 45 to 64, and deaths of people 65 years and older was then up to about 52.6%. This is a huge reversal from 1900 (U.S. Bureau of the Census, 1950).

THE CHANGING ROLE OF FUNERAL DIRECTORS FOLLOWING WORLD WAR II

In this dramatically changed social and demographic environment, it is not surprising that funeral directors came to evaluate their changing role. The old, established traditional funeral practices with dark drapes surrounding the casket and other funeral paraphernalia that once had played an important role in helping people and communities deal with the deaths of younger people, now seemed dismal, not fulfilling, and less satisfying. After the war, the social and demographic changes forced an eventual reevaluation of just how appropriate time-honored funeral practices could be in a demographically altered contemporary society. In spite of the changes, there remained efforts to honor the fallen military who had been killed or died as a result of the war.

Following the war, the National Funeral Directors Association (NFDA) began to adapt to changing times. The Association, which had been founded in 1881, had a long history as a trade association whose primary focus was providing funeral directors, undertakers, embalmers, and others in the field exposition-like annual conventions to show new products, including caskets, vaults, memorial products, hearses, limousines, stretchers, chemical products, and emerging embalming techniques. Starting in 1951, the annual convention began to include an educational component. Initially, postwar educational programs were aimed primarily at technical proficiency in embalming, restorative treatments, and similar matters.

In the early 1950s, NFDA was led by the visionary Howard C. Raether, who had recently become the Association's executive director. One of his initial goals was to heighten funeral director awareness of the social–psychological importance of death and the value of the funeral. Raether was a committed proponent of the benefits of public ceremonial activities. He recognized that there were important functional aspects of funeral practices that went far beyond embalming the dead and "undertaking" the attendant activities. Raether sought scholars, clergy, and academics who were doing research and writing about the funeral and the changing role of the funeral director in postwar American society.

SCHOLARSHIP ABOUT FUNERALS, DEATH, GRIEF, AND BEREAVEMENT

Among early scholars of death were individuals who recognized and extolled the therapeutic value of the funeral both for individuals and for society. Early on, there were the lectures, seminars, and writings of noted academics and authors of books and articles on death, such as Edgar N. Jackson, Paul E. Irion, and Robert L. Fulton. All three had studied aspects of dying, death, funerals, and the role of the funeral director in contemporary American society.

Furthermore, all of them were familiar with the writings of the intellectual giants of the early 20th century and the World War II era, including Malinowski (1948), Freud (1917/1957), and Lindemann (1944). In their works were many crucial bits of knowledge and observations about funerary behavior spanning the fields of psychiatry, anthropology, psychology, and sociology. Many of the ideas developed by Freud were well known to Jackson, Irion, and Fulton, all of whom encouraged funeral directors to become familiar with some of his principal theories. In Freud's writings were references to the psychosocial elements of mourning and grief in funerary behaviors that he thought were normal and therapeutic.

From the anthropological literature, there was the early work of the Polish anthropologist Bronislaw Malinowski who examined grief and bereavement in a cross-cultural milieu. Malinowski's (1948) collection of essays in the book *Magic, Science, and Religion* focused on his work with native cultures, how they deal with death in their own particular society, and how many of the specifics exist in some related form across societies. Malinowski emphasized that mourning behavior serves to demonstrate the emotions of the bereaved and the loss experienced by the whole group. The rituals of death reinforce as well as reflect the natural feelings of the survivors. Therefore, it is partly through funeral rituals that a social cohort comprehends death.

Deriving from Malinowski were the works of one of his leading students. Anthropologist Raymond Firth (1964) explained in his book *Elements of Social Organization* that there are societal practices that help resolve ambivalent feelings about death. Firth states that the funeral provides three elements to the living. The first element is the resolution of uncertainties in the behavior of the immediate kin. The funeral provides relatives an opportunity to display their grief publicly and establishes a time for mourning and providing the bereaved social support.

Firth's second element is the fulfillment of social consequence. To do this, the ceremony helps to reinforce the appropriate attitudes of the members of society to each other. Although it focuses on the dead person, the funeral emphasizes the value of the living. The third element is the economic aspect. Firth explains that every funeral involves the expenditure of money, goods, services, and/or other assets. In this sense, the exchange process is important to the bereaved on a tangible social and economic level. Bereaved people may feel the need to make restitution to the deceased by purchasing such nonabstract items as funeral feasts, funeral merchandise, religious services, memorial items, dedicated buildings, and other legacies.

Because of the important insights of psychiatrist Lindemann (1944) in his classic article, "Symptomatology and Management of Acute Grief," Jackson, Irion, and Fulton used many of his concepts to help assist funeral directors to realize the value of their work. Although he did not write any known treatises about funerals per se, Lindemann expressed a belief in the therapeutic symbolic value of funeral ceremony. In his clinical practice near the end of World War II and then afterward, if Lindemann encountered a patient who was experiencing unresolved grief or apparently absent grief following a traumatic or war-related death or relationship with a soldier who was missing in action in which there was no dead body, he would take that person to a funeral mass of an unconnected military decedent. Often, while at the mass, the patient would become overwhelmed by feelings of grief and loss, and Lindemann would use this experience as the start of a symbolic step toward trying to resolve the grief for the lost loved one.

Noted pastoral psychologist Edgar N. Jackson (1957) was the author of an influential book entitled *Understanding Grief: Its Roots, Dynamics, and Treatment*. Jackson's intellectual and erudite analysis of grief and its many dimensions was highly readable because of his extensive use of concrete examples of individuals who had serious grief-related issues. His writing style was less formidable than that of either Freud or Lindemann, and readers could understand his observations and illustrations with ease. Moreover, Jackson was a superb public speaker who could enthrall an audience of funeral directors, as well as captivate a congregation of churchgoers who came to hear his Sunday sermons.

Jackson became a clergy consultant for NFDA in the late 1950s, and he dedicated many hours explaining his practical approaches to resolving grief to funeral directors as well as to the elected leadership of NFDA. Drawing from his academic book, Jackson wrote a trade version with the simple title *You and Your Grief* (1962) that was a self-help guide to comfort people going through the painful process of grieving over the death of someone loved. Many funeral directors not only read Jackson's books, but they also bought them in bulk and gave complimentary copies to bereaved families to help them face the grief process with guidance.

Theologian Paul E. Irion (1954) published *The Funeral and the Mourners*, which raised questions about the place and value of the funeral in modern society, especially given the early emerging evidence of trends that showed opposition to traditional religious and sacred funeral customs and practices, many of which were abstract and not "helpful" compared with being "proper." He looked at the funeral as it relates to the particular needs of a mourning person. Irion's approach initially was questioned by some funeral directors who were hesitant to change their practices. However, many existing funeral customs and practices did not deal with the shifting demographic patterns in which those who died were "elderly" rather than young or middle aged.

Irion (1966) wrote another book entitled *The Funeral, Vestige or Value?* His major thesis was that the funeral, as a vehicle for comforting bereaved people, would have "value" for people if it addressed several important dimensions. Contrarily, too many traditional aspects of the funeral remained little more than remnants of long-ago practices that once held value for people but are today mere "vestiges" of past customs. Irion identifies anthropological, social-psychological, psychological, and theological dimensions that interact to make funerals meaningful. These dimensions have become increasingly important as recent authors weighed in on the funeral as a ceremonial, celebratory event that can specifically address the particular needs of bereaved people. As with Jackson, Irion also became a clergy consultant for NFDA and a well-known speaker to funeral directors, enlightening them about the value of ceremony and the concept of celebration.

Irion (1971) contributed another important book to the intellectual and professional growth of funeral directors entitled *A Manual and Guide for Those Who Conduct a Humanist Funeral*. This book provided instructions that many funeral directors shared with clergy who provided funerals at their funeral establishments. As with Irion's earlier works, part of his creative genius lay in establishing a meaningful dialogue within the funeral industry. Through his programs for NFDA, his views and opinions helped shape the professional development of countless funeral directors willing to consider contemporary adaptations to the traditional funeral.

RESEARCH FOCUSED ON FUNERAL DIRECTING

In the early 1950s, Raether had identified two scholars whom he encouraged to carry out a research project to trace the history of the American funeral director. Robert W. Habenstein was a sociologist/anthropologist with an interest in studying death customs in different ethnic groups. William M. Lamers was an educator/historian whose interest in death grew out of his studies of the Civil War. In 1953, Habenstein and Lamers (1955) began their collaborative efforts to research, study, and describe the history of the funeral director in America, leading to the publication of their book *The History of American Funeral Directing*. This fact-filled volume is historically fascinating and informative, and it helped solidify the growth of the funeral director as a professional.

Continuing their collaborative research throughout the 1950s, Habenstein and Lamers (1960) published their study of multicultural funeral customs in the book *Funeral Customs the World Over*. Because of the scholarly style and informed analysis of the two topics, funeral directors in general were considerably more likely than in years past to explore the many faces of death customs and practices. It was the beginning of a long process of trying to make death's ceremonies relevant and meaningful to the emerging social demands of the nation.

In the mid-1950s, sociologist Robert L. Fulton was carrying out studies with a focus on death in American society. Collaborating with Faunce, Fulton (1958) coauthored a provocative article entitled "The Sociology of Death: a Neglected Area of Research." In this seminal paper, they point out that even though death is an institutionalized phenomenon with many cultural characteristics, sociologists had largely ignored it. They urged that more research be directed to aspects of death and its social manifestations.

Fulton continued to pursue studies in the specialty field that by the early 1960s was being called the sociology of death. Fulton (1961) examined "The Clergyman and the Funeral Director: A Study in Role Conflict," a study sponsored by NFDA. He attributed the reported conflict to three points: the basic distinction that religions usually make between that which is spiritual or clergy, focused from that which is physical- or body-focused, that is, the funeral director's domain; the inconsistency of the funeral director's role as a business person as well as a kind of counselor; and the clergy's fear of the funeral director's role as an indiscriminant server of all religious faiths as being religiously "unclean" unless of the same faith as those served.

As was the case with Jackson and Irion, Fulton served as an advisor/consultant to NFDA on a wide range of important conceptual and practical matters. Because of the unique and unusually close relationship all of the consultants had with Raether and with each other, there was multidisciplinary cross-fertilization of concepts, evidence, and conclusions. This was the case with Fulton's (1965) major contribution to the study of death in his edited book *Death and Identity*. Wide ranging in his selection of essays and articles by scholars from many intellectual traditions, one of his goals was to illuminate the many problems that death presents to each of us. The collection of essays contained articles by several of the emerging death scholars, including Lindemann (1944), Weisman (1972), Feifel (1959), and Kalish (1981). The preparation of the book was funded in part by a grant from NFDA, and in the acknowledgments Fulton personally thanks "Howard C. Raether . . . whose courage and foresight made this book possible." The book came to be of great value to funeral directors and has been influential in their further education in the field.

Another scholar who emerged in the late 1950s in the seminars and speaking programs of many funeral director associations was rabbi/author Earl A. Grollman, whose scholarship included in-depth study of the works of Freud and Lindemann, both of whose work was important in Grollman's writings. He also shared an interest in the theological dimensions of funeral behavior and became a friend and confidant of Jackson, Irion, and Fulton. Today, Grollman remains a prolific writer on a vast array of topics.

An early notable publication of Grollman's (1967) was the edited book titled *Explaining Death to Children*. Each chapter in the book focuses on a particular facet of how death can be explained to children in a society that has difficulty facing the subject, let alone talking about it with other adults. With chapters by Fulton, Kastenbaum, Jackson, and Grollman himself, the material is clear and easily accessible to a wide audience. It became well known to funeral directors and was found to be helpful in assisting bereaved people to communicate with their children.

Grollman (1974) edited another book entitled *Concerning Death: A Practical Guide for the Living*, which became popular with funeral directors. This book contained chapters by authors with different areas of expertise and included presentations by Jackson, Irion, and Raether. The ever-growing intellectual and academic domain of funeral directors was again expanded. Grollman successfully strove to make death-related information both accessible and relevant, and his work has had a long-lasting effect on the professionalization of funeral directors, helping them to encourage greater personalization in funeral practices.

As a sociologist, I had written an article entitled "Comparative Funeral Practices," which analyzed the death practices in five diverse cultures (Pine, 1969). Although the actual practices differed from one society to another, I found that there were six common features of funerals: social support, confrontation with the dead body, a death ceremony, sanitary disposition of the dead body, a funeral procession, and funeral expenditure. The particular activities of each society reflected the dominant religious beliefs, social structure, degree of cohesiveness, and geographical location of each, but the unifying theme was that death gave rise to similar behaviors.

I coauthored with sociologist Derek L. Phillips a study entitled "The Cost of Dying: A Sociological Analysis of Funeral Expenditures" (Pine & Phillips, 1970). We found that funerals selected varied according the social status of the deceased, gender of the arranger, and the arranger's relationship to the dead person. This article, which later was reprinted in the second edition of Fulton's (1976) *Death and Identity: Revised Edition*, was the basis for the numerous studies of funeral expenditure I conducted through research sponsored by NFDA.

During the 1970s, I edited the books *Responding to Disaster* (1974a) and *Acute Grief and the Funeral* (1976) and wrote the book *Caretaker of the Dead: The American Funeral Director* (1975). I wrote many articles and essays about dying, death, grief, and bereavement. I also spoke to thousands of funeral directors through association and organization meetings about the professional aspects of death, grief, and bereavement. I hope the aggregate of these has had a lasting influence on the funeral directors who found them useful at the time.

Psychotherapist J. William Worden (1976) published the book *PDA (Personal Death Awareness)*. The goal of the book was to enhance life for readers by helping them understand death at the personal level. He extolled the benefits of funerals, encouraging readers to give thought to their own funerals and actually to plan what they would wish for their own service. He hoped people would get beyond the oft-stated idea that "I don't want anything when I die," as he felt this sentiment provides poor instructions to the bereaved who may try to honor this comment, much to their own detriment. Worden recognized that an appropriate funeral is more for the living than it is for the dead and that the individual should convey his or her own suggestions to the person most likely to arrange the funeral. Worden encouraged the use of music, selected readings, religious remarks if appropriate, and other activities that would reflect the deceased's goals, values, and lifestyle.

Worden's exposure to funeral directors was greatly enhanced by his service on the board of trustees of a funeral service school. In this capacity, he encouraged funeral directors to address the importance of being grief facilitators in their professional activities. He also came to understand some of the unique dimensions of a funeral practice. In his writings on grief counseling, Worden makes a strong case for the important role that funeral directors can play in facilitating grief at the time of the funeral.

Worden (1982), in *Grief Counseling and Grief Therapy*, explains that "the funeral service, if it is done well, can be an important adjunct in aiding and abetting the healthy resolution of grief" (p. 50). He goes on to point out four reasons why: (1) it helps make real the fact of the loss by having family members see the body of the dead person, (2) it provides an opportunity to express thoughts and feelings about the dead person and helps the grief process as it lets the bereaved talk about the dead person, (3) it provides a reflection on the life of the dead person, and (4) it assists in drawing a social support network around the bereaved family.

Starting in the mid-1970s, sociologist/gerontologist Kenneth J. Doka began studying death. As an ordained Lutheran clergyman, Doka brought a unique perspective to the sociological analysis of issues of dying and death. He had studied dying and death in his academic career, plus he attended relevant seminars in which he studied under a number of the early death scholars. Doka's (1982) first publication specifically dealing with funerals was entitled "The Funeral Service: Grace in

Grief," in which he extolled the value of assuring that the funeral should address the personal needs of the bereaved.

Over the years, Doka has been a prolific author and a very popular speaker and lecturer to funeral director associations and organizations. He has exerted a powerful positive influence on funeral directors in terms of helping them understand disenfranchised grief (1989), spirituality (Doka & Morgan, 1993), and how bereavement counseling can be a helpful augmentation to the funeral process. Doka recognizes that funeral directors often are the first postdeath professionals with whom the immediately bereaved are in contact. This allows a sensitive funeral director to provide situational counseling and solace to the bereaved and encourages creating arranger-centered funerals.

Clinical psychologist Therese Rando has been a highly regarded contributor to the field since she emerged in the late 1970s. She has been a dedicated and productive author, and her writings on grief (1984) and anticipatory grief (1986) have been beneficial to funeral directors, especially when dealing with deaths following long illnesses. Her personal life history with death and her extensive research experiences have contributed to her special talent for understanding and assuaging grief, not just to her clinical patients but to other professionals in the field. Because of her clear writing style and use of clinically relevant examples, her writings have been important in the emerging professional development of funeral directors. For example, Rando's (1988) book *Grieving: How To Go On Living When Someone You Love Dies* often is given to bereaved families by funeral directors as a practical guide to facilitate their grieving.

William G. Hoy is a pastoral counselor who brings many years of experience as a congregational minister and student of bereavement to his work as a clinical educator in medical humanities. He is the author of a recent book entitled *Do Funerals Matter? The Purposes and Practices of Death Rituals in Global Perspective* in which he uses a multidisciplinary approach to study death rituals from a worldwide perspective (Hoy, 2013). One of his central arguments is that funerals should be a personal reflection of the deceased. Tracing the history of funeral beliefs, customs, and ceremonies, Hoy explicates the value of ritual behavior for individuals, families, and communities. He provides counselors with ideas and suggestions for how to weave sensitive rituals into their professional practices. Hoy has conducted many seminars that have had a powerful positive impact on funeral directors throughout the United States.

Hoy (2013) enumerates the myriad options that are available for funerals today and into the future. In laying out the many ways rituals and practices can be used by bereaved people, he puts it this way:

> A dizzying array of "options" is available for people endeavoring to orchestrate a meaningful ceremony. . . . [There are] . . . "celebrations of life," home funerals, personalized music selections, video tributes, internet broadcast services, and green funerals are just a few of the choices available to today's funeral consumer (p. 5).

Clearly, as Hoy and other active death scholars continue working with and for funeral directors, the collective imagination of the field of funeral service will continue to grow. This will be a good thing for those who seek individualized and personal ceremonial services and observances to commemorate death. These fairly new creative approaches to life's final chapter have their roots in the scholarly study of dying, death, grief, and bereavement.

Alan Wolfelt is a widely known inspirational educator and grief counselor whose writings and seminars have been important to many funeral professionals. His interest in death education is long-standing, and he has many unique ideas about the process of grief and its resolution. He has been successful in teaching funeral directors how they can assist bereaved people by "companioning" them through the process. Over the years, many people have attended his seminars and have studied his writings and found the information to be of considerable help in increasing their own personal ability to counsel about death.

Through the writings and seminars of the death scholars and the educational programs provided to funeral associations and organizations, funeral directors have inexorably been moving toward a more professional level, with many having become qualified, licensed therapists, specializing in grief and bereavement counseling. Many others, have embraced the value of therapeutic modalities and have made such services available to the people they serve.

As it has evolved over the years, funeral service continues to go through many changes. In general, funeral directors have been held to higher professional standards and have striven for more professionalism within the industry. An increasing number of professionals in the field are going on to graduate work or training in fields such as aftercare specialists, bereavement counselors, and as funeral celebrants. It is anticipated that with the decline in religious affiliation, there will be a continued increase in the use of celebrants. There already are several celebrant training programs of which many funeral directors have availed themselves.

One of the critical transformations has been in the changing of funeral practices from director-centered to arranger-centered events. Greater emphasis was, gradually at first, but more fully later, placed on funeral directors to seek ways to draw out creative ideas and thoughts about funeral practices that would honor the dead person in a fitting and unique fashion. This was far different from funeral directors telling arrangers what was "customary and expected." Old-time funeral directors often tended to be paternalistic in the sense that they "knew" what was good for funeral arrangers. The contemporary approach is more a celebration of life that focuses on the experiences and aspirations of the deceased, while keeping in mind the needs and desires of the bereaved in a setting where "anything" is possible.

CRITICISM OF FUNERAL DIRECTORS AND FUNERAL PRACTICES

For some people today, the idea of having a "funeral with the dead body present" is repugnant and undesirable. Even so, many people do feel that having a commemorative farewell event is a good idea. In many parts of the United States, "memorial services" have become more widely practiced, developing partly out of the formation of memorial societies. According to humanist counselor Ernest Morgan (1962), the initial creation of memorial societies traces its roots to the Progressive era of the early 20th century and the Farm Grange movement in the American northwest. At that time, the rural cooperatives were led by Protestant clergy who preferred group planning for funerals of their parishioners. Church leaders spread the idea to the West Coast. Seattle was the first city to have a memorial association, which was founded in 1939. Memorial societies soon began to emerge in other West Coast cities of the United States and parts of Canada.

These organizations were committed to bringing postdeath activities to their members in a cooperative manner wherein caskets and services were made available for low costs. By the late 1950s, there were more than 1,000 memorial associations nationwide, most on the West Coast and upper midwest in Iowa, Minnesota, and Wisconsin. "Memorial" associations were so named because of the prevailing negative attitude their founders had about the term "funeral." By their use of the word "funeral," they meant "the traditional funeral with the body present" rather than the process of having a funeral ceremony.

In 1963, the Continental Association of Funeral and Memorial Societies was founded, and it continues to serve as a clearinghouse for information and to assist new societies in forming. Further encouragement for funeral reform was provided by the publication of Mitford's (1963) *The American Way of Death.* Some of the same issues had been raised by Bowman (1959) and then almost simultaneously with Mitford they were repeated by Harmer (1963). Their works focused on American funeral practices and the commercialization of them, as well as their high cost. Of the three, only Mitford's satirical, popular paperback became a true bestseller, and it did draw public scrutiny to funeral simplicity and funeral pricing.

Often aggregated with the memorial service movement is the trend toward cremation. Part of this tendency reflects the perception that cremation is less expensive than earth burial. However, there is not a direct relationship between the two. Many cremations are preceded or followed by a memorial service, and, increasingly, burials also are followed by some sort of memorial service. It is also common for traditional funerals to be followed by a cremation as the means of final disposition. According to the Cremation Association of North America (CANA) statistics, the confirmed percentage of cremations represented about 43.5% of the deaths in 2012. This can be compared with 36% in 2008, 29% in 2003, 17% in 1990, 10% in 1980, and about 5% in 1950. It is estimated that by 2017 approximately 49% of all deaths in the United States will result in cremation, and by 2020 the percentage of cremations nationwide is projected to be more than 50%.

Historically, cremations often have been less expensive than traditional funerals and burials. However, the principal cost difference between a funeral followed by cremation versus a funeral followed by burial is the cost of buying a cemetery plot and opening and closing the grave versus the cost of the cremation itself. It is true that some people who choose cremation tend to select a less expensive casket or an alternative container, making the overall selection less expensive. However, it is not a one-to-one relationship. Another variable that must be considered is embalming. It is not required by law for either type of funeral unless there will be a delay until the final disposition. Embalming is the temporary preservation of the body to enable viewing or to accommodate a delay; the cost of embalming must be factored in.

THE IMPACT OF THE BABY BOOM ON THE FUNERAL INDUSTRY

The baby boom generation refers to the period from 1946 through 1964, during which approximately 76,000,000 babies were born in the United States. The impact of this cohort, now between the ages of 50 and 68, has been profound in terms of American politics, human rights, secondary and higher education, sexual behavior, and even the rites of passage. Specifically, many boomers who decided to marry often did so in unique, self-satisfying ways, with popular music, personally written vows, and nontraditional ceremonies. Not surprisingly, many of these boomers may want a unique funeral experience.

As they grew older, baby boomers increasingly questioned the traditional funeral. Some decided to have no funeral or ceremony at all, avoiding any outward manifestation of death. Many others decided to create their own rituals and invent practices that would satisfy their personal needs with ceremonies "celebrating" the lives that had been lived. This is distinctly different from the traditional mourning of a child's or young person's death as an irretrievable loss.

The jury remains out and no real verdict has emerged as to what the future of funeral service may bring, but it is clear that the later part of the 20th century and the first decade of the 21st century has brought a multitude of substantive changes. Many boomers continue to seek answers to questions about the value of the social norms, customs, and traditions of the funeral. One such question that has a long history has once again emerged, namely, how much do funerals cost? And, why? Though the questions are not new, the baby boom generation has taken them to a new level. The concern with the cost of a funeral gives impetus to the issue of today's changes in terms of seeking value for what price is paid for a funeral.

Following World War I, Americans in general manifested a sense of community. In the early 1920s, the majority of bereaved American families desired a relatively "standard" funeral that included embalming the dead body, a set period of hours or days for visiting the bereaved and viewing the dead body, a funeral ceremony with the clergyman of the decedent's church, and a reception after the ceremony. The pattern of the "standard" funeral was not just common in terms of funeral practices, but it also helped establish the pricing of the funeral as a standard amount. In this package style of pricing, there was a standard charge in which the price of a given funeral was for a fixed fee, including all services, use of the funeral establishment, other facilities, and the casket. Typically, the only difference between the price of one funeral from another was the casket the bereaved selected. That uniformity in services and the single unit-pricing style lasted until well into the 1980s.

In 1984, the Federal Trade Commission (FTC) enacted the Funeral Trade Rule regarding the itemization of funeral prices, specifying that funeral directors must enumerate 17 separate items each with a distinct price. Over time, there have been modifications to the Rule some of which allow alternative methods depending on state laws, but the result after 30 years is that nationwide funeral directors use some form of itemized pricing, allowing a funeral arranger to have many choices when arranging a funeral. Today, "itemized" funeral pricing is the norm.

THE FUTURE

Predicting the future is always risky business, but the proverbial handwriting has begun to appear on the wall. I believe that because of the ongoing study of dying, death, grief, and bereavement, and the insights this provides, funeral behavior will continue to evolve during the next decade. There will be an ongoing demand for creativity in developing appropriate ceremonial events to suit the changing needs and desires of bereaved people. Much has been written about the general business trends toward being an experiential era. I believe that the funeral is no exception and will continue its shifting status, with more and more bereaved people seeking to create a memorable experience as they say their final goodbyes, even if the deceased is an elderly person. Gathering favorite mementos of the deceased and displaying pictures and other life memories will help bereaved people and their relatives and friends reflect on the life they are honoring and celebrating.

Today, the handling of illness, dying, and death continue to be the responsibility of institutions other than the family. Furthermore, the reduction of infant and child mortality and increased control over the diseases of adolescence and midlife have combined to concentrate death to the ranks of the elderly. Finally, even with television news reports, there still is an absence of direct contact with the deaths resulting from war. The result is that the average American still has very little exposure to actual death and its consequences.

As is so evident in the shifting duties and responsibilities of funeral directors, funeral practices will continue to evolve in the direction of ceremonies that focus on the conclusion of a life well lived rather than somberly focusing on a young person's death as cutting off a life too soon. Funeral directors will continue to be part of this demographic revolution, whether they choose to be voluntarily or not. These demographic and social changes plus increased institutionalization have shifted the contemporary American funeral into the hands of family members and a funeral director. This shift makes death a private matter for the family rather than a public matter for the society. In light of this, death, especially of children and younger adults, can be thought of as less present in American society than in many other cultures or than it was in our past.

As the presence of death in our society has diminished, so have our ceremonial observances for the dead. For example, we no longer use special "black-edged" mourning stationery, mourning clothes are no longer expected, there is less formal cancelation of social engagements for a predetermined period, visits to the home of mourning are less common, the respectful viewing of the dead body has declined, and participation in funerals increasingly involves just family members and close friends rather than the larger community. As a result of these and other diminishing ceremonials, family members shoulder a greater emotional burden than in the past.

At the same time, individual deaths have become less disruptive to society in general. However, the consequences of death in some ways have become more serious for the individual. Given the many noted changes, one fact remains, sooner or later, most of us will experience death's presence when someone close dies, such as a parent, a spouse, a child, another close relative, or a friend. Moreover, bereaved people today experience grief less frequently, but often more intensely, because their emotional involvements generally are not spread throughout an entire community, but rather they are usually concentrated on just one or a few people.

For Americans, then, without a definite way to mourn, death has become less disruptive for society, but it has become a more serious problem for the immediately bereaved. The future of funerary behavior, whether it involves a traditional funeral with the body present or a memorial service without the dead body, or whether final disposition be by earth burial, entombment, cremation, or body donation, will be influenced by funeral directors who must strive to assist individual mourners in saying their final goodbyes in ways that help them grieve in a healthy fashion.

REFERENCES

Bowman, L. (1959). *The American funeral: A study in guilt, extravagance, and sublimity.* Washington, DC: Public Affairs Press.

Doka, K. J. (1982). The funeral service: Grace in grief. *Currents in Mission and Theology, 9,* 235–238.

Doka, K. J. (Ed.). (1989). *Disenfranchised grief: Recognizing hidden sorrow.* Lexington, MA: Lexington Books.

Doka, K. J., & Morgan, J. D. (Eds.). (1993). *Death and spirituality.* Amityville, NY: Baywood.

Faunce, W. A., & Fulton, R. L. (1958). The sociology of death: A neglected area of research. *Social Forces, 36*(3), 205–209.

Feifel, H. (Ed.). (1959). *The meaning of death.* New York, NY: McGraw-Hill.

Firth, R. (1964). *Elements of social organization.* Boston, MA: Beacon.

Freud, S. (1957). Mourning and melancholia. In J. Strachey (Ed. & trans.), *The standard edition of the complete works of Sigmund Freud* (Vol. XIV, pp. 275–300). London, UK: The Hogarth Press and the Institute of Psycho-analysis. (Original work published 1917)

Fulton, R. L. (1961). The clergyman and the funeral director: A study in role conflict. *Social Forces, 39*(4), 317–323.

Fulton, R. L. (1963). *The sacred and the secular: Attitudes of the American public toward death.* Milwaukee, WI: Bulfin.

Fulton, R. L. (Ed.). (1965). *Death and identity.* New York, NY: Wiley.

Fulton, R. L. (Ed.). (1976). *Death and identity* (rev. ed.). Bowie, MD: The Charles Press.

Glaser, B. G., & Strauss, A. L. (1965). *Awareness of dying.* Chicago, IL: Aldine.

Gorer, G. (1965). *Death, grief, and mourning.* New York, NY: Doubleday.

Grollman, E. A. (Ed.). (1967). *Explaining death to children.* Boston, MA: Beacon.

Grollman, E. A. (Ed.). (1974). *Concerning death: A practical guide for the living.* Boston, MA: Beacon.

Habenstein, R. W., & Lamers, W. M. (1955). *The history of American funeral directing.* Milwaukee, WI: Bulfin.

Habenstein, R. W., & Lamers, W. M. (1960). *Funeral customs the world over.* Milwaukee, WI: Bulfin.

Harmer, R. M. (1963). *The high cost of dying.* New York, NY: Crowell-Collier.

Hoy, W. G. (2013). *Do funerals matter? The purposes and practices of death rituals in global perspective.* New York, NY: Routledge.

Irion, P. E. (1954). *The funeral and the mourners.* New York, NY: Abingdon.

Irion, P. E. (1966). *The funeral: Vestige or value?* Nashville, TN: Parthenon.

Irion, P. E. (1971). *A manual and guide for those who conduct a humanist funeral.* Baltimore, MD: Waverly.

Jackson, E. (1957). *Understanding grief.* New York, NY: Abingdon.

Jackson, E. (1962). *You and your grief.* New York, NY: Abingdon.

Kalish, R. A. (1981). *Death, grief, and caring relationships.* Monterey, CA: Brooks/Cole.

Lindemann, E. (1944). The symptomatology and management of acute grief. *American Journal of Psychiatry, 101,* 141–148.

Malinowski, B. (1948). *Magic, science, and religion.* Garden City, NY: Doubleday.

Mitford, J. (1963). *The American way of death.* New York, NY: Simon and Schuster.

Morgan, E. (Ed.). (1962). *A manual of death education and simple burial.* Burnsville, NC: Celo Press.

Pine, V. R. (1969). Comparative funeral practices. *Practical anthropology, 16*(2), 49–62.

Pine, V. R. (Ed.). (1974a). *Responding to disaster.* Milwaukee, WI: Bulfin.

Pine, V. R. (1974b). Grief work and dirty work: The aftermath of an aircrash. *Omega, 5*(4), 281–286.

Pine, V. R. (1975). *Caretaker of the Dead: The American Funeral Director.* New York, NY: Wiley.

Pine, V., Kutscher, A. H., Peretz, D. & Slater, R. (1976). *Acute grief and the funeral.* Springfield, IL: Charles C Thomas, V. Pine, A. H. Kutscher, D. Peretz, & R. Slater.

Pine, V. R., & Phillips, D. L. (1970). The cost of dying: A sociological analysis of funeral expenditure. *Social Problems, 17*(3), 405–417.

Rando, T. A. (1984). *Grief, dying, and death: Clinical interventions for caregivers.* Champaign, IL: Research Press.

Rando, T. A. (1986). *Loss and anticipatory grief.* Lexington, MA: Lexington Books.

Rando, T. A. (1988). *Grieving: How to go on living when someone you love dies.* Lexington, MA: Lexington Books.

U.S. Bureau of the Census, Statistical Abstract of the United States: 1900 (22nd edition) Washington, D.C. 1900.

U.S. Bureau of the Census, Statistical Abstract of the United States: 1950 (72nd edition), Washington, D.C. 1950.

Weisman, A. D. (1972). *On dying and denying: A psychiatric study of terminality.* New York, NY: Behavioral Publications.

Worden, J. W. (1976). *Personal death awareness.* Englewood Cliffs, NJ: Prentice-Hall.

Worden, J. W. (1982). *Grief counseling and grief therapy: A handbook for the mental health practitioner.* New York, NY: Springer Publishing Company.

Charles A. Corr

15

DEATH EDUCATION AT THE COLLEGE AND UNIVERSITY LEVEL IN NORTH AMERICA

This chapter examines the development and some aspects of the history of formal offerings of courses on death, dying, and bereavement at the college and university level in the United States and Canada. The chapter reflects what I have experienced or know about this type of what is popularly called "death education." This chapter does not consider death education at the precollege level, formal education programs for health professionals, workshops, conference presentations, or other adult programs of study.

Although the phrase "death education" correctly points to the death-related subject matter of this type of education, actually these courses are about life and living as viewed from the perspective of death-related issues. That is, death education considers what Kastenbaum (2004, p. 19) has called "the study of life—with death left in." Some aspects of the development of death education in its early years were examined in two articles by Pine (1977, 1986) and in an encyclopedia article by Corr and Corr (2003), but I believe this chapter is the first to offer a retrospective reflection on more than 50 years in this field.

In brief, this chapter describes how I came to be involved in these educational ventures, identifies some early initiatives in the field, provides examples of some of the early pedagogical resources that were created to support and foster those initiatives, and sketches more recent developments as regards survey courses in this field, other death-related courses, and programs in thanatology. The chapter concludes with some thoughts about what we have learned from and about death education.

MY INVOLVEMENT IN THIS FIELD

Some people originally came to death education as a result of a personal encounter with death or bereavement. More recently, they might have been guided to this work by a graduate advisor or through their choices of a thesis or dissertation topic. By contrast, it wouldn't be completely unfair to say that I almost stumbled into teaching in this area. In the early 1970s, during a comprehensive revision of its General Education program, my former university created a requirement that every student take an interdisciplinary course at the junior level. Not surprising, no such courses had previously existed, so the requirement encouraged faculty to propose new interdisciplinary courses. In response, a colleague who was a developmental psychologist and I proposed a course on death and dying. We offered a number of apparent reasons for making this initiative. For example, we noted correctly that developmental psychologists have natural interests in end-of-life issues involving both children and older adults, whereas someone with academic training in philosophy might appropriately be interested in ethical issues related to euthanasia and suicide, as well as concerns about the meaning of life and beliefs in relation to a possible afterlife. Looking back on our original proposal many years later, however, it is clear that our joint backgrounds left large gaps in the topics that an introductory college course on death education would need to cover. For example, neither of us had had any direct involvement in caring for dying or bereaved persons. In short, it wouldn't be too far wrong to say that in reality we had little idea about what we were getting ourselves into.

On a later occasion, we were asked why we were teaching such courses. Before we could answer, one student cleverly suggested that we were doing so because we wanted to be in charge and thus be able to control the discussion. Our adroit response was to quickly switch the topic of the conversation. In retrospect, if that student's suggestion had been accurate, our desire to tiptoe up to these topics and then move on when we became uncomfortable would likely have been buried so deeply in our unconscious that we would have been unaware of it. As it was, our reasons for proposing and then teaching courses on death education were multiple and, I think, not at all sinister.

As we gained experience in teaching courses of various types to diverse audiences on different topics in the field of death, dying, and bereavement, both in class and most recently online, it quickly became evident that this was and continues to be a stimulating experience. When we began, like many others we had no direct professional training for teaching such courses because there simply was no such training available. In addition, there were few obvious resources to draw on, what was available was scattered and uneven, and there were few ready-to-hand textbooks.

In my case, I benefited from team teaching, something I had never done previously, which was a requirement for the university's new interdisciplinary courses. Over the years, I taught with colleagues who had expertise in such fields as psychology, nursing, health education, and medical ethics. Teaching with a nursing faculty member and talking with my nurse wife, who later became a nursing faculty member at a local community college, exposed obvious gaps in my competencies, especially in regard to care of the dying. With that in mind, I worked to enhance my competencies in this field by volunteering in the first hospice program in the metropolitan area and arranging to spend a summer in 1978 as a volunteer in a well-established British hospice. That summer at St. Luke's in Sheffield, England, was a life-changing experience for me both professionally and personally. Rather unexpectedly, it also led to arrangements for me to lead 2-week work/study groups back to the hospice each summer for 9 years and to many other contacts with organizations and individual professionals in England that resulted in our first edited book in the field (Corr & Corr, 1983).

Throughout the 1980s, I also pursued growing interests in death-related issues that involve children and/or adolescents. That led to a series of coedited books that have continued into the 21st century (Balk & Corr, 2009; Corr & Balk, 1996, 2010; Corr & Corr, 1985, 1986; Corr & McNeil, 1986; Wass & Corr, 1984). I also developed a special interest in death-related literature for children and adolescents that is reflected in a special issue of *Omega, Journal of Death and Dying* (Corr, 2004). Later, I had opportunities to visit and learn from the work of several child and adolescent bereavement support programs, most notably The Dougy Center in Portland, Oregon, and Winston's Wish in Cheltenham, England.

An invitation to become a professional advisor to a new Compassionate Friends chapter and later to join the Executive Committee of the National Donor Family Council expanded my understanding of and sensitivity to issues in adult bereavement.

Finally, over the last 4 years, I have had the opportunity to teach an online "Survey of Thanatology" course for a Canadian university. Interacting with those students and considering differences between the Canadian and U.S. situations has given me new perspectives and new learning experiences in death education. We never stop learning and growing in this field.

All of these initiatives indicate that I and many others who teach in the death education field had much to learn from ill, dying, and bereaved individuals who allowed us to benefit from their personal experiences, often at very difficult times in their lives. Frankly, in the 1970s and 1980s we were all learning our way in this field. We had much to learn from guest speakers and from students in our classes, as well as from a wide variety of professionals who shared their expertise with us. Our job as educators was and continues to be to draw on all such experiences and communicate their lessons in effective ways to those who take part in our classes.

EARLY INITIATIVES

The first courses on death education at the university level in North America were taught by Robert Fulton at the University of Minnesota in 1963 and by Edwin Shneidman at Harvard University in 1969. That led Fulton to edit (with Robert Bendiksen) an anthology entitled *Death and Identity* (1965/1994) and, with other coeditors (Fulton, Markusen, Owen, & Scheiber, 1978), a reader for a Course by Newspaper project in this field. In turn, Shneidman published an article, "Can a Young Person Write His Own Obituary?" (1972a), edited a collection of papers written by college students (1972b), and contributed a chapter on "The College Student and Death." (1977) Of course, there were other educators who made significant contributions to the field during the late 1960s and throughout the following decade, including Richard Kalish and Robert Kastenbaum.

Around the same time, some instructors began to share syllabi for their courses (e.g., Bloom, 1975; Corr, 1978; Gurfield, 1977; Leviton, 1975; Lonetto, Fleming, Gorman, & Best, 1975; Margolis, Cherico, O'Connor, & Kutscher, 1978; White, 1970). Somewhat later, some attendees at annual conferences of the Association for Death Education and Counseling [ADEC] arranged some sharing of course syllabi, but that effort gradually dissipated, and there have not been many published articles in recent years on the pedagogy of death education at the college and university levels (one exception might be Buckle, 2013).

Over the years, many authors published articles that attempted to show whether and/or how death education courses might or actually do alter death-related attitudes of participants, although those efforts go beyond the concerns of this chapter. More to the point, even in the early years of death education some writers initiated a critical reflection on what we were doing in these courses (e.g., Leviton, 1977; Stillion, 1979). Perhaps the most imaginative of these self-critiques appeared in an article entitled "We Covered Death Today" (Kastenbaum, 1977), which reflected on the roles actually being played by this form of death education. The article asked whether this was an open and disciplined inquiry into our relationship with death or merely another, perhaps more sophisticated, form of denial. Did we think we could open discussions of death-related subjects and complete educational analyses of them as we might in teaching multiplication tables? Were instructors aware of social pressures to make death education merely comforting?

EARLY PEDAGOGICAL RESOURCES

During these early years, there was a rush to identify and describe resources that instructors could draw on in shaping and implementing their courses. Reflecting on those efforts can tell us a good deal about the status of death education during that period. In the first place, unannotated lists of pedagogical resources for death education, some quite lengthy, were circulated. These were soon found not to be very helpful because they were often uneven, indiscriminate, and not specific as to how the listed resources could actually be located. Much more useful were two large volumes of annotated guides to print, audiovisual, organizational, and community resources, along with reprints of some key documents touching on this field, developed and published by Wass Corr, Pacholski, and Forfar (1985) and Warr, Corr, Pacholski, and Sanders (1980).

In the second place, among a plethora of books with varying emphases, two edited volumes by Feifel (1959, 1977) and the widespread popularity of *On Death and Dying* (Kübler-Ross, 1969) contributed greatly to interest in matters of death and dying. For some instructors, these and other books, some articles, and/or extracts from other published materials that offered personal stories of encounters with dying, loss, and grief were sufficient to serve as primary resources for their courses. For example, early books on coping with dying included *Anatomy of an Illness as Perceived by the Patient* (Cousins, 1979), *Autobiography of Dying* (Hanlan, 1979), *Death of a Man* (Wertenbaker, 1957), and *How Could I Not Be Among You?* (Rosenthal, 1973). Some more recent books in this genre are *At the Will of the Body* (Frank, 2002), *The Last Lecture* (Pausch, 2008), and *Tuesdays with Morrie* (Albom, 1997). Another enduring title is the classic *The Death of Ivan Ilych* (Tolstoy, 1884/1960). Books by adults who recount personal encounters with loss, bereavement, and grief that have been used in death education courses include *A Grief Observed* (Lewis, 1961/1976), *A Widow's Story: A Memoir* (Oates, 2011), *Motherless Daughters* (Edelman, 1994), *The Year of Magical Thinking* (Didion, 2005), and *Widow* (Caine, 1975). Another distinctive book with significant pedagogical value is *Voices of Death* (Shneidman, 1980/1995).

In the third place, for many instructors, early purpose-designed textbooks like *Death: Current Perspectives* (Shneidman, 1976/1980) and *Dying: Facing the Facts* (Wass, 1979) offered more direct practical utility for instructional purposes with most general college audiences. Similar books offered strong nursing (Quint, 1967), social work (Prichard et al., 1977), sociological (Fulton, 1965/1994), or theological and pastoral (Mills, 1969) slants. At first, faculty were attracted to the quality of previously published materials brought together in these texts or to the new materials in contributing authors' books. In time, however, many found that students were dissatisfied with the lack of coherence and multiple voices in books of these types, whereas instructors became concerned about the burdens placed on them to weave together disparate materials in an effective pedagogical manner.

In the fourth place, pedagogical resources for death education became more focused when a book like *Death, Society, and Human Experience* (Kastenbaum, 1977/2012) offered the thoughts of a single author, already well respected in the field. It also drew on what Kastenbaum (1972) called the interplay between the individual and the "death system," a concept that he had developed earlier and by which he meant a "socio-physical network by which we mediate and express our relationship to mortality" (p. 310). The important point is that every society has some type of death system and each will have its own constitutive elements and characteristic functions.

Death, Grief, and Caring Relationships (Kalish, 1981/1985) is another introduction to dying, death, and bereavement by an early and insightful pioneer in the field. It contains the memorable allegory, "The Horse on the Dining-Room Table," now perpetuated in *Death & Dying, Life & Living* (Corr & Corr, 2013).

Publications that had more of a supplementary character included some books (e.g., Knott, Ribar, Duson, & King, 1989; Meagher & Shapiro, 1984; Neale, 1973) and an article on the "Do-It-Yourself Death Certificate" (Sabatini & Kastenbaum, 1973) that described exercises that some instructors employed to encourage students to enter into a personal and educational reflection on death and life. Asking students to write eulogies or fill out personal death certificates might indicate this was a rather wild time in death education. In many instances, experience showed that because one would never be alive to complete such documents in real life, these exercises sometimes tended to promote fantasy unless students were pressed to be honest about what they believed people would have to say about them if they were to die in the near future. The obvious educational goal here was to encourage participants to take the prospect of their own mortality seriously. An alternative tactic we discovered for such exercises was to ask students to complete these documents in advance for a loved one; that often had a significant personal impact.

MORE RECENT DEVELOPMENTS: SURVEY COURSES ON DEATH, DYING, AND BEREAVEMENT

Survey or overview courses in death education are typically identified as "Death and Dying," "Introduction to Thanatology," or "Survey of Thanatology" courses. Whatever their title, these courses have become extremely popular in many diverse settings. For example, before his retirement and death, Leviton taught death and dying classes with enrollments in the several hundreds at the University of Maryland, while Attig taught similar classes of 150 to 180 students each semester from 1983 through 1995 at Bowling Green State University. Among current examples, multiple sections of death education courses are offered each term at the University of Akron (a "Death & Dying" course housed in Summit College, the university's technical college; this course is a social science elective in the university's general education program, an elective for majors in such fields as nursing, allied health, social work, psychology, and sociology, and part of the curriculum for the undergraduate Certificate in Gerontology, offered by the Institute for Life-Span Development and Gerontology, housed within the College of Arts and Sciences) and at the University of Central Oklahoma (housed in the Department of Funeral Service Education; offering 10 sections of "The Psychology of Grief" in fall and spring terms, along with summer and intersession sections, that serve as a university core elective).

Instructors and audiences for these courses have come from such widely different backgrounds as counseling, funeral service, health education, nursing, philosophy, psychology, religious studies, social science, social work, and sociology. Often it is the initiative of a particular instructor that leads to the initial offering of a course in this field. On the one hand, sometimes it is the success of these instructors in attracting enthusiastic enrollments that leads administrators to recruit additional or replacement faculty to schedule and staff such courses. On the other hand, when courses depend on the presence and energies of individual instructors, they may be downgraded or even disappear when such instructors retire or are otherwise no longer available to teach them.

In terms of participants, experience has shown that there are many different motivations or concerns among those who come to formal courses on death education at the college level.

- Some are interested in these subjects because of work they are already doing or are preparing to do in a profession or vocation in which they expect to be asked to help people who are coping with death-related issues. These include students or those working in fields like counseling, education, funeral service, nursing, medicine, the ministry, social work, and individuals who volunteer in hospice organizations.
- Others seek out courses in death education for personal motivations, such as a desire to cope more effectively with a current encounter with someone who is dying or with their own grief and mourning after a significant other has died.
- Some people seek out death education courses because they are trying to prepare for a personal experience that might arise in the future (e.g., the anticipated death of aging parents or grandparents). People like this often say things such as "No important person in my life has yet died, but I know it can't continue this way."
- Finally, some individuals are simply curious about some issue in this field (e.g., physician-assisted suicide, media reports about homicide, or how one might be able to talk to children about dying and death) or are simply seeking to fill a gap in their academic schedules.

This diversity of participants requires that instructors be both competent in the subject matter in this field and attentive to the needs of individual participants in their courses. Even though a classroom or online setting is not really an appropriate setting for individual counseling, some participants may simply need to talk out their concerns with a sympathetic instructor. Further, some individuals who are having difficulty coping with death-related challenges may need to be referred to appropriate resources for personal assistance. In all cases, as Attig (1981) reminded us, instructors need to demonstrate that they care for the uniqueness, individuality, and special concerns of those in their classes.

Because death education courses can be of many different types, experience has shown that it is important to be clear about their goals in each particular case. For example, although college courses in death education are fundamentally academic in nature, they are not confined solely to cognitive issues. As Attig (1981, p. 169) observed, "[D]eath educators dare not pretend that death education can take place on a purely intellectual or academic plane." There undoubtedly are factual matters to explore and theories to examine that can help to provide new understandings of issues in this field. However, there are also other dimensions that are inescapable in such courses, such as: affective dimensions involving feelings, emotions, and attitudes; behavioral dimensions relating to how people do, could, or should act in death-related situations; and valuational dimensions in which death education can help identify, articulate, and affirm the basic values that govern human life.

One way to address these many dimensions of death education courses is to ground courses in the basic academic concerns of encouraging critical thinking in order to help individuals judge for themselves the value, meaning, and validity of the subjects they address. Beyond that, instructors need to pay attention to the following six goals that have emerged over time as specific aims of death education:

- To enrich the personal lives of participants, for example, by helping them to understand themselves more fully and to appreciate their strengths and limitations as finite human beings

- To inform and guide individuals in their personal transactions with society, for example, by making them aware of services and options they might have in end-of-life care and funeral practices or memorial rituals
- To prepare individuals for their public roles as citizens, for example, by clarifying important social issues, such as advance directives in health care, assisted suicide or euthanasia, and organ or tissue donation
- To help prepare and support individuals in their professional and vocational roles, for example, in caring for the dying or counseling the bereaved
- To enhance the ability of individuals to communicate effectively about death-related matters, for example, by showing how excessive reliance on euphemisms is unhelpful and how, as the guru says in "The Horse on the Dining-Room Table" (Corr & Corr, 2013, p. xxxiii), "[I]f you speak about the horse, then you will find that others can also speak about the horse—most others, at least if you are gentle and kind as you speak."
- To assist individuals in appreciating how development across the human life course interacts with death-related issues, for example, by showing how children, adolescents, and older adults often face dissimilar issues and cope with them in different ways even though they all share in a common humanity

In support of these goals, efforts have been made over time to provide some degree of structuring for instructors and students in college courses on death education. For example, ADEC has developed what it calls a "Body of Knowledge" matrix and has implemented its concerns both in a certification program and in the publication of a *Handbook of Thanatology* (Meagher & Balk, 2013). For more immediately pedagogic use, leading textbooks in the field seek to organize materials in ways that are directly helpful to students and instructors. Such textbooks include *Death & Dying, Life & Living* (Corr & Corr, 2013); *Death, Society, and Human Experience* (Kastenbaum, 2012); and *The Last Dance: Encountering Death and Dying* (DeSpelder & Strickland, 2010), which are in their 7th, 12th, and 9th editions, respectively, as this is being written. These textbooks also provide supplementary materials, such as instructor's guides and test banks to enhance their utility in death education offerings. In addition, my recent experiences in an online survey course for a Canadian university have shown that a book on *Dying and Death in Canada* (Northcott & Wilson, 2008) very well fills its designed role as an excellent supplementary text, one that reminds us not to focus too narrowly on issues limited to the United States. The goal in using these textbooks and, indeed, in all of the pedagogy in death education, must be to offer something more than an eclectic jumble of diverse factual materials, personal stories, and academic theories, while still providing freedom for individual faculty to organize their own courses in view of their particular interests and competencies, the needs of their students, and the goals established for their courses.

Our experience has shown that one way to do this is to focus, initially, on the central components of death-related experiences, that is, encounters with death, attitudes toward death, and death-related practices. Attending to these principal features of death-related experiences can lead to an appreciation of the characteristics of the "death system" in every society. In particular, this framework can help students identify the elements and functions of the death system in our own society, refute the superficial claim that ours is little more than a "death-denying society," and permit comparisons both with other societies and with distinctive cultural and ethnic patterns within our society. With that in hand, both the central topics of dying and bereavement can be illuminated through a focus on the many efforts—including tasks, adaptive strategies, lifelong adjustments, and even accommodating to mystery—as we seek to understand how individuals actually cope with these experiences, how others can help such individuals, and how communities can and do offer assistance (e.g., through hospice programs and bereavement support groups). Another important way to consider death-related issues is to explore them through a developmental perspective that considers the distinctive experiences of children, adolescents, young and middle-aged adults, and older adults. Finally, examination of legal, moral, ethical, religious, and spiritual values as they help determine issues like advance directives, organ and tissue donation, suicide and assisted suicide, and the meaning and place of death in life can reinforce the conviction that education in this field is not just about death, it also offers important lessons about life and living. There are, of course, other topics that individual instructors might wish to include in their courses, such as matters of social justice, abortion, capital punishment, and global challenges.

MORE RECENT DEVELOPMENTS: OTHER DEATH-RELATED COURSES

I would like to think that I developed and offered the first full-term, college-level, credit-bearing course on children and death in 1977 (Corr, 1984, 1992, 2002). Of course, I cannot prove that claim. Nevertheless, courses that focus on death-related issues involving children and adolescents are of great interest to many audiences, and I was able to offer them in different formats for 22 years before taking early retirement from my former university. For example, in the summer of 1985, we first offered this course in a format of five day-long, Saturday sessions scheduled at 2-week intervals. When a diverse enrollment of nearly 50 participants appeared (to the great surprise of many of our academic administrators), we realized that this format served several important purposes. First, it did not exclude traditional students regularly enrolled at the university. Second, and perhaps more important, this innovative arrangement attracted nontraditional participants, both those who lived at a distance from our campus and those who worked during the week. We adapted this format without difficulty to six day-long, Saturday sessions in 1995 when the university converted from a quarter system to a semester system. In each case, the Children and Death course was open to: traditional students enrolling for academic credit at either the undergraduate or the graduate level, participants who sought formal recognition of their involvement in the form of continuing education unit (CEU) credits, and members of the general public (sometimes called lifelong learners) who paid a small fee under the university's Educard program to obtain permission to sit in on the course and have access to its textbooks without a requirement to undertake normal academic work and with no record kept of their enrollment. Bringing together different audiences in this way with diverse backgrounds and concerns did not pose any pedagogical difficulties. In fact, we learned that courses on children and death attracted self-selected, interested, and well-motivated participants, many of whom were midlife adults and midcareer professionals with personal and vocational experiences that they contributed to enriching our courses.

Since the mid-1980s, many other college- and university-level courses in the field of death education have been developed on subjects such as: end-of-life care; hospice or palliative care; grief and bereavement; grief counseling and support; grief and trauma; suicide; spiritual and philosophical issues in death, dying, and bereavement; ethical concerns in end-of-life care; developmental perspectives; historical and multicultural perspectives; and specialized topical seminars. In the programs described in the next section, these courses are often supplemented by practicum or internships related to death education, as well as by independent research projects.

MORE RECENT DEVELOPMENTS: THANATOLOGY PROGRAMS

In recent years, programs in thanatology or the organized study of death-related topics have been developed at several colleges and universities. Prominent examples include the programs at Brooklyn College in New York City; Madonna University in Livonia, Michigan; King's University College of Western University (formerly, the University of Western Ontario), in London, Canada; Hood College in Frederick, Maryland; and Marian University in Fond du Lac, Wisconsin. Each of these programs offers a distinctive set of educational opportunities and forms of recognition for those who enroll. Most often, these programs provide certificates of completion in various thanatological areas and academic minors or majors leading to some type of degree, which may be at the undergraduate or graduate levels. Courses include a variety of death-related subjects and may be offered on campus, online, or in a combination of both, depending on the program.

- The thanatology program at Brooklyn College (http://academic. brooklyn.cuny.edu/hns; tel. 718-951-4197 or 718-951-5026; e-mail: dbalk@brooklyn.cuny.edu) originated from a series of courses that Dr. David Meagher developed in response to requests from some nurses and others who were seeking postbaccalaureate educational opportunities in this subject area. A package of those courses became a master's degree in 1982, where it was and still is housed in the Department of Health and Nutrition Sciences. This program is described as "The first of its kind in the United States." The program currently offers a concentration in thanatology in the Master of Arts in Community Health degree, as well as an Advanced Certification in Grief Counseling. Courses in this program are offered in various venues: three of the courses are fully online, asynchronous courses (Children and Death, Bereavement, Heath and Medical Dilemmas); each semester, at least two courses are offered on weekends, meeting five separate Saturdays (or Sundays) from 9 a.m. to 5 p.m.; and each semester, one or more courses are offered that meet over the duration of a full semester, in the evening, once a week, 6:30 to 9:00 p.m.
- The Department of Hospice and Palliative Studies (originally, the Hospice Education Department) at Madonna University in Livonia, Michigan (e-mail: krhoades@madonna.edu; tel. 734-432-5478), is housed in the College of Nursing and Health. Beginning with courses for an academic minor and a certificate of completion in 1984, the department developed both a Bachelor of Science and Associate Degree in Hospice in 1992, moved on to add a Master's of Science in Hospice and Palliative Studies in 1996, included a Post-Master's Certificate in Bereavement in 2000, and changed its name to the Department of Hospice and Palliative Studies in 2008. Certificate programs at both the graduate and undergraduate levels are currently offered completely online, and future online degree offerings are in the planning stages.
- The Thanatology Program at King's University College, Western University (formerly University of Western Ontario), in London, Ontario, Canada (http://www.kings.uwo.ca/academics/interdisciplinary-programs/thanatology/; tel. 800-265-4406; 519-433-3491, ext 4374) has been built on the individual courses and

a series of annual, international conferences spearheaded by Dr. John (Jack) Morgan before his retirement and subsequent death in 2005. Currently, this program is housed in the Department of Interdisciplinary Studies. Since 1994, Kings has offered a Certificate in Palliative Care and Thanatology (later renamed as a Certificate in Grief and Bereavement Studies) (http://wcs.uwo .ca/postdegree/grief/index.html). In 2007, the program developed an academic minor in thanatology, followed by a major and honors specialization in thanatology in 2008. These latter are described as "the first undergraduate degree program in Thanatology in North America." Most of the courses in this program are offered both on campus and online.

- The thanatology program at Hood College in Frederick, Maryland (http:// www.hood.edu/academics/academic-catalogs/current-catalog/graduate-catalog/graduate-programs/thanatology, -m-a-.html; tel. 301-696-3892), was inspired by the work of Dr. Dana Cable before his death in 2010 and remains housed in the Department of Psychology. Beginning with independent courses in 1972, this program first offered a Thanatology Certificate that was later followed by a Master of Arts degree in 2001. The program also offers a Summer Institute in Thanatology, which allows students to earn their certificate over the course of a single summer. All courses in this program are currently offered in a face-to-face format in the evening or on weekends, but it is planned to offer an Introduction to Thanatology course in a fully online format in spring of 2014.
- Marian University in Fond du Lac, Wisconsin, offers a program formerly designated as Grief and Bereavement (http://www.marianuniversity.edu/ Academic-Programs/Adult-and-Graduate/Grief-and-Bereavement/;tel.920-923-8938) housed in the School of Nursing and Health Professions. Recent changes describe this program as currently offering a Master of Science degree in Thanatology, as well as undergraduate and graduate Certificates in Thanatology. All courses in this program are now delivered fully online.

WHAT HAVE WE LEARNED FROM AND ABOUT DEATH EDUCATION?

If we could predict the future, it might be interesting to forecast how death education at the college and university level in North America might develop in years to come. Perhaps we can content ourselves by noting that individual survey or introductory courses in death, dying, and bereavement, along with courses in related subjects, have clearly shown themselves to offer significant educational experiences that have a well-earned record of attracting a wide range of interested participants. Further, the thanatology programs of the types described here appear to be well recognized and firmly established in their respective roles. That said, we may have to wait to see whether introductory courses at this level continue to spread across North America and whether additional or enhanced thanatology programs present themselves.

In the meantime, perhaps we can note that commentators who do not have much direct experience with death education have sometimes described it as "morbid." In fact, that word means "unhealthy." But even the most cursory acquaintance with death education as it is actually implemented demonstrates that it is a vital and healthy enterprise. Death education is a serious but not necessarily grim endeavor; classes are often punctuated with laughter. After all, like death itself, much of humor trades on limitation and the absurdity of many aspects of life.

In fact, experience has amply shown that education about dying, death, and bereavement has much to teach about life and living. For example, we can learn from this form of education about:

- **Control and limitation.** Specifically, we learn that we humans are finite, limited beings, which means that although we can control many things in our lives, there are many other things that we cannot control as we seek to come to terms with or learn to live with the great mysteries of life, death, and suffering; in other words, death education reveals some specific things we can control or at least influence even as it shows many of the limitations that make our control less than complete.
- **Individuals and communities.** Specifically, because no one else can die our death or experience our grief, we learn that death-related events are indisputably marked by their unique individuality. Nevertheless, being human means being members of communities and being inescapably linked to other persons who are and will be involved in and impacted by whatever happens to us as regards death, dying, and bereavement.
- **Vulnerability and resilience.** Specifically, although we may often try to ignore our mortality, death-related events make our vulnerability to pain and suffering all too obvious. At the same time, this vulnerability is not the same as helplessness. Most human beings have powerful coping capacities and are amazingly resilient, some responding to death-related challenges in ways that can be ennobling and even awe inspiring.
- **Quality in living and the human search for meaning.** Specifically, studying death-related events reveals the importance of incorporating the motto "make today count" (the title of a book by Kelly, 1975) in our daily lives, of striving to maximize the quality of our own lives right now, and of appreciating that life can be good even though it is transient. At the same time, death education shows that when death challenges the value of life, humans work hard to find or create sources of inspiration and religious or philosophical frameworks within which enduring meaning can be established.

Some observations from experienced faculty in this field can also teach us about death education. For example, Dr. Angela Knight wrote recently, "We have the privilege of teaching a subject devoted to the importance of a life well lived. I do enjoy working with students in this area of study and I am touched each semester by the comments from students regarding the importance of what we teach" (Angela Knight, personal communication, July 29, 2013). Dr. Elizabeth Kennedy added that death education "is a truly rewarding course to teach and, most importantly, such a wonderful opportunity to engage students of all ages and all backgrounds in what is the quintessential human quest, the meaning of life and death" (Elizabeth Kennedy, personal communication, July 30, 2013).

Death education is alive and well in many colleges and universities across the United States and Canada! It has much to offer to all who take part, including both students and faculty.

REFERENCES

Albom, M. (1997). *Tuesdays with Morrie: An old man, a young man, and life's greatest lesson.* New York, NY: Doubleday.

Attig, T. (1981). Death education as care of the dying. In R. A. Pacholski & C. A. Corr (Eds.), *New directions in death education and counseling* (pp. 168–175). Arlington, CA: Forum for Death Education and Counseling.

Balk, D. E., & Corr, C. A. (Eds.). (2009). *Adolescent encounters with death, bereavement, and coping.* New York, NY: Springer Publishing Company.

Bloom, S. (1975). On teaching an undergraduate course on death and dying. *Omega, Journal of Death and Dying, 6,* 223–226.

Buckle, J. L. (2013). University students' perspectives on a psychology of death and dying course: Exploring motivation to enroll, goals, and impact. *Death Studies, 37,* 866–882.

Caine, L. (1975). *Widow.* New York, NY: Bantam Books.

Corr, C. A. (1978). A model syllabus for death and dying courses. *Death Education, 1,* 433–457.

Corr, C. A. (1984). A model syllabus for children and death courses. *Death Education, 8,* 11–28.

Corr, C. A. (1992). Teaching a college course on children and death: A 13-year report. *Death Studies, 16,* 343–356.

Corr, C. A. (2002). Teaching a college course on children and death for 22 years: A supplemental report. *Death Studies, 26,* 595–606.

Corr, C. A. (Ed.). (2004). Death-related literature for children [Special issue]. *Omega, Journal of Death and Dying, 48*(4), 399–414.

Corr, C. A., & Balk, D. E. (Eds.). (1996). *Handbook of adolescent death and bereavement.* New York, NY: Springer Publishing Company.

Corr, C. A., & Balk, D. E. (Eds.). (2010). *Children's encounters with death, bereavement, and coping.* New York, NY: Springer Publishing Company.

Corr, C. A., & Corr, D. M. (Eds.). (1983). *Hospice care: Principles and practice.* New York, NY: Springer Publishing Company.

Corr, C. A., & Corr, D. M. (Eds.). (1985). *Hospice approaches to pediatric care.* New York, NY: Springer Publishing Company.

Corr, C. A., & Corr, D. M. (Eds.). (1996). *Handbook of childhood death and bereavement.* New York, NY: Springer Publishing Company.

Corr, C. A., & Corr, D. M. (2003). Death education. In C. D. Bryant (Ed.), *Handbook of death & dying* (Vol. 2, pp. 292–301). Thousand Oaks, CA: SAGE.

Corr, C. A., & Corr, D. M. (2013). *Death & dying, life & living* (7th ed.). Belmont, CA: Wadsworth.

Corr, C. A., & McNeil, J. N. (Eds.). (1986). *Adolescence and death.* New York, NY: Springer Publishing Company.

Cousins, N. (1979). *Anatomy of an illness as perceived by the patient: Reflections on healing and regeneration.* New York, NY: Norton.

DeSpelder, L. A., & Strickland, A. L. (2010). *The last dance: Encountering death and dying* (9th ed.). New York, NY: McGraw-Hill.

Didion, J. (2005). *The year of magical thinking.* New York, NY: Knopf.

Edelman, H. (1994). *Motherless daughters: The legacy of loss.* Reading, MA: Addison-Wesley.

Feifel, H. (Ed.). (1959). *The meaning of death.* New York, NY: McGraw-Hill.

Feifel, H. (Ed.). (1977). *New meanings of death.* New York, NY: McGraw-Hill.

Frank, A. W. (2002). *At the will of the body: Reflections on illness (new afterword).* Boston, MA: Houghton Mifflin.

Fulton, R. (Ed.). (1994). *Death and identity.* (3rd ed.) Bowie, MD: The Charles Press. (Original work published 1965)

Fulton, R., Markusen, E., Owen, G., & Scheiber, J. L. (Eds.). (1978). *Death and dying: Challenge and change.* Reading, MA: Addison-Wesley.

Gurfield, M. (1977). On teaching death and dying. *Media and Methods, 13,* 56–59.

Hanlan, A. (1979). *Autobiography of dying.* Garden City, NY: Doubleday.

Kalish, R. A. (1985). *Death, grief, and caring relationships* (2nd ed.). Monterey, CA: Brooks/Cole. (Original work published 1981)

Kastenbaum, R. (1972). On the future of death: Some images and options. *Omega, Journal of Death and Dying, 3,* 306–318.

Kastenbaum, R. (1977). We covered death today. *Death Education, 1,* 85–92.

Kastenbaum, R. J. (2004). *On our way: The final passage through life and death.* Berkeley, CA: University of California Press.

Kastenbaum, R. J. (2012). *Death, society, and human experience* (11th ed.). Upper Saddle River, NJ: Pearson. (Original work published 1977)

Kelly, O. (1975). *Make today count*. New York, NY: Delacorte Press.

Knott, J. E., Ribar, M.C., Duson, B. M., & King, M. R. (1989). *Thanatopics: Activities and exercises for confronting death*. Lexington, MA: Lexington Books.

Kübler-Ross, E. (1969). *On death and dying*. New York, NY: Macmillan.

Leviton, D. (1975). Education for death, or death becomes less a stranger. *Omega, Journal of Death and Dying, 6*, 183–191.

Leviton, D. (1977). Death education. In H. Feifel (Ed.), *New meanings of death* (pp. 254–272). New York, NY: McGraw-Hill.

Lewis, C. S. (1961/1976). *A grief observed*. New York, NY: Bantam.

Lonetto, R., Fleming, S., Gorman, M., & Best, S. (1975). The psychology of death: A course description and some student perceptions. *Ontario Psychologist, 7*, 9–14.

Margolis, O. S., Cherico, D. J., O' Connor, B. P., & Kutscher, A. H. (Eds.). (1978). *Thanatology course outlines* (Vol. 2). New York, NY: MSS Information Corporation.

Meagher, D. K., & Balk, D. E. (Eds.). (2013). *Handbook of thanatology* (2nd ed.). New York, NY: Routledge.

Meagher, D. K., & Shapiro, R. D. (1984). *Death: The experience*. Minneapolis, MN: Burgess.

Mills, L. O. (Ed.). (1969). *Perspectives on death*. Nashville, TN: Abingdon.

Neale, R. E. (1973). *The art of dying*. New York, NY: Harper & Row.

Northcott, H. C., & Wilson, D. M. (2008). *Dying and death in Canada* (2nd ed.). Peterborough, Ontario, Canada: Broadview Press.

Oates, J. C. (2011). *A widow's story: A memoir*. New York, NY: Ecco.

Pausch, R. (with Zaslow, J.). (2008). *The last lecture*. New York, NY: Hyperion.

Pine, V. R. (1977). A socio-historical portrait of death education. *Death Education, 1*, 57–84.

Pine, V. R. (1986). The age of maturity for death education: A socio-historical portrait of the era 1976–1985. *Death Studies, 10*, 209–231.

Prichard, E. R., Collard, J. Orcutt, B. A., Kutscher, A. H., Seeland, I., & Lefkowitz, N. (Eds.). (1977). *Social work with the dying patient and family*. New York, NY: Columbia University Press.

Quint, J. C. (1967). *The nurse and the dying patient*. New York, NY: Macmillan.

Rosenthal, T. (1973). *How could I not be among you?* New York, NY: George Braziller.

Sabatini, P., & Kastenbaum, R. (1973). *The do-it-yourself death certificate as a research technique. Suicide and Life-Threatening Behavior, 3*, 20–32.

Shneidman, E. (1972a). Can a young person write his own obituary? *Life-Threatening Behavior, 2*, 262–267.

Shneidman, E. (Ed.). (1972b). *Death and the college student*. New York, NY: Behavioral Publications.

Shneidman, E. (1977). The college student and death. In H. Feifel (Ed.), *New meanings of death* (pp. 68–86). New York, NY: McGraw-Hill.

Shneidman, E. S. (1980). *Death: Current perspectives* (2nd ed.). Palo Alto, CA: Mayfield. (Original work published 1976)

Shneidman, E. S. (1980/1995). *Voices of death*. New York, NY: Harper & Row/Kodansha International.

Stillion, J. M. (1979). Rediscovering the taxonomies: A structural framework for death education courses. *Death Education, 3*, 157–164.

Tolstoy, L. (1884/1960). *The death of Ivan Ilych and other stories* (A. Maude, Trans.). New York, NY: New American Library.

Wass, H. (Ed.). (1979). *Dying: Facing the facts*. Washington, DC: Hemisphere.

Wass, H., & Corr, C. A. (Eds.). (1984). *Childhood and death*. Washington, DC: Hemisphere.

Wass, H., Corr, C. A., Pacholski, R. A., & Forfar, C. S. (1985). *Death education II: An annotated resource guide*. Washington, DC: Hemisphere.

Wass, H., Corr, C. A., Pacholski, R. A., & Sanders, C. M. (1980). *Death education: An annotated resource guide*. Washington, DC: Hemisphere.

Wertenbaker, L. T. (1957). *Death of a man*. New York, NY: Random House.

White, D. K. (1970). *An undergraduate course in death. Omega, Journal of Death and Dying, 1*, 167–174.

Allan Kellehear   **16**

DEATH EDUCATION AS A PUBLIC HEALTH ISSUE

In 1998, I established Australia's first academic palliative care unit devoted to a public health approach to end-of-life care. In academic terms, this palliative care emphasized the application of health promotion, community development, and death education to clinical services in palliative care. The unit is located in the School of Public Health at La Trobe University in Melbourne, Australia.

Although like all sections within a "research intensive" university this unit conducts research and supervises research postgraduates, an important role for the unit was and remains social activism—to encourage social and professional changes in palliative care services and also in the broader community. In other words, one of the main purposes of this palliative care unit was to reorient conventional clinical services in palliative care toward community engagement and partnerships and public death education. The unit is also active in encouraging all sections of a community to take an interest and to play a modest role in end-of-life care—to foster a view that end-of-life care is everyone's responsibility, not simply health services.

The initial steps in encouraging different groups and communities to discuss dying, death, loss, or long-term care encountered the usual and expected forms of resistance. The phrase "death education" was and remains a difficult one, and the case for making death education a public health priority is not well understood. People commonly view "death education" as a rather morbid affair. This is an understandable reaction—especially as for a good many people the idea of death is frequently linked to funerals, cremations, burials, or memorials—all sad things, dark reminders of grief, and all too commonly sources of fear and social avoidance. In this connection, death education has substantial overlap with human reactions to a visit to the dentist or the dreaded annual medical check-up. But in all these examples, we too often forget that 99% of dental or medical health is far more than visits to the doctor, dentist, and in the case of death education, a funeral event or a bereavement.

Few people reduce their own understanding of health and well-being to a visit to a health professional. Most people know that health promotion is the best way to prevent illness, reduce harm, or the time needed for recovery when you do fall ill. Education about nutrition, the benefits of protected/safe sex, the avoidance of harmful substances—such as tobacco or asbestos—keeping fit with exercise, wearing sunblock, avoiding too sedentary a lifestyle, wearing your vehicle seatbelt or bike helmet are just some of hundreds of ways we are able to live longer and aspire to a good quality of life. In these ways, modern health education in schools, workplaces, in media campaigns, or on food packaging has helped change attitudes, behaviors, and even laws. This is a recent understanding about health and its relationship to illness that most of us appreciate. In terms of the history of public health, then, death education is about where health education was in the 1940s.

This chapter outlines the case for the need to make death education a public health priority, taking its place alongside all other public health campaigns that contribute to national health and well-being. I will argue that death education is both a necessary professional responsibility and community action if we are to successfully tackle the increasing and frequently anxiety-inducing national death-related issues from euthanasia, palliative care, or the determination of death to aging, dementia, or organ donation. Only by increasing the education level, and therefore the quality of community engagement about death and loss, are we able to bring a more informed public to the table so that they may willingly and soberly address these important topics and reduce the level of hysteria and public anxiety.

THE CASE FOR DEATH EDUCATION AS A PUBLIC HEALTH ISSUE

There are at least nine good reasons to implement death education as part of a wider public health approach to national health and well-being. These can be described as: (1) encouraging a normalization of death and loss; (2) building on, learning from, and consolidating personal and community experience; (3) promoting a public understanding that there is more to death and dying than palliative care or grief work; (4) restoring a social context to (the often frightening) problem-focused professional images of death, dying, and loss; (5) keeping abreast of the latest research about death, dying, and loss as informed consumers of related health services; (6) minimizing personal and community anxiety, fear, and hysteria; (7) maximizing an informed sense of hope and control—knowledge is power and encourages mastery; (8) combating personal and community ignorance—major sources of fear and prejudice that always hobble, narrow, even hide our full range of human choices and responses; and (9) reducing the morbidity and mortality rates associated with, but underrecognized as associated with, death, dying, and loss. I will elaborate on each of these public health objectives.

Encouraging a Normalization of Death and Loss

To meet this aim, it is important to connect individual experiences with the experiences of others, for it is a fact that most people have their own experiences of dying, death, loss, or care and that to swap stories of those experiences with other people is important in reducing a sense of isolation. Reducing a sense of isolation that comes from a sad or terrible experience prevents its recipient from developing an overblown sense of self-blame, guilt, or unfairness. In this way, providing a broader context for one's sad experiences encourages harm reduction of the negative impacts of believing this is a trouble entirely unique to you. This also maximizes the possibilities of social support from others who have had similar losses. Such principles of prevention and harm reduction can be actualized in public health practices, such as creating opportunities for people to share these experiences of death and loss on regular occasions.

For example, palliative care professionals can organize an annual round-table event in which they meet to discuss and share their experiences of death and loss with colleagues in a similar end-of-life-care field. Accident and emergency personnel (e.g., paramedics), nursing home professionals, or bereavement care colleagues can meet annually with palliative care colleagues to discuss and swap personal experiences and practice wisdom when dealing with professional issues that affect all of them. In this way, annual round-table events help normalize professional end-of-life care by connecting previously isolated professional efforts with other fields and colleagues in related areas. This can serve as an important professional support alone or as an adjunct support alongside professional supervision and counseling.

For people not professionally involved in end-of-life care, for example, in schools, an annual school-wide effort to work on a policy for death, dying, and loss can serve the same purpose. Parents, teachers, and students can help create a school guidance or policy document that helps these three groups openly discuss and develop practical responses to experiences of death and loss in their school community. As their joint experiences accumulate from year to year, the guidance document becomes a living document that chronicles the practice wisdom of that community. In this way, death and loss become routinized as parts of the proper work of the school alongside health and safety.

Both of these above strategies have two principles in common (see Kellehear, 2005). First, they encourage the use of informal social supports rather than assuming that a professional response is an appropriate first response. In this way, they encourage a reskilling of the broader community in matters to do with death and loss while reserving professional response for complex cases. Second, they foster openness toward death and loss that helps normalize this subject area, laying the groundwork for future receptivity to discussions about death (e.g., advance care planning) more likely.

Building on, Learning From, and Consolidating Personal and Community Experience

The attempt to build practice bridges between services that work in death and loss or to encourage policy developments in workplaces or schools recognizes three major insights into human learning about health and well-being. First, experience does not automatically translate into learning. People often sort their experiences through the lens of their own life or work priorities and prejudices. Or they may not always have time to process and debrief from their experiences, especially exceptional experiences. Or they may not have frameworks of related experience that they can readily identify to see how those other experiences or ways of seeing might be related to their current experience. Whatever the reason, these barriers apply to the end-of-life care professions just as much as they might for ordinary communities, such as schools, workplaces, businesses, or churches/temples. The second principle to recognize, then, is that the formal business of death education, as it is for health education, is a task for everyone.

Third, all learning programs require a two-pronged approach—to build on an absence of experience for some and to build on pre-existing experiences for others. For health professionals in end-of-life care, this may mean guiding these colleagues through their earlier or previous experience with community health, health promotion, or health education to see how the ideas of morbidity and mortality, prevention, harm reduction, or early intervention apply to experiences of dying, death, loss, and long-term care. For lay communities, this might mean encouraging people to join up previously unrelated experiences to their current experiences of death and loss, for example, to link experiences of growing old and infirm with cancer or HIV, or experiences of human bereavement to experiences of loss of companion animals or job loss or forced migration. Experiences of racial prejudice or discrimination can be pushed into reflective service to help understand other experiences of stigma, rejection, or isolation in matters to do with aging, serious illness, or bereavement. Connection of related experiences and their application to new experiences can bring insight and learning. This is key to experiential-based learning.

Promoting a Public Understanding That There Is More to Death and Dying Than Palliative Care or Grief Work

It is essential to remember that addressing our needs in death, loss, and end-of-life care is a multisector task that involves more than palliative care. We must recognize that hospice and palliative care workers are only *one* player in this field. Collaboration with others is crucial, not only for palliative care workers' own professional development and self-care but, equally important, in the task of continuity of care for their patients and families. Coronial workers, aged care workers, those working in disaster management, funeral and cemetery workers, bereavement care professionals, accident and emergency workers, and those working in intensive care are just some of the central professions working in end-of-life care. And they are only the obvious ones! Veterinarians, for example, are commonly de facto bereavement workers because much of their work involves euthanizing animal companions and living and working with the emotional aftermath experienced by pet owners.

Each of these professions has its own practice wisdom in matters to do with personal and community supports and education; ways to tackle communication of bad news as well as aftercare; strategies it employs in self-care; and networks into the community that probably differ substantially from other end-of-life care sectors. In these ways, the different sectors in end-of-life care offer collaborative opportunities in the broader public health system in matters to do with research, professional development and practice, and in pathways to community development that might enhance everyone's efforts to raise awareness and change behavior for the better around dying, death, loss, and care.

Restoring a Social Context to (the Often Frightening) Problem-Focused Professional Images of Death, Dying, and Loss

Adopting a public health approach to dying, death, loss, and care also permits a shift in thinking about these experiences as mere problems. Dying and loss, like love and work, are a mixture of complex and changing experiences. A public health gaze identifies the problem in the context of the normal and usual, commonly by use of social science perspectives. On the other hand, the professional is expected and socialized to be sensitive to problems that he or she is usually asked to "fix," "cure," "manage," or "treat." The emphasis is firmly on the unusual, not the usual. A broad public health approach to death and loss allows us to see the major transitions in life and death as patterns of experience and response in a broad context. When I conducted my first study of the experience of dying (of 100 people with a short life expectancy in a regional cancer unit) and asked people about their negative experiences, I found only 10% of those asked reported social stigma, social rejection, or loss of friends since the time of their diagnosis (Kellehear, 1990). On the other hand, and balancing these negative experiences, were another 10% of respondents who reportedly gained friends, whose existing friends redoubled their support, and who reported closer social intimacy at this time. About half the total of the study's respondents reported no change, and most of the other half reported positive changes to their relationships. In other words, although social stigma and rejection remains a problem for the dying *it is not the whole picture*. An overall view of the public health of dying people's social relationships suggests positive support is normal—not negative experiences. This is quite a different image of dying from the received wisdom of the clinical, case-based literature of cancer and end-of-life care.

In a later study I examined the cross-cultural and historical data on near-death experiences (NDE; Kellehear, 1996). In modern versions of these experiences, people who recover from resuscitation often report out-of-body experiences, tunnel sensation, life review, and sometimes meetings with a bright light or deceased relatives. An examination of existing medical and neuropsychology literature strongly suggests that these experiences are anomalies that arise from oxygen deprivation of the brain. However, a study of precisely these psychological characteristics of modern near-death experiences in the broader transcultural and historical context demonstrates that *all* of those features (i.e., out-of-body experiences, tunnel sensation, life review, and meetings with deceased relatives) do occur to people while fully conscious—in examples from trapped miners, castaways at sea, shamanic initiates, the bereaved, or those in personal crises, to name only a few. Although oxygen deprivation may play a role in some of these examples, a study of near-death experiences that proffers this as a sole explanation is nothing but mere biological reductionism.

In these above examples—stigma while dying and the medicalization, even pathologizing of experiences near death—we see how a sociological approach to the study of death provides a context for the problematizing gaze of clinical work we often associate with dying or death. The far smaller "size" of the problem of public stigma helps reduce people's anxiety about what to expect from others while dying. For near-death experiences, a public understanding that people who experience these NDEs are not mentally ill, their brains not necessarily "malfunctioning," can reduce anxiety in those who experience them first hand or must react to them when told about them from dying friends or patients. This "big picture" approach is also characteristic of a public health approach. These larger frames of seeing help inform, educate, and facilitate new lines of thinking by contextualizing problems. This in turn allows us to control a sense of anxiety about some of these matters by encouraging us to literally see things "in perspective." Problems are not allowed to assume exaggerated importance beyond their size and context. In this way, death education—knowing all the facts—is essential not only in gaining a sober perspective, but also in controlling unnecessary hysteria and myth making.

Keeping Abreast of the Latest Research About Death, Dying, and Loss as Informed Consumers of Related Health Services

The two examples in the fourth purpose of death education highlight the need to keep abreast of the latest research about death, dying, loss, and care as informed consumers of related health services. Just as it is vital that we understand why we need to eat right and understand the benefits of that lifestyle, so we need to understand why we need advanced care planning and why this needs to be performed regularly, as in making legal wills, because our aspirations and attachments keep changing.

But an interest in death education is not simply an interest in health or medical education. Dying, death, loss, and long-term care are not simply matters of learning about the body and how to enhance its health and well-being. Dying, death, loss, and care are multidimensional experiences with major and sometimes competing understandings from religious studies, philosophy, social sciences, psychoanalysis, history, cultural and legal studies, as well as medicine and the social care professions. Death education as a public health issue must be embraced as a multidisciplinary, multidimensional topic. This is a key reason why journals of death studies are multidisciplinary—*Omega: Journal of Death and Dying, Death Studies, Mortality,* or the *Journal of Near-Death Studies.* These journals are key resources not only for professional in-service education but also for public education. For these two audiences, then, for professionals and lay communities, these academic sources are major public health resources.

Minimizing Personal and Community Anxiety, Fear, and Hysteria

Another key purpose of death education as a public health priority is that such education can minimize personal and community anxiety, fear, or hysteria. Remember that away from end-of-life care professions, most people's exposure to dying or death is low, and frequently late in life. With low exposure to dying and death, information is limited, understanding is poor, and reactions are often equally poor. Poor reactions can range from being disabled by anxiety that interferes with usual work or recreational cycles to more severe sexual "acting out"; phobic or avoidance reactions to any associations or people related to serious illness, death, or loss; to social withdrawal and personal isolation.

All of these reactions are preventable or, at the very least, subject to harm reduction by death education. If information and discussion opportunities are provided during the life course, in schools, workplaces, recreational sites, or in the social media, people have a broad opportunity to learn about the realities of dying, death, or loss well before these events or experiences affect them directly (Kellehear, 1999). Alternatively, such opportunities permit them to explore, discuss, and contextualize their own experiences with support from others and with information that extends beyond their own previously limited experiences. The targeting of personal and community fears about dying, death, loss, and care are key aims of any death education.

Maximizing an Informed Sense of Hope and Control: Knowledge Is Power and Encourages Mastery

Although dying, death, and loss are certainties in all our lives, what happens inside those experiences is not certain. Dying may be difficult but nevertheless a rewarding social experience, or it may simply be an experience of abandonment and suffering. When we die, we may go to another and better place in the afterlife, or simply lose all consciousness and become worm fodder. Loss creates grief, and grief can destroy a life or redirect it, reinforce it, inspire it (Kellehear, 2002). Although the outcomes in the story of mortality are certain, the processes within it are not. All things are possible, good and bad. Death education offers an opportunity to explore the positive uses of uncertainty, for it is inside the experience of uncertainty that opportunities for hope and control also find their possibilities.

In this way, it is not merely information that is important in the matter of death education but participation—the sheer involvement in the process of exploration, evaluation, and judgment, of coming to fresh insights and conclusions for oneself that death education can bring. This aspect of death education can free participants from the passive circumstance of being "victim" to partial information about dying, death, and loss and hence to be vulnerable to myth, distortion, and misunderstanding. Death education as part of the school, work, or play environments permits both active consideration of information from several angles through group discussion and learning but, more important, by mere fact of participation—a process that encourages a sense of control and hence mastery of one's own ignorance and anxieties. One of the central public health aims—and benefits—of death education, therefore, is a participatory approach to learning that brings personal ownership to learning. A didactic, passive, or paternalist approach to learning does not encourage lifelong learning because it fails to instill process. Death education as a public health issue is participatory.

Combating Personal and Community Ignorance

The eighth purpose of death education as a public health concern is that most of our education efforts must focus on community. This underlines the fact that the longer part of dying and grieving occurs in community contexts, so the major challenges of change lie there. Contact with health services is usually episodic, whereas the longer periods of care come from family, friends, coworkers, or simply people encountered on the street. It is in these broader social relationships that dying and grieving people are able to observe and experience the major social reactions to themselves, so it is these relationships that are crucial to target in death education terms.

Ignorance about matters to do with dying, death, loss, or long-term care breeds fear and misunderstanding, and these will and do lead to ignorant and fearful social responses from others toward the dying, grieving, and carers. In this way, an important aim of death education as a public health issue is *social marketing*. Just as we must "sell" the benefits of health, exercise, smoking cessation, or safe sex, it is equally important that we sell the value of social support, long-term support, practical support, or the pursuit of multiple understandings about death itself. Each of these modes of support and understanding increases the quality of life of those living with serious illness, loss, or long-term care by reducing their potential isolation, sharing their losses, and encouraging and fostering resilience in those most at risk. But these ideas and benefits must be "sold" to communities that may not have thought about exactly how these things can help and also how these modes of support and understanding might be built into their everyday relationships with each other. Death education must not only be part of schools, workplaces, or churches/temples but must be integrated into a community's social media—television, newspapers, radio, and websites. Public health education is not solely about attempting to change behavior to make people healthy but also about selling people on the idea that being healthy has real benefits. People must *want to be health and safety-wise*. In death education terms, this means that people must *want to learn to be mortality-wise*. We must first sing the benefits of this particular approach to the life cycle.

Reducing the Morbidity and Mortality Rate Associated, but Underrecognized to Be Associated, With Death, Dying, and Loss

The final aim of death education—and the most important aim of all public health initiatives—is to reduce the morbidity and mortality associated with any threats to health and well-being. It is important to note at the outset that it is *not* the aim of any public health campaign to prevent death. Biologically speaking, death is not preventable. The history of public health has been to prevent *unnecessary and early death* and to reduce the burden of suffering and disability caused by preventable disease or injury. In this way, death education as a public health concern is designed to identify the unnecessary causes of death or suffering caused by living with a life-limiting illness, living with bereavement and loss, and living with long-term care.

There are significant social and psychological morbidities and deaths associated with spousal death (Charlton, Sheahan, Smith, & Campbell, 2001; Raphael, 1984; Stroebe, Schut, & Stroebe, 2007) as well as those living with life-limiting illness (Smith et al., 2008; Wilson et al., 2010). The medical and psychological effects of serious loss and bereavement are known to cause early deaths. Furthermore, the negative toll from depression, anger, or anxiety about dying, death, loss, and long-term care on marriages, friendships, or on sexual behaviors is well known. Stigma, isolation, loneliness, fear, social withdrawal or the physical symptoms associated with these social and psychological experiences—insomnia, cardiac arrhythmias, headaches, gastrointestinal disorders, hypertension, or anxiety disorders—are all documented to be associated with the stresses and strains of living with a life-limiting illness, loss and bereavement, or long-term caring. All of these problems and risks are subject to prevention, harm reduction, and early intervention by educating the people at the center of these experiences of the risks and hazards as well as the potential solutions *and* by educating the support networks of those people so that they may offer strategic and timely support for people at risk, including themselves some day.

TWO CURRENT INTERNATIONAL EXAMPLES

The above social, psychological, and medical factors and circumstances are the key reasons why several countries have now implemented programs of death education. Mostly led by hospice and palliative care interests in the two following examples, death education is seen as essential to supporting a country's end-of-life care system. Palliative care is widely defined as whole person care—addressing the physical, psychological, social, and spiritual well-being of patients and their families. Most palliative care services provide a primary health response to these needs (first contact with service, e.g., general practitioners) or a specialist response (services accessed through referral to specialist doctors or hospitals). In either case, the health care service attempts to address these needs through a professional response, that is, by offering social work, counseling or pastoral services along with the usual medical and nursing services. The limitations of this services-only approach are threefold: (1) Many of the psychological, social, and spiritual needs or problems that people with life-limiting illness, bereavement, or long-term care experience are embedded, derived from, or mediated by their wider families and communities, and are mostly inaccessible to professional intervention. (2) Most of the time that people spend living with their illness, loss, or care experiences is with their families or communities outside the narrow time band of episodic care provided by health care professionals. In other words, time with health care professionals is very minimal, in contrast to the time spent without them; that is, most of the time is spent, for most people in palliative, bereavement, or respite care, with family, friends, and community. Finally (3), it is not financially possible or sustainable for health services to provide continuity of care from diagnosis to death or to the aftercare needed in long-term bereavement. Most services simply do not have the resources to be there for patients and family most of the time.

In these circumstances of formal end-of-life-care services, only by working in partnership with community to build resilience and continuity of support can communities and families begin to take more informed and active roles in end-of-life care. To do this effectively, families and communities need to know, understand, and continue to learn about dying, death, bereavement, and long-term care. In this public health approach, end-of-life care becomes everyone's responsibility (Kellehear, 2013). Only through means of community-based death education programs are we able to begin the work of building genuine capacity in communities to care for themselves at the end of life. Death education not only builds knowledge and confidence, but it is also instrumental in building trust, empathy, and support in what public health theorists describe as "building social capital" (Lomas, 1998).

Scotland

The Scottish government has commenced a program of death education through its organization The Scottish Partnership for Palliative Care (SPPC). This was enshrined in its end-of–life-care policy in 2008. Since that time, the SPPC has developed and implemented community-based death education programs throughout Scotland in both urban and rural areas (see http://www.goodlifedeathgrief.org.uk). This includes the creation of a national website with over 800 members, a national awareness week campaign in 2013, and numerous single-site projects across diverse communities in Scotland. The website introduces its approach to death education with the first sentence asserting that "Death is normal," and elaborates by describing the reasons why death education is crucial for the health and well-being of professionals but also their patients, families, and supporting communities. It describes its "key messages" by declaring:

We believe that:

Being more open about death is a good thing
Death is normal
Planning for death when you're healthy means there is less to think about if you get sick
We can all help each other with death, dying and bereavement
Coming to terms with your own mortality can help you to live life to the full
There are things individuals and communities can actively do to help others through difficult times relating to death, dying and bereavement
Death is happening all around us, causing sadness and difficulties that people often don't share
Death can be upsetting, and people need to take the time to grieve

Projects that palliative care services have led across Scotland include: (1) Creating a "Before I Die" wall in several public sites, including construction sites, so that people might take time to think about what they would really like to do before they die and to share this publicly on a blackboard for others to see and get inspired to participate with their ideas. (2) Offering a Master Class on death and dying for occupational therapists. (3) Implementing a "Let's Talk" seminar in collaboration with the Church of Scotland to assess the role and needs of congregations in matters to do with their experiences of dying, death, and bereavement. (4) One Glasgow-based hospice setting up a "conversation stall" in the middle of a shopping mall to encourage passersby to speak with them about dying, death, and bereavement. (5) One school organizing a drop-in lunchtime session for teachers and other staff to discuss issues of dying, death, and bereavement that concerned them. (6) Several hospitals in collaboration with hospices holding death information events to encourage people to raise questions; to seek information and hold practical conversations about will-making, funeral planning, advance care directives; and to participate in Before I Die Blackboards. (7) Another hospice developing a special iPhone app—the Legacy Organizer —to enable "users to store their life history as well as their intentions and wishes for all aspects of their funeral, farewell and will."

Australia

In Australia, similar projects of death education are an integral part of health-promotion campaigns by hospices and palliative care services. Public health approaches that include death education are part of the practice guidelines of Palliative Care Australia—the national professional body for palliative care (Palliative Care Australia, 2000). The major Australian academic public health palliative care unit established by myself in 1998 has, among other tasks, a role to promote death education in palliative care services and in the communities that those services support (Kellehear, 1999). Among the many approaches taken by services in that country are the facilitation and implementation of school policies on dying, death, and loss—helping schools to hold ongoing conversations about dying, death, and loss and to commit some of their experiences to forming school guidance documents to help them prepare for future crises and losses in their own school community (Kellehear & O'Connor, 2008).

Other services have led "World Café Conversations" in communities that they have served. In these cases, restaurants are booked and topics or questions about dying, death, or loss discussed and recorded on disposable tablecloths between meal courses (Kellehear & Young, 2007). Questions commonly discussed are: "If I had only 6 months to live, what would I like to do for me—and for others?" "What are the best ways to help a grieving friend?" and "Should one prepare for death—Why? Why not?" These café conversations have also been popular in England and Scotland as ways to engage communities in death education, providing both information and a safe (and often humor-filled?) community context in which to become accustomed to speaking about potentially threatening topics.

FUTURE CHALLENGES

In the United States, addressing death education as a community public health issue is in its infancy. Most death education is confined to universities and colleges. Much of palliative care remains clinically oriented, emphasizing bedside care in the hospital, hospice, or at home. Education work in the community tends to emphasize information about the benefits of hospice/palliative care and not the broader issues of dying, death, and loss. Education programs remain didactic—led, content-controlled, and delivered solely by health care professionals. Too often, end-of-life care is *performed on* people rather than *with* them. In this developing context, it might be useful for U.S. interests in hospice and palliative care to seek out and examine international programs in death education in the United Kingdom, Canada, Australia, Africa, or Asia (see Sallnow, Kumar, & Kellehear, 2012), and to learn and adapt these existing programs for local American use and experiment.

At the same time, it will also be important for hospice and palliative care workers to learn new ways of working with resistance, cultural diversity, and fear in groups that are not their usual patient populations, or in families that are connected to current or past service use. *Working with healthy populations* who have little or no interest in dying, death, or bereavement is testing work with different challenges than working with patient populations. Partnerships with public health colleagues working in community health, HIV/AIDS, abuse and trauma, or migrant health populations can be beneficial in facilitating exchange of practice wisdom in working with groups with particular sensitivities and resistances.

This last point also highlights the overall importance of the need for training, supportive partnerships, and mentoring in the public health methodologies, especially health promotion, community development, and health education strategies and theories. Although it is true that public health professionals have little experience in matters to do with dying and death, it is equally true that palliative care colleagues have little formal training in health promotion, health education, or community development. These gaps in training in the respective health fields complement each other and can lead to important in-service training programs and exchanges that can be valuable to both.

However, although it is easier to see how palliative care professionals might see the value of death education for their own future work with patients and families, it is more difficult for public health professionals to understand the links between death education and health and well-being. Today, public health encyclopedias and journals are filled with concerns about smoking cessation, obesity, industrial accident prevention, work stress, or child health. Dying and death are portrayed as targets of prevention—they are destinations to be avoided. Academic public health does not see dying or bereavement as particular life journeys that bring their own lifestyle-related hazards that can benefit from prevention and harm-reduction interventions. An ironic challenge for those of us who work in end-of-life care is to help reorient our public health colleagues to these facts about dying, bereavement, and long-term care so that we can have a useful and powerful ally in the task of delivering death education as a public health good.

Finally, although death education programs are currently proliferating around the world, and we can expect to see more of these in the future, we have yet to see major examples of their evaluation. Much of the current research-based evaluations are in the so-called "grey literature"—postgraduate dissertations, government or private organization reports, or in conference presentations and abstracts. More work remains to be done to establish the evidence base for the effectiveness, limitation, or benefits of death education as a public health good. The practice of death education in health services is recent, and many of its methodologies are new and novel. The pace of death education has so far outstripped attempts to evaluate it, but this cannot be sustained. If national associations and governments are to take the value of death education seriously in their future policy ruminations and developments, we must have a robust evidence base to persuade them.

Self-evidently, modern death studies, the hospice movement, and the "new" public health movements are all recent developments. Many would argue that these fields really only came into their own in the 1960s and 1970s. The issues of advanced care planning, organ donation, the debates about the determination of death or the public health debates about the limits to health services contributions to life expectancy or compressing morbidity at the end of life have achieved public and media attention only in the last 20 years or so. In this historical context, the idea of death education as a public health issue may seem novel to many observers in health service and policy circles.

However, unless death education does become widely adopted and adapted to the culture-specific needs of all countries, the need to address end-of-life care issues in an intelligent and informed manner, without a significant sense of social threat, will remain illusive when we deal with future patients and their families. This is a set of circumstances that benefits no one. Death education therefore remains the single most important public health challenge for the future if we dare to hope for informed public discussion and rational policy development in end-of-life care.

REFERENCES

Charlton, R., Sheahan, K., Smith, G., & Campbell, I. (2001). Spousal bereavement—Implications for health. *Family Practice, 18*, 614–618.

Kellehear, A. (1990). *Dying of cancer: The final year of life.* Chur, Switzerland: Harwood Academic.

Kellehear, A. (1996). *Experiences near death: Beyond medicine and religion.* New York, NY: Oxford University Press.

Kellehear, A. (1999). *Health promoting palliative care.* Melbourne, Australia: Oxford University Press.

Kellehear, A. (2002). Grief and Loss: Past, present and future. *Medical Journal of Australia, 177*(4), 176–177.

Kellehear, A. (2005). *Compassionate cities: Public health and end-of-life care.* London, UK: Routledge.

Kellehear, A. (2013). Compassionate communities: End of life care as everyone's responsibility. *Quarterly Journal of Medicine (UK), 106*(12), 1071–1075.

Kellehear, A., & O'Connor, D. (2008). Health promoting palliative care: A practice example. *Critical Public Health (UK), 18*(1), 111–115.

Kellehear, A., & Young, B. (2007). Resilient communities. In B. Monroe & D. Oliviere (Eds.), *Resilience in palliative care: Achievements in adversity* (pp. 223–238). Oxford, UK: Oxford University Press.

Lomas, J. (1998). Social capital and health: Implications for public health and epidemiology. *Social Science & Medicine, 47*(9), 1181–1188.

Moore, D. J., & Posada, C. (2013, January). HIV and psychiatric co-morbidities: What do we know and what can we do. *Psychology and AIDS exchange Newsletter.* Retrieved from http://www.apa.org/pi/aids/resources/exchange/2013/01/comorbidities.aspx

Palliative Care Australia. (2005). *A guide to palliative care service development: A population-based approach.* Canberra, Australia: Palliative Care Australia.

Raphael, B. (1984). *The anatomy of bereavement.* New York, NY: Basic Books.

Sallnow, L., Kumar, S., & Kellehear, A. (Eds.). (2012). *International perspectives on public health and palliative care.* Abingdon, VA: Routledge.

Smith, A. W., Reeve, B. B., Bellizzi, K. M., Harlan, L. C., Klabunde, C. N., Amsellem, M.,. . . Hays, R. D. (2008). Cancer, comorbidities, and health related quality of life of older adults. *Health Care Financial Reviews, 29*(4), 41–56.

Stroebe, M., Schut, H., & Stroebe, W. (2007). Health outcomes of bereavement. *Lancet, 370*, 1960–1973.

Wilson, M. G., Chambers, L., Bacon, J., Rueda, S., Ragan, M., & Rourke, S. B. (2010, December 7). *Issues of comorbidity in HIV/AIDS: An overview of systematic reviews.* Toronto, Ontario, Canada: Ontario HIV Treatment Network.

Part III: Practice Developments

Kenneth J. Doka

17

SPIRITUALITY: *QUO VADIS?**

The earliest writings of humans were essentially spiritual treatises on death. *The Epic of Gilgamesh*, one of the earliest surviving pieces of literature, is the story of Gilgamesh's search for the secret of immortality. Similarly, The Egyptian *Book of the Dead* is a self-help manual on what to do when one is dead—including magical spells and incantations to facilitate the journey through the afterlife. Other early scriptures from all the major faiths address death and the afterlife. This is not unexpected. As Becker (1973) noted, humans have always been troubled by the paradox of mortality. That is, humans have both the conceptual ability to recognize their mortality and the survival instinct to resist that knowledge. Spirituality remains an effective mechanism to resolve that paradox.

As in other areas, as death became a subject for the medical and social sciences, the spiritual dimension lost prominence. Freud, in his classic article, *Mourning and Melancholia* (1917/1957), an article that arguably represents the first beginnings of a modern psychology of death, ignores any spiritual component to mourning. In many ways, this trend of secularization reaches its zenith in Moody's *Life After Life* (1975). Here, Moody offers "scientific proof" of an afterlife—devoid of any overt notion of faith. In essence, it is a secular vision of afterlife wrapped in scientific guise.

However, with the rise of the hospice movement, led by openly spiritual Dame Cicely Saunders, spirituality reemerged as a critical aspect of hospice care. In recent years, varied initiatives, such as the National Consensus Project, emphasized the value of spirituality as an aspect of palliative care, The ACE (Achieving Clinical Excellence) project offering training in palliative care to chaplains and psycho social professionals, and The Hospice Foundation of America's Teleconference on spirituality at the end-of-life, all stressed the importance of spiritual care in death and bereavement.

On a personal note (Doka, 2011), this subject has always been a personal interest of mine as it is at the intersection of two of my critical roles—as a professor of counseling with a specialty in thanatology and as a Lutheran clergyman. I have also always been gratified by the interest in spirituality that seemed always to be an undercurrent in the field. I remember an early conference of ADEC (the Association for Death Education and Counseling) at which a group proposed a breakout session on spirituality. The conference committee assigned a small breakout room on the assumption of limited interest in the topic. Twice, though, the room had to be changed to accompany the crowd, which included nearly two thirds of the conference attendees. Out of that conference came the book *Death and Spirituality* (Doka, 1993b). In this chapter, I explore what has been learned about spirituality in palliative and bereavement care—considering the ways that spirituality affects health, coping with

---

*Portions of this work were drawn from previous pieces published by the author and noted in the references.

dying and bereavement, as well as critical issues in the delivery of spiritual care. Yet, despite considerable progress, significant challenges remain. A concluding section reviews these continuing concerns.

RELIGION, SPIRITUALITY, HEALTH, AND GRIEF

Research has indicated that religion and spirituality can both facilitate and complicate responses to life-threatening illness and grief. In reviewing this research, both terms may be linked as the operational definitions of spirituality and religion vary considerably among the researchers. Nonetheless, this research has indicated that spirituality and religion can have positive roles in assisting individuals who struggle with life-threatening illness or grief.

For example, research has supported the fact that religion and spirituality can assist persons in coping with illness by providing a sense of meaning in the illness (Siegel & Schrimshaw, 2002). Others have noted that spiritual support and spiritually based faith can facilitate a sense of resilience and hope even in the face of devastating illness (Pentz, 2005). Often, the diagnosis of a life-threatening illness challenges an individual's assumptive world as the person struggles with attempting to make sense of the illness. Later in the illness, individuals may seek to make sense of their suffering, their death, or their life. Throughout this existential endeavor, religious and spiritual perspectives can offer meaning. Religious and spiritual perspectives may reassure persons with life-threatening illness that their illness is part of a larger plan or that the illness experience may offer lessons to self or others. In some spiritualities, suffering may offer a cosmic connection to humankind. Even with death, there is some evidence that religious and spiritual beliefs may minimize fear and uncertainty (Siegel & Schrimshaw, 2002). In short, spiritual and religious perspectives can assist individuals in making sense of the illness.

It may also allow a sense of a larger connection. Even in the inherent existential isolation of an illness, there may be a sense that God or some Higher Power will sustain and protect. This connection may be more tangible as well. Many individuals may benefit from the social support available through the ministries of a chaplain, clergy, spiritual advisor, ministry team, or even within the larger faith community. The sense that one is not alone and others are caring, visiting, and praying seems to provide benefit (Siegel & Schrimshaw, 2002; Townsend, Kladder, & Mulligan, 2002).

Religious and spiritual practices and beliefs may even enhance health. Most spiritual belief systems suggest either abstinence or moderation in certain behaviors, such as alcohol or tobacco use. Such practices and beliefs may discourage inappropriate coping techniques throughout the course of the illness or subsequent grief. Spiritual and religious beliefs may also enhance coping by encouraging self-esteem. Most religious and spiritual systems stress the inherent worth of the individual. Such beliefs may be especially important in a life-threatening illness or in grief where self-blame may loom large and self-acceptance is threatened. There is also some speculation that spiritual and religious beliefs may have physiological benefits, such as lowering blood pressure or enhancing immune function, though here the research has shown some inconsistency (Dane, 2000; Lin & Bauer-Wu, 2003; Miller & Thoresen, 2003; Olive, 2004; Sephton, Koopman, Shaal, Thoresen, & Spiegel 2001; Stefanek, McDonald, & Hess, 2005).

Religious and spiritual beliefs may also influence an individual's sense of control. In a time of life-threatening illness, an individual may feel that he or she has little or no control. Religious and spiritual beliefs may reaffirm a sense of personal control. This can be expressed in a number of ways. Individuals may have a sense of interpretive control—the ability to find meaning or benefit from the experience. They may have a sense of vicarious control—leaving the illness in the hands of a Higher Power. In some cases, the control may be of a predictive nature; perhaps believing that God will cure them or be with them throughout this experience.

Yet, this discussion also demonstrates the ways that religious and spiritual beliefs may complicate the response to a life-threatening illness or grief. For example, a person with life-threatening illness may be convinced that he or she may be cured by a divine intervention. If death ensues, such an individual or other family members may become immobilized, unrealistic in decisions, or even despondent. In other cases, the illness may be viewed as a punishment for prior acts.

Certain religious or spiritual beliefs may serve to increase rather than decrease death anxiety or complicate grief. For example, fears over divine judgment or uncertainty in an afterlife may not offer comfort to a dying person. The certainty with which religious and spiritual beliefs are held as well as the nature of such beliefs is a factor in the reasons that the relationship of religiosity and spirituality to death anxiety is inconsistent (Neimeyer, 1994). Moreover, religious and spiritual perspectives can sometimes conflict with medical practices and advice. For example, some spiritual systems, such as Christian Science, may eschew any medical treatment, whereas others, such as Jehovah's Witnesses, may prohibit certain medical practices such as blood transfusions or blood-based therapies. In other cases, a fatalistic spirituality may inhibit health-seeking behaviors or adherence to a medical regimen. It is little wonder that Pargement, Koenig, Tarakeshwar, and Hahn (2004) found in a longitudinal study that certain types of religious coping, such as seeking spiritual support or believing in a benevolent God, were related to better health, whereas other spiritual coping behaviors and beliefs, such as a perspective of a punishing God or religious discontent, were predictive of declines in health.

Religious and spiritual beliefs may also be evident in reactions to illness. For example, anger could be directed toward God. There may be anger that one has the disease or that the disease has come at an inopportune or unfair time. Guilt may be clouded by moral guilt —a belief that this illness is a punishment for some transgression. Fear and anxiety, as mentioned earlier, can also have a religious or spiritual root, as one may fear the wrath of God in this world or the next. There may even be an existential sense of abandonment—a sense that one is facing the crisis alone, alienated from God. In all of these cases, religious and spiritual beliefs may intertwine with psychological and affective reactions to the illness.

SPIRITUAL TASKS IN LIFE-THREATENING ILLNESS

Throughout the course of an illness, an individual may have to cope with distinctly spiritual tasks. In an earlier work (Doka, 1993a), I proposed, building on the work of both Pattison (1978) and Weisman (1980), that life-threatening illness can best be viewed as a series of phases. These phases are the prediagnostic, diagnostic, chronic, terminal, and recovery phases. In any particular disease, individuals may jump from one phase to another. For example, in some cases, a successful removal of a tumor may place an individual right into a recovery phase with virtually no chronic phase. In another disease, diagnosis may be immediately followed by a steep and inexorable decline toward death. In each phase, there are distinct medical, psychological, social, and spiritual tasks.

For example, in the first two phases, the prediagnostic and diagnostic phases, individuals had to deal with the diagnosis of a life-threatening illness. As Weisman (1980) noted, even when the diagnosis is expected or feared, it still comes as a shock, creating a sense of "existential plight" in which one's very existence is threatened. Often it is a life divide. Even if the person survives the encounter, he or she will often talk about this as a turning point fraught with implications that follow for the rest of life.

Here, the spiritual issue is incorporating the present reality of illness into one's sense of past and future. Questions such as, "Why did I get this disease now?" loom large here. An individual now struggles to make sense of the disease and of the new reality of his or her life. Spiritual and religious beliefs may offer an answer to these questions or at least provide direction for further quest.

The chronic phase centers around the time of treatment. Here, the individual must cope not only with the disease but also with the burdens and side effects of treatment. Often, as persons continue such treatment, they may resume some of their prior roles—returning to work or functioning within their families. Often, this is a lonely time. The crisis of the diagnosis is now past, so family, friends, and other social support may not be as available. This phase can also be a time of great uncertainty as individuals cope with the ambiguities of both the disease and the treatment.

In the chronic phase, suffering may become a major spiritual issue. "Why am I suffering through this disease and treatment?" "Is it all worth it?" Persons will often look to their religious or spiritual beliefs to make sense of this suffering. Their beliefs may vary. Again, some may see the suffering as retribution for sins in this or another life. Some may even find comfort in that thought, believing that suffering now may offer recompense or even purification that will mollify God or better prepare him or her for an afterlife. Others may see suffering as random. Still others may see their suffering as a learning experience allowing greater empathy. Others may see it as sacrifice, offering it as a way to gain a greater connection to God or others. Such beliefs can strongly influence patients' receptiveness to pain management (Doka, 2006).

Not everyone dies from life-threatening illness. Many individuals may fully recover, resuming their lives, and others may face long, even permanent, periods of remission. Yet the encounter with disease leaves all types of residues. Individuals may have an enhanced sense of their fragility, feeling that they are living under a sword that can strike at any time (Koocher & O'Malley, 1981).

There is also spiritual residue. Individuals may struggle with a sense of "the bargain." It is not unusual for persons to make spiritual commitments and promises in a cosmic deal to surmount the illness. Now that they have recovered from this threat, individuals may now feel they have to fulfill their promises. A failure to fulfill such commitments may loom large should a person experience a relapse or even encounter another disease.

There may be other spiritual changes as well. Some individuals may move closer to their religion or become more spiritually aware and active. Others may feel alienated either from their God or their spiritual community. Some may actively seek a new spirituality, perceiving that their past beliefs did not serve them well in this crisis.

During the course of a life-threatening illness, patients and their families will have to make critical ethical decisions about care. How long should active medical treatment persist even if it is perceived as futile? When should treatment cease, and who should be empowered to make such determinations? Should the patient receive artificial hydration and nutrition? Can treatments be withheld or, if administered, withdrawn? Is assisted suicide ever a valid ethical choice in life-threatening illness?

Health professionals have long realized that religious and spiritual systems play a significant role in the ways that patients and their families make end-of-life decisions and resolve ethical dilemmas (Koenig, 2004). As patients and their families struggle with these decisions, they often turn to their religious and spiritual values, and even to their clergy or spiritual mentors, for guidance.

In the terminal phase, the goals of treatment move from extending life or curing the individual to a strictly palliative goal. In this phase, individuals often struggle with three spiritual needs (Doka, 1993a, 1993b). The first is to have lived a meaningful life. Individuals may assess their life to find a sense of meaning and purpose. Here, individuals may struggle, seeking forgiveness for tasks unaccomplished or for hurtful acts that they may have committed. Therapeutic approaches, such as life review, reminiscence therapy, and dignity therapy (Chochinov, 2012) can assist individuals in achieving a sense of meaningfulness. Individuals may struggle with a second goal—to die an appropriate death, however that is individually defined. A final spiritual need is to find hope beyond the grave. This means that the individual needs a sense that life will continue—in whatever appropriate way is supported by the person's spirituality. This can include living on in the memories of others, in the genes of family members, within one's community, in the creations and legacies left, in a sense of "eternal nature" (that is, that one returns to the cycle of life), in some transcendental mode, or in an afterlife (Doka 1993a; Lifton & Olsen, 1974).

SPIRITUALITY AND GRIEF: AFTER THE DEATH

Families, too, may cope with similar spiritual issues. Even after the individual dies, the family may still struggle spiritually, trying to reconstruct their own faith or spiritual system, which may have been challenged by that loss (Doka, 1993b). There may be very significant spiritual issues as individuals experience grief. Bereaved individuals may experience a number of spiritual reactions. There may be a loss of faith. Individuals who are grieving may have a spiritual or cosmic anger—alienating them from sources of spiritual strengths, such as their beliefs, rituals, faith practices, or their faith community. They may experience a sense of "moral guilt"—or a belief that the death of the deceased is due to some moral failing or sin that is now being punished.

As in illness, spirituality can be both facilitating and complicating. It may allow a sense of meaning—that this loss fulfills some purpose or is part of a cosmic plan. Spirituality can offer a sense of connection—a belief that the deceased is now safe or happy, or a belief that even entertains a possibility of future contact or reunion. Spiritual beliefs and practices can even allow a continuing connection—through, for example, prayer, veneration of ancestors, or some other form of contact.

Yet not all beliefs or practices may be facilitating. Some beliefs may disallow or disenfranchise the normal feelings of grief as indicating a lack of faith. Other beliefs may trouble the bereaved. For example, a survivor of a completed suicide who feels the person who commits suicide faces eternal damnation may find such a belief complicates grief.

ASSISTING INDIVIDUALS AND FAMILIES AT THE END OF LIFE: USING SPIRITUALITY

Because spirituality is so central as individuals and their families struggle with later life, it is important that holistic care include spiritual assessment. Although there are a variety of tools available to assist assessment (Hodge, 2005; Ledger, 2005), the key really is to engage both the individual and family in an exploration of their individual and collective spiritual histories. The goal is to understand these collective and individual spiritual journeys. Do they identify with a particular faith? Do they actively practice that faith—engaging in public and private rituals and practices? Do they belong to a church, temple, synagogue, or mosque? How important is their faith system in making decisions?

However, such an assessment should go beyond religious affiliation. It might be worthwhile to explore with individuals when and where they feel most spiritually connected. What practices do they use when they're stressed, anxious, or depressed? What are the stories, prayers, or songs that offer spiritual comfort? Such approaches may allow a larger exploration of the very distinct ways that individuals find meaning and hope. An assessment may yield information on spiritual strengths that an individual possesses, themes within an individual's spirituality (such as grace, karma, fate, or retribution), and experiences that have tended to challenge that person's spirituality. Occasionally, such an assessment may uncover forms of spiritual abuse—spiritual beliefs or practices or behaviors of spiritual mentors that have resulted in a sense of spiritual alienation.

Once an assessment of spirituality is made, an individual can be encouraged to connect with their spiritual strengths. Often, this may involve clergy, chaplains, spiritual mentors, or members of their faith community. Clergy, chaplains, and other spiritual mentors can play an important supportive (and sometimes an unsupportive) role as an individual responds to a life-threatening illness, death, or grief. Their visits throughout the illness may be valued. Clergy, chaplains, and other spiritual advisors may be sought as an individual or family member responds to the spiritual questions inherent in the experiences of grief and illness. Despite the importance of ministry to the ill, the dying, and bereaved, many clergy reported little formal seminary education on dealing with dying patients and their families (Abrams, Albury, Crandall, Doka, & Harris, 2005; Doka & Jendreski, 1985).

Although clergy, chaplains, and other spiritual mentors play an important role, faith communities also can play a critical role. Often, such communities can offer spiritual comfort and connection; visits, calls, cards, and letters that show support and ease isolation; and assistance with tangible tasks, such as cooking, home maintenance, transportation, and caregiving.

Spiritual beliefs and practices may also be sources of strength. A person's spiritual beliefs may be critical in making meaning throughout an illness, and for family, after the death. Often, a simple question, such as "How do your beliefs speak to you in this situation?" can engage the person in spiritual exploration. It may also be useful to investigate the ways that the individual's beliefs assisted and helped the person make sense of the experience in earlier crises. There may be situations in which the individual's beliefs seem inadequate or dysfunctional.

Spiritual practices, such as prayer and meditation, may also have a role in the illness. At the very least, intercessory prayer (that is, the prayer of others) is a tangible sign that the individual is not facing this crisis alone. It offers family and friends a tangible thing to do—reaffirming a form of vicarious control in an unsettled time. Individuals who are struggling with physical illness often use prayer as a form of coping (Ribbentrop, Altmaier, Chen, Found, & Keffala, 2005). There is some evidence that prayer and meditation do affect physical health in a number of ways, including lowering stress levels and blood pressure (Mayo Clinic Health Letter, 2005). Schroeder-Sheker (1994) has even pioneered the field of musical thanatology, using spiritual music as a way to ease the transition to death.

THE POWER AND USE OF RITUALS

Rituals also can be a source of comfort to both the ill or dying patient as well as family. Many faith traditions have rituals for the sick and the dying, such as the Roman Catholic Rite for Anointing of the Sick (popularly known as "Last Rites") or rituals at the time of death, such as washing or preparing the body.

In addition, for individuals struggling with issues of guilt, spiritual traditions often offer rituals or beliefs that encourage and offer forgiveness, of either self or others, such as the Roman Catholic Ritual of Confession and Reconciliation. However, it is important to remember that forgiveness should be addressed by and not imposed on dying or bereaved clients. Imposing such beliefs by impressing, for example, that a client ought to forgive someone is a form of spiritual countertransference. As Shneidman (1978) once wisely said, "no one has to die in a state of psychoanalytic grace" (p. 211).

Individuals who do not have distinctive rituals as part of their tradition may be invited to create one at the time of death. Lighting a candle, anointing the dead person, joining in prayer or meditation, singing a spiritual hymn or song, or in other, individual ways, saying a final goodbye can mark the transition from life to death. Rituals work well in these liminal or transitional moments—offering participants a way to acknowledge loss and transition.

Certainly, rituals after the death, such as funerals, can be critically important to families and others as they cope with loss. Funerals can allow mourners a sense of the reality of death, they offer a chance to ventilate feelings, to provide meaninful actions in a disorganized time, present opportunities to remember the deceased, foster a coming together of supportive others, and create an interpretation of the death according to their own philosophical or spiritual background (Rando, 1984).

The value of funerals can be enhanced when mourners have opportunities to plan and participate in the ritual (Doka & Jendreski, 1985). Although funeral rituals can be exceedingly therapeutic, there is much that can be done to enhance the salutary significance of the rite. Early evidence has emphasized the value of planning and participating in funeral ceremonies (Doka, 1984). There are numerous opportunities and ways that this can be done. Family members can serve as pallbearers, readers, and eulogists. Dependent on the religious service, there may be other opportunities to participate. For example, in liturgical churches, such as Anglican, Lutheran, and Roman Catholic Services, there may be other possibilities. Adolescents may be employed as crucifers, acolytes, or altar boys. Even younger children can participate—perhaps handing out programs.

There are also a wide range of ways to personalize the funeral. Memory boards, photograph displays, and media presentations can highlight the life of the deceased—reaffirming the meaning and significance of life. Eulogies, personally selected music and readers also enhance the individual quality of the rite.

In planning meaningful funerals, it is important to acknowledge the diversity of cultural and spiritual backgrounds among participants in the funeral ritual. Few participants are likely to share the same cultural and spiritual roots. This calls for cultural and spiritual translation—that is, explaining what is occurring to those of different cultural or spiritual traditions.

Moreover, rituals can be used therapeutically throughout the mourning process. In some cases, there may be rituals beyond the funeral that allow for the continued commemoration of the deceased and reaffirmation of a continuing bond with the deceased within the survivor's spiritual traditions and practices. For example, the wide-ranging rituals in Japanese Buddhism associated with ancestor worship offer reassurance of a continuing bond, mitigate grief, and reinforce family ties and national identity (Klass, 1996). Judaism, as well, has multiple rituals and observances, especially in the first 12 months after a death (Lamm, 1969). Christianity too has such opportunities to use rituals in the course of the mourning process. In the Roman Catholic tradition, for example, masses for the deceased are often offered at significant times, such as the birthday of the deceased or on the anniversary of the death. In many spiritual traditions, altar flowers can be dedicated to the deceased on such occasions. In addition, certain Feast Days, such as All Souls Day (November 2), can be a time to commemorate the deceased. Other churches have begun "Longest Night" services on the Winter Solstice to comfort people who are bereaved, acknowledging their loss in a generally festive time.

We incorporate the elements of ritual in the therapeutic process. Such rituals focus on specific therapeutic goals and reaffirm specific therapeutic messages (see Doka, 2013; Doka & Martin, 2010). Such rituals may be performed by individuals and larger groups, such as the intimate network of survivors. They can be a bridge to an individual's culture or spirituality by incorporating elements of that culture, faith, or philosophy into the rite.

Therapeutic rituals have a specific message. One such message may be one of continuity. *Rituals of continuity* reaffirm a continuing bond with the deceased—recognition that the relationship is retained even in death. In many ways, these are relatively common rituals that may be undertaken in a wide variety of settings. Participation in an anniversary mass, toasting a deceased individual on a birthday, or lighting a candle are all examples of such a ritual.

Rituals of transition are designed to indicate movement within the process of grief. One of the most powerful rituals of transition that I participated in was with a middle-aged widow whose husband had died of a progressive illness about 5 years earlier. The presenting issue was that she wanted to start to date again—ready for new relationships within her life. There were issues about this with her adult children—in fact they were unthreatened, even encouraging. The issue was that she still wore her wedding ring. She realized she could not date with it but was ambivalent about removing the ring. In therapy, we spoke about the ring's significance. It had much meaning. She remembered her vows when the ring was placed on her finger. Throughout the illness, the demands of caregiving often strained their relationship. Yet, every night, in bed together, they would touch their rings together and repeat their vows—*in sickness and in health*. Given that the ring was placed on her finger in a ritual, the meaning of the ring reinforced by ritual, I invited her to consider a ritual for removing the ring. She returned to the church where she made her marriage vows. After Mass, the priest called her up to the altar and repeated the vows—now in the past tense. *Were you faithful in sickness and health?* She could affirm that she had been. The priest then asked for the ring. As she later said, the ring came off easily—as if magically.

Rituals of reconciliation allow mourners to finish business. Such rituals can permit the mourner to give or to receive forgiveness. Often, for illustration, the Vietnam Memorial offers a space for such rituals. In one, an unknown medic left a note attached to a name on the wall. "*I want you to know, I did everything possible to save you. You're here. It was not enough. I'm sorry.*" In another such ritual, a young client's mother was an IV drug user who eventually died of HIV/AIDS. The child had a difficult relationship with her mother—often bouncing back and forth into foster care. The positive aspect of this was the girl's foster parent was her godmother. The girl had a highly positive relationship with her godmother and the godmother's husband—her foster father. In fact, they watched over the girl and maintained a relationship when she returned to her biological mother—encouraging the mother's abstinence. When her mother died, her foster parents adopted her. At that time, I asked her where her mother was. The girl explained that her mother was now a ghost. In the girl's singular spirituality—good people went to heaven becoming angels. Bad people descended to hell, burning up into skeletons. People in between became ghosts. The question to determine their final fate was whether they would be bad or good ghosts. In therapy, we worked on her ambivalent relationship with her mom. Over time, she was able to resolve that ambivalence. The young girl announced that her mother was ready to go to heaven. Together we created a ritual recognizing her mother's ascension to heaven. We took a picture of her mom and placed angel wings on it. The girl suggested we then burn it so it could go with her mother to heaven. I thought it interesting that the mother still had to burn something, even if it was a purging flame!

Rituals of affirmation complement rituals of reconciliation. Here, the message is to affirm the person of the deceased or the relationship. A ritual of affirmation fundamentally thanks the deceased for his or her legacies. When a good friend died, he asked me to look out for his young son, my godson, after his death. A number of years later, my godson and I decided to create a small ritual to thank his dad for putting us in each other's lives.

In creating therapeutic rituals, a few principles should be employed. First, the ritual should emerge from the narrative. That is, each ritual has to be individually constructed—arising from the client's individual story. There is no single template for any therapeutic ritual.

Second, the ritual should include tangible objects that also have symbolic significance. Rituals revolve around objects. They offer a focal point for the rite. The medals, photograph, or letter remind participants of the qualities and message they wish to confer in the ceremony.

These therapeutic rituals also have to be planned and processed. The planning needs to be both therapeutic and practical. From a therapeutic context, the counselor should ask questions clarifying the message of the ritual and affirming the significance of the acts and objects that will comprise the rite. The client may wish to consider whether this is a private or public ceremony as well as whether there may be others who will participate or witness the event. There may need to be practical issues that have to be considered. For example, in the ritual of affirmation described earlier, the mother was asking her sons and their families to be part of this ritual. This led to other questions, such as the timing of the ritual, as well as details as to whether she would serve a meal to the family, what the menu would be, and what accommodation would be made for a daughter coming from a distance.

The counselor also needs to process the ritual with the client following the experience. *How did the client react during the rite? Did the ritual accomplish the client's goals and expectations? What worked well? What might have been done differently? Are there other things the client needs to do?*

Finally, in preparing a ritual, there are lessons to be learned from faith communities. Rituals all take on a special character when they are encased in the primal elements of fire (candles), wind (music, chimes, etc.), water, and soil (flowers).

THE CHALLENGE OF SPIRITUAL SUPPORT

Spiritual support can be a challenge. Many health professionals have little specialized training in spirituality. Moreover, there may be concern lest one impose his or her own spirituality on a patient or family member. Sometimes out of respect for the diversity and individuality of a person's spiritual beliefs, health professionals may be reluctant to enter into conversations involving religion or spirituality. Thus, there often is temptation to leave these issues to chaplains, clergy, or other spiritual mentors. This is unlikely to suffice. Spiritual concerns arise throughout the entire experience of the illness. Patients and families will choose when, where, and with whom they will share these spiritual concerns. These choices may not always fit into neat organizational charts or job descriptions. They are the responsibility of the team.

Nor can these spiritual concerns be neglected. Holistic care entails that spiritual concerns are both acknowledged and validated. A true respect for spirituality means that such concerns and spiritual struggles need to be addressed by every professional. Spirituality, therefore, cannot be ignored. Death, after all, may be the ultimate spiritual journey.

QUO VADIS

The 1951 "sword and sandal" epic movie *Quo Vadis* was based on the Christian tradition that the disciple Peter was challenged when fleeing possible martyrdom in Rome by a vision in which Jesus asks him, *"Quo Vadis?"* or "Where are you going?" As a result of that vision, Peter returns to continue his ministry in Nero's Rome. In many ways, the question is an apt conclusion to the chapter.

The importance of spirituality as a component in care for the dying and bereaved is finally being recognized as something beyond the province of clergy and chaplains. Yet challenges remain.

Some challenges are basic. Until there is a commonly accepted definition of *spirituality* that clearly differentiates it from *religion*, research will be compromised. In addition, given the complexity of spirituality and religion, it seems that research might well focus more on the content of spiritual beliefs rather than simply their presence. For example, what is the impact of dying on someone whose spirituality emphasizes grace and mercy compared with spiritualities that focus on judgment.

Practical problems remain as well. Although there is a general recognition of the importance of spiritual care, as the hospice benefit indicates, it remains an unfunded mandate. As spiritual care continues to be acknowledged as an important component of holistic care, such policies may need to be revisited. Only then will we fully acknowledge the wisdom of the Catholic mystic Pierre Teilhard de Chardin's comment that "We are not human beings having a spiritual experience; we are spiritual beings having a human experience" (Teilhard de Chardin 1955, p. 47).

REFERENCES

Abrams, D., Albury, S., Doka, K., Crandall. L., & Harris, R. (2005). The Florida Clergy end-of-life education enhancement project: A description and evaluation. *American Journal of Hospice & Palliative Medicine, 22*(3), 181–187.

Becker, E. (1973). *The denial of death.* New York, NY: Simon and Schuster.

Chochinov, H. M. (2012). *Dignity therapy: Final words for final days.* New York, NY: Oxford University Press.

Dane, B. (2000). Thai women: Mediation as a way to cope with AIDS. *Journal of Religion and Health, 38,* 5–21.

Doka, K. J. (1984). Expectation of death, participation in planning funeral rituals and grief adjustment. Omega: Journal of Death and Dying, 15,119–130.

Doka, K. (1993a). *Living with life-threatening illness: A guide for patients, their families, and caregivers.* Lexington, MA: Lexington Books.

Doka, K. (Ed.). (1993b). *Death and spirituality.* Amityville, NY: Baywood Press.

Doka, K. (2006). Social, cultural, spiritual, and psychological barriers to pain management. In K. Doka (Ed.), *Pain management at the end of life: Bridging the gap between knowledge and practice.* Washington, DC: The Hospice Foundation of America.

Doka, K., & Jendreski, M. (1985). Clergy understandings of grief, bereavement and mourning. *Research Record, 2,* 105–114.

Doka, K. J. (2011). Religion and spirituality: Assessment and bereavement. *Journal of Social Work in End-of-Life & Palliative Care, 7,* 99–109.

Doka, K. J. (2013). Sacred ceremonies, sacred space: The role of rituals and memorials in grief and loss. In K. Doka & A. Tucci (Eds.), *Improving care for veterans: Facing illness and loss.* Washington, DC: The Hospice Foundation of America.

Doka, K. J., & Martin, T. (2010). *Grieving beyond gender: Understanding the ways men and women grieve* (rev. ed.). New York, NY: Routledge.

Freud, S. (1957). Mourning and melancholia. In J. Strachey (Ed. & Trans.), *The standard edition of the complete psychological works of Sigmund Freud* (Vol. XIV, pp. 239–260). London, UK: The Hogarth Press. (Original work published 1917)

Hodge, D. (2005). Developing a spiritual assessment toolbox: A discussion of the strengths and limitations of five different assessment methods. *Health & Social Work, 30,* 314–323.

International Work Group on Death, Dying, and Bereavement (Spiritual Care Work Group). (1990). Assumptions and principles of spiritual care. *Death Studies, 14,* 75–81.

Klass, D. (1996). Grief in Eastern cultures: Japanese ancestor worship. In D. Klass, P. Silverman, & S. Nickman, (Eds.), *Continuing bonds: New understandings of grief.* Bristol, PA: Taylor & Francis.

Koenig, H. (2004). Religion, spirituality, and medicine: Research findings and implications for clinical practice. *Southern Medical Journal, 97,* 1194–1200.

Koocher, G., & O'Malley, J. E. (1981). *The Damocles syndrome: Psychological consequences of surviving childhood cancer.* New York, NY: McGraw-Hill.

Lamm, M. (1969). *The Jewish way in death and mourning.* New York, NY: Jonathon David Publishers.

Ledger, S. (2005). The duty of nurses to meet patients' spiritual and/or religious needs. *British Journal of Nursing, 14,* 220–225.

Lifton, R., & Olsen, G. (1974). *Living and dying.* New York, NY: Bantam Books.

Lin, H., & Bauer-Wu, S. (2003). Psycho-spiritual well being in patients with advanced cancer: An integrative review of the literature. *Journal of Advanced Nursing, 44,* 69–90.

Mayo Clinic Health Letter. (2005). *Meditation, 23*(3), 3–4.

Miller, J. (1994, November). *The transforming power of spirituality.* Presentation to a conference on transformative grief, Burnsville, NC.

Miller, W., & Thoresen, C. (2003). Spirituality, religion, and health: An emerging research field. *American Psychologist, 58,* 1–19.

Moody, R. (1975). *Life after life: The investigation of a phenomenon – Survival of bodily death.* New York, NY: Harper One.

Neimeyer, R. (Ed.). (1994). *Death anxiety handbook: Research, instrumentation, and application.* Washington, DC: Taylor & Francis.

Olive, K. (2004). Religion and spirituality: Important psychosocial variables frequently ignored in clinical research. *Southern Medical Journal, 97,* 1152–1153.

Pargament, K., Koenig, H., Tarakeshwar, N., & Hahn, J. (2004). Religious coping methods as predictors of psychological, physical, and spiritual outcomes among medically ill elderly patients: A two-year longitudinal study. *Journal of Health Psychology, 9,* 713–730.

Pattison, E. M. (1978). The living-dying process. In C. Garfield (Ed.), *The psychosocial care of the dying patient.* New York, NY: McGraw-Hill.

Pentz, M. (2005). Resilience among older adults with cancer and the importance of social support and spirituality-faith: "I don't have time to die." *Journal of Gerontological Social Work, 44*(3–4), 3–22.

Rando, T. A. (1984). *Grief, dying, and death: Clinical interventions for caregivers.* Champaign, IL: Research Press.

Ribbentrop, E., Altmaier, E., Chen, J., Found, E., & Keffala, V. (2005). The relationship between religion/spirituality and physical health, mental health, and pain in a chronic pain population. *Pain, 116,* 311–321.

Schroeder-Sheker, T. (1994). Music for the dying: A personal account of the new field of music thanatology – History, theory and clinical narratives. *Journal of Holistic Nursing, 12,* 83–99.

Sephton, S., Koopman, C., Shaal, M., Thoresen, C., & Spiegel, D. (2001). Spiritual expression and immune status in women with metastatic cancer: An exploratory study. *Breast Journal, 7,* 345–353.

Shneidman, E. (1978). Some aspects of psychotherapy with dying persons. In C. Garfield (Ed.), *Psychosocial care of the dying patient* (pp. 201–218). New York, NY: McGraw-Hill.

Siegel, K., & Schrimshaw, E. (2002). The perceived benefits of religious and spiritual coping among older adults living with HIV/AIDS. *Journal for the Scientific Study of Religion, 41,* 91–102.

Stefanek, M., McDonald, P., & Hess, S. (2005). Religion, spirituality and cancer: Current status and methodological challenges. *Psycho-Oncology, 14,* 450–463.

Teilhard de Chardin, P. (1955). *The phenomenon of man.* New York: Harper Collins.

Townsend, M., Kladder, V., & Mulligan, T. (2002). Systematic review of clinical trials examining the effects of religion on health. *Southern Medical Journal, 95,* 1429–1434.

Weisman, A. (1980). Thanatology. In O. Kaplan (Ed.), *Comprehensive textbook of psychiatry.* Baltimore, MD: Williams & Williams.

Sandra Bertman

18

USING THE ARTS AND HUMANITIES WITH THE DYING, BEREAVED, . . . AND OURSELVES

Poets, artists, and writers have always illustrated and illuminated death, dying, and grief. This chapter documents how the arts and humanities have played a critical role in educating both medical personnel and budding thanatologists. The chapter also includes a brief discussion of art therapy and an introduction to specific techniques used with children and adults. Attempting to demonstrate the richness involved in this process to multiple audiences over a half century, I hope this chapter provides substance and inspiration for all who work in the field.

WHERE AND HOW IT ALL BEGAN

My 53-year-old mother was diagnosed with liver and pancreatic cancer in 1969, when I was 33. Immediately after the operation the doctors pronounced, "Nothing more can be done." After my father insisted, "She couldn't take it . . . she'll be destroyed," the physicians conspired with him not to tell her. Yet, on the eve of her operation, this serious, thoughtful woman who was terrified of hospitals, who was the caretaker of the entire family, three to four generations worth, and whose husband was in the midst of salvaging a business disaster, rose to her stature of barely 5 feet, looked me in the eye, and said in a soft voice, "Sandra, if it is cancer. . ." "Only hepatitis," she was reassured.

I felt impotent and angry. What sense did it make to tell her everything was fine? It just did not compute. Would this still be the refrain as her pain increased and she became sicker and more debilitated? Her body was and would continue to be telling her something. She knew something. (Years later, I discovered there was, in fact, a term: she had what Avery Weisman named "middle knowledge.") It seemed to me an act of deliberate cruelty to wait until she was weaker to face the reality of the diagnosis that she clearly suspected. A part of her was bracing herself for the truth in the very phrasing of those words to a daughter "If it is cancer. . ." My mother didn't need the physician's response to look beyond her dis-ease. Her head was already racing with the hypotheticals and with the real questions.

Kind physician friends gave me journal articles to read while my mother was dying. "Why are you giving me all this psychological stuff to read?" I asked in frustration. "You're acting like the only ones who know anything about suffering are the credentialed 'professionals,' the psychiatrists. Read Tolstoy's *The Death of Ivan Ilych*; read Tillie Olsen's *Tell Me a Riddle*; read John Gunther's autobiographical account of his son's brain tumor—or John Donne's poem—both titled *Death Be Not Proud*; read Simone de Beauvoir's chronicle of her mother's dying, anything but, as its title suggests, *A Very Easy Death*; read *The Notebooks of Rilke*, the poetry of Emily

Dickinson, Edna St. Vincent Millay, Donald Hall; see the plays or films *I Never Sang for My Father, Ikiru, Hamlet, Sunshine.*" These books and others opened a door for me; a door to understanding the totality of death. And I walked through that door, armed with my background in teaching English, and began a 30-year career teaching prospective doctors how to begin to work with dying and bereaved people.

My mother's situation was reminiscent of the responses in Tolstoy's novel *The Death of Ivan Ilych* (1886/1960) to the physicians' assurances of hepatitis: "This deception tortured him—their not wishing to admit what they knew and what he knew, but wanting to lie to him concerning his terrible condition, and wishing and forcing him to participate in that lie." (p. 137). To Ivan Ilych (and to my mother) only one question was important: "Was my case serious or not? But the doctor ignored that inappropriate question" (p. 121; Figure 18.1).

In video clips—as in a physician's real experience—authenticity is immediately apparent. Humanities materials could be used to sharpen observational and critical-thinking skills. Stories, film, and cartoons vicariously present the encounters with illness, mortality, ethical challenges, and bereavement through shrewd eyes and, ideally, before one has to do so in actuality with patients and families. Things normally unseen are so small—might they not benefit from a close-up so big they must be taken in? The question Mr. Watanabe asks the physician in Akira Kurosawa's 1960 film *Ikiru* is almost the same one my mother asked (or rather, told) me: "Is it cancer?" What an opportunity for practice/rehearsal in viewing such a film clip: (1) Interactions can be witnessed firsthand as opposed to "reported" as was the custom in rounds and conferences. (2) Difficult moments can be honestly explored by freezing the frame, for example, and grappling with the situation before, during, and after viewing the actual sequence. (3) Scenarios can be instantly replayed for language cues (e.g., "All tumors aren't malignant, are they doctor?"), attention to nonverbal behaviors, complexities, ambiguities, and other discomforts.

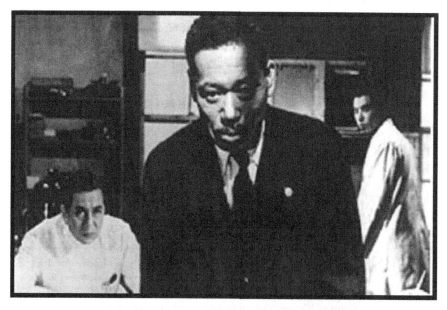

FIGURE 18.1 Still from Akira Kurosawa's film *Ikiru* (1960).
Source: Bertman (1991). Used with permission.

What's to "update" about Ivan Ilych's experience? Were my mother's agonies any different from his, or from Mr. Watanabe's ("It's only an ulcer"). Isn't his facial expression proof of or an unmistakably excellent example of "inner knowledge"? Moreover, note the physicians' behaviors. How comfortable were they in their roles? How skilled were they in creating containers where healing might begin to take place?

About that time (the late sixties), forums to bring together those interested in the field of death, dying, and bereavement were being organized in Boston (The Equinox Institute) and Philadelphia (*Ars Moriendi*, which eventually became the International Work Group on Death, Dying, and Bereavement in 1974).

THE EQUINOX INSTITUTE (1969–1971)

By the time my mother died in February 1970, an oncologist, Melvin J. Krant, who cared as much about suffering as about tumors, had enlisted a group of three psychiatrists (Avery Weisman, Ned Cassim, and Jerry Adler), a rabbi (Earl Grollman), a nurse, and a social worker (Ruth Abrams) to meet evenings initially at his home to plan how to effect change in the care and treatment of the terminally ill and the bereaved. Because of my teaching experience, belief in ways of knowing other than the biomedical, and conviction that adult education and the public—not just health care professionals—have a stake in these issues, I was invited to participate in these colloquia and in the subsequent formation of Equinox Institute. Our mission then read not so differently from the one of the Open Society Institute's, particularly its Project on Death in America (2001–2003), which supported initiatives in research, scholarship, the humanities, and the arts "to transform the culture and experience of dying and to foster innovations in the provision of care, public education, professional education and public policy."

Offerings for teachers and counselors in the Newton, Brookline, and Belmont school systems ("Coping with Crisis and Loss") and periodic lectures ("On Ethics and Decision Making") at Tufts Medical School preceded the course offerings at University of Massachusetts, Boston campus ("Death, Dying, and Other Lethal Behaviors" created by Robert Kastenbaum and later my own field-study course for students who wished to work in nursing homes, on suicide hotlines, etc.) and the Medical Center in Worcester. The first course in the Boston–Cambridge area, "Perspectives on Death," offered at the Adult Education Center, Cambridge, had paved the way and set the syllabi content. The catalogue description read: "The American people have been characterized as death-denying when dealing with death and loss experiences. In an effort to become more comfortable with the subject of death, grief and bereavement, we shall explore attitudes and feelings expressed in the written, visual, and lyrical arts (especially story, film, music) as well as in documents such as Patients' Rights and Living Will. Materials ranging in tone from Tolstoy, Brel, and Beatles shall be viewed against the theories of professionals Kübler-Ross, Weisman, Farberow, and Feifel and shall provide the points of departure for reflecting on such topics as terminal illness, sudden death, isolation ('person' vs. 'patient'), a 'meaningful' death; repercussions (creative and non) that accompany loss, *carpe diem*, and talking about death with children." For the public, early media credits included the films *Death: The Great American Dream Machine* (Public Broadcast System [PBS], 1971) and *Dying* (WGBH-TV, 1976); and the United Press International award-winning radio show "Sing a Song of Dying" (WCAS, 1971).

FAILPROOF TECHNIQUES FOR ALL AGES

The ultimate goal of all art is relief from suffering and the rising above it.
—Gustav Mahler

One technique that is infallible for novice or experienced professional is expressive therapy. Expressive therapy is predicated on the assumption that people can heal through use of the imagination and various forms of creative expression in the arts—literary, musical, dramatic, and visual. Expressive therapy, also known as creative arts therapy, differs from traditional art expression in emphasizing the creative process rather than the final product or work (Figure 18.2).

Even the most insignificant sketch, a performance charade, four-line poem, aims boldly and blindly at the impossible, at striving for totality, an attempt to enclose chaos in a nutshell (adapted from Hesse, 1974). Why write? Why draw? More than catharsis, something as simple as taking pen or crayon to paper magically defuses stress, evokes curiosity, and inspires creativity. Research has shown the benefits of expressive writing. The very act of changing emotions and images into words affects the way a person organizes and thinks about an experience. "If it's mentionable, it's manageable," Mr. Rogers reassured the youngsters in the TV series, *Mr. Rogers' Neighborhood*. It would seem that only by making visible that which was invisible do we allow the healing process to begin. One might ask a group to add cartoon balloons to each of the figures in the drawing shown in Figure 18.2. For example, the youngster in front might ask, "Why did he die?" And the mother or person behind him might reply, "Because he was very *very* old and his body stopped working." Or "Sweetheart, everyone has to die" or "Why do you think he died?" or "_____." Or one might ask about the nails in the coffin, or the antennae on the tombstone.

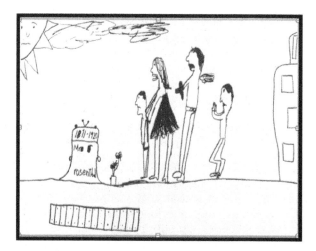

FIGURE 18.2 From *Death Education in the Face of a Taboo* (Grollman, 1974). Reprinted with permission.

For a quarter of a century, as professor of humanities in medicine at the University of Massachusetts Medical Center, I invited medical students, health care professionals, and therapy groups to reveal their worst-case scenarios or most stressful situations in coming to grips with dying, death, and grief. I might be accused of going for the jugular vein. My instructions were "Please devise an image of any sort relating to your thoughts and feelings as you anticipate the dissection experience, giving bad news, or supporting a terminal patient." For those who are more comfortable with writing, variations on the assignment include visual poetry (Bertman, 2011); 6- or 9-word stories; and haikus on hope, love, and grief or the current 55-word story exercise (Fogarty & Gross, 2011), which helps us to understand or to appreciate something about a patient or about a counseling incident. It's all about encouraging reflective practice, taking a conscious look at our emotions, experiences, actions, and responses, and using that to add to our existing knowledge base to draw out new knowledge, meaning, and to attain a higher level of understanding (Paterson & Chapman, 2013).

Another technique to use is the visual case study. The images offered in this chapter, for example, are nothing if not instantaneous visual case studies with an amazing capacity to ignite our therapeutic imaginations, creating a space where we can grapple with morality, mortality, and the relational aspects of our practices (Bertman, 2002, 2003, 2008). These images differ from the traditional medical case studies delivered in grand rounds in graciously/sensitively removing the practitioner's and patient's identities and potential for emotional vulnerability in disclosing thoughts and feelings about a particular experience (Figure 18.3).

A twist on the visual case study technique for using art is to provide the participants with masks. "Give a man a mask," the wry Irish writer Oscar Wilde (Ellman, 1968) tells us, "and he will tell the truth about himself." Poet Emily Dickinson (1830–1886) suggests addressing truth obliquely: "Tell all the Truth, but tell it slant" (Dickinson, 1890). Educator Parker Palmer calls this "the third thing." "Mediated by a third thing—a poem, a piece of music, a painting—truth can emerge from, and return to, our awareness at whatever pace and depth we are able to handle—sometimes

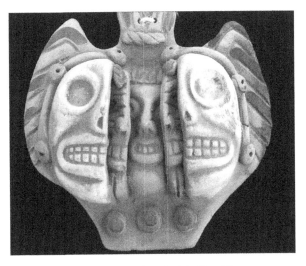

FIGURE 18.3 Clay-painted mass-produced .50″× 6″× 2″ artifact.
Source: Bertman, Multicultural and Visual Case Study Projects, Ward Street Studio Archives.

inwardly in silence, sometimes aloud in community—giving the shy soul the protective cover it needs" (Palmer, 2009).

For several decades before the computer came into being (or before I became aware of the digital age), I presented double-slide presentations to classes, conferences, and other gatherings. I invited audiences to select and comment on a Most Memorable Image (Bertman, 1991, pp. 101–163) from those that I projected. In them, I always tried to point out that choice is a critical variable. Several medical schools and residencies are now routinely using an adaptation of this technique in their training, accompanying their learners in visits to art museums. There, they are given instructions or tasks, such as: "Find an image that. . . . is difficult to look at. . . . says something about loss. . . . finds order in chaos. . . . and give reasons for your choice" (Gaufberg & Batalden, 2007, Miller, 2009, 2012; Brooks, 2013; Williams 2009, 2012). Art educator and curator Ray Williams explains how students benefit from being in a different learning environment than the classroom, citing David Carr's thinking (*The Promise of Cultural Institutions*, 2003) of the museum as a place that supports visitors in their "process of becoming." For most of us limited to a constrained lecture or workshop session, 5 to 10 minutes is usually ample time for participants to think of immediate responses or ideas, generate and write sketchy notes, and compose brief reflections—just a few pertinent phrases or sentences. I encourage the act of literally writing one's thoughts as a way of discovering what you think, what you see, what it means, and a way of stimulating—finding the words—for what you want to say. The excitement in sharing responses, particularly diverse responses to a single image, immediately builds community as it provides safety and tolerance for viewpoints other than one's own, all the while reminding us there is always more to see.

Thus, engaging in the arts, as participant or observer (in itself a creative act), is often catalyst enough not only to arouse our senses but also to stimulate our imaginations, causing us to wonder, to analyze, to feel connected (or disconnected), and to be inspired. The engagement with art, whether through reading or writing, viewing or drawing, listening or enacting, involves attention, analysis, identification, catharsis, and insight. The beauty of the process is its openness to interpretations, to the way any of us—therapist, nurse, patient, client, colleague—takes it in and uses it for oneself, in personal and professional contexts (adapted from Bertman, 1999).

Our role—the doctor, therapist, teacher, fellow human being—is less a question of treatment than of developing the creative potential within the client, patient, or person we are serving (adapted from Jung, 1954). Looking again at some of the images presented and to come (Figures 18.1, 18.4, 18.6), they seem to suggest we are moving from a paternalistic relationship to a patient-centered one, Martin Buber's "I and Thou." Are we ready—vulnerable enough to meet thou to thou? Soul to soul?" Remen (1996) challenges us as she puts this into perspective:

> There is a distance between ourselves and whatever or whomever we are fixing. Fixing is a form of judgment. All judgment creates distance, a disconnection, an experience of difference. In fixing there is an inequality of expertise that can easily become a moral distance. We can't serve at a distance. We can serve only that to which we are profoundly connected, that which we are willing to touch. (Remen, 1996, p. 24)

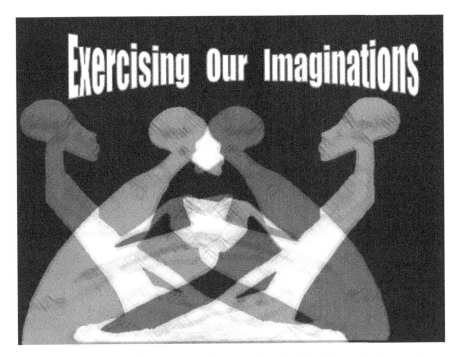

FIGURE 18.4 Copyright image from Bertman, *Exercising Our Therapeutic Imaginations* presentations, 1998.

FAST FORWARD: FROM DISSECTION TO PALLIATIVE CARE—SOUL PAIN, AESTHETIC DISTANCE, AND THE TRAINING OF PHYSICIANS

The Very First Patient

It is commonly known that medical students dissect the bodies of the dead; it is less commonly realized that these same dead do a great deal of cutting, probing, and pulling at the minds of their youthful dissectors.
—Alan Gregg, MD

Perhaps it is fortuitous that the first patient a medical student meets is a dead one. Absent in this inaugural encounter are the awkward introductions, the uncomfortable silences, and the embarrassments (for both parties) that always accompany the first laying on of hands. Although a measure of comfort can be derived from knowing that neither can pain be inflicted on nor can harm be done to this patient, there is no getting around the fact that he or she is dead. Yet, there is no escaping the gnawing thought that this could be my mother, my father, or me.

Medical students and practicing physicians alike make compelling arguments for early and ongoing "vaccinations" of education and training having to do with emotional armor. Physician writer Selzer (1996) reminds us that when the surgeon cuts into the patient, he himself must not bleed; he must find the appropriate, protective clinical distance. In *A Parting Gift*, pediatrician Sharkey (1982)

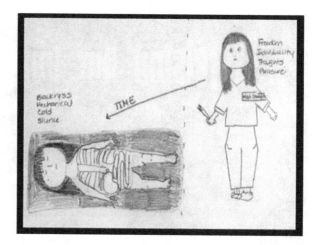

FIGURE 18.5 Medical student's identification with cadaver (1994) as intimated by Gregg
quotation in *One Breath Apart: Facing Dissection* (Bertman, 2009), p. 50.
Source: Bertman (2009). Used with permission.

traces the development of her own "emotional detachment" as she makes her way
through medical education, from her dissection experiences to the discomfort she
has at deaths of patients she has attended. She vividly recounts how frequently
she dreamed about her cadaver: "He was always very much alive in the dreams. I
never told this to my fellow students. We didn't talk about the effects our cadavers
had on us; nor did we talk about death" (Sharkey, 1982, p. 16).

Patients often find themselves looking to the physician for "metaphysical"
expertise. "Just as he orders blood tests and bone scans of my body, I'd like my
doctor to scan me, to grope for my spirit as well as my prostate" (Broyard, 1992,
p. 46). So how do we train physicians to know when to treat aggressively, to be
action oriented, and when (and how) to shift gears to grope for the soul instead
of the prostate? How do we educate them to tolerate discomfort, ambiguity, and
uncertainty when they are programmed to obtain answers? How do we teach
them their job is not to provide ultimate answers but to manifest ultimate commitment? How do we teach them to feel comfortable sharing their own humanity
with patients on the examining table who are grappling with the manifestations of
soul pain—loneliness, hopelessness, valuelessness, meaninglessness?

Seeing Patients

In fact, what doctors do most of the time presupposes visual and auditory
observation. A good diagnostician needs to be alert to body language, tone of
voice, eye contact, blushes, and sudden flushes of embarrassment or shame. The
white coat is no vaccination or immunization against irritation, antipathy, arousal,
or discomfort. The good doctor needs to be aware of his or her own reactions so
they do not interfere with this sacred relationship between two human beings,
one who happens to be in this moment a doctor, the other, a patient. There is a
shared self-consciousness in the doctor–patient relationship; the visible and invisible elephants (the uncomfortable silences and the embarrassments), is there not?

When I first began to work with medical students, I wanted an armamen-
tarium of pictures, stories, photographs, poems, nonfiction accounts of sharply
focused vicarious encounters for engagement, reflection, and discussion of the

unmentionables and unmeasureables in health care. We meaning-making, mean-ing-seeking creatures cannot look at images or symbols or arrangements of letters or words or sounds without trying to make sense of them. What do I see? What do I think? Feel? Why do I think/feel that? What else do I see? How might I change that image? These "triggers" invite close inspection, while still taking responsibility for propriety and granting us permission to stare without having to avert our eyes or "modify" without feeling guilt or shame.

Medicine is and always has been a deeply spiritual profession. The earliest recorded images portray physicians as priests and priestesses. In an illumination from a 14th-century manuscript, "Treatise and Commentary of Medicine" in the Biblio-theque Municipale, Rheims, one could easily mistake the scene, which depicts a medi-cal consultation, for a private confessional. So too in the contemporary painting *Mr. S. Is Told He Will Die.* Artist Robert Pope, a fellow cancer patient, portrays the moment during which two physicians present Mr. S. with his devastating prognosis. Pope says of his painting, "The cross symbolizes religion, and the doctors, in their white lab coats, symbolize science. The man is grasping onto both, and neither one can save his life and he knows this" (from Pope, *Illness & healing: Images of cancer, p. 90, 1991,* Figure 18.6).

I see quite a different scene: compassion incarnate. The two physicians are seated with the patient on *his* bed, *his* turf. Whatever their personal beliefs—or those of Mr. S.— the physicians are sharing his suffering, deliberately touching yet allowing space for their patient to absorb the import of the moment. Seated beside the patient on his hospital bed, they are literally buttressing him with their bodies as they reveal their news. Comfortable with the silence, willing to suspend their busy schedules for as many moments as are necessary, they are fully present. The inti-macy of the scene, the human relatedness, seems almost sacramental, the essence of soul, an earthly embodiment of love. At bottom, no equipment is necessary but the human heart. I see genuine connection. Sacredness has not so much to do with the content the physicians are imparting, but with the process they're igniting. As

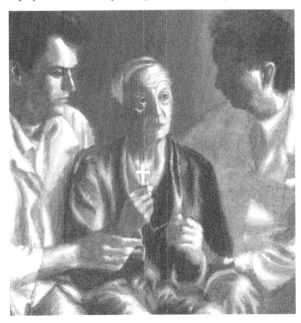

FIGURE 18.6 *Mr. S. is Told He Will Die,* acrylic on canvas (1989).
Source: Copyright 2005 by the Robert Pope Foundation. Used with permission.

Dr. Brad Stuart reminds us, "Despair can only be treated by meeting the pain that often aches deep and unnoticed inside the bone metastasis . . . the kind of pain that morphine cannot reach and that only can be treated by meeting soul to soul" (B. Stuart, personal communication, February 17, 2013).

Rx: An Image a Day

Art washes away from the soul the dust of everyday life.
—Pablo Picasso

Each of us needs periodic reinspiration to invigorate our imaginations and souls. An image a day—a painting, poem, lyric, cartoon—used as preamble or to pepper the most didactic medical conference may be just the prod to shake us out of the ruts of ordinary perception in medical practice and to approach what we cannot bear to look at—admit to—or interact with—in a fresh and strangely bracing way. In this light, it makes sense to change the basic motto for training physicians to "see one, do one, teach one, use one."

CHANGING IDEAS ABOUT HEALTH CARE

Art in health care is a diverse, multidisciplinary field that humanizes the health care experience for patients, families, and caregivers. Although each program and creative endeavor is unique to the community it serves, this rapidly growing field applies a multitude of art forms to a wide variety of health care settings for therapeutic, educational, or recreational purposes to enhance the well-being of patients and caregivers. Not only does creative self-expression provide solace, strength, and affirmation that alleviate personal stress, but it also contributes to self-awareness, understanding of patients and their families, and ultimately to forging stronger communities through support and empowerment. Our entire society is finding new ways to use the expressive arts in health care. The following section reviews but a few of these.

Holistic Care

Holistic care is predicated on the belief of the wholeness in one serving the wholeness in another. "The Arts and Humanities in Health Care and Education" (International Work Group on Death, Dying, and Bereavement [IWG], 2000) is a document of assumptions and principles ultimately adaptable to any culture, clinical practice, or educational setting. Created by the International Workgroup on Death, Dying, and Bereavement, this detailed statement of assumptions and principles underscores how the arts and humanities reflect the existential, inspirational, and transcendent realms of experience and can contribute to creating an aesthetic, nurturing, and healing environment.

Narrative Medicine

What's most thrilling now is the plethora of courses in narrative, visual, and spiritual studies in health professionals' clinical training. Charon (2006, p. 4) defines narrative medicine as "medicine practiced with these skills of recognizing, absorbing, interpreting, and being moved by the stories of illness." Caregivers who possess "narrative competence" are able to bridge the "divides" of their relation to mortality; the contexts of illness; beliefs about disease causality; and emotions of shame, blame, and fear. In her training and supervision, Dr. Charon has devised a "parallel chart" for interns and residents that allows them to record their own stories of their experiences in caregiving and to share and explore them with their colleagues for purposes of enhancing self-understanding and improving their effectiveness in responding to the whole persons in their care.

Bioethics and Humanities

With the growing interest in clinical ethics, the Society for Health and Human Values morphed into the American Society for Bioethics and Humanities (ASBH). The purpose of ASBH is to promote the exchange of ideas and foster multidisciplinary, interdisciplinary, and interprofessional scholarship, research, teaching, policy development, professional development, and collegiality among people engaged in all the endeavors related to clinical and academic bioethics and the health-related humanities. The founding documents maintain that these purposes shall be advanced by the following kinds of activities: (1) encouraging consideration of issues in human values as they relate to health services, the education of healthcare professionals, and research; (2) conducting educational meetings dealing with such issues; (3) stimulating research in areas of such concern; (4) contributing to the public discussion of these endeavors and interests, including how they relate to public policy (ASBH, n.d.).

ASBH members have created an amazing resource developed to be an accessible, comprehensive, dynamic online compendium for teaching and research in medical humanities. The Literature, Arts and Medicine Database is an annotated multimedia listings of prose, poetry, film, video, and art. It not only summarizes specific works (poems, novels, paintings, films, theatre) but also adds commentary and suggestions for their use in a number of settings (litmed.med.nyu.edu).

American Academy of Hospice and Palliative Medicine

Founded in 1988, the American Academy of Hospice and Palliative Medicine (AAHPM) is a professional organization primarily for physicians whose motto is to advance the science of comfort and affirm the art of caring (AAHPM, n.d.-a). The mission of the Humanities SIG (special interest group) is to infuse educational activities and publications with works from the humanities and arts. Visit (1) *End of Life: Visions and Voices* (AAHPM, n.d.-b), which showcases PDIA-funded humanities projects; (2) a *Staying Soulful* (AAHPM, n.d.-c) column; and (3) the *ArtSpace, Phoenix, 2004* (AAHPM, 2004) video of interacting with the creative process in the Healing Space (Figure 18.7).

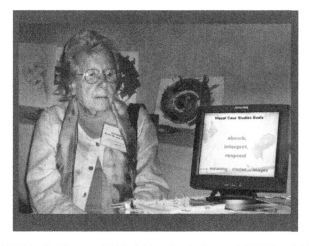

FIGURE 18.7 (a): Dr. Florence Wald visiting the ArtSpace, AAHPM and APNA First Annual Conference, Phoenix (2004).

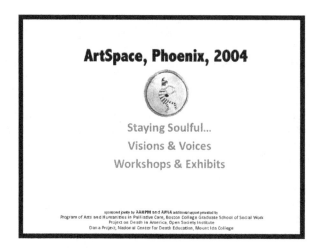

FIGURE 18.7 (b): *Art Space, Phoenix, 2004 video.*
Source: View Quicktime movie at http://www.sandrabertman.com/files/publications
.html

The Global Alliance for Arts and Health

The Global Alliance for Arts and Health (formerly Society for the Arts in Health-care founded in 1991) is dedicated to advancing arts as integral to health care by (1) demonstrating the valuable roles the arts can play in enhancing the healing process; (2) advocating for the integration of the arts into the environment and delivery of care within health care facilities; (3) assisting in the professional development and management of arts programming for health care populations; (4) providing resources and education to health care and arts professionals; and (5) encouraging and supporting research and investigation into the beneficial effects of the arts in health care.

Music Therapy

Using live harp music at the bedside of acutely dying patients in 1973, Therese Schroeder-Sheker pioneered the use of terms such as "music thanatology," "music vigil," and "prescriptive music" (The Chalice of Repose, n.d.). Music therapists have much to teach the world about the interrelationship of music and breath in their strategies to help patients, family, friends, and those of us who care for them lift the spirits and cope with the pain and distress that accompanies loss and that ends life. Musical memories (Berger, 2006) and the use of music to stimulate recall can be an enjoyable and emotionally engaging part of life review, at the same time providing a comforting background when words just aren't needed. The clinical use of music-facilitated breathing techniques at the first and last breaths of life and with people who have cancer is explored (Hanser, 1996, 1999).

Thankfully there is new respect for and inclusion of these expressive therapies. There now is an enormous range and diversity of programs and settings. One doesn't have to be a certified therapist. Volunteers, too, are trained to man music and art carts, which not only provide distraction and solace but often facilitate grief, healing, and moving on in life.

WHERE WE ARE GOING

T. S. Eliot's (1952) profound poetic insight in his poem "Little Gidding" comments on the circularity of life and death and the increase in our understanding of life as we move toward and think about death: "We shall not cease from exploration/And the end of all exploring/Will be to arrive where we started/And know the place for the first time" (p. 145). In his novel *Siddhartha,* the German writer Hermann Hesse assures us that "we are not going in circles, we are going upwards and that the path is a spiral; we have already climbed many steps" (Hesse, 1992, p. 27).

The future is so promising. Thanks to technology (I hate to admit it), health services combat ageism and functional loss in ways that open us up to coping with all challenges. To cite just two examples: The Music Maker is an interactive human–computer interface that uses a set of cameras to convert body movements into real-time auditory feedback, providing patients with sensory feedback as a reward for correct actions. Playing the Music Maker does not require special musical talent and is possible for patients with very limited movement (Lahav, 2007). Even carmakers are using the new technology as some brands of cars are equipped with medical alert systems that keep seniors safe. And, I truly believe, though not in my lifetime, perhaps, it will be discovered that we are all born with two genes heretofore undiscovered: a creative gene and a spiritual gene.

Looking back, the joy for me is seeing the relevance and use of the arts and humanities materials. I'm still addicted to the multidisciplinary approach, and I'm noticing that the rest of the world is becoming more and more inclusive. It is no longer only the traditional silos (MD, nurse, social worker, chaplain) but also collaborations and inclusions (integrative therapist and practitioners, volunteers, artists, musicians, lay persons). Medical humanities, for example, is being broadened to health care humanities. As our field has changed from thinking of grief as pathologic or an illness, so too, there is a strong movement from the disease model to the wellness model, to one of well-being and healthy aging.

What is relevant to our world, besides an appreciation for the vast resources of literature and the humanities, is a deep respect for the intuitive, intelligent, creative potential within every human being—and, perhaps, a healthy skepticism for divisions by disciplines, experts, and curators of culture. I rest my case with this lovely quotation from Liz Lerman (2010), founding artistic director of Liz Lerman Dance Exchange, Takoma Park:

> Sometimes art achieves what therapy, medication or the best care cannot. These moments can feel like little miracles when they happen, but they are usually instances of art functioning as it normally does: inspiring motivation, engaging parts of people's bodies or brains that they haven't been using, or allowing them to transcend their environments for a little while.

REFERENCES

American Academy of Hospice and Palliative Medicine. (2004). *ArtSpace, Phoenix.* Retrieved from http://www.sandrabertman.com/files/publications.html

American Academy of Hospice and Palliative Medicine. (n.d.-a). Retrieved from http://www.aahpm.org

American Academy of Hospice and Palliative Medicine. (n.d.-b). *End of life: Visions and voices.* Retrieved from www.sandrabertman.com/files/outreachcontent.html

American Academy of Hospice and Palliative Medicine. (n.d.-c). *Staying soulful.* Retrieved from http://www.aahpm.org/pdf/win02.pdf

Association for Bioethics and Humanities. (n.d.). Retrieved from http://www.asbh.org

Berger, J. S. (2006). *Music of the soul: Composing life out of loss.* New York, NY: Routledge.

Bertman, S. (1991). *Facing death: Images, insights and interventions: A handbook for educators, healthcare professionals and counselors.* New York, NY: Taylor & Francis.

Bertman, S. (Ed.). (1999). *Grief and the healing arts: Creativity as therapy.* New York, NY: Baywood.

Bertman, S. (2002). Visual case studies: A practice tool for dialogue about HIV. *Journal of HIV/AIDS & Social Services: Research, Practice & Policy, 1*(2), 79–86.

Bertman, S. (2003). Staying present with suffering—Images still and moving. *Journal of HIV/AIDS & Social Services: Research, Practice & Policy, 2*(2), 65–80.

Bertman, S. (2008). Visual art for professional development. In G. Bolton (Ed.), *Dying, bereavement, and the healing arts* (pp. 51–56). London, UK: Jessica Kingsley.

Bertman, S. (2009). *One breath apart: Facing dissection.* New York, NY: Baywood.

Bertman, S. (2011). Expressive arts and thanatology: An image a day. *ADEC Forum, 37*(1), 1,3–4,7.

Brooks, S. (2013). *Art museum visits help doctors understand feelings.* Retrieved from http://www.news.wisc.edu/22286

Broyard, A. (1992). *Intoxicated by my illness.* New York, NY: Clarkson Potter.

Carr, D. (2003). *The promise of cultural institutions.* Lanham, MD: Altamira Press.

Charon, R. (2006). *Narrative medicine: Honoring the stories of illness.* New York, NY: Oxford University Press.

Chalice of Repose. (n.d.). Retrieved from www.chaliceofrepose.org

Cummings, R. (n.d.). Retrieved from http://blog.blantonmuseum.org/2012/07/meet-ray-blantons-new-director-of.html

Dickinson, E. (n.d.). *Tell all the truth but tell it slant—Ret.* Retrieved August 2, 2014, from http://en.wikisource.org/wiki/Tell_all_the_Truth_but_tell_it_slant_—ret

Eliot, T. S. (1952). Little Gidding. In *The complete poems and plays: 1909–1950* (p. 145). New York, NY: Harcourt, Brace.

Ellman, R. (1968). (Ed.). *The artist as critic: Critical writings of Oscar Wilde* (p. 389). New York, NY: Random House, 1968.

Fogarty, C., & Gross, N. (2011). 55-Word stories: Small jewels for staying alive. *AAHPM Bulletin, 12* (1), 18.

Gaufberg, E., & Batalden, M. (2007). The third thing in medical education. *Clinical Teacher, 4*, 78–81.

The Global Alliance for Arts and Health. (n.d.). Retrieved from www.thesah.org

Grollman, E. (1974). *Concerning Death: A Practical Guide for the Living.* Boston: Beacon Press.

Hanser, S. B. (1996). Music therapy to reduce anxiety, agitation, and depression. *Nursing Home Medicine, 4*(10), 286–291.

Hanser, S. B. (1999). Relaxing through pain and anxiety at the extremities of life: Applications of music therapy in childbirth and older adulthood. In T. Wigram & J. deBacker (Eds.), *Clinical applications of music therapy in psychiatry* (pp. 158–175). London, UK: Jessica Kingsley.

Hesse, H. (1992). *Siddhartha, demian and other writings.* New York, NY: Continuum.

International Work Group on Death, Dying, and Bereavement. (2000). The arts and humanities in healthcare and education. *Death Studies, 24*(5), 365–375. Retrieved from http://iwgddb.com/documents/pubfiles/arts2000.pdf

Jung, C. G. (1954). *The practice of psychotherapy.* Princeton, NJ: Princeton University Press.

Lahav, A. (2007). *The medical benefits of music making: A musical human-computer interface for stroke rehabilitation.* Presentation at Annual Society for Arts in Healthcare Conference.

Lerman, L. (2010). Retrieved from http://danceexchange.org/projects/metlife-foundation-healthy-living-initiative/

Miller, A. (2009). Retrieved from http://www.artspractica.com

Palmer, P. (2009). *A hidden wholeness: The journey toward an undivided life.* Hoboken, NJ: John Wiley.

Paterson, C. and Chapman, J. (2013). Enhancing skills of critical reflection to evidence learning in professional practice. *Physical Therapy in Sport, 14*(3), 133–138.

Pope, R. (1989). *"Mr. S. is Told He Will Die,"* acrylic on canvas. (Reprinted from Pope, R., *Illness & healing: Images of cancer*, p. 90, 1991, Hantsport, Nova Scotia, Canada: Lancelot Press.)

Project on Death in America. (2001–2003). Retrieved from http://www.opensocietyfoundations.org/death

Public Broadcast Service. (1971). *Death: The great American dream machine.* New York, NY: Author.

Remen, R. (1996). In the service of life. *Noetic Science Review, 37,* 24–26.

Selzer, R. (1996). The knife. In *Mortal lessons: Notes on the art of surgery.* New York, NY: Harcourt Brace.

Sharkey, F. (1982). Ingmar Wollenstrum. In *A parting gift.* New York, NY: St. Martin's.

Thompson, B., & Berger, J. (2012). Expressive arts therapy and grief. In R. A. Neimeyer, H. R. Winokur, D. L. Harris, & G. F. Thornton (Eds.), *Grief and bereavement in contemporary society: Bridging research and practice.* New York, NY: Routledge.

Tolstoy, L. (1960). *The death of Ivan Ilych and other stories.* New York, NY: The New American Library. (Original work published 1886)

WCAS-740. (1970). *Sing a song of dying* [radio show]. Cambridge, MA: Sandra Bertman and Tony Cennamo.

WGBH-TV. (1976). *Dying* (Documentary film). New York, NY: Filmmaker's Library.

Williams, R. (2009). Retrieved from http://blog.blantonmuseum.org/2012/07/ meet-ray-blantons-new-director-of.html.

Williams, R. (2012). Retrieved from http://blog.blantonmuseum.org/2012/07/ meet-ray-blantons-new-director-of.html

David W. Kissane **19**

FAMILY SUPPORT FOR THE DYING AND BEREAVED

Like birth, death is a family affair. Whether death is familiar or a feared and unaccustomed event, the death of a loved one has always impacted the family as key caregivers to the dying and eventually those most affected by bereavement. Yet curiously, the dominant paradigm in studying the experiences of both dying and of mourning has been through the individual lens. This is not surprising given the common research methodologies of the psychological sciences and the usual focus of clinical care providers. Nevertheless, the systemic approach is crucial to achieving a comprehensive understanding of all that occurs and often serves as the most pragmatic care model for those left bereaved.

In this chapter, I trace the central elements of this family-centered model of care, from the early work that laid a foundation in the twentieth century to recent studies that have consolidated this approach, before considering the challenges that can limit further development and the hopes for future expansion.

THE DEVELOPMENT OF FAMILY-CENTERED CARE

Let me begin by considering who constitutes the family, what potential exists for caring for a family during a serious illness and in bereavement, the various stages of the life cycle, and whether emotionally connected people can find collective meaning in loss and death? These aspects set the stage intellectually to consider family-centered care.

Who Is the Family?

When an individual meets a clinician, the first question that develops as one considers family-centered care is who belongs to the patient's family? The best response might be "Whoever the patient says the family is." Although the notion of kinship suggests either vertical connection through blood relationships or horizontal union via marriage, families are clearly flexible and varied social entities. Processes of industrialization, urbanization, migration, and even reproductive technology have steadily impacted the nature of the family within our communities. Loyalty varies by cultural tradition. The growth of the no-fault divorce, rates of female employment, and ease of global mobility have further impacted the changeability of who is family.

In the clinical setting, Boss (1992) has placed helpful emphasis on the "psychological" family, a group of like-minded people who share both a history and a future together. This might include members of the nuclear and extended family, neighbors in a residential village, colleagues from work, parishioners from a place of worship, and so on. There is no place for rigidity in considering who might be included within the notion of family. Often the therapist works with whoever is available, and the size of the circle grows as people appreciate the value that such meetings deliver to the group.

Why Be Interested in Family-Centered Care?

It is worth pausing to consider this question. I have long considered the family to be the primary context of human development and maturation. Because we, as human beings, are tribal creatures, significant meaning develops in our lives through the roles and relationships we experience within our families. A parent's influence in shaping a child's personality, coping abilities, interpersonal style, and, eventually, marital outcomes is substantial. Furthermore, the home environment has been shown to impact significantly adaptation to mental illness.

At a personal level, whenever I treat a patient, I have found it rewarding to meet his or her family and, as needed, nurture this group as a vital source of support for each patient. The time invested with a family magnifies the beneficial outcomes considerably. It has thus always made sense to me to include the family, yet it is surprising within medicine how often clinicians do not do this regularly. Given this reality, I was drawn to devote time academically to study families and examine an empirical model that facilitated appropriate intervention that includes the family. Having completed training as a young psychiatrist, I undertook my doctoral studies observing bereaved families and examining the nature of family grief. Much of what follows has developed from that beginning.

The Continuity of the Family's Experience of Illness, Dying, and Bereavement

From the perspective of a death and dying movement, which is the subject of this book, what is most noteworthy is the potential continuity of care provision initiated during the illness of the identified patient with progressive disease, through to care of the family alongside the patient as dying becomes certain, and eventually to support of the survivors in bereavement. The hospice and palliative medicine movements quickly recognized the importance of this continuum within their conceptual models of the goals of treatment. Axioms, such as "bereavement support begins during palliative care" were thus coined (Kissane & Bloch, 1994).

Whenever bereavement care is viewed as an add-on after the death of the patient, and a psychological postmortem seeks to then identify who might be at risk, clinical services can struggle to make an adequate connection with the bereaved, and preventive models can be challenging to instigate. In contrast, when the psychosocial care team meets the patient and family together in the setting of disease progression, and delivers support throughout this final illness, then continuity can follow smoothly into bereavement as therapeutic alliances have been firmly established. Furthermore, when the psychosocial clinician—be he or she psychologist, social worker, psychiatrist, or other allied health team member —has met the family with the patient expressing his or her views within the circle, these comments are readily recalled during therapy sessions. An empty chair can signify the lost relative and empower observation of the continuing bonds of relationship despite death.

Families at Different Phases of the Life Cycle

Some families will have children facing the death of one parent, others adolescents losing a grandparent, yet others will comprise adult offspring caring for their elderly parents while also bringing up their own children. These families will have different needs and potentially address a wide variety of concerns as they meet together (Kissane & Bloch, 1994). Cultural differences may impact their comfort in discussing death and dying, access to medical treatments, and acceptance of palliative care in the home. Moreover, the relational functioning of each unit will influence its openness of communication, ease of sharing thoughts and feelings, patterns of mutual support and tolerance of differences of opinion among the members (Kissane et al., 1996). As a result, clinicians who respond in a family-centered manner will address the needs and concerns that each individual family brings, no matter at what stage of the life cycle he or she is.

How has the family managed to acknowledge the reality of illness and subsequent death, and participate together to commemorate the deceased relative and share their grief? How will they reorganize their system to cover the roles and responsibilities that have been disrupted by the loss and then move forward with new relationships and life pursuits? These tasks are common to all phases of the life cycle. Zaider (2014) describes these agendas as the roadmap that a clinician explores in making sense of how a family is adapting following a death. Families that communicate openly, prove cohesive in their mutual support, and resolve conflict constructively tend to successfully negotiate these experiences and construct together new meaning as time unfolds.

How the Family Perceives Meaning in the Death

As the story of illness and narrative of the family unfolds, the clinician is both scribe and editor in making sense of and reframing the coping responses of the members (White, 1989). The family's capacity to discover new and richer meanings in the life of their relative and the nature of their shared relationships governs their ability to complete their mourning process and adapt to new challenges moving forward (Nadeau, 2008). Families can carry multiple and potentially contradictory stories that they need to share about the journey, what happened, and how it can be understood. When parents have lost a child, for instance, this meaning-making is often very difficult and yet proves central to the restoration of equanimity in their lives.

Positive growth and transformation can develop within families despite traumatic loss, ambiguous and stigmatized deaths, or ongoing stress and apparent hardship (Tedeschi & Calhoun, 2004). For others, the experience of death from homicide, suicide, or natural disasters may be shocking and leave the family reeling from dismay at what has happened. The needs of the family can be very great in these circumstances. For mourning to achieve resolution so that generativity returns to life, recognition of the meaning of the life lived and the continued benefit that this life brings to the bereaved family proves central to adaptation. The family's capacity to share this meaning ensures that the grief of all involved heals so that creativity in life can continue.

THE FOUNDATIONS OF FAMILY-CENTERED CARE

Let us consider the empirical work that initiated family-centered care in bereavement, the tension between approaches focused on deficits versus those built on resilience, and the outcomes of interventions using family therapy.

Early Observations

Building on Freud's brief reflection about the difference between grief and depression, psychoanalysts established the normality of mourning as a necessary coping response to loss (Deutsch, 1937; Klein, 1940) and encouraged the emotional expression of grief as a pathway to the resolution of mourning.

In 1965, psychologists Norman Paul and George Grosser first lamented the relative inattention that had occurred clinically to family reactions to loss. They described a therapeutic model whereby the emotional expression of grief was actively shared with the family (Paul & Grosser, 1965). In their pioneering study, families were encouraged to reflect together on their loss, share their feelings, and attempt to understand the impact of this death on them. Denial of the loss, inflexibility in attitudes about how to react, and the influence of the coping style of prior generations were noticed to impact on the coping behaviors of family members.

As a social worker in 1974, Lily Pincus further emphasized the importance of the family to any comprehensive consideration of the impact of bereavement, highlighting the value of working with the family as a whole as a clinical approach. In her seminal book, *Death in the Family*, she contrasted, for instance, how a bereaved spouse might regress, whereas their adult offspring displayed growth-oriented outcomes following the death of their parent (Pincus, 1974).

As family therapists began to define their capacity to contribute to bereavement care, in 1976 Murray Bowen highlighted how crucial the consideration of the role of the dying member was to the family's life together. When this role was emotionally or financially vital, greater disruption invariably followed (Bowen, 1976). When a primary breadwinner is lost, the very foundations of the family may be shaken at its core. As another example, an especially painful void might follow the loss of an only child or one with special needs.

These early contributions by Paul and Grosser, Pincus, and Bowen made it clear how grief was metabolized by the family, whose members modeled for one another how to deal with and respond to the loss. Families differed considerably in how well they did this. Systemic understanding of the nature and impact of the loss would empower the clinician to address the many and varied reverberating influences of death on the family as a whole, as well as on any symptom-bearing individual member.

Family Deficits

As family therapy developed as discipline, early theorists speculated that the family might play an etiological role in the development of mental illness (Bateson, Jackson, Haley, & Weakland, 1956). Disordered family communication, for instance, was seen to create mixed and confusing messages for its members, termed a "double bind," and as such it was thought to precipitate illnesses like schizophrenia, placing the blame squarely on the family. These hypotheses proved destructive to families and remind us of the potential harm that well-intended but misguided psychotherapy can cause (Dixon & Lehman, 1995).

With some similarity to the deficit model, the contribution of critical comments by family members to the development of a relapse of psychiatric disorders—the so-called high "expressed emotion" model—was seen empirically to be linked to readmission to hospital (Vaughan & Leff, 1976). Gradually less intrusive, psychoeducational models took the place of the early deficit theories (Falloon, Boyd, & McGill, 1984), but this historical background throws further light on why systemic models of care might have been slow in gaining currency within thanatology.

Family Strengths

Movement from viewing the family as carrying deficits to one in which their contribution became harnessed as a resource proved seminal to refocusing the direction of family-centered care (Wynne, McDaniel, & Weber, 1986). As the family's strengths were brought into sharper focus, therapists moved to a more collaborative role in their support for the family. Greater allowance was made for the impact of the illness on the family and for the resultant burden of caregiving. Recognition of the family's resilience created a clearer pathway for the therapist to foster each family member's mutual support of one another (Walsh, 1996). When applied to the family's experience of medical illness, death, dying, and bereavement, a family-centered approach to care began to make an important contribution to the death and dying movement (Walsh & McGoldrick, 1991).

Early Family Therapy Interventions

A mixed picture of outcomes was found among early grief interventions that used family therapy. Two studies reported by Lieberman (1978) and Rosenthal (1980) suggested that involvement of the family was crucial to overcome contributory factors that otherwise perpetuated mourning as complicated grief. Two other studies failed to find benefits. In the first of these, Williams and Polak (1979) intervened immediately upon the occurrence of a motor vehicle accident. Families experienced this as intrusive and unhelpful. A second study, led by Black and Urbanowicz (1987), involving younger families in which a parent had died showed initial promise at 1 year, but no sustained benefit by 2 years. This inconsistent picture called for further studies to evaluate the systemic contribution that a family model of care could offer.

Meta-analytic evidence has subsequently emerged that bereavement interventions delivered to everyone fail in formal randomized controlled trials to show definitive outcome benefits (Currier, Neimeyer, & Berman, 2008; Rosner, Kruse, & Hagl, 2010). The selection of distressed subjects (or families for that matter) has been seen as the appropriate focus of scarce clinical resources. This raised the question of how one identifies families "at greater risk" from those resilient families that are likely to do well and not need clinical intervention.

CLINICAL ORGANIZATION OF FAMILY-CENTERED CARE TODAY

In considering where we are in applying family-centered care during palliative care and bereavement, I draw on the work of key research teams that have helped mature this approach: my own family focused grief therapy (FFGT) model for adult families, care models for children facing the death of a parent, and family care when a child dies. Let us take each circumstance in turn.

Family Focused Grief Therapy for Adults and Adolescents

In examining the way families share their grief, early observational studies in Australia revealed that the quality of relational functioning of families was highly predictive of bereavement outcome (Kissane et al., 1996). Cluster-analytic work was able to discern a typology of family functioning that separated well-functioning, supportive, and resilient families, who experienced adaptive outcomes during bereavement, and families with reduced communication, cohesion, and conflict resolution, who carried high rates of clinical depression and poorer social adjustment over time. This typology has been subsequently replicated in the United States,

Japan, and a range of European countries (Ozono et al., 2005). For instance, among 1,809 American patients with advanced cancer, 45% viewed their families as supportive and 23% conflict resolving, whereas 21% were low communicators, 5.5% less involved, and 5.5% highly conflictual (Schuler et al., 2014).

The Family Relationships Index (FRI) is a 12-item, true–false questionnaire about family relational life that has been derived from the longer 90-item Family Environment Scale (FES) originally developed at Stanford and used in thousands of studies of families (Moos & Moos, 1981). The FRI has good sensitivity in palliative care populations to identify families at risk of poorer outcomes in bereavement (Edwards & Clarke, 2005). Families are never labeled, lest this prove harmful; rather, the potential benefits of a family meeting about a relative's illness form the basis of an invitation to meet with the clinician.

Two randomized controlled trials have demonstrated the efficacy of 6 to 10 sessions of FFGT that is started preventively during the treatment of a relative for advanced cancer, when the patient's family is deemed to carry a greater risk of a morbid outcome, based on screening with the FRI (Kissane et al., 2006; Kissane, Zaider, Li, & Del Gaudio, 2013). In following the bereaved across 13 months postdeath, those most distressed at baseline have significantly reduced rates of clinical depression and improved social functioning as a result of enhanced family support compared with families receiving usual care. In the first randomized controlled trial, measures of family functioning did not change, perhaps because they reflected trait rather than state characteristics. In the second study, family perceptions of their communication were examined session by session, demonstrating not only significant improvement but also that this, in turn, facilitated a greater sense of life completion for the ill family member (Zaider & Kissane, 2010). Families gaining a sense of improved communication from meeting felt more engaged, emotionally connected, shared a greater sense of purpose, and felt safe in being together (Zaider & Kissane, 2012).

When the initial meeting is set up, the therapist identifies an agenda of talking about the illness and related care provision. As the first meeting unfolds, communication, cohesion, and conflict resolution are reviewed, and the family is invited to consider the benefits of focus on any of the domains about which they share concerns. A genogram is used to examine any patterns of relating and coping with illness, death, or grief across the generations. Families move to a nonshameful acceptance of patterns of coping when these are perceived to have been transmitted as behavioral scripts from one generation to the next (Byng-Hall, 1988). When such a pattern (e.g., avoidance of sharing feelings) constricts family connection, the therapist is generally able to guide the family to reach consensus that more work together on such an issue is worthwhile. Thus, the focus of brief yet continued therapy with the family is established. Therapy generally occurs monthly until progress is evident, when its frequency is reduced. Typically, three to five sessions occur predeath and three to five in bereavement, most families having contact with their therapist over approximately 18 months.

FFGT aims to support coping in the family, while palliative treatments continue for the ill patient's cancer and, in doing so, seeks to optimize their communication, teamwork, and care provision of their sick relative. Strengths of the family are affirmed as a pathway to foster optimal functioning. Sessions can occur in the clinic or the home, depending on the family's availability. Therapists take responsibility to facilitate a safe discussion of themes, avoiding frank disagreements or conflict that would interfere initially with building a therapeutic alliance with the family. Families often prefer to avoid open discussion of death, dying, or the seriousness of prognosis to protect their relative from loss of hope. The therapist's naming of such existential concerns, gently helping the family to discuss them, proves liberating for many and results in outcomes that most families appreciate (Kissane & Bloch, 2002; Kissane & Parnes, 2014).

Efforts are now maturing to disseminate this model of support within hospice and palliative care programs. Training workshops for therapists to acquire practical skills to undertake such a model of therapy have been held in many countries.

Family Bereavement Care for Younger Children

When children face bereavement as a result of the death of one parent, psychoeducational models for families have been tested to assist the subsequent adjustment of these children. Christ, Raveis, Seigel, Karus, and Christ (2005), for example, randomized 88 families to a parental guidance intervention or a supportive-reflective intervention. Group comparison outcomes were not clear, but the qualitative data showed the benefits of preparation, with facilitated visits near the end of life, and open communication about the illness and what was expected (Christ et al., 2005). Muriel, Rauch, and other colleagues in Boston have developed a measure of parenting confidence in the setting of serious illness and shown that single parents and mothers carry greater needs for support and guidance (Muriel, 2014; Muriel et al., 2012). The pursuit of aggressive anticancer therapies makes these parents less likely to develop advanced care plans (Nilsson et al., 2009).

A more detailed and manualized group program of 12 2-hour sessions was tested by Sandler and colleagues (2003), who randomized a community-based sample of families with children aged 8 to 16 years who were between 4 and 30 months post the death of a parent. The control-arm families were given a book about grief each month for 3 months, along with an educational syllabus covering aspects of child, adolescent, and parental grief. In the group-intervention arm, there were four conjoint parent–child sessions and eight separate group sessions for parents, adolescents, and children. The parent groups were taught ways to strengthen the parent–child relationship while sustaining appropriate limit setting, promoting positive activities, and guiding the children in active problem solving. The child and adolescent groups focused on validating the emotions of grief, supporting coping efficacy, optimizing self-esteem, reframing negative thoughts, and using active problem solving. The group arm demonstrated improved parenting and better overall coping, with greater gains for the more distressed youth and less confident parents. Clear benefits follow from such psychoeducational approaches, which affirm normal grief and support parents in their roles.

Family Bereavement Care After the Death of a Child

Parental grief after the loss of a child can be intense and enduring (deCinque et al., 2006), with different responses occurring for mothers and fathers, and siblings sometimes being recognized as the silent mourners. Factors that foster an optimal outcome include excellent communication with the child's medical team, close and supportive family relationships, strong religious faith, and an ability to find meaning despite death (Kreicbergs, Lannen, Onelöv, & Wolfe, 2007). Evidence that siblings are coping poorly includes behavioral disturbance and acting out, conflict and deteriorating family relationships (Davies, 1999; Weiner & Gerhardt, 2014).

Severe parental distress after the death of their child, especially maternal depression, increases the risk of negative parent–child interactions and poorer adaptation for the surviving children (Foster et al., 2008; Garber & Cole, 2010).

Reciprocal interactions clearly occur between parents and surviving children, calling for a family-centered approach to care. Although some marriages may become strained, many have been noted to grow closer and stronger following the loss (Pai et al., 2007). When the family as a whole can make sense of the loss and find meaning in the life of the deceased child (Keesee, Currier, & Neimeyer, 2008), growth and improved family experiences can result from such worthwhile commemoration of the deceased.

When engaging with these families in therapy, therapists must meet them where they are emotionally and tailor what follows to their needs (Kazak & Noll, 2004). Use of art, music, puppets, and storytelling can bring metaphor and symbolism to the communication, whereas the creation of commemorative family rituals can prove very helpful.

Moving From Individual to Family Therapy in Bereavement Care

Patients may be referred individually for bereavement care; however, they can be invited to bring accompanying support persons with them. Expansion of both the voices that recall and the range of stories told about the deceased opens up opportunities that these diverse perspectives will enrich understanding more deeply (Kissane & Hooghe, 2011). In this manner, family therapy can complement both group and individual approaches to bereavement care. The simple prompt for the bereavement counselor is "How could the family assist here?"

CHALLENGES FOR THE FUTURE OF FAMILY-CENTERED CARE

The implementation of models of family-centered care depends on staff having the necessary skills and experience. Sustaining safe therapy, engaging ambivalent families, and optimizing therapeutic processes to consolidate benefits remain as challenges for the future.

Dose and Optimal Processes in the Safe Conduct of Therapy

Future research might profitably explore the dose and length of therapy alongside strategies, as stated, that optimize the process and safety of the therapy. One challenge is for therapists to integrate, through the use of reflective summaries, a deeper understanding by family members of what has been discussed and how it impacts their life together. Another need is knowing when to intervene with a more conflictual family to sustain a constructive orientation and contain very contentious issues for discussion later. A third challenge is to assist each family to find meaning in their relationships, roles, care provision, and connection with one another. When this meaning can be channeled into a fresh sense of purpose and commitment, the family's energy is harnessed to pursue collective goals and priorities.

Change or Acceptance

A paradox for all systemic therapies is whether to pursue a "change" or "acceptance" agenda. In the FFGT model, we have avoided use of the term "problem" lest this appear in some way to be critical in stance; instead, we ask families to identify their "concerns." Our goal is to stimulate reflective functioning as the family considers its issues and thus allow the agenda for change to arise from within the family's circle.

Engagement of the Ambivalent

With a preventive model, we respect a family's wishes not to meet. Distance can be chosen as a preferred solution by a family that has found itself too readily conflict ridden. There is no place for omnipotence in a therapist seeking a miracle. On the other hand, our studies have shown a 75% likelihood that families considered by their clinicians to be very difficult will in fact be helped to relieve clinical depression among their members and deliver benefits for the family as a whole.

Ethical Issues in Family Therapy

The competing needs of family members might be seen to create an ethical dilemma for the thoughtful clinician who is concerned for both the patient and his or her family. This is grist for the mill, and typically dealt with by the stance of neutrality, through which the clinician avoids taking sides and inadvertently aligning himself or herself with a person who invites collusion. Feminist ethics would place emphasis on the relationships and the goals of care (Gilligan, 1982). Yet the complexity of reciprocally interacting systems of distress, angst, and suffering can make this issue of unmet needs challenging for therapists engaging with this work.

Training as a Path to Dissemination

Services seeking to deliver palliative care or bereavement programs often lack staff trained as family therapists. Much of this rests on tradition, where family-centered care has not been on offer. As a result, any dissemination of family grief therapy necessitates creation of a vision for a more comprehensive service, with training workshops to equip staff with skills and more senior therapists to provide ongoing supervision.

Family work requires a different skill set from that needed for individual psychotherapy. Techniques for engaging with a family, setting an agenda, unpacking several perspectives about a story, and freeing up the family's dynamics to operate constructively to their benefit are specific skills for running family meetings. Questions move from a linear orientation used in one-on-one therapy to circular questions, where each person is invited to step into the shoes of another to consider how the other thinks and feels. The science of this interventive questioning has matured within family therapy: see, for example, the work of Tomm (1987) or Dumont and Kissane (2009). As families progress through FFGT, we have seen steady growth in the number of reflexive and strategic questions used in place of initial joining questions that may be linear in orientation (Dumont & Kissane, 2009).

Use of the summary, as an integrative and pacing strategy, is an essential tool ideally employed at junction points in family meetings, when the direction of therapeutic inquiry or theme is about to change (Del Gaudio, Zaider, Brier, & Kissane, 2012). The therapist's summary ensures consensus by a process of taking stock and leads to permission to move ahead to another agenda. Observation of the process of therapy reveals that this is a mature skill seen in experienced therapists, who appear more confident of their work and understanding of the family and its needs.

Generic Versus Specialist Skills

Many clinicians were never trained to run a family meeting, let alone conduct therapy with a family. A considerable educational agenda exists to build basic skills in staff if family-centered care is to be truly disseminated. Differentiating between a generic skill set used by clinicians to conduct an initial family meeting, define agendas, and effect referral to family clinics (where specialist skills are employed) is one model of dissemination that allows for graduated abilities within service providers. Workshops training clinicians through facilitated role play with simulated family members are one means to develop a generic set of skills within palliative care services. Communication skills training programs have begun to run such workshops over the past decade. Many universities and centers of clinical excellence in family therapy run degree courses and formal training programs that accredit clinicians as family therapists for more specialist work.

Supervision

Irrespective of the training and experience of a family therapist, the existential themes in end-of-life and bereavement care are challenges for therapists. The process of peer group supervision is extremely beneficial to help clinicians deepen their insight and monitor their countertransference responses to themes relating to death and dying. We invite each clinician to take their turn in presenting a family using the genogram as a way to understand the patterns of relating across generations and response styles to loss or change. As this formulation of family dynamics unfolds, the discussion helps therapists to strategize about what will help the family, where the therapeutic goals are best targeted, and sometimes what circular questions will assist the family to address its concerns. Across the past 20 years, I have found this method enriching and rewarding for all concerned.

Workforce Issues

Any clinical service that is sincere in its desire to offer family-centered care must employ a credentialed family therapist as a senior member of its team to help educate and provide supervision of others, alongside care delivery to families that might otherwise be perceived as difficult.

Family support for the dying and bereaved is a now an established model of care with proven outcome benefits that make it cost-effective and often optimal within any comprehensive program of clinical care delivery. The palliative care movement adopted this philosophy in a very early phase of its development. The bereavement world has moved more slowly because of its historical focus on individual and group models of treatment. Yet the literature is replete with examples in which attention to the family is essential to deal with confounding and perpetuating influences that would, if neglected, contribute significantly to relapse or prolongation of illness and suffering. Today, it is a central and vital component of both palliative and bereavement care programs, but it remains underdeveloped or poorly done in many parts of the world. It will be a key signifier of the maturation of these programs in the decades ahead. A service's model of family-centered care ought to be consistently appraised by accreditation reviews seeking to certify that the clinical service is providing optimal care.

CONCLUSION

In the Introduction to this book, Judith Stillion and Thomas Attig reviewed the emergence of thanatology as a multidisciplinary field of study, and asserted that the work of this death and dying movement remains unfinished. It does continue to mature. One of its bright hopes in this ongoing development is family-centered care focused on the dying and the bereaved, for the family is both context and center stage, at risk and in need, vulnerable and yet full of potential and resilience. When we harness the creative forces of the family, we optimize powerful pathways toward healing as a most natural and containing form of embrace. If we can bring the strength of love in a family to the fore, we can promote life in its fullness and continuity, despite death.

REFERENCES

Bateson, G., Jackson, D., Haley, J., & Weakland, J. (1956). Toward a theory of schizophrenia. *Behavioral Science, 1*, 251–264.

Black, D. & Urbanowicz, M. (1987). Family intervention with bereaved children. *Journal of Clinical Psychology and Psychiatry, 28*, 467–476.

Boss, P. (1992). Primacy of perception in family stress theory and measurement. *Journal of Family Psychology, 6*, 113–119.

Bowen, M. (1976). Family reactions to death. In P. J. Guerin (Ed.), *Family therapy: Theory and practice* (pp. 335–348). New York, NY: Gardner Press.

Byng-Hall, J. (1988). Scripts and legends in families and family therapy. *Family Process, 27*, 167–180.

Christ, G. H., Raveis, V. H., Seigel, K., Karus, D., & Christ, A. E. (2005). Evaluation of a preventive intervention for bereaved children. *Journal of Social Work in End-of-Life & Palliative Care, 1*, 57–81.

Currier, J. M., Neimeyer, R. A., & Berman, J. S. (2008). The effectiveness of psychotherapeutic interventions for bereaved persons: A comprehensive quantitative review. *Psychological Bulletin, 134*, 648–661.

Davies, B. (1999). *Shadows in the sun: The experience of sibling bereavement in childhood*. Philadelphia, PA: Bruner/Mazell.

deCinque, N., Monterosso, L., Dadd, G., Sidhu, R., Macpherson, R., & Aoun, S. (2006). Bereavement support for families following the death of a child from cancer: Experience of bereaved parents. *Journal of Psychosocial Oncology, 24*, 65–83.

Del Gaudio, F, Zaider, T. I., Brier, M., & Kissane, D. W. (2012). Challenges in providing family-centered support to families in palliative care. *Palliative Medicine, 26*, 1025–1033.

Deutsch, H. (1937). Absence of grief. *Psychoanalytic Quarterly, 6*, 12–22.

Dixon, L., & Lehman, A. (1995). Family interventions for schizophrenia. *Schizophrenia Bulletin, 21*, 631–643.

Dumont, I., & Kissane, D. W. (2009). Techniques for framing questions in conducting family meetings in palliative care. *Palliative & Supportive Care, 7*, 163–170.

Edwards, B., & Clarke, V. (2005). The validity of the Family Relationships Index as a screening tool for psychological risk in families of cancer patients. *Psycho-Oncology, 14*, 546–554.

Falloon, I., Boyd, J., & McGill, C. (1984). *Family care of schizophrenia*. New York, NY: Guilford.

Foster, C. E., Webster, M. C., Weissman, M. M., Pilowsky, D. J., Wickramaratne, P. J., Talati, A., . . . King, C. A. (2008). Remission of maternal depression: Relations to family functioning and youth internalizing and externalizing symptoms. *Journal of Clinical Child & Adolescent Psychology, 37*, 714–724.

Garber, J., & Cole, D. A. (2010). Intergenerational transmission of depression: A launch and grow model of change across adolescence. *Developmental Psychopathology, 22*, 819–830.

Gilligan, C. (1982). *In a different voice*. Cambridge, MA: Harvard University Press.

Kazak, A. E., & Noll, R. B. (2004). Child death from pediatric illness: Conceptualizing intervention from a family/systems and public health perspective. *Professional Psychology: Research and Practice, 35*, 219–226.

Keesee, N. J., Currier, J. M., & Neimeyer, R. A. (2008). Predictors of grief following the death of one's child: The contribution of finding meaning. *Journal of Clinical Psychology, 64*, 1145–1163.

Kissane, D. W., & Bloch, S. (1994). Family grief. *British Journal of Psychiatry, 164*, 728–740.

Kissane, D. W., & Bloch, S. (2002). *Family focused grief therapy: A model of family-centred care during palliative care and bereavement*. Buckingham, UK: Open University Press.

Kissane, D. W., Bloch, S., Dowe, D. L., Snyder, R. D., Onghena, P., McKenzie, D. P., & Wallace, C. S. (1996). The Melbourne Family Grief Study, I: Perceptions of family functioning in bereavement. *American Journal of Psychiatry, 153,* 650–658.

Kissane, D. W., Bloch, S., McKenzie, M., O'Neill, I., Chan, E., Moskowitz, C., & McKenzie, D. (2006). Family focused grief therapy: A randomized controlled trial in palliative care and bereavement. *American Journal of Psychiatry, 163,* 1208–1218.

Kissane, D. W., & Hooghe, A. (2011). Family therapy for the bereaved. In R. A. Neimeyer, D. L. Harris, H. R. Winokuer, & G. F. Thornton (Eds.), *Grief and bereavement in contemporary society: Bridging research and practice* (pp. 287–302). New York, NY: Routledge.

Kissane, D. W., & Parnes, F. (Eds.). (2014). *Bereavement care for families.* New York, NY: Routledge.

Kissane, D. W., Zaider, T., Li, Y., & Del Gaudio, F. (2013). Family therapy for complicated grief. In M. Stroebe, H. Schut, & J. van den Bout (Eds.), *Complicated grief: Scientific foundations for health care professionals* (pp. 248–262). New York, NY: Routledge.

Klein, M. (1940). Mourning and its relation to manic-depressive states. *International Journal of Psychoanalysis, 21,* 125–153.

Kreicbergs, U., Lannen, P., Onelöv, E., & Wolfe, J. (2007). Parental grief after losing a child to cancer: Impact of professional and social support on long-term outcomes. *Journal of Clinical Oncology, 25,* 3307–3312.

Lieberman, S. (1978). Nineteen cases of morbid grief. *British Journal of Psychiatry, 132,* 159–163.

Moos, R. H. & Moos, B. S. (1981). *Family Environment Scale Manual.* Stanford, CA: Consulting Psychologists Press.

Muriel, A. C. (2014). Care of families with children anticipating the death of a parent. In D. W. Kissane & F. Parnes (Eds.), *Bereavement care for families* (pp. 220–231). New York, NY: Routledge.

Muriel, A. C., Moore, C. W., Baer, L., Park, E. R., Kornblith, A. B., Pirl, W., & Rauch, P. K. (2012). Measuring psychosocial distress and parenting concerns among adults with cancer: The Parenting Concerns Questionnaire. *Cancer, 118,* 5671–5678.

Nadeau, J. W. (2008). Meaning-making in bereaved families: Assessment, intervention, and future research. In M. S. Stroebe, R. O. Hansson, H. Schut, & W. Stroebe (Eds.), *Handbook of bereavement research and practice: Advances in theory and intervention* (pp. 511–530). Washington, DC: American Psychological Association.

Nilsson, M. E., Maciejewski, P. K., Zhang, B., Wright, A. A., Trice, E. D., Muriel, A. C., . . . Prigerson, H. G. (2009). Mental health, treatment preferences, advance care planning, location, and quality of death in advanced cancer patients with dependent children. *Cancer, 115,* 399–409.

Ozono, S., Saeki, T., Inoue, S., Mantani, T., Okamura, H., & Yamawaki, S. (2005). Family functioning and psychological distress among Japanese breast cancer patients and families. *Supportive Care in Cancer, 13,* 1044–1050.

Pai, A. L., Greenley, R. N., Lewandowski, A., Drotar, D., Youngstrom, E., & Peterson, C. C. (2007). A meta-analytic review of the influence of pediatric cancer on parent and family functioning. *Journal of Family Psychology, 21,* 407–415.

Paul, N., & Grosser, G. (1965). Operational mourning and its role in conjoint family therapy. *Community Mental Health, 1,* 339–345.

Pincus, L. (1974). *Death and the family.* New York, NY: Pantheon.

Rosenthal, P. A. (1980). Short term family therapy and pathological grief resolution with children and adolescents. *Family Process, 19,*151–159.

Rosner, R., Kruse, J., & Hagl, M. (2010). A meta-analysis of interventions for bereaved children and adolescents. *Death Studies, 34,* 99–136.

Sandler, I. N., Ayers, T. S., Wolchik, S. A., Tein, J. Y., Kwok, O. M., Haine, R. A., . . . Griffin, W. A. (2003). The family bereavement program: Efficacy evaluation of a theory-based prevention program for parentally bereaved children and adolescents. *Journal of Consulting and Clinical Psychology, 71*, 587–600.

Schuler, T. A., Li, Y., Zaider, T. I., Hichenberg, S., Masterson, M., & Kissane D. W. (2014). Typology of perceived family functioning in an American sample of advanced cancer patients. *Journal of Pain and Symptom Management*, doi:10.1016/j.jpainsymman.2013.09.013.

Tedeschi, R. G., & Calhoun, L. G. (2004). Posttraumatic growth: Conceptual foundations and empirical evidence. *Psychological Inquiry, 15*, 1–18.

Tomm, K. (1987). Interventive interviewing: Part II. Reflexive questioning as a means to enable self-healing. *Family Process, 26*, 167–183.

Vaughan, C. E., & Leff, J. P. (1976). The influence of family and social factors on the course of psychiatric illness. *British Journal of Psychiatry*, 129, 125–137.

Walsh, F. (1996). The concept of family resilience: Crisis and challenge. *Family Process, 35*, 261–281.

Walsh, F., & McGoldrick, M. (1991). *Living beyond loss: Death in the family.* New York, NY: Norton.

Weiner, L., & Gerhardt, C. A. (2014). Family bereavement care after the death of a child. In D. W. Kissane & F. Parnes (Eds.), *Bereavement care for families* (pp. 197–219). New York, NY: Routledge.

White, M. (1989). Saying hello again: The incorporation of the lost relationship in the resolution of grief. In M. White (Ed.), *Selected papers* (pp. 29–35). Adelaide, Australia: Dulwich Centre.

Williams, W. V. & Polak, P. R. (1979). Follow-up research in primary prevention: a model of adjustment in acute grief. *Journal of Clinical Psychology*, 35, 35–45.

Wynne, L., McDaniel, S., & Weber, T. (1986). *Systems consultation: A new perspective for family therapy.* New York, NY: Guilford.

Zaider, T. I. (2014) Assessing bereaved families. In D. W. Kissane & F. Parnes (Eds.), *Bereavement care for families* (pp. 79–91). New York, NY: Routledge.

Zaider, T. I., & Kissane, D. W. (2010). The association between family relationships and caregivers' end of life experiences. *Psycho-Oncology, 19*(Suppl. 2), S1816-5, S9.

Zaider, T. I., & Kissane, D. W. (2012). Therapeutic pathways to improved family communication in palliative care. *Asia Pacific Journal of Clinical Oncology, 8*(Suppl. S3), 183.

Linda Goldman

20

SUPPORTING GRIEVING CHILDREN

In the field of childhood bereavement, honoring and respecting past achievements that have withstood the test of time assures a solid foundation for present concepts, as well as a clear path toward future understandings. This chapter presents a narrative on the growth of literature and resource materials, research and education, and important concepts involving children and grief over the past decades. It traces a time that begins with the lack of words to address grieving youngsters to the present wealth of information on the many loss and grief issues young people face. Important understandings and practical information are included, highlighting a major shift from television to modern digital technology that has helped anchor and disperse concepts, techniques, and materials important to bereaved children and families.

MY EARLY YEARS IN THE FIELD

Working with grieving children has been my life's work and passion. Personal experiences with children and loss began after college in 1968. I entered the field of teaching, where I would remain for 20 years as a first-grade, second-grade, kindergarten, reading teacher, and guidance counselor.

My first class was a group of 22 second-grade repeaters. Being a novice educator, I was given a class labeled "throw away children," those children no one wanted to teach, and placed in an aluminum trailer far removed from the rest of the school body. At the onset of the school year, these girls and boys looked sad, withdrawn, and disinterested. During this time in the field of education, many children repeated a grade when they could not achieve academic standards, without insight into the factors that may have inhibited their learning and school performance.

Luckily I was given free rein in my approach to teaching. I decided on a twofold plan. The first step was to start at the beginning of the first-grade curriculum and reteach what the children may not have absorbed in order to create a uniform foundation for learning. The next step was to enhance self-esteem by creating positive learning experiences and allowing children time each day to process their life issues. These simple steps became the seed point for my future work. This first attempt introduced the paradigm that children's grief and loss issues deeply impact their school performance and potential and influence their ability to learn and grow.

We worked together with these guidelines in mind, each day building concepts on the basis of what the children knew and each day creating a safe space for sharing life issues. Many of these children had experienced death, divorce, multiple moves, and family issues such as alcoholism and abuse. I began to realize that as these young people shared emotional issues, their learning capacity increased. Our principal visited the classroom that spring and marveled at the academic progress and the enthusiasm for learning he witnessed. "How did you do this?" he remarked. And the answer became my life's work to develop and share.

The second major influence propelling my work into the field of child bereavement was the death of our stillborn daughter, Jennifer. My husband, Michael, and I had never known such a tragedy. We questioned a clergy for advice and counsel. "What can we do for Jennifer? Should we have a funeral, a burial, a memorial?" He responded, "You don't need to worry about that. In this religion we do not consider her a life." However, Michael and I did consider Jennifer a life and decided to seek council within ourselves and do what we felt was the right path for us. We held Jennifer for hours, created a service for her, and memorialized her in many ways. This overwhelmingly deep, profound death experience influenced the rest of my life and opened the doors to explore working with children and death and dying.

I decided to attend a 5-day *Life, Death, and Transition Workshop* in 1991 with the Elisabeth Kübler-Ross Foundation and continued to participate in Elisabeth's trainings through the years. Corresponding often, she became my mentor and support. This workshop was quite experiential, spontaneously sharing my journey about Jennifer with over a hundred people. Others openly communicated a myriad of life issues ranging from abuse to AIDS, suicide, homicide, and more as the suffering of humanity was expressed on every level in touching and greatly meaningful ways. The love, understanding, and healing generated from this experience expanded my mind to the possibility that the same transformation could take place for children.

I left Elisabeth's workshop with a new vision that permeated my awareness: creating programs in schools and universities to work with grieving children. I became the liaison to school systems with Children's National Medical Center Educational Program, Washington, DC, giving the first of many courses spanning 30 years for teachers, counselors, and health care professionals, and I acquired credentialing to become a grief therapist with children and families.

When I explained to a friend my newfound vocation, she questioned adamantly, "Why would you ever want to work with grieving children, and what do you do to stop them from crying?" My response became the foundation for a life-long career: My goal was not to stop bereaved children from crying, but to create a safe oasis where they could share all of their feelings freely and without judgment.

CHILDREN'S CONCEPTS OF DEATH

Much has been written over the years concerning children's concepts of death. There is not space here to review that literature. However, it is important to note that children's concepts of death and mourning change over time. Wadsworth (1989) summarized Jean Piaget's theory of cognitive development as it relates to children's understanding at different developmental stages. Applied to their perceptions about death, in the sensorimotor stage (approximately 0–2), a child's concept of death is characterized as "out of sight, out of mind." The preoperational stage (approximately 2–7) presents a child's concept as including magical thinking, egocentricity, reversibility, and causality. In the concrete operations stage (approximately 7–12), a child is curious and realistic. The child knows death is not reversible and looks for the facts about what happened. The last stage, formal operations (approximately 13 and up) describes adolescents as self-absorbed. Teens usually see death as remote, relying on their peers for support. Although later research cast doubt on the age ranges, the sequence of developing a mature understanding of death seems reliable. The following examples illustrate young children's thinking about death and heaven.

On death (preoperational): Even though 5-year-old Tucker had gone to the funeral, the gravesite, and felt his mom was in heaven, he still wrote her a letter, mailed it, and waited for a response, magically thinking death was reversible.

On heaven (concrete operations): "This is what heaven is to me. It's a beautiful place. Everyone is waiting for a new person, so they can be friends. They are also waiting for their family. They are still having fun. They get to meet all the people they always wanted to meet (like Elvis). There are lots of castles where only the great live, like my mom. There's all the food you want and all the stuff to do—There's also dancing places, disco. My mom loved to dance. I think she's dancing in heaven. Animals are always welcome. (My mom loved animals.) Ask her how Trixie is. That's her dog that died. Tell her I love her" (Michelle, age 11) (Figure 20.1).

On suicide (early concrete operations): One taboo topic for children is discussion of suicide. Often issues involving children and suicide have been steeped in secrecy and shame, resulting in a secondary loss of trust of the child's emotional environment. The following drawings illustrate suicidal precursors in children and convey a picture (an archetype) of a young person disconnected from his soul.

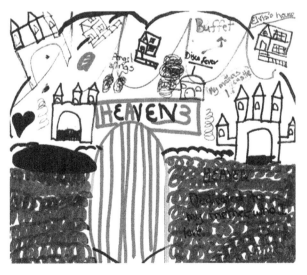

FIGURE 20.1 Michelle's drawing of heaven.
Source: Goldman, 2014, p. 71.

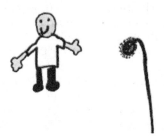

This is me and this is my soul.
The pain is in the center of my soul.
It's kind of like a disease.
Sometimes I feel like killing myself so I'll disappear
and not have pain.

FIGURE 20.2 Seth's drawing of his pain.
Source: Goldman, (2001a).

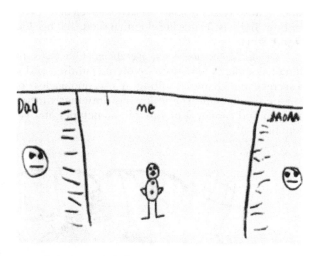

FIGURE 20.3 Seth's drawing of walls closing in.
Source: Goldman, 2001a.

Seth was 8 when his sister died from a drug overdose. The family was in deep grief. He drew this picture and explained, "This is me and this is my soul. The pain is in the center of my soul. It's kind of like a disease. Sometimes I wish I could kill myself so I'll disappear and not have pain." Yet his picture shows this pain is masked with a smile, common with children (Figure 20.2).

Seth continued, "Sometimes when I am in school, I feel like the walls are closing in on me." "If you could draw those walls and give them a name, what would that be?" "Mom and Dad" he replied, drawing another picture of a child grieving in isolation within his family (Figure 20.3).

RESOURCES FOR CHILDREN

Anything that's human is mentionable, and anything that is mentionable can be more manageable.
—Fred Rogers

As more and more people became aware of children's changing concepts about death and their need to grieve, the field of working with children and grief burgeoned. Our culture had been a death denying one . . . especially with children. Throughout the mid-20th century into the 21st century, we witnessed a change of thought ranging from silence to openly discussing these issues with children and creating words to use and information to access. From the loss of a tooth to the death of a parent, to the crumbling of a building, the concept that *children grieve what they miss and can't have back* began to unfold and develop. Children's literature became a valuable tool for dialogue and comfort.

As a child, I realized most friends I knew rarely attended funerals. Adults did not seem to talk to children about death or include them as recognized mourners. *Charlotte's Web* (White, 1952) was one of the first books for young people to speak on issues of life and death, as farm animals share poignant feelings for the young reader to process and relate to. Surprisingly honest dialogues like the following between Wilbur, the pig, and Charlotte, the spider, exemplify this hallmark book: "The thought of death came to him and he began to tremble. 'Charlotte?' he said softly. 'Yes Wilber?' 'I don't want to die.' 'Of course you don't,' said Charlotte in a comforting voice" (White, 1952, p. 62). Sixty years later, it still stands strong as a beloved resource on grief and loss for every generation with the sixth-anniversary edition issued in 2013.

Another classic resource was *The Dead Bird* (Brown, Charlip, & Eichenberg, 1958), the story of young children preparing a funeral and commemoration for a dead bird. One of the first books for young children that spoke of the word "death" was *About Dying* (Stein, Kliman, & Frank, 1974). Stein described what death looks and feels like, including real photos of a storyline about children finding a dead bird and coming together with rituals to memorialize the death. Tommie DePaola's celebrated *Nana Upstairs and Nana Downstairs* (1973) explores the losses involved with aging and the death of a grandparent. *The Fall of Freddie the Leaf* (Buscaglia, 1982) became a classic story about the change in seasons and the understanding that death is a part of life. Freddie, the leaf, and his companions share changes that occur in passing seasons and their falling to the ground with winter's snow, illustrating the delicate balance between life and death. *Lifetimes* (Mellonie & Ingpen, 1983) again addressed life changes for older children. *The Tenth Good Thing About Barney* (Viorst & Blegvad, 1971) was a groundbreaking story about the death of Barney the cat, the sadness surrounding his death, Barney's funeral, and the ways children try to think of 10 good things about Barney. The little boy telling the story can only think of nine, but his father helps him discover the tenth good thing: Barney is buried in the ground and is helping the plants to grow.

The Hurt (Doleski & McNichols, 1983) is a book that gave children permission to express hurt feelings. It is a special story about a boy who is troubled because a friend called him a name. He harbored *the hurt* inside until it got too big to live with. He decided to talk to his dad. Then he could let the hurt go. *When Dinosaurs Die* (Brown & Brown, 1996) explains through age-appropriate language that dying is very much a part of life. *When a Pet Dies* (Rogers & Judkis, 1988) shares photographs and words about the death of a pet. This treatment of pet death was expanded in an exceptional book for young children, *Goodbye Mousie* (Harris & Ormerod, 2001), which served as a teaching tool to allow children to actively commemorate a pet's death. After Mousie died, a little boy placed his dead body in a box with food in case he gets hungry, crayons in case he is bored, and a picture so he won't be lonely. After reading this book, 7-year-old Chad had the idea of placing a picture of himself and his grandfather in Grandpa's coffin at Grandpa's funeral service.

Recognition of children's development in thinking has been reflected, not only in books, but also in action centers for children in grief. A shift in consciousness from ignoring children's grief to creating peer support has come about through the creation and growth of grief centers, peer-support groups, and grief camps. Mental health educator and pioneering author of *The Grieving Child* (1992), Helen Fitzgerald, laid the framework for working with children and grief as coordinator of the Grief Program for Mental Health Services, conducting therapeutic group sessions for young grieving children.

The Dougy Center (n.d.), founded in 1982, was the first center in the United States to provide peer-support groups for grieving children. Thirteen-year-old Dougy had died of an inoperable brain tumor. Dougy wrote a poignant letter to Dr. Kübler-Ross asking why no one would speak to him about dying and his own death. Beverly Chappell supported Dougy during his treatment and observed his ability to bond with other teens facing serious medical issues. Inspired by Dougy's wisdom, Chappell led the first grief-support group in her home. This grassroots effort grew to become a year-round child-centered program offering peer-support groups to grieving families (The Dougy Center, 2014).

TAPS, The Tragedy Assistance Program for Survivors, was founded in 1994, as a "good grief" camp for children who had suffered the loss of a military loved one. Its work has been extended into many grief camps for military children throughout the country, helping grieving girls and boys and their families from the wars in Iraq and Afghanistan.

This shift of thinking from protecting children from painful loss issues to openly including them as recognized mourners has been extraordinary, from the first Dougy Center support group in 1982 to the emergence of numerous grief facilities supporting children's involvement with others in their grief process. Saint Lewis reports, "There are now more than 300 of these non profit counseling centers" and "at least 150 more peer-to-peer programs nationwide that serve a similar function" (Schuurman, as quoted in Saint Lewis, 2012, p. 1). Children's grief-support centers, groups, and camps are now playing a major role in providing children an oasis of safety and comfort to share grief with others.

CHILDREN'S GRIEF AND THE DIGITAL AGE

The digital world has also produced many vehicles that can support children's knowledge about death as well as their ability to grieve in positive ways. In 1970, Fred Rogers introduced youngsters to the world of television as a vehicle for learning about death and dying. *Mister Rogers' Neighborhood*, "Episode 1101: The Death of the Goldfish" (1970) sensitively approaches a goldfish's death and the feelings associated with finding a dead goldfish in his aquarium. Using age-appropriate language, Rogers conveys the heavy sadness surrounding death and suggests that these feelings won't last forever. Television was the first step on the long road to today's hi-tech world and played an integral role in transmitting understandings involving bereaved kids.

Working as a child bereavement advisor, I collaborated with *Sesame Street* in their project When Families Grieve (Sesame Workshop, n.d.) designed to reach children throughout the globe and support their families when a parent dies. It serves as a model of what can be accomplished on a grand scale to provide information and resources for grieving children on television and via the Internet, video, downloadable materials, and two customized bilingual (English and Spanish) resource kits. This program recognized that the death of a parent influenced every aspect of a child's life, acknowledged the need for children to identify and express emotions, and empowered adults to feel comfortable with children on the topic of death.

Young people have access to technology as never before. Face-to-face contact and online interaction seems to blend as one and the same. One mom shared the new challenges of raising her children with this advanced technology. "They don't talk to each other. They go to Facebook." Creative approaches to aid children's expression of grief are found in tablet computers equipped with "apps" that engage children. Moody Monster Manor (McClam & Varga, 2011, p. 31) is an app that allows young children to create a monster that portrays their immediate emotions and gives adults an indication of how to dialogue with them. Online grief-support groups and virtual memorials have grown in the past decade as young people commemorate friends and family and pay tribute to those they admired but had not known.

The death of Apple creator Steve Jobs had a huge impact on many young people. Memorials and tributes by children spontaneously appeared at Apple stores throughout the world, generating *a teachable moment* for girls and boys whose lives were forever changed by his inventiveness. His death inspired children to express feelings and gratitude through the very social media he helped create. Children became active participants as recognized mourners in commemorating this icon through letters and e-mails to Apple, expressing a range of grief feelings and a tribute to his life. One letter spoke to many of this generation born into the digital age: "Thank you for making computers. You changed my life" (Figure 20.4).

"How do grief and loss and the world of technology intersect the lives of children? Not only is bereavement and the computer age intertwined, they cannot be separated" (Goldman, 2014, p. 114). The information explosion in the digital age has remarkably transformed earlier ideas into the current wealth of literature in the field of child bereavement. Technology has progressively played a major role in childhood bereavement. Young people use sophisticated communication to blog their emotions about intimate personal issues, find websites that support challenges associated with grief and loss, create memory chat rooms with friends, and instantly message 24/7 about thoughts and feelings. The Internet and its social media, cell phones, and even iTunes allow children of this new electronic age instant communication, companionship, and information. Some funerals are posted online for young people to access and continually review. Families are often given a DVD of the service as well.

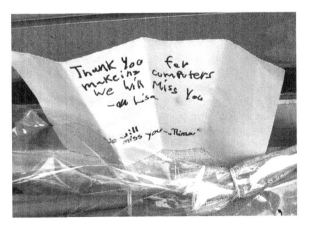

FIGURE 20.4 Child's letter remembering Steve Jobs.
Source: Goldman, (2014).

Children have fresh ways to combat isolation and loneliness with the new social media technology as their constant buddy. Its value is unquestionable in a global community in accessing immediate data, news, and intimacy. These innovative resources and many more have led the way to today's expansion of children's bereavement resources, ranging from issues of death to suicide, homicide, and terrorism. Today's message includes children in rituals and memorializing, dispels myths past generations were raised on, and incorporates child-oriented activities to include children as recognized mourners.

GRIEF WORK WITH CHILDREN

Although the resources available to grieving children have proliferated in the last half century, nothing takes the place of face-to-face contact with them. Silverman (2000) clarified the goal of grief work with children as follows: "The goal of helping children of all ages to cope with death is to promote their competence, facilitate their ability to cope, and recognize that children are active participants in their lives" (p. 42). Children and adults can work toward this goal using many techniques, including memory work, projection, role-play, and expressive arts techniques for grief work.

Memory work is an important component of grief work that allows children to release their hurt and express feelings. It includes memory books, memory projects, memory boxes, and even memory e-mails and memorials. Marge Heegaard wrote several creative children's memory books using art therapy techniques, beginning with *When Someone Very Special Dies* (1988). *Fire in My Heart, Ice in My Veins* (Traisman, 1992) was a memory journal for teens. Karen Carney originated interactive storybooks for young children and grief in her series *Barclay and Eve* (1997), including often unspoken topics such as death, funerals, hospice, pet death, cremation, organ and tissue donation, cancer, and Shiva. *Changing Faces* (O'Toole, 1995) was a practical memory book for preteens. *Bart Speaks Out on Suicide* (Goldman, 1998) was the first interactive child's story/memory book on suicide, followed by *Children Also Grieve* (Goldman, 2005b), the first child's interactive story/memory book translated into Chinese.

Therapists using projective play can invite youngsters to work with complex issues including their grief process through play. Play allows them to use their imagination to safely express thoughts and feelings. Girls and boys may have a restricted verbal ability for sharing feelings and a limited emotional capacity to tolerate the pain of loss. They communicate their feelings, wishes, fears, and attempted resolutions to their problems through play (Webb, 2002).

Puppet play, sand play, telephones, dishes, and dollhouses are props suggested by Gil (1991, p. 64). Nurturing props, including dolls, baby bottles, and blankets, permit a safe space for the symbolic nurturance children can no longer give or receive from the person who died. Children use drama and imagination with props like a toy telephone to create a private role-play conversation with a loved one. For example, Amy was 6 years old when her mom died. "I really miss my mom," she explained. She picked up the toy telephone and began an ongoing dialogue with Mom. "Hi Mommy. How are you? I love you. Are you OK? Let me tell you about my day." This toy telephone allowed Amy to work through challenging spaces through role-play. A magic wand can also serve as a useful object for projective play. For example, Olivia's mom had died of cancer. I asked her, "If you had one wish, what would it be?" She waved the magic wand and said, "I would bring my mom back from the dead and never let nice people die." What may appear to be a frivolous play activity may actually be a profound avenue for young people to work through these complex issues.

Providing props, such as helping figures, costumes, and building blocks, allows children to recreate their loss experience and role-play what happened. Girls and boys can recreate a disaster setting with doctors, nurses, fireman, and policeman by using projective play props. In one instance, Gabrielle (age 6) pretended to be a nurse helping those hurt at the Pentagon crash while Kyle (age 5) put on the fire hat and gloves and said, "Don't worry I'll save you. Run for your lives." The children felt "empowered to take action and control over the difficult experience they had witnessed" (Goldman, 2005a, p. 122).

Puppets and stuffed animals are another way for children to express feelings and work through challenging spaces that they can't verbalize. Therapists can prompt, "I wonder what Max the puppet would say? Let's hear Max's story." "This play allows and provides an outlet for thoughts and feelings and helps participants adapt to their life situation" (Goldman, 2001a). Some books that may stimulate young children to interact in therapy include *Brave Bart* (Sheppard, 1998), *A Terrible Thing Happened* (Holmes & Mudlaff, 2000), and *Children Also Grieve* (Goldman, 2005b). These stories use animals as a safe vehicle for projection of emotions surrounding grief.

Projective drawing can help children place unresolved feelings outside of themselves and onto paper. In one case, Chase was an 8-year-old boy when he came to grief therapy after his father's murder. His mom explained he had previously witnessed her mental and physical abuse by his dad, which had left her physically ill. Chase kept much inside, and his moods fluctuated from hyperactivity to withdrawal. He often could not or would not express feelings. One day he came into a grief therapy session, sat down, and did not speak.

After a few minutes, I invited him to draw a scribble picture. "If you can see something inside the scribble color, can you give it a name?" Chase drew the following picture and wrote "A Tornado" on top. I continued, "If that tornado could talk, what would it say?" "Help me" Chase replied. This projective technique became a tool to explore feelings and discuss what would be helpful (Figure 20.5).

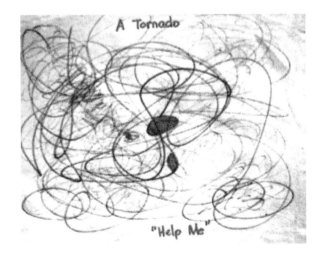

FIGURE 20.5 Projective scribble drawing.
Source: Goldman, 2001a.

GRIEF EDUCATION FOR ADULTS

At the same time that resources for children were proliferating, authorities were presenting helpful resources for adults. *The Way of Dialogue on Death Between Parents and Children* (Grollman, 1976) began to educate parents on creating a dialogue with grieving children. *The Private Worlds of Dying Children* (Bluebond-Langner, 1978) opened a previously closed window on insights into a child's processing of his or her illness and dying and created increased understanding of children's stages of awareness, which range from closed awareness, mutual pretense, to open awareness.

O'Toole (1999) developed a pioneering curriculum to work with schools and established associated childhood loss categories that included relationships, environ- ronment, skills and abilities, external objects, self, and routines and habits. The loss of the future and protection of the adult world and privacy were added in *Life and Loss* (Goldman, 2001b, 2014).

The Children's Loss Inventory Checklist for educators, which is found in *Life and Loss* (Goldman, 1992, 2001b, 2014), underscores the emerging realization that communication through all the grades to all school personnel is essential in seeing the whole child. It maintains a shared history as students progress in their education and focuses awareness of loss issues children face in life, which range from death, illness, divorce, moving, and losses in the family before a child is born.

As the awareness of children's developmental understandings related to death and loss emerged, grief educator Alan Wolfelt founded the Center for Loss & Life Transition (1983) and authored *Helping Children Cope With Grief* (1984). Wolfelt pioneered educating professionals and grieving people on working with children and grief.

Great strides in understanding adolescent bereavement appeared with trusted books, such as *Adolescence and Death* (Corr & McNeil, 1986), the *Handbook of Adolescent Death and Bereavement* (Corr & Balk, 1996), and *Living with Grief: Children, Adolescents, and Loss* (Doka, 2000). Each highlights the unique attributes of adoles- cents and parental relationships and the support that influences their grief process.

Another innovator, Sandra Fox, in her book *Good Grief* (1985), built on Wor- den's four tasks of grief (understanding, grieving, commemorating, and going on) as they related to children (Worden, 1982). These tasks were an integral part in children's successfully working through grief. Topics included understanding, grieving, commemorating, and going on, explored in *Life and Loss* (Goldman, 1992).

As I began to share my first book, *Life and Loss* (1992), with family, my dad requested I not bring it out, as the topic would upset everyone. That statement deep- ened my awareness of how fearful adults were at the time to talk about these issues, and how many felt it was unthinkable to address death with children. I began to develop words to use and creative communication to be used with children to open the topic of suicide by writing *Bart Speaks Out on Suicide* Goldman, (1998) and give voice to a grandparent's death in *Children Also Grieve* (Goldman, 2005b).

These words crossed cultural barriers and extended internationally through- out the years to include the children of many cultures. My translated works included *Life and Loss* (Goldman, 2005d [in Japanese]), *Breaking the Silence* (Goldman, 2002 [in Chinese]), *Children Also Grieve* (Goldman, 2005c [in Chinese]), *Great Answers to Difficult Questions About Death* (Goldman, 2012 [in Polish]; Goldman, 2013a [in Korean]), and *Helping the Grieving Child in the School* (Goldman, 2013b [in Hebrew]), Goldman [in Czech, in press, 2015]. What was once a resource hidden from frightened family members has become an accepted template for adults work- ing with grieving children globally.

In an effort to prepare adult professionals who will come into contact with children experiencing death and grief, undergraduate and graduate courses on children, death, and grief began to be offered in colleges and universities in the late 1970s. For example, as an adjunct faculty member at Johns Hopkins University, Counseling and Education, I developed and began teaching the graduate course on working with children and grief, continued in the University of Maryland School of Social Work in 1997, and today I teach in many schools and universities, including Johns Hopkins Graduate School and Kings College in Canada.

BASIC UNDERSTANDINGS FOR ADULTS

In spite of the many resources now available to them, parents and professionals may still feel inadequate to speak to children about death. As a result, they might consciously or unconsciously restrain emotions in children. The myth that adults should avoid topics that might make a child cry only inhibits the grief process. In order to reduce anxiety and fear, it is essential for adults to become familiar with the following basic understandings about bereaved children. Knowing fundamental paradigms involving childhood losses, myths about grieving children, tasks of grief, and common signs of grieving in children establish a needed structure for working with bereaved children.

One basic insight often overlooked by caring adults is that children experience multiple losses in childhood. Such losses include the loss of relationships as children enter school or move; the loss of the secure environment of their primary home as they move out in ever-larger circles; possible loss of skills and abilities in the face of accident or trauma; loss of routines and habits as more demands are placed on them; loss of external objects, such as blankets and other security symbols; and loss of adult protection as they assert their independence. Recognizing these losses and the need to grieve them can open communication between adults and children.

Another area of adult education involves dispelling past myths about grief. These include the following (Goldman, 2014):

- Grief and mourning are the same experience.
- Adults can instantly give explanations to children about death and spirituality.
- The experience of grief and mourning has orderly stages.
- The grief of adults does not impact on the bereaved child.
- Adults should avoid topics that cause a child to cry.
- An active, playing child is not a grieving child.
- Infants and toddlers are too young to grieve.
- Parents and professionals are always prepared and qualified to explain loss and grief.
- Children need to "get over" their grief and move on.
- Children are better off not attending funerals.

Attending funerals creates a structure for allowing children to participate in the grief process. We can prepare young people, invite them but not force them, and offer choices. Research findings by Silverman and Worden (1992) conclude, "attendance helped them to acknowledge the death, provided an occasion for honoring their deceased parent, and made it possible for them to receive support and comfort" (p. 319). Justin's drawing, age 13, illustrates how comforted he felt attending a funeral (Figure 20.6).

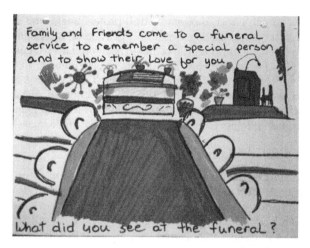

FIGURE 20.6 Drawing of funeral.
Source: Goldman, (2014).

Recognizing that there are four basic psychological tasks of grief can give guidance to adults. These include understanding, grieving, commemorating, and going on (Fox, 1985, Worden, 1982). Caring adults can help children come to grips with the meaning of death, give permission to grieve, find ways to memorialize, and reassure them that life will continue.

It is also important to create a language to use with young children in order to increase comfortable dialogue. We can say: "Death is when the body stops working. Usually someone dies when they are very, very old or very, very sick, or their bodies are so injured that the doctors and nurses can't make their bodies work again" (Goldman, 2009, p. 106).

The use of common clichés can inhibit the grief process *and should be avoided.* Children often take language literally and need direct and simple explanations. For example, "Grandfather went on a long trip." The child might respond, "Why didn't he take me?" "Amy lost her mom." The child might respond, "How could she lose her mom, she was so big?" "Dad is watching over you." The child might respond, "That could be very embarrassing." "We put your dog Max to sleep and he died." The child might respond. "Will I die if I sleep?" "God loved Dad so much he took him to heaven." The child might respond, "Why didn't God take me? Can I go too? Doesn't God love me?"

Adults need to recognize common signs of grieving children, including the following (Goldman, 2014):

- The child retells *events* of the deceased's death and funeral over and over.
- The child dreams about the deceased.
- The child idolizes or imitates behaviors of the deceased.
- The child feels the deceased is with him or her in some way.
- The child speaks of his or her loved one in the present.
- The child rejects old friends and seeks new friends with a similar loss.
- The child wants to call home during the school day.
- The child can't concentrate on homework or class work.
- The child bursts into tears in the middle of class.
- The child seeks medical information on death of deceased.

- The child *worries excessively* about his own health.
- The child sometimes appears to be unfeeling about loss.
- The child becomes the "class clown" to get attention.
- The child is overly concerned with caretaking needs.

These signs don't necessarily indicate that children are grieving abnormally. Nevertheless they may alert adults to spend more time or communicate more clearly with a grieving child.

Alan Wolfelt (2006, p. 2) has published a document that should be helpful to adults working with grieving children. Entitled "Ten Healing Rights for Children," it reads as follows:

- I have the right to have my own unique feelings about the death.
- I have the right to talk about my grief whenever I feel like talking.
- I have the right to show my feelings of grief in my own way.
- I have the right to need other people to help me with my grief.
- I have the right to get upset about normal, everyday problems.
- I have the right to have "griefbursts"—sudden, unexpected feelings of sadness.
- I have the right to use my beliefs about my God to help me deal with my feelings of grief.
- I have the right to try to figure out why the person I loved died.
- I have the right to think and talk about my memories of the person who died.
- I have the right to move forward and feel my grief and, over time, to heal. www.centerforloss.com

A fundamental understanding about parentally bereaved children is their tendency to reconstruct a dead parent through means of connection that include locating the deceased, experiencing the deceased, reaching out, waking memories, and linking objects. Research findings by Silverman, Nickman, and Worden (1992) explain: "In facilitating mourning . . . work with children (we) may need to focus on how to transform connections and place the relationship in a new perspective, rather than on how to separate from the deceased" (p. 502).

An example of this ongoing connectivity was seen in 6-year-old Ashley. She arrived at grief therapy with tears in her eyes. It was Mother's Day and no one had mentioned her mom. I invited her to write a letter to her mother. Ashley clearly illustrates her ongoing relationship, reaching out, experiencing and locating Mom, and seeking a linking object. After sharing the letter, I asked Ashley if she wanted to buy a balloon for her mother. She chose a red heart balloon and wrote "I Love You." She felt much better (Figure 20.7).

Adults also must recognize that not all deaths bring about the same grieving patterns. For example, sudden or traumatic death brings shock to everyone and can be overwhelming for children. Multiple losses can strain even the best developed coping skills. Deaths that cause shame or stigma (e.g., suicide and homicide) can impede grieving and grief therapy. The grief processes of the adults in a child's life, if unhealthy, can further affect a child's grief. In addition, the relationship that the child has had with the deceased, especially if it has been troubled, can be a challenge.

With the increase of violence, natural disasters, and terrorism, our children face the challenge of a world in which traumatic events increasingly impact their day-to-day lives. The following are a few examples.

Jared survived hurricane Katrina. He used the sand table to place figures of himself, Mom, and Dad, and his dog, Scruffy. "I couldn't find my dog, my house

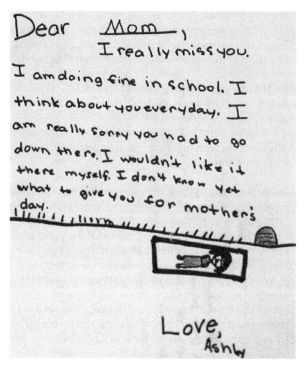

Dear Mom,
    I really miss you.
I am doing fine in school. I
think about you everyday. I
am really sorry you had to go
down there. I wouldn't like it
there myself. I don't know yet
what to give you for mother's
day.

Love,
Ashley

FIGURE 20.7 Ashley's letter to Mom.
Source: Goldman, (2014).

was gone, and all of my stuff was missing. Me and my mom and dad were scared. We didn't know if help would ever come."

Shen (2002) conducted a statistical study on the effectiveness of child-centered play therapy after the Taiwanese earthquake. His work demonstrated a significant reduction of anxiety and suicidal ideation, which supports the effectiveness of play therapy.

Tanya, age 4, watched with her family in their car, when dad was murdered at a convenience store. She constantly replayed the murder through play, creating "good guy–bad guy" scenarios and reenacting the crime over and over again. Practical experience as a grief therapist with complex grief issues involving children, such as suicide and homicide, has revealed that isolation and detachment exist in young children. Once again, play may be the key to reaching them. "Play allows children to use symbolic expression, so that they often feel safer to reveal difficult feelings. . . . Children who are considered to have avoidance symptoms may be more able to articulate their traumatic experiences in a play therapy setting" (Ogawa, 2004, p. 25).

Today there is renewed emphasis on raising resilient children. *Raising Our Children to Be Resilient: A Guide to Help Children With Traumatic Grief* (Goldman, 2005a) was inspired by the 9/11 terrorist attacks. One example of a child's misperception that might lead to difficulty in grieving occurred after the Pentagon terrorist attack, which killed 5-year-old Kim's mother. As if telling a secret, Kim whispered in my ear. "It's my fault Mommy died. She had a cold and I didn't make her stay home from work that day." Kim couldn't integrate the overwhelming facts of the day. I replied, "You did not make your mom die. Mommy was killed when some people flew a plane into the building where she was working and destroyed it. You couldn't have known that was going to happen."

My goal as children's bereavement advisor with the TAPS, Tragedy Assistance Program for Survivors was to help identify children's traumas and support their natural attributes of resilience after a death in the military. This objective was achieved through individual work with parents and children across the country, trainings for military parents, and grief camps for kids.

JOINING AS A GLOBAL GRIEF COMMUNITY FOR CHILDREN

The advent of our digital age allows children vicariously, if not directly, by the click of a TV remote or computer mouse, to image these events over and over and imprint them in their minds. I realized we are sometimes "powerless to control the losses and catastrophic events our children may need to face. But by honoring their inner wisdom, providing mentorship, and creating safe havens for expression, we can empower them to become more capable, more caring human beings" (Goldman, 2005b, p. 72).

It is my hope and prayer that we join together with alacrity as cocreators of a global grief community, understanding the unique, yet universal ways children process grief and loss. A shared vision and renewed commitment to honor young people in their grief process is mandatory. By advocating in homes, schools, neighborhoods, cities, and countries, we can help solidify a safe journey for our grieving girls and boys.

As a wife, mom, daughter, friend, teacher, therapist, educator, and pet owner, my personal and professional experience with children's bereavement runs a broad spectrum of life issues. Open communication, expression of feelings, and access to age-appropriate techniques and materials are time-tested practices that empower children by acknowledging and respecting their process, creating recognized mourners, and providing safe havens for sharing. By becoming more knowledgeable on issues involving child bereavement and gaining comfort in exploring them, adults can reduce the fear and denial often accompanying children's grief work.

The challenge of modernity was also the challenge of antiquity . . . to view children as individuals to be seen and heard as valued mourners. Our charge is to learn and understand the nuances of children's grief processes and the explosion of resources available. The digital age has solidified the presence of a global grief team—instantaneously sharing traumatic events that bring into consciousness the awareness of how powerfully interconnected we are in life and death. Within this framework, children can express thoughts and feelings, communicate with others, and support peers in fresh and caring ways. We can step forward into a future that holds clear acceptance of useful paradigms and expels outdated myths on children's grief, creating an original blend of new insights coupled with the rich heritage of past contributions.

> If we can envision each universal child having the support of caring adults . . .
> If we share the conviction that we can join together to help our children everywhere . . .
> We can create a light to lead the way through grief with understanding and compassion for all. (Goldman, 2014, p. 20)

REFERENCES

Bluebond-Langner, M. (1978). *The private worlds of dying children*. Princeton, NJ: Princeton University Press.

Brown, L. K., & Brown, M. (1996). *When dinosaurs die*. Boston, MA: Little, Brown.

Brown, M. W., Charlip, R., & Eichenberg, F. (1958). *The dead bird*. New York, NY: W. R. Scott.

Buscaglia, L. F. (1982). *The fall of Freddie the leaf*. Thorofare, NJ: C.B. Slack.

Corr, C. A., & Balk, D. (1996). *Handbook of adolescent death and bereavement*. New York, NY: Springer Publishing Company.

Corr, C. A., & McNeil, J. N. (1986). *Adolescence and death*. New York, NY: Springer Publishing Company.

DePaola, T. (1973). *Nana upstairs & nana downstairs*. New York, NY: Putnam.

Doka, K. J. (2000). *Living with grief: Children, adolescents, and loss*. Washington, DC: HFA.

Doleski, T., & McNichols, W. H. (1983). *The hurt*. New York, NY: Paulist Press.

The Dougy Center. (2014). *About us*. Retrieved from http://www.dougy.org/about-us/

Fitzgerald, H. (1992). *The grieving child: A parent's guide*. New York, NY: Simon & Schuster.

Fox, S. S. (1985). *Good grief: Helping groups of children when a friend dies*. Boston, MA: New England Association for the Education of Young Children.

Gil, E. (1991). *The healing power of play: Working with abused children*. New York, NY: Guilford.

Goldman, L. (1992). *Life and loss: A guide to help grieving children* (1st ed.). New York, NY: Routledge.

Goldman, L. (1998). *Bart Speaks Out on Suicide*. California, WPS Publishers.

Goldman, L. (2001a). *Breaking the silence* (2nd ed.). New York, NY: Routledge.

Goldman, L. (2001b). *Life and loss: A guide to help grieving children* (2nd ed.). New York, NY: Routledge.

Goldman, L. (2002). *Breaking the silence* (2nd ed.), Chinese translation. New York, NY: Brunner-Routledge.

Goldman, L. (2005a). *Raising our children to be resilient: A guide to help children with complicated grief*. New York, NY: Brunner-Routledge.

Goldman, L. (2005b). *Children also grieve: Talking about death and healing*. London, UK: Jessica Kingsley.

Goldman, L. (2005c). *Children also grieve: Talking about death and healing*. Chinese Translation. London, UK: Jessica Kingsley.

Goldman, L. (2005d). *Life and loss: A guide to help grieving children* (2nd ed.), Japanese translation. New York, NY: Routledge.

Goldman, L. (2009). *Great answers to difficult questions about death: What children need to know*. London, UK: Jessica Kingsley.

Goldman, L. (2012). *Great answers to difficult questions about death: What children need to know* (Polish translation). London: UK: Jessica Kingsley.

Goldman, L. (2013a). *Great answers to difficult questions about death: What children need to know* (Korean translation). London: UK: Jessica Kingsley.

Goldman, L. (2013b). Helping the grieving child in school. In H. Shanun-Klein, S. Kreitler, & M. Kreitler (Eds.), *Thanatology—The study of loss, dying and bereavement: Selected topics* [Hebrew] (pp. 379–390, chap. 18). Haifa, Israel: Pardres.

Goldman, L. (2014). *Life and loss: A guide to help grieving children* (3rd ed.). New York, NY: Routledge.

Goldman, L. (in press 2015). *Great answers to difficult questions about death: What children need to know* (Czech translation). London: UK: Jessica Kingsley.

Grollman, E. (1976). The way of dialogue on death between parent and child. *Religious Education, 69*(2), 123–124.

Harris, R. H., & Ormerod, J. (2001). *Goodbye Mousie*. New York, NY: Margaret K. McElderry Books.

Heegaard, M. E. (1988). *When someone very special dies*. Minneapolis, MN: Woodland Press.

Holmes, M. M., & Mudlaff, S. J. (2000). *A terrible thing happened*. Washington, DC: Magination Press.

McClam, T., & Varga, M. (2011). Connecting college students and grieving children. *ADEC Forum, 37*(4), 31–33.

Mellonie, B., & Ingpen, R. (1983). *Lifetimes.* Toronto, Ontario, Canada: Bantam.

Ogawa, Y. (2004). Childhood trauma and play therapy intervention for traumatized children. *Journal of Professional Counseling, Practice, Theory, & Research, 32*(1), 19–29.

O'Toole, D. R. (1995). *Facing change.* Burnsville, NC: Mountain Rainbow.

O'Toole, D. R. (1999). *Growing through grief.* Burnsville, NC: Compassion Press.

Rogers, F. (1970). Death of a goldfish [Television series episode]. In *Mister Rogers' neighborhood.* Arlington, TX: The Public Broadcasting Service.

Rogers, F. (2005). *Life's journey according to Mr. Rogers* (Audio CD.). New York, NY: Hyperion.

Rogers, F., & Judkis, J. (1988). *When a pet dies.* New York, NY: Putnam.

Saint Lewis, C. (2012, September 19). Letting children share in grief. *New York Times.* Retrieved from http://www.nytimes.com/2012/09/20/garden/letting-children-share-in-grief.html?pagewanted=all&_r=0

Sesame Workshop. (n.d.). *When families grieve.* Retrieved from http://www.sesameworkshop.org/what-we-do/our-initiatives/when-families-grieve/

Shen, Y. (2002). Short-term group play therapy with Chinese earthquake victims: Effects on anxiety, depression and adjustment. *International Journal of Play Therapy, 11*(1), 43–63.

Sheppard, C. H. (1998). *Brave Bart: A story for traumatized and grieving children.* Gross Pointe Woods, MI: Institute for Trauma and Loss.

Silverman, P. R. (2000). *Never too young to know: Death in children's lives.* New York, NY: Oxford University Press.

Silverman, P. R., Nickman, S., & Worden, J. W. (1992). Detachment revisited: The child's reconstruction of a dead parent. *American Journal of Orthopsychiatry, 62*(4), 494–503.

Silverman, P. R., & Worden, J. W. (1992). Children's understanding of funeral ritual. *Omega: Journal of Death and Dying, 25*(4), 319–331.

Stein, S. B., Kliman, G., & Frank, D. (1974). *About dying.* New York, NY: Walker.

Traisman, E. S. (1992). *Fire in my heart, ice in my veins.* Portland, OR: Centering Corporation.

Viorst, J., & Blegvad, E. (1971). *The tenth good thing about Barney.* New York, NY: Atheneum.

Wadsworth, B. J. (1989). *Piaget's theory of cognitive and affective development* (4th ed.). New York, NY: Longman.

Webb, N. B. (2002). *Helping bereaved children* (2nd ed.). New York, NY: Guilford.

White, E. B. (1952). *Charlotte's web.* New York, NY: Harper.

Wolfelt, A. (1983). *Helping children cope with grief.* Muncie, IN: Accelerated Development.

Wolfelt, A. D. (2006). *Ten healing rights for grieving children.* Washington, DC: U.S. Department of State, Center for Loss and Life Transition. Retrieved from http://www.state.gov/documents/organization/90523.pdf

Worden, J. W. (1982). *Grief counseling and grief therapy.* New York, NY: Springer.

Worden, J. W. (1996). *Children and grief: When a parent dies.* New York, NY: Guilford.

Phyllis R. Silverman

21

HELPING EACH OTHER: BUILDING COMMUNITY

What was helpful to me is that I don't feel so alone.
I am with other children whose parent died.
—A 9-year-old boy at the Children's Room

Why do people find it so helpful to meet others who have similar problems or life-changing experiences? Why does finding others like ourselves give us a sense of hope, of being understood, and often a direction to a solution to our problem? Coming together in this way often takes place in what we call mutual help groups. This chapter offers some understanding of how these groups come about, what they do for those who participate, and the kind of settings in which they take place with a special focus: when there is a death in the family.

BACKGROUND

As populations have increased and the geography of where people live has changed, the concept of what constitutes a community has also changed. Extended family, neighbors, and friends once provided help as a matter of personal obligation and concern. People were there to share their common knowledge, to teach each other what they had learned from their own experience (Silverman, 1977). They were sometimes recipients, sometimes helpers. Most human life would be barren without these exchanges, without this sense of community (Kropotkin, 1902/1972). However, as we moved through the 20th century, as cities grew, as populations became more diverse and more industrialized, these informal exchanges became less frequent. People move about more easily, greater distances often separate families, core units of these exchanges. It can also be difficult to easily find people with similar problems. Such information has become centered in specialized groups that are represented by experts. These experts offer help to those in need in the context of what have become formal organizations (McKnight, 1995). Mutuality and the exchange of care are less available or missing. This is true of issues related to normal life-cycle events, such as childbirth and death. To these we now add more complex social and health problems, as people live longer, owing to advances in science and medicine. The focus is no longer on survival but on the quality of life.

As help has become more specialized and formal, we are witnessing the professionalization of services once performed by citizens for each other. This focus on professionalization has led to what is called the medicalization of human experience (Conrad, 2007; Horwitz & Wakefield, 2007). Professionals often see themselves as repositories of "the right way" to remedy difficulties. What is learned from lived experience, as opposed to professional training, has often not been valued. Normal life events become medical crises. Forman (2009), in her syndicated news column on health, reported on a study by mental health professionals of the level of stress people experienced after receiving news that they have a life-threatening illness. She reports that these reactions met the criteria for a significant psychiatric diagnosis, such as major depression or posttraumatic stress disorder. Forman asks if it is really news that a serious medical diagnosis can shake a person to the core?

When a person's response to a serious change in their sense of well-being is assigned a psychiatric diagnosis, the focus turns to another dimension of what is wrong with them. Are we talking about treating symptoms of pathological problems, or should we be focusing on social competence building, that is, promoting people's adaptive capacities even in the face of devastating news (Silverman, 1985, 2007)? Promoting adaptive capacities, even while facing life-threatening situations, very often requires learning many new skills, and many new ways of looking at the world, and at oneself. It requires considering the stress as appropriate and normal under the circumstances. How is learning in this kind of a situation facilitated? Today, friends and family are often hesitant to offer help in times of stress. This is in part due to their concerns that they lack the credentials to do so, and fear that they may cause more harm than good by "intruding."

McKnight (1995) writes about the negative consequences for society when "care" becomes a commodity. He points to the destruction of a sense of community as people rely more and more on experts and the experts' knowledge and technology. McKnight's concern is how to restore a sense of community that involves the ability to extend care and help to its citizens. He sees caring as the work of a community.

Looking at end-of-life care, Kellehear (2005) describes the need to rebuild what he calls "compassionate cities." He recommends that people need to differentiate between times when professional care is truly required and helpful, and when friends and relatives might rely on their own experience to provide care and offer help. Kellehear's goal is to raise people's awareness of their own abilities and skills. His main concern is how communities care for the dying. He sees the employment of available support systems, problem solving, and communicating with each other as the work of the community. He wants to see a return to people helping people at times of stress and change in their lives, to counter what he sees as a threat from professional and medical dominance.

How is the help found in a return to caring communities different from that offered by professionals? What is special about help offered in a compassionate or caring community? How can we create them? Finding others who may have had a similar experience can be part of what is needed. What is it about finding others like oneself that is so important, especially at times of crisis and loss in our lives. Such opportunities can occur spontaneously as people meet in the normal course of living, or they can occur in planned encounters.

In this chapter I focus on my experience with the Widow-to-Widow Program (Silverman, 1969, 2004, 2013) and what I have come to call "mutual help" rather than "self-help." (Silverman, 1976a, 1976b, 2010). The Widow-to-Widow program stood out as an interesting experiment focusing on the value of help from one widow to another widow (1966). There were very few groups at the time that were based on the assumption that help from people sharing common problems was very valuable. Alcoholics Anonymous was the best known. The Widow-to-Widow program demonstrated the value of helping based on personal experience. Since then, we have learned that problem solving among peers creates a different kind of dynamic from what is found in professionally led support groups. Borkman (1999) reminds us that experience changes "victims" into "helpers." We are witnessing a growing movement of groups that were formed and are being formed by people grieving many types of losses, and many suffering from life-cycle and medical issues. I hypothesized (Silverman, 1980a, 1980b) that this growth was in response to people living longer, and seeking ways to build communities (groups) that would help them live with these difficulties. As they met others with the same difficulties, they found that solving their difficulties was easier when they learned from each other (Silverman, 1980a, 1980b). This chapter describes what we have learned from the Widow-to-Widow program, and then looks at why this program became an example of an effective way to assist the bereaved and to build caring communities.

THE WIDOW-TO-WIDOW PROGRAM

The original Widow-to-Widow program was a demonstration research project that began in 1966 and ended in 1973. It was sponsored by the Laboratory of Community Psychiatry at Harvard Medical School (Silverman, 2004, 2013). At the time, research (Parkes, 1965) pointed to the widowed being at high risk of developing emotional problems. The original goal of the study was to find a way to try to prevent this outcome. Problems associated with the death of a critical person in the mourners' life were seen as signs of emotional problems that could be "prevented" or "cured." To some extent this is still true. This view can be seen as a consequence of most research in the area being conducted by psychiatrists and psychologists who were more likely to see problem behavior as something to treat and to cure rather than an expected part of the life cycle. In planning a program, we were influenced by this research and guided by a public health perspective. Because we had no way of knowing in advance who was at risk, it seemed necessary to reach out to every newly widowed person in the target community. When there is danger of a disease spreading in a community, everyone is inoculated. We had no vaccine, so we focused on the helpfulness of a human contact.

If a physician, nurse, or social worker reached out, we believed that the newly widowed would get the impression that they were seen as ill. This was not the message we wanted to send at that time. Other research at the time (Maddison & Walker, 1967) pointed to the widowed they had studied who identified other widowed people as most helpful. The work of the New Career for the Poor program in New York City (Pearl & Reissman, 1965) pointed to a way of reaching the newly widowed. The experience, of the New Career's Program, in reaching out to low-income families proved that people from their own neighborhood serving as helpers were most effective in encouraging potential clients to participate in the service program they were developing. Reaching out would have to be done in the daytime, and because most widowers worked, we decided to focus on widows who were less likely to be working then. We also considered that we were more likely to find widows who were not working at that time of day who might be interested in doing the outreach. A grant from the National Funeral Directors Association made it possible for these women to earn a small salary that did not jeopardize the money they received from Social Security (Silverman, 2004).

We chose a neighborhood that was geographically easy to identify. Like most of Boston, the population was largely Catholic with a small Protestant minority. In addition, there was a small population of African Americans and a community of older Jewish people. As a social worker I had learned a good deal about community organization and visiting in the homes of clients. This experience served me well in developing this program. I recruited a group of clergy who were willing to provide us with some support and help in recruiting the widow helpers. Because we were associated with Harvard Medical School, we could get death certificates for this community. For our target population we decided to recruit women under the age of 65 whose husbands had just died. We assumed that a senior center would reach out to women over 65. We were wrong, although today many such centers have Widow-to-Widow programs that include widowers as well.

We recruited five women who lived in or near the neighborhood; an African American woman, a Jewish woman and three Catholic women who were comfortable reaching out to Protestant women as well as Catholic women. We learned the religion of the newly widowed from the funeral home that conducted the funeral. We were not sure what these women would have to offer, nor were they. The women, whom we called "aides," decided to send a brief letter to the new widow offering to come to visit and giving their phone number. The names of the clergy who were working with us were on the stationery, so that the newly widowed could see that we had the support of people they recognized. The aides reached out to every newly widowed woman under 65 in the target community. Using their own experience, these women offered neighbor-to-neighbor support in the widow's own home. Once they made contact, conversation came easily. The newly widowed woman wanted to know about the aide's widowhood and how she had managed (Silverman, 2004).

The original program was active for 2 ½ years. It reached 300 widows in the first year and a half. Of these, 61% accepted the offer of help (Silverman, 2004). Those who accepted were most likely to be women whose husbands had been ill for an extended period, women who did not work, and those with dependent children at home. Another demonstration program followed, sponsored by the Jewish Family Service. It employed an aide from the original project to reach older Jewish women in this same community (Silverman & Cooperband, 1975).

In both projects, we reached families that, regardless of their background, had similar experiences as they coped with the death of their husbands. A very small number had serious and long-standing financial, physical, or emotional problems, were accustomed to asking for help, and had established relationships with social agencies, public welfare, or psychiatric clinics. Most, however, had never had any contact with an agency or received assistance from anyone outside the family. The project was able to compile a profile of every widow in the target community and demonstrate the value of what I came to call "a little help from a friend" (Silverman, 2004).

WIDOWS WHO ACCEPTED HELP

The widows who participated in these projects had similar needs. They needed to talk with someone who would understand their feelings. They wanted information about how others had managed. Many women simply needed reassurance that they would weather the crisis successfully. Many of the women were not employed (as was much more common at the time) and had depended on their husband's wages. They now had difficulty covering living expenses. Women with children at home and those over 60 received some assistance from Social Security. Some women asked for advice about or support in getting a job or going back to school. Others wanted specific advice about managing what money they had, and many needed help with benefit claims. Older women who couldn't drive needed transportation to get medical care. Some of the younger women learned to drive for the first time.

We planned several meetings in various homes of these women, and they discovered that they had neighbors who were in similar situations but were unaware of each other. They began to plan various group activities using their own resources and their own imaginations. They discovered a social program for the widowed in a Catholic Center in Boston. One of the new drivers in the group agreed to take some of the women to these meetings. As a result, one woman whose dream it had been to visit Ireland learned that the church group was planning such a trip, and to her delight she had enough money to join them. For these women, their horizons were broadening, and it was possible to see it at our meetings.

Some women had difficulties with relatives who did not understand their new situation. Some had children who were misbehaving and who had problems at school. These mothers did not understand that these actions were related to the child's grief (Silverman & Englander, 1975). As I looked at it then, I thought these children seemed to be even more at risk than their mothers for developing serious emotional problems. This awareness led me to seek funding for a study of children whose parent had died and led to the Massachusetts General Hospital/ Harvard Child Bereavement Study (Silverman, 2000; Silverman & Nickman, 1996; Silverman & Worden, 1992). A closer examination of the families studied in the Child Bereavement Study, with children who were seen as having a high risk for developing emotional problems, revealed that these were families who had difficulties before the death (Silverman, Baker, Cait, & Boerner, 2002–2003).

Some of the widows we got to know had adult children at home. For some this was a blessing, and for others this created tension. The children were protective of their mothers and wanted to be sure that we had their mothers' interests at heart. They were suspicious of what we were trying to do to the extent of even making it difficult for their mother to come to a meeting at a neighbor's house.

As we got to know the women we met, we learned that four of them had histories of alcoholism and four others had histories of depression and schizophrenic episodes. These women were getting help from mental health agencies, and there was little more the project could do to prevent these problems from reoccurring. In some instances, it seemed that it had been the now-deceased husband who had kept the family together. On the whole, this was not a population that sought psychiatric help unless the problem was very severe, nor was this a time historically when counseling was sought for problems associated with mourning.

WIDOWS WHO REFUSED HELP

The widows who refused help fell into two groups (Silverman, 2004): those who never became involved in any way, and those who initially responded favorably on the phone but subsequently refused any contact. Thirty-five of these women, representing both groups, agreed to be interviewed after the project ended. They reported that they refused, because, in descending order of frequency: (1) they were too busy with work, family, or setting their husbands' affairs in order; (2) they received plenty of support from family and friends; (3) their grown children refused on their behalf (some of these women said that they should have stood up to their children); or (4) they were independent and did not need support. Several of these women were not the first to be widowed in their family or among their friends and were benefiting from the experience of others already in their network.

THE WIDOWED SERVICE LINE

In the early 1970s, the idea of telephone hotlines was receiving a good deal of attention. We developed the Widowed Service Line, which was staffed by two of the women who worked as aides in the original project, and volunteers to answer the phones were recruited from those served by the original program. They were now, in turn, helpers. This is a typical transition made in mutual help groups. During the line's first 7 months of operation, 750 widowed people called. The calls fell into three main categories: (1) they wanted someone to listen to them, (2) they wanted to meet other widowed people, and (3) they needed specific practical information. Most who called spoke of their loneliness and desire to meet others. Many were happy to find others to listen to them (Silverman, 2004).

The people most likely to call were those who lived alone and those who had children under the age of 16. Occasionally, callers lived in the same neighborhood but did not know each other. For example, two women called who were newly widowed, and both were pregnant. Another woman called who talked about her baby being born after her husband died. With their permission, we put them in touch with each other, and they formed their own informal support group. We were careful about callers who presented serious problems far beyond the capabilities of the service line, and we referred them to professional caregivers in their community. Talking to another widowed person would not have met their needs.

The line also had silent consumers. We assumed that there were many more people who read our advertisements than actually called. A widow I met socially several years later told me that she kept the phone number by her bed. She never called, but found it comforting to know that someone was available. I assume that she was not unique.

OTHER PROGRAMS

The Widow-to-Widow program demonstrated the value of mutual help and was a model for the AARP's Widowed Persons Service (AARP no longer maintains a national office for the service). Compassionate Friends, an active national and international organization with roots in Great Britain, started at about the same time as our project (Stephens, 1973). Other independent programs have developed in cities and towns across the United States and abroad in which the widowed themselves take the lead. The Widow-to-Widow program coincided with and perhaps added some stimulus to the growing self-help movement, from which many programs for the bereaved developed (Madera & White, 1997; Silverman, 1978, 2000). The Widow-to-Widow program stimulated the imagination of clergy and funeral directors, who compiled a workbook on how to set up similar community programs (Silverman, 1976a, 1976b).

Vachon replicated our program in a demonstration research project in Toronto, Canada, that led to a community-based program that existed for many years. Vachon's research documented the value of social support and of another widowed person as helper (Vachon et al., 1980). Lund (1989), stimulated in part by the original Widow-to-Widow findings, examined the consequences for elderly widows and widowers of participating in social support groups led either by peers or by professionals. His findings supported the special value of another widowed person as helper. Lieberman and Borman (1979) studied the effect of participating in a self-help/mutual aid organization and confirmed its positive impact on the widowed members. In particular, they found that the greatest benefits often accrued to the helpers. Overall, this work has had an impact on the way services to the bereaved are provided in this country and abroad, although with almost none of the outreach that characterized the original Widow-to-Widow program, and often with convenors who are unaware of the connection of these ideas to the original project. There is still some discussion in the professional community about whether facilitators should be professionally trained. Organizations such as Compassionate Friends have limited the involvement of professionals in programs when members felt they were intruding on what they wanted from the organization. When there is a national office, such as the one supported by Compassionate Friends, members are more likely to maintain control of how groups are run and who can facilitate them.

A VIEW OF GRIEF

Over the years, research has provided new insights into the needs of the widowed person and a new understanding of what it means to be bereaved (Silverman, 2013). The Widow-to-Widow project contributed to these changes. The program led to the questioning of bereavement as a simple time-limited process that could lead to serious emotional problems. The widows who worked with me told a different story when they said their experience did not always coincide with the theory I was describing. They said they did not think of themselves as recovering; rather, they thought there was "hope" when they were able to look ahead (usually about 2 years after their husbands died). They began to see the world in a different way than they had seen it before, and there was a marked *change* in how they felt (Silverman, 2004, 2013). They did not leave behind their feelings about their husbands, but they looked at themselves in a different way and saw their place in the world differently.

To understand grief, it was apparent that we had to look at the social context in which the mourner is embedded, that is, to look at the world in which the widowed person lives as well. When we started the Widow-to-Widow program, we were trying to find ways of preventing the widowed from developing serious mental health problems. But what we found gave us little real evidence that the death of a spouse raised the mourners' danger of developing a mental illness that did not exist before. What was it about widowhood that might lead to what appeared to be a mental illness? Could it be related to people losing their place in society? The role of marriage in these women's lives, in the mid-1960s, was central to their sense of who they were and their sense of well-being. As we met more widows, over time, we discovered that they were indeed emotionally distressed, but unless they had been psychologically ill before the death of their spouse, what they needed most was to expand their ways of coping with this stress. We could not prevent the stress, but we could help them understand what they were experiencing and find effective ways of dealing with their new role as widows. They needed to find ways to redefine themselves after the loss of the role of spouse. They learned that they had lost a way of life as well as a spouse, and they learned how to develop new roles, new relationships, and new ways of living in the world (Silverman, 1987, 1988). They grieved and felt pain, but they learned how to manage the pain. They found comfort in new friends and in building a different kind of relationship with the deceased, with themselves, and with the world around them (Silverman, 1987; Silverman & Klass, 1996).

Van Gennep (1909) described the change and transformations that take place when people move from one social status or condition to another as a rite of passage. He described this rite in three phases. The first phase, separation, involves the individual moving away from an earlier fixed point in the social structure. The second stage is the liminal phase (threshold), a period between states, and its attributes are necessarily ambiguous. The final stage is reincorporation with a new role and a new status. Turner (1969) introduced the concept of *communitas* to refer to the ties that people develop with each other as they go through the changes involved, and how, in many ways, they form a new community and become reintegrated into the larger society in new roles and in new ways.

Tyhurst (1958) and Bowlby (1961), both of whom had an impact on my thinking (Rolfe, 1966), described this as a time of transition, and, as I later learned, they were describing a rite of passage that Van Gennep had described many years before. A widow moves from the role of married woman to that of widow and to a new sense of who she is and how she will move in her world. Indeed, a "rite of passage" is an appropriate way of describing this time in a widowed person's life, and provides a meaningful perspective in understanding the bereavement process.

Grief is not an illness that can be cured. We cannot prevent a widowed person's pain or protect that person from the disruption the death causes. We know that the rest of this person's life will not look the way it would have if the death had not occurred. The death becomes part of the person's life story and of who that person is. Bereavement changes people and forces them to look at their life differently, which in many ways leads them to behave differently and to, in part at least, develop a new sense of self. The widowed helper can be integral in this process. I learned from the Widow-to-Widow program that the goal is to promote the ability of bereaved persons to cope with their pain and with these changes (Silverman, 2013). In a sense, experience is not what happens to you but what you do with what happens to you. The help offered in this situation is not an effort to prevent grief or stress but to help people cope in ways that enhance their competence to deal with this new situation.

MUTUAL HELP

In 1964, mutual help or self-help was primarily associated with such organizations as Alcoholics Anonymous and programs established by parents for their retarded children. Recovering alcoholics helped other alcoholics, and parents helped other parents. Although it has been common practice throughout the ages for the bereaved to help each other, formal mutual-help programs as we have come to know them were rare.

A mutual-help exchange, as the term is used here, involves people who share a common problem, with which some of the participants have coped successfully. The helping persons have expertise based on personal experience rather than the formal education that is the professional helper's base of expertise. Borkman (1999) distinguishes between two sources of information: professional knowledge, which comes from formal learning, and experiential knowledge, which comes from personal experience. In the latter, Borkman writes, self-help is the first step: the person becomes aware of the problem and tries to do something about it. Once the person engages someone else in sharing experiences, it becomes mutual help. A mutual-help experience limits its participants to those with a specific common problem; their purpose in coming together is to offer one another help and guidance in coping with the problem or predicament. "You alone can do it, but you cannot do it alone" is an often-quoted saying in the literature on self-help and mutual aid . . . "[It] produces a special form of interdependence in which the individual accepts self-responsibility within a context of mutual aid—that is, giving help to others and receiving help from others" (Borkman, 1999, p. 196). These are settings in which rites of passage take place.

Informal mutual exchanges go on all the time, as people discover common experiences that until that moment they believed were theirs alone. Informal encounters may develop into formal organizations, if people believe they have a mission to extend the exchange to others like themselves. The literature on mutual help and bereavement concentrates on the formal encounters. However, it is the informal encounters that need to be encouraged; in many ways they are the major influence on the way a community responds to grief and helps bereaved persons.

To maintain its character as a formal mutual-help organization, a group must develop a sustainable organizational structure with officers, a governing body, and procedures for continuity (Silverman, 1980a, 1980b). The members determine policy and control resources, and they are both providers and recipients of service. Mutual-help organizations are distinguished from voluntary philanthropic organizations, such as the American Cancer Society, in which volunteers join to help others, not to solve a common problem.

Mutual-help organizations sometimes develop when there is no match between people's needs and the help offered in their communities (Silverman, 1977). In the case of bereavement, such organizations may be a response to the community silence that grieving people often face. When friends and family distance themselves from the pain and needs of mourners, mourners seek out each other. Even in communities that offer resources for coping with grief, there is no substitute for sharing with peers who have been there. When people in this context say, "I understand," they really do. The purpose of these groups is to help bereaved people negotiate a transition, to get from here to there; for example, from being a married woman, to being a widow, and finally a formerly married, now single, woman (Silverman, 1987, 1988). For widowed persons, the goal is to go from feeling lost and overwhelmingly sad to finding new direction and meaning in life. The same may be true for widowers as well.

The essence of mutual help is the exchange that takes place among people as they cope with a common problem. The relationships available in a mutual-help exchange can be seen as linking opportunities or, in Goffman's (1963) words, a place to learn "the tricks of the trade." We identify with our peers throughout the life cycle. At each new stage or phase of life, we seek to learn from others who have gone before us. If bereaved persons cannot find anyone in their existing network to meet this need, they look outside their own network for people who can serve as a bridge between the past and the future. This is the *communitas* that Turner referred to.

As we look at the grieving process, we recognize the changes that take place as mourners cope with their grief. With time, the new situation may become more real and painful, and we can see how groups can respond to these changing needs. In the beginning, another widowed person can provide validation for feelings and for discovering new ways of living in the world. The widowed find validation of the pace of their progression through grief in contrast to those around them who have not experienced grief and who often expect them to "recover" more quickly. To meet the various needs of the participants and of new members who may join the group, groups can have a life span of a year or more. They are not necessarily in a great hurry. People talk of developing a new sense of optimism and finding new ways of living in the world. There are new people in their lives; they are part of a new community and begin to think that they may have something to offer as a helper in this context. There is a beginning of an integration of a new sense of identity and an interest in helping others, in sharing their experience and what they have learned.

CURRENT PROGRAMS AND PRACTICES

The Internet has changed the way people approach problems or periods of transition in their lives and how services are located and offered (Colon, 2004; Madara & White, 1997). The web provides a new way for people to find each other. An Internet search finds two main kinds of resources. One is chat rooms—for example, the Young Widow chat room—where people can sign on and engage in an ongoing exchange with others. Help is also available for particular groups, for example, for parents who have lost their only child or for grandparents whose grandchild has died. The other resource is mutual-help or self-help organizations—such as Compassionate Friends, Mothers Against Drunk Driving, and To Live Again—that have local chapters where members come together on a regular basis to support each other and to participate in various programs and activities. These local chapters survive over the years as new members join and give new life to them. Organizations that have a national office are more likely to flourish, as a central office can provide direction and support to local chapters.

Malkinson and Geron (2006) describe an initiative in Israel for parents whose children have died in automobile accidents. What began as a professionally led support group evolved into a mutual-help group, with members meeting on their own and using their own experience to help each other. Hospice programs often provide support groups for grieving families they have served as a family member was dying. Several are providing educational training for participants to lead groups that want to continue after the formal program has ended. Caserta and Lund (1996) describe a health-promotion program for older widowed people in Salt Lake City—preliminary data showed that about two thirds of the participants maintained contact with each other outside the class and that half noted the continuing value of getting new information and learning new skills from their peers. These relationships extended long after the formal program ended. The role of the mental health professional in this situation is to relinquish control to the group's members and recognize their experiences. The resulting transitional relationships can become a permanent part of a friendship network. A professionally led program can thus create an environment in which participants are encouraged to continue to meet on their own after the professionally led group ends.

It is not unusual for professionals to question the work of volunteers using their own experience in helping and to insist on a supervisory relationship with the volunteers or limit what volunteers can do. As there is a growing focus on bereavement as something that is time limited and curable, the focus on helpers is assigned to professionally trained people. If grief is seen as an expected life-cycle issue that all of us will experience, from which there is no cure, we need to ask what is appropriate help and delivered by whom? Because this is an experience we will all have, it would seem that we all need to be experts.

There is a growing number of centers directed by professionals where much of the work is done by volunteers, many of whom come after having dealt with a death in their own lives and with a desire to help others. The most extensive center of this type serves families with children in which either a parent or a child has died (see Dougy Center for Grieving Children, in Silverman, 2000). These centers provide an opportunity for grieving persons to meet others like themselves, to be in an environment where their loss is understood and where they can learn from each other. The quote at the beginning of this chapter is from a child in the Children's Room: Center for Grieving Children and Their Families. The website for a network of similar centers in various parts of the United States and Canada is www.allianceforgrievingchildren.com. Performing acts of caring and concern for our fellow human beings is the cornerstone in the foundation of most societies. We are social creatures, and we need each other. How can we express our needs and care for others? One way is to make available to those in need the lived experience of others like themselves. Borkman (1999) reminds us that experience changes "victims into helpers." In the context of a mutual-help group, the effect is on promoting members' abilities to live positively with the disabling or life-changing consequences of long-term "problems" that could not be prevented.

CONCLUSION

Death, dying, and grieving must be part of community discourse. Coping with life and death invariably happens in a community of others with whom we are linked in many ways. The nature of these links determines the kinds of communities we build, and how each of us understands our part in caring as professionals or as citizens.

REFERENCES

Borkman, T. (1976). Experiential knowledge: A new concept for analysis of self help groups. *Social Service Review, 50*, 445–456.

Borkman, T. (1999). *Understanding self-help/mutual aid: Experiential learning in the commons.* Camden, NJ: Rutgers University Press.

Bowlby, J. (1961). Processes of mourning. *International Journal of Psychoanalysis, 42*, 317–340.

Caserta, M., & Lund, D. (1996). Beyond bereavement support group meetings: Exploring outside social contacts. *Death Studies, 29*, 537–556.

Colon, Y. (2004). Technology-based groups and end-of-life social work practice. In J. Berzoff & P. R. Silverman (Eds.), *Living with dying: A handbook for end-of-life healthcare practitioners* (pp. 534–547). New York, NY: Columbia University Press.

Conrad, P. (2007). *The medicalization of society: On the transformation of the human condition into treatable disorders.* Baltimore, MD: Johns Hopkins University Press.

Forman, J. (2009, January 22). How to cope with the shock of cancer diagnosis. *Boston Globe*, p. C3.

Goffman, E. (1963). *Stigma: Notes on the management of spoiled identity.* Englewood Cliffs, NJ: Prentice Hall.

Horowitz, A., & Wakefield, J. C. (2007). *The loss of sadness: How psychiatry transformed normal sorrow into depressive disorder.* New York, NY: Oxford University Press.

Kellehear, A. (2005). *Compassionate cities: Public health and end-of-life care.* New York, NY: Routledge.

Kropotkin, P. (1972). *Mutual aid.* New York, NY: New York University Press. (Original work published 1970).

Lieberman, M. A., & Borman, L. D. (1979). *Self help groups for coping with crisis: Origins, processes and impact.* San Francisco, CA: Jossey-Bass.

Lund, D. A. (1989). *Older bereaved spouses: Research with clinical applications.* New York, NY: Taylor & Francis/Hemisphere.

Madera, E. J. (2008). Self help groups: Options for support, education and advocacy. In P. G. O'Brien, W. Z. Kennedy, & K. A. Ballard (Eds.), *Psychiatric mental health nursing: An introduction to theory and practice* (pp. 151–168). Sudbury, MA: Jones and Bartlett.

Madera, E. J., & White, B. J. (1997). *Online mutual support: The experience of a self-help clearing-house information and referral*. New York, NY: Brunner/Routledge.

Maddison, D., & Walker, A. (1967) Factors affecting the impact of conjugal bereavement. *British Journal of Psychiatry, 113*, 1057–1067.

Malkinson, R., & Geron, Y. (2006). Intervention continuity in post traffic fatality, from notifying families of the loss to establishing a self help group. In E. K. Rynearson (Ed.), *Violent death: Resilience and intervention beyond crisis* (pp. 217–232). New York, NY: Brunner/Routledge.

McKnight, J. (1995). *The careless society: Community and its counterfeits*. New York, NY: Basic Books.

Parkes, C. (1965). Bereavement and mental illness. Part I: A clinical study of bereaved psychiatric patients; Part 2: A classification of bereavement reactions. *British Journal of Medical Psychology, 38*(1), 1–26.

Pearl, A., & Reissman, F. (1965). *New careers for the poor: The non-professional in human services*. New York, NY: Free Press.

Rolfe, P. (1966). Services for the widowed during the period of bereavement. In *Social work Practice* (pp. 170–189). New York, NY: Columbia University Press.

Silverman, P. R. (1969). The Widow to Widow Program: An experiment in preventive intervention. *Mental Hygiene, 53*(3), 333–337.

Silverman, P. R. (1976a). The widow as caregiver in a program of preventive intervention with other widows. In G. Caplan & M. Killilea (Eds.), *Support systems and mutual help: Multidisciplinary explorations* (pp. 233–243). New York, NY: Grune & Stratton.

Silverman, P. R. (with Musicant, A. & Richter, S. C.). (1976b). *If you will lift the load I will lift it too*. New York, NY: Jewish Funeral Directors of America.

Silverman, P. R. (1977). Mutual help groups for widowhood. In D. Klein & S. Goldstston (Eds.), *Primary prevention: An idea whose time has come* (DHEW Publication No. 9 ADM, pp. 77–447). Washington, DC: U.S. Government Printing Office.

Silverman, P. R. (1978). Mutual help: An alternate network. In *Women in mid-life-security and ful-fillment* (U.S. House of representatives Select committee on aging, Committee Publication No. 955-170, pp. 254–270). Washington, DC: U.S. Government Printing Office.

Silverman, P. R. (1980a). *Mutual help groups and the role of mental health professionals* (NIMH, DHEW Publication No. ADM 78-646). Washington, DC: U.S. Government Printing Office.

Silverman, P. R. (1980b). *Mutual help: Organization and development*. Beverly Hills, CA: SAGE.

Silverman, P. R. (1985). Preventive intervention: The case for mutual help groups. In R. K. Conyne (Ed.), *The groups workers handbook: Varieties of group experience* (pp. 237–258). Springfield, IL: Charles C Thomas.

Silverman, P. R. (1987). Widowhood as the next stage in the life cycle. In H. Z. Lopata (Ed.), *Widows: Vol. 2 North America* (pp. 171–190). Durham, NC: Duke University Press.

Silverman, P. R. (1988). Research as process: Exploring the meaning of widowhood. In S. Reinharz & Rowles, G. D. (Eds.), *Qualitative gerontology*. New York, NY: Springer Publishing Company.

Silverman, P. R. (2000). *Never too young to know: Death in children's lives*. New York, NY: Oxford University Press.

Silverman, P. R. (2004). *Widow-to-widow: How the bereaved help one another*. New York, NY: Bruner-Routledge.

Silverman, P. R. (2007). Resilience and bereavement: Part 2. In B. Monroe & D. Oliviere (Eds.), *Resilience in palliative care: Achievement in adversity* (pp. 167–180). New York, NY: Oxford University Press.

Silverman, P. R. (2010). Mutual help groups: What are they and what makes them work? In R. K. Conyne (Ed.), *The oxford handbook of groups counseling* (pp. 511–519). New York, NY: Oxford University Press.

Silverman, P. R. (2013). Lessons I have learned. *British Journal of Social Work, 43*(2), 216–232.

Silverman, P. R., Baker, J., Cait, C. R., & Boerner, K. (2002–2003). The effects of negative legacies on the adjustment of parentally bereaved children and adolescents. *Omega, 46*(4), 335–352.

Silverman, P. R., & Cooperband, A. (1975). Mutual help and the elderly widow. *Journal of Geriatric Psychiatry, 8*(1), 9–26.

Silverman, P. R., & Englander, S. (1975). The widow's view of her dependent children. *Omega, 6* (1), 3–20.

Silverman, P. R., & Klass, D. (1996). Introduction: What's the problem? In D. Klasss, P. R. Silverman, & S. Nickman (Eds.), *Continuing bonds: New understanding of grief* (pp. 3–27). New York, NY: Taylor & Francis.

Silverman, P. R., & Nickman, S. (1996). Children's construction of their dead parent. In D. Klasss, P. R. Silverman, & S. Nickman (Eds.), *Continuing bonds: New understanding of grief* (pp. 73–86). New York, NY: Taylor & Francis.

Silverman, P. R., & Worden, J. W. (1992). Children's reactions to the death of a parent. In M. Stroebe, W. Stroebe, & Hansson (Eds.), *Handbook of bereavement* (pp. 300–316). New York, NY: Cambridge University Press.

Stephens, S. (1973). *When death comes home.* New York, NY: Morehouse-Barlow.

Turner, V. W. (1969). Liminality and communitas. In *The ritual process: Structure and anti-structure.* Chicago, IL: Aldine.

Tyhurst, J. (1958). *The role of transition states, including disasters in mental illness.* Symposium on preventive and social psychiatry conducted at Washington, DC.

Vachon, M. L. S., Sheldon, A. R., Lancie, W. J., Lyall, W. A. L., Rogers, J., & Freeman, S. J. (1980). A controlled study of self help interventions for widows. *American Journal of Psychiatry, 137*, 1380–1384.

Van Gennep, A. (1909). *The rites of passage* (M. B. Vizedon & G. L. Caffee, Trans.). London, UK: Routledge and Kegan and Paul.

22

TREATING COMPLICATED BEREAVEMENT: THE DEVELOPMENT OF GRIEF THERAPY

When my father took his life on a cold January morning in Ohio, 10 days before my 12th birthday, one world ended, and another began. Awakening to the panicked voice of our mother—*Boys, boys, I can't wake up your father!*—my little brother and I scrambled confused from beneath the cowboy comforters on the matching beds in our shared bedroom and peered afraid around the door jamb of our parents' adjacent room as our mother tried once more to shake our father into wakefulness. The shriek that emerged from our mother's small frame as she withdrew her hand from his lifeless body shattered the life story we had lived until that day and launched us into another teeming with questions about the meaning of his suicide and the meaning our lives would have from that day on. In a certain sense, my career in thanatology represents a lifelong response to that traumatic tear in the fabric of our family narrative, embroidered as it has become with many other losses before and since.

And so, in the seemingly random but ultimately meaningful way that Jung termed "synchronicity," I entered college 6 years later primed to hear the call of thanatology when that path presented itself. And it soon did, in the form of training for a paraprofessional position at the Suicide and Crisis Intervention Center in Gainesville, Florida, and as I became a research assistant to Seth Krieger, a doctoral student pursuing dissertation research in personal construct theory and the threat posed by one's own mortality.[1] Although it would take another 20 years before this long engagement in death-anxiety research (Neimeyer, 1994) would begin to mature into a deeper engagement with bereavement, the course was set. The confluence of these various personal and professional tributaries continues to configure my current concern with meaning reconstruction in the context of grief therapy as I enter my fifth decade of research and practice in thanatology. This chapter places my own involvement in this work in the broader context of other contemporary approaches to grief therapy, as well as the models of mourning that help inspire them. But first, let's consider the historical backdrop against which the mid-20th century field of bereavement studies emerged into prominence, in order to appreciate its subsequent evolution and probable future.

A BACKWARD GLANCE

In the Beginning: The Psychoanalytic View

As detailed in Chapter 7 (by Bill Worden) of this book, the scientific attempt to understand the responses of bereaved people dates to Freud's (1917/1957)

Mourning and Melancholia, published in the midst of World War I. In it he posited that, just as death was a universal fact of life, there were also universal dynamics involved in grieving the death of a loved one. Freud defined mourning as the nonpathological response to such bereavement. Its distinguishing features include painful dejection, withdrawal of interest in the outside world, loss of the capacity to love, and inhibition of all activity. The work of mourning is accomplished gradually as the mourner's psychic energy or *libido* once invested in the attachment to the lost person or "object" is systematically recalled, reexperienced, and then released, resulting in detachment from the lost object. This concept of emotional disconnection or *decathexis* as the natural end-point of mourning has had an enduring impact on the practice of bereavement counseling through the 20th century, as reflected in decades of emphasis on *Trauerarbeit* or "grief work," in the form of painful review of the relationship, *catharsis* through emotional expression, and the saying of a final "goodbye" to a loved one as the goal of grieving (Stroebe, Gergen, Gergen, & Stroebe, 1992).

Freud's second major contribution was his effort to delineate how processes of mourning can go awry and become unhealthy. *Melancholia* was defined as a pathological outcome marked by an insistent narcissistic identification with the lost object, in effect, a refusal to "let go." Instead, the mourner's self or *ego* incorporates the lost object into itself as a way of warding off the loss, while denying its reality (Freud, 1917/1957). This suspicion about the pathological implications of identification and "holding on" to the lost love object was carried over by subsequent psychodynamic theorists and researchers (Lindemann, 1944) and is only recently being contested by newer models. Thus, although Freud's grim realism about the need to mourn one's losses and "move on" can be seen as an understandable response to the catastrophic loss of life in World War I, it continued to shape practices in grief therapy for most of the 20th century.

A Thoroughly Modern Model of Mourning: Stage Theory

With the advent of the death awareness movement at midcentury (see especially the Introduction and Chapters 1 and 2), popular and professional culture in the United States was ripe for a reconsideration of bereavement understood as a psychosocial transition, especially in the context of keen interest in end-of-life care. The most influential theory of grief to emerge from this focus stemmed from Elisabeth Kübler-Ross's (1969) book, *On Death and Dying*. From consultation interviews with patients hospitalized for terminal illnesses, she derived her framework, featuring five *stages* in the dying process: denial, anger, bargaining, depression, and acceptance (Kübler-Ross, 1969). Her concepts subsequently were generalized to describe how the reality of death—even for the bereaved, as well as the dying themselves—is assimilated gradually, rather than all at once, and then only after a series of psychological protests, delaying tactics, and mourning. As such, stage theory captures some of the ambivalence of accepting one's own death or that of another, while at the same time providing a simple framework for organizing the turbulent emotional responses that can be experienced in the process. Almost inevitably, given its fit with a modernist emphasis on clarity, efficiency, and positive outcomes, it soon became the dominant, if not the only, model of grief informing professional and medical education (Downe-Wambolt & Tamlyn, 1997), as well as hospice-based bereavement programs.

The intuitive appeal of stage theory notwithstanding, serious criticisms of Kübler-Ross's work have been lodged from several quarters. Critics argue that its "one-size-fits-all" approach constitutes too narrow a formula to explain individual and cultural variations in bereavement experiences and that it focuses on emotions to the near exclusion of cognitive and behavioral responses to loss (Corr, 1993; Neimeyer, 2013). Most serious, it simply receives little support from studies of the actual adaptation of bereaved people, most of whom report high levels of "acceptance" from the earliest weeks of grieving, particularly when the loss is from natural, as opposed to violent, death (Holland & Neimeyer, 2010). As a result, bereavement professionals have turned to a new generation of theories to inform their research and practice (Neimeyer, Harris, Winokuer, & Thornton, 2011).

THE CONTEMPORARY LANDSCAPE OF LOSS

Coping With Bereavement: The Dual-Process Model

Rather than emphasizing universal stages or tasks, the dual-process model (DPM) put forward by Margaret Stroebe and Henk Schut proposes that people deal with loss dialectically, oscillating between *loss-oriented coping* and *restoration-oriented coping* (Stroebe & Schut, 1999, 2010). The former process entails experiencing and managing the negative emotions of grieving triggered by the death, missing and longing for the lost person, and reorganizing the attachment relationship with the deceased. Significantly, coping in this way entails temporarily denying or distracting oneself from the demands of the external world that has been changed by the loss. Restoration-oriented coping, on the other hand, entails attending to the many life changes required to adjust to one's world after the loss of a close person. These can include learning new skills, assuming new roles, reengaging changed relationships, and forming new ones. It is important to note that this sort of outwardly focused coping involves denying or distancing from the pain of grief in order to "learn to live again."

One of the distinctive features of the DPM is its implication that individuals normally self-regulate their bereavement by confronting their loss at times and, alternately, avoiding the emotional pain of grieving. Rather than proposing a phasic progression through grief, this model posits waxing and waning, an ongoing flexibility over time with loss-oriented coping dominant early on in bereavement and restoration-oriented coping more prevalent later. Finally, Stroebe and Schut argue that their model provides a means of understanding gender differences in bereavement, as women tend to be more emotion focused, and hence more loss oriented, whereas men tend to be more problem focused, and hence more restoration oriented in their coping behaviors. The DPM has proven attractive to grief therapists as well as researchers, suggesting that counselors help clients take a "time out" from preoccupation with their grief through greater restoration coping and mitigate brittle emotional avoidance through greater confrontation with the loss (Zech & Arnold, 2011). The development of a preliminary measure of this process of oscillation, the Inventory of Daily Widowed Life (IDWL), should contribute to both clinical assessment and substantive research in light of the model (Caserta & Lund, 2007).

A straightforward example of the clinical application of the DPM arose in my second and third sessions with a young widow named Cheryl,[2] who consulted me 1 month following the suicide of her husband, Jeff. Although Cheryl had been remarkably stoic in managing this traumatic loss—made more horrific still by Jeff's having shot himself in their bed while his wife was at work and his two young children were at school—she struggled with the conflicting emotions of grief and anger, as well as with her withdrawal from the social world out of a sense of shame and fear of stigmatization. Balancing attention to her conflicting feelings with the growing importance of reengaging extrafamilial relationships and work (as she was now the sole breadwinner), I first invited Cheryl to tell me the story of their family prior to Jeff's troubling descent into an agitated depression, perhaps bringing photographs to "introduce" him to me.[3] Cheryl readily accepted the invitation to lift the veil of silence that had descended over discussions of her husband since his death, and in the next session brought in her iPad to share a remarkable series of professional photographs showing him lovingly relating to his family, taken only 2 weeks before his tragic death. Responding to my earnest interest in coming to know Jeff in both his brighter and darker moods, she began to disentangle her own guilt and anger at him for his fatal decision from her genuine grief for the terrible loss of the man she deeply loved. Tracking her sensed need to reach out to others for both emotional and instrumental support, we then shifted attention in the following week to her selective engagement with friends and coworkers, considering which ones specifically would be able to offer practical advice or a simple break from the seriousness of her predicament and which could provide a compassionate willingness to hear the troubling questions and emotions that others might not.[4] Thus, in keeping with the DPM, we alternated attention naturally between loss-oriented processing of Cheryl's tragic experience and restoration-oriented rebuilding of a viable social world.

Reworking the Continuing Bond: The Two-Track Model

At the heart of bereavement is an existential conundrum: *we are wired for attachment in a world of impermanence.* Scholars have long recognized that humans have evolved as social beings whose sense of felt security depends critically on bonds with caregivers—typically their parents—in early life (Bowlby, 1980). From these early patterns of interaction, children develop "internal working models" that implicitly shape expectations regarding the availability of others as sources of security and support, and regarding their own resourcefulness and lovability in later relationships (Parkes & Prigerson, 2009). Given the powerful challenge to conservation of an attachment bond posed by the death of a loved one, it is not surprising that older widows and widowers who display an insecure and dependent attachment on their spouse tend to fare poorly across the first 4 years of bereavement (Bonanno, Wortman, & Nesse, 2004). Interestingly, however, avoidant attachment—essentially maximizing one's sense of self-reliance and minimizing one's dependence on others—seems to mitigate grief-related distress, at least until challenged by traumatic and violent losses (Meier, Carr, Currier, & Neimeyer, 2013). In general, however, insecure attachment seems to be one empirically established risk factor for complicated bereavement (Burke & Neimeyer, 2013).

The related continuing bonds perspective extends attachment theory by focusing specifically on the reformulation of the relationship to the deceased in the aftermath of bereavement. Once considered patently pathological by the psychoanalytic tradition, the retention rather than relinquishment of such attachment to the loved one is now regarded as normative (Klass, Silverman, & Nickman, 1996) and commonly associated with more favorable bereavement outcomes (Datson & Marwit, 1997; Hedtke, 2012). There is also some evidence that the character of the continuing bond evolves across the course of grieving, as frequently resorting to "continuing bonds coping" (e.g., consciously reminiscing about the deceased throughout the day) seems to be associated with higher levels of *negative* emotion in the early months of widowhood, whereas similar processes are also linked to reports of more *positive* emotion after 2 years of bereavement (Field & Friedrichs, 2004).

One contemporary theory that accommodates such findings is the two-track model of bereavement (TTMB), which posits that grief proceeds along two avenues simultaneously, the first concerned with the mourner's *biopsychosocial functioning*, such as disruptions in mood, social behavior, physical health, and capacity for work, and the second focused on one's *relationship to the deceased*, not only before the death, but also in one's ongoing life (Rubin, 1999; Rubin, Malkinson, & Witztum, 2003). In the latter case, for example, the bereaved may access or avoid memories of times spent with the deceased, carry out public or private rituals of remembrance, pursue projects that extend the essential purposes of the loved one, or feel compelled to grieve as a sign of loyalty to him or her. The development of the Two-Track Model of Bereavement Questionnaire (Rubin, Malkinson, Koren, & Michaeli, 2009), which measures both symptomatic and relational tracks through grief as well as a third concerned with traumatic responses, helps operationalize the model for research and clinical application. One advantage of the TTMB is its capacity to conceptualize difficulties in adaptation that arise on one or both tracks of the model, serving as a useful guide to clinical assessment and intervention (Rubin, Malkinson, & Witztum, 2011), as illustrated in the following case study.

At the age of 71, Carl was the quintessential family man, devoted to his wife, Beth, of more than 40 years, as well as his two grown children and their families, to all of whom he had passed on his love of the great outdoors. When tragedy struck in the form of the accidental drowning deaths of both his son Gary (38) and youngest grandson, Ben (7), when the small boat in which they were fishing somehow capsized in a sudden and violent storm, he fell into a deep, if silent, grief. Finally, after several months, Carl accepted Beth's encouragement to seek therapy to try to get his own life "back on an even keel."

In our first few sessions of therapy, we worked with the manifest biopsychosocial disruptions in Carl's life: his insomnia and nightmares, his ruminative preoccupation with the boating accident, his need to find some way to modulate the shared grief that would be triggered by his wife's evident distress, and their attempts to provide mutual soothing to one another. But the most therapeutic and memorable dimension of our work followed the relational track of the TTMB, as Carl conceived of and ultimately implemented a unique legacy project that both honored his son and grandson and sought to prevent similar tragedies in the future. Drawing on the drive and organization that had characterized him over the course of a long and successful career, he became a "crusader" for boating safety, beginning with the large state park bordering the lake in which his family members had drowned. Over a period of months in the course of our later therapy, extending to years following its completion, Carl tirelessly goaded park service administration, lobbied lawmakers, and spearheaded a substantial fundraising and publicity campaign. Ultimately these efforts garnered the permits and resources to let him install unique and eye-catching signage throughout the park featuring smiling images of his son and grandson holding up their catch, emblazoned with the headline, "Kids don't float," and briefly telling the story of their lives and deaths. The same signage featured special hooks for life-jackets in several sizes, offered in a free loaner program for all boaters, an intervention that was reinforced with public safety announcements, flyers to park users, and routine warnings by park rangers. Gradually Carl's mission expanded to lakes throughout the popular fishing region, as he continued to "work the circuit" of public lectures, school programs, and media appearances to promote boating safety. In

Carl's words, spoken tearfully in session, these efforts represented his "personal pact" with Gary and Ben to continue "working with them to spare other families the needless pain we have suffered." Keeping this pact across time helped him restore a sense of purpose and direction in his life, give voice to his grief in a way it could be heard, partner with his wife on the safety campaign, and in an important sense maintain a living bond with his son and grandson so that their deaths would not be entirely in vain.

The Search for Significance: A Meaning-Reconstruction Approach

A final contemporary perspective on bereavement is not so much a theory about grief as it is a metatheory, that is, an approach that can inform a variety of models by emphasizing that *a central process of grieving is the attempt to reaffirm or reconstruct a world of meaning that has been challenged by loss* (Neimeyer, 2002). In this meaning-reconstruction view advanced by Robert Neimeyer and his associates, the death of a loved one is seen as posing two narrative challenges to the survivor: (1) to process the *event story* of the death in an effort to "make sense" of what has happened and its implications for the survivor's ongoing life and (2) to access the *back story* of the relationship with the loved one as a means of reconstructing a continuing bond (Neimeyer & Sands, 2011). (See Tables 22.1 and 22.2 for typical questions that the bereaved implicitly engage in in each of these domains, both in the context of grief therapy and in their daily lives.) In a sense, then, the bereaved are prompted to "rewrite" important parts of their life story to accommodate the death and project themselves into a changed, but nonetheless meaningful future, one that retains continuity with the "back story" of a past shared with the loved one. Such an emphasis on "relearning the self" and "relearning the world" in the wake of loss (Attig, 1996, 2000) is consonant with the narrative therapy approach to bereavement support championed by Hedtke (2012).

A good deal of research has demonstrated a link between an inability to find meaning (whether spiritual or secular) in the loss and intense, prolonged and complicated grief in groups as varied as bereaved young people, parents, older adults, and survivors of homicide, suicide, and other violent deaths (Neimeyer, 2014). Conversely, higher levels of sense making about the loss have been found to prospectively predict higher levels of well-being among widowed persons (e.g., interest, excitement, accomplishment) 1 to 4 years later (Coleman & Neimeyer, 2010), and success over time in integrating the loss into one's meaning system

TABLE 22.1 Sample of Implicit Questions Entailed in Processing the "Event Story" of the Death

- How do I make sense of what has happened, and what is the meaning of my life now in its wake?
- What do my bodily and emotional feelings tell me about what I now need?
- What is my role or my responsibility in what has come to pass?
- What part, if any, did human intention, inattention, or wrongdoing have in the dying?
- How do my spiritual or philosophic beliefs help me accommodate this transition, and how are they changed by it in consequence?
- How does this loss fit with my sense of justice, predictability, and compassion in the universe?
- With what cherished beliefs is this loss compatible? Incompatible?
- Who am I in light of this loss, now and in the future? How does this experience shape or reshape the larger story of my life?
- Who in my life can grasp and accept what this loss means to me?
- Whose sense of the meaning of this loss is most and least like my own, and, in the latter case, how can we bridge our differences?

TABLE 22.2 Sample of Implicit Questions Entailed in Accessing the "Back Story" of the Relationship to the Deceased

- How can I recover or reconstruct a sustaining connection to my loved one that survives his or her physical death?
- Where and how do I hold my grief for my loved one in my body or my emotions, and how might this evolve into an inner bond of a healing kind?
- What memories of our relationship bring pain, guilt, or sadness and require some form of redress or reprieve now? How might this forgiveness be sought or given?
- What memories of our relationship bring joy, security, or pride and invite celebration and commemoration now? How can I review and relish these memories more often?
- What were my loved one's moments of greatness in life, and what do they say about his or her signature strengths or cherished qualities?
- What lessons about living or loving have I learned in the course of our shared lives? In the course of my bereavement?
- What would my loved one see in me that would give her or him confidence in my ability to survive this difficult period?
- What advice would my loved one have for me now, and how can I draw on his or her voice and wisdom in the future?
- Who in my life is most and least threatened by my ongoing bond with my loved one, and how can we make a safe space for this in our shared world?
- Who can help me keep my loved one's stories alive?

is associated with a significant reduction in complicated grief symptomatology (Holland, Currier, Coleman, & Neimeyer, 2010).

A variety of carefully constructed scales have been devised to help researchers and clinicians map meaning-making processes as well as to reliably discern themes in the content of the specific meanings that result. For example, the Integration of Stressful Life Experiences Scale or ISLES (Holland et al., 2010) assesses the extent to which the bereaved respondent finds *comprehensibility* in the loss and retains or regains a secure *footing in the world* in light of it. A short form of this same instrument also has been shown to share its psychometric strengths, including its incremental validity in predicting health and mental health outcomes even after demographic factors, relationship to the deceased, cause of death, and complicated grief symptoms are taken into account (Holland, Currier, & Neimeyer, 2014). In addition, the Inventory of Complicated Spiritual Grief (Burke et al., 2014), a specialized scale assessing struggles in religious meaning-making following a loss, has been validated in a Christian context, with subscales bearing on Insecurity With God and Disruption in Religious Practice. Finally, investigators have constructed detailed and reliable coding systems for categorizing the meanings made by mourners (e.g., Valuing Life, Impermanence, Personal Growth) to study their relation to bereavement adaptation (Gillies, Neimeyer, & Milman, 2014; Lichtenthal, Currier, Neimeyer, & Keesee, 2010). A meaning-reconstruction view has also extended the range of creative strategies incorporated within grief therapy (Neimeyer, 2012c; Thompson & Neimeyer, 2014), as illustrated in the case study that follows.

Several months after the tragic overdose of her 29-year-old son, Daniel, Susan sought therapy, as she anguishingly acknowledged that the "stages of grief" that she "knew in her head" failed to describe the deep and preoccupying grief in which she had been encased since the loss. From the opening moments of therapy, it was clear that she struggled both with the manner of her son's dying and with complications in the strong emotional bond that she maintained with him, carrying his ashes in her purse wherever she went. I therefore invited her to take a step back, in a sense, from the trauma of his dying, and to introduce me to Daniel by sharing something of the boy he had been, and the young man he became (Hedtke, 2012). In response, Susan shared a compelling, if ambivalent, narrative of his life and place in the family, from the moment when "he came out of womb screaming" through a childhood of special intimacy with her in which he clearly "understood her in ways that even her husband did not." The story darkened with the advent of unsubstantiated sexual abuse of Daniel by a neighbor in middle school, introducing a troubled adolescence that was nonetheless marked by athletic achievement. Gradually, this pattern of vacillation coalesced into a stormy young adulthood of "working hard and drinking hard," with increasingly serious drug abuse interrupted but never overcome through his participation in a series of treatment programs. As Susan in her first session neared the conclusion of this story of maternal pride and despair, she stood at the brink of his dying, sobbing, "God, why did I have to find him dead?" She opened our second session explicitly asking us to "pick up where we left off last time, with going in to see him, find him," in his bedroom in their home, that fateful morning when the great rupture in her life narrative occurred.

Following procedures for retelling the narrative of the death (Neimeyer, 2012b), I first asked her where that tragic chapter in the story began. She immediately painted for me the scene of Daniel's car wreck the evening before his death, in which he had totalled his small sedan against a roadside railing, to be picked up, apparently unhurt, by his father as Susan herself was at work. Questions abounded regarding what had happened: Had he fallen asleep at the wheel? Was he high on cocaine? Using opiates? When she arrived home she saw her son doubled up in abdominal and psychological pain and "out of it," unable to answer the questions that still burned inside her. Tacking to the "back story" of their special mutual understanding, I invited her, eyes closed, to imagine what was going through his mind at that time. Instantly she gave it voice, ventriloquizing her son, and perhaps herself: "Why am I suffering like this? Why does God do this to me? What am I supposed to learn from this?" No easy answers were to be found, and returning to the slow, measured retelling of the story, Susan described how she had suggested "Let's all go to bed and get some rest." Turning in for a night of exhausted but fitful sleep, it was the last time she saw her son alive.

As the session continued, we shifted systematically between telling, witnessing, and gradually mastering the troubling imagery and events of that night and the still more horrific morning that followed, and interludes of imaginal dialogue (Jordan, 2012; Neimeyer, 2012a) with Daniel, prompted by Susan's dramatically ambivalent feelings toward him. For example, after giving voice to her sadness, compassion, and anger at him, she visualized him at my invitation in the empty chair opposite her, and asked, "You had it all. Why did you do this to yourself?" Taking Daniel's place and loaning him her voice, she replied, "I didn't care . . . no one gets it, the dark pain of my cravings. There was no hope."

Shifting once again to the critical scene of Susan's knocking first on her son's bedroom door, and hearing no response, entering the room, I metaphorically stood beside her as she related what she saw: his body, twisted in the sheets, torso trailing off the bed to the floor, with blood, blood, congealing from his mouth, spilt out upon the white sheets and carpet. Again I slowed her down into the moment, encouraged her to take a few deep breaths with me, inhaling and releasing slowly, while remaining in the scene. Resuming the story when she was ready, she related her panicked but futile attempt to find a pulse, and the anger that rose up in her, and had scarcely subsided in the intervening months. "A reservoir of anger," I reflected, to which she responded, "That's a good image; there is such a great amount of energy behind that wall . . . I guess it tells me that I am still alive." "What would ease it?" I asked with hope. "That comes with an assumption," she slowly and reflectively answered, "that I *want* it to ease. Maybe I want to *punish* myself for not saving him. Maybe I'm not *ready* to be happy."

Susan's phrasing alerted me to what my constructivist colleague Bruce Ecker refers to as a *pro-symptom position* (or PSP), that is, a construction of the *meaning* of problem—in this case, Susan's great reservoir of anger and unreadiness to let in any form of happiness—that makes it compellingly important to maintain, despite the real suffering associated with it (Ecker, Ticic, & Hulley, 2012). In the presence of such a meaning, initially held with minimal awareness, Ecker's approach is *noncounteractive*: simply to articulate the "emotional truth" of the client's position, with no attempt to change it. Asking Susan's patience, I simply wrote out the essence of what she had just told me on a blank sheet of paper: *I'm keeping my anger because it lets me know that I am still alive. If I let it go, I'd have to replace it with joy, and I'm not ready for that.* Handing the PSP to her and asking her to read it aloud, I listened rapt as Susan did so, with explicit permission to alter it as needed to make it more emotionally true. With tears in her eyes, she affirmed the spoken statement, adding, after a pause, a single word—*yet*. We then followed this with another written statement that she also read aloud: *The anger serves me because it helps me punish myself for mistakes I made—including in raising my son.* With a voice broken by painful sobs, she also affirmed that this captured her deep knowing, adding, "Yes. That is so true." I then drew on a technique Ecker calls *symptom deprivation*, simply asking her to close her eyes and imagine awakening to a day that did not begin in anger, that moved forward normally, but without sensing the press of that emotional reservoir. Wrinkling her brow, Susan slowly whispered, "Without the anger. . . I'd feel. . . naked. . . and vulnerable. . . ." "To?" I prompted. "The *unknown*," she responded, adding emphatically, "I'd feel *powerless*. . . . And if I woke up happy, I would have betrayed my son." In my own work with complicated grief, I often discover that the *meaning of mourning*—whether this takes the angry form that predominated for Susan, or any of a variety of other forms of desolation—suggests that it serves deep, if initially unconscious, purposes, which make it essential to retain, rather than relinquish, even if at very great expense.[5] Like Ecker (2012), I have found that simply holding these emotional truths consciously rather than unconsciously tends to promote their transformation, with no therapist interventions to "dispute" their rationality, as in more cognitive behavioral forms of therapy (Neimeyer, 2009a). In Susan's case, she spontaneously returned to the image of the "reservoir of anger," saying, "That's a great word . . . it fits me where I am. But it takes so much energy to keep that wall up." Glancing quickly to "Daniel's chair," she continued, "I see Daniel and me in those two chairs, just *two lost souls*," elaborating on the pain and struggle of her own early life as an unwanted child, "pulsating with anger." "Something about that anger is very old, very familiar," I reflected. "Yes," Susan replied, "but I never *languaged* that before. . . . I am the wall of the reservoir, the locks, the water behind it." Looking over toward "Daniel," she continued, "Even in your death, your physical death, the loss of you is helping me touch pieces of myself I haven't languaged." As I encouraged the continuation and deepening of this spontaneous dialogue, Susan went on to express tearfully her deep regret that she could not save her son, "touching his cold body to find his energy gone." Taking her son's chair, she then extended genuine understanding for the limits of her power to save him, and, from each position, extended a touching statement of their "imperfect love," each for the other. In the remaining four sessions of our six-session therapy, Susan reported "making the choice to give up some of the anger," and with this, felt an uncanny sense of closeness to Daniel, in which she "felt him say that he was okay . . . at peace." Smiling, she commented on the character of our position work together: "It was smart of you to know that I wouldn't trust anyone's words but my own. Writing those down, speaking them, and talking to Daniel was a wonderful way to make things clear. I realize now that I am in charge of the reservoir." Though we continued our work to clarify the essential self-protective role of anger in her life, and the courage it would take to relinquish it, Susan had begun a process of change that now seemed irresistible, and her grieving for the sadness of her son's life and death began to move forward in more adaptive ways.

A SCIENTIFIC CODA

As has been true for me, many of those professionals who are drawn to the field of grief therapy have been animated in part by the impulse to come to terms with the losses in their own lives as they attempt to help their clients do likewise. Thus it is not surprising that the resulting sense of "calling" that we feel does not, at first blush, easily accommodate the evidence that the majority of bereaved persons do not require professional grief therapy for uncomplicated bereavement. That is, when grief therapy is offered "universally," when the only criterion is that recipients have lost a loved one, there is very little evidence that they benefit more than those receiving no assistance, as most members of the latter group improve of their own accord, drawing on their personal resilience and that of their families and communities (Currier, Neimeyer, & Berman, 2008). However, this is not to deny that bereavement counseling and support might be an entirely humane and appropriate service to offer when the bereaved seek it (Schut, 2010). In light of these findings, and the reality of human resilience, it may be more respectful to ask the bereaved some version of the simple question, "Are you having trouble dealing with the death?" or "Are you interested in seeing a grief counselor to help with that?" (Gamino, Sewell, Hogan, & Mason, 2009–2010). When the answer to either question is positive, there is a high probability that the bereaved respondent will find grief counseling helpful.

Similarly, when specialized grief therapy is "selectively" offered to high-risk groups, such as parents who have lost children, or to survivors of a loved one's death by inherently troubling causes, such as suicide or homicide, reliable differences favoring treatment begin to emerge. But the clearest evidence for the efficacy of grief therapy derives from its application to "indicated" clients, that is, those who are demonstrably distressed at clinically significant levels for a prolonged period (Currier, Neimeyer, & Berman, 2008; Neimeyer & Currier, 2009). Such clients are often recognized, of course, by providers of bereavement support who see that some people need assistance beyond what they offer. Taken in conjunction with research indicating that approximately 10% to 15% of bereaved persons suffer from prolonged, complicated grief reactions (Prigerson et al., 2009), it therefore seems that contemporary grief therapists have something of value to offer to the significant minority of grieving people who truly need professional therapy.

But what more does research teach us about the sort of practices that have been found effective in mitigating the distress associated with complicated bereavement? Writing from attachment, coping, cognitive behavioral, and constructivist perspectives, Shear, Boelen, and Neimeyer (2011) recently reflected on their various evidence-based approaches to grief therapy and concluded as follows:

> Notwithstanding differences in the three approaches, we were struck by convergence in: (1) fostering confrontation with the story of the death in an attempt to master its most painful aspects and integrate its finality into the mourner's internalized models of the deceased, the self and the world, (2) encouraging engagement with the image, voice or memory of the deceased to facilitate a sense of ongoing attachment while allowing for the development of other relationships, (3) gradually challenging avoidance coping[6] and building skill in emotion modulation and creative problem solving, and (4) encouraging the bereaved to review and revise life goals and roles in a world without the deceased person in it. We believe these commonalities can serve as principles to guide clinicians and that the differences in our three approaches indicate that there is not just one way to follow these principles. (pp. 158–159)

In short, the evolution of bereavement studies in the half century following the advent of the death awareness movement has begun to generate demonstrably effective practices, which continue to grow in their variety and evidence base (Neimeyer, 2012c). As this fund of grief theory and therapy develops in richness and relevance, it gives us reason to hope that we may offer something of genuinely therapeutic value when clients struggle greatly in the wake of life-altering loss.

NOTES

1. For an account of my personal participation in this work, and the research program on death anxiety to which it gave rise, see Neimeyer (2009b) and Neimeyer, Wittkowski, and Moser (2004), respectively.
2. All cases discussed in this chapter have been redacted to protect client confidentiality, and all names replaced with pseudonyms.
3. For more detail on use of family photo albums in the context of grief therapy, see Gamino (2012). Readers interested in a broader discussion of "re-membering" the deceased as a counseling practice can consult Hedtke (2012).
4. For a simple technique used to facilitate a client's identification of support figures who represent a mix of "doers," "respite figures," and "listeners" in the context of bereavement counseling, see Doka and Neimeyer (2012).
5. For a video demonstration of accessing and beginning to transform a pro-symptom position with a bereaved mother, see my work with Darla, whose "suffering" offered the most compelling connection to her son, Kyle, following his death from cancer (Neimeyer, 2004).
6. Recent controlled research on behavioral activation as an antidote to behavioral avoidance in bereavement further supports this point (Papa, Sewell, Garrison-Diehn, & Rummel, 2013).

REFERENCES

Attig, T. (1996). *How we grieve: Relearning the world.* New York, NY: Oxford University Press.

Attig, T. (2000). *The heart of grief.* New York, NY: Oxford University Press.

Bonanno, G. A., Wortman, C. B., & Nesse, R. M. (2004). Prospective patterns of resilience and maladjustment during widowhood. *Psychology and Aging, 19,* 260–271.

Bowlby, J. (1980). *Attachment and loss: Loss, sadness and depression* (Vol. 3). New York, NY: Basic Books.

Burke, L. A., & Neimeyer, R. A. (2013). Prospective risk factors for complicated grief: A review of the empirical literature. In M. Stroebe, H. Schut, P. Boelen, & J. Van den Bout

(Eds.), *Complicated grief: Scientific foundations for health care professionals* (pp. 145–161). Washington, DC: American Psychological Association.

Burke, L. A., Neimeyer, R. A., Holland, J. M., Dennard, S., Oliver, L., & Shear, M. K. (2014). Inventory of Complicated Spiritual Grief: Development and validation of a new measure. *Death Studies, 38*, 1–12. doi:10.1080/07481187.2013.810098

Caserta, M. S., & Lund, D. A. (2007). Toward the development of an Inventory of Daily Widowed Life (IDWL): Guided by the Dual Process Model of coping with bereavement. *Death Studies, 31*, 505–535.

Coleman, R. A., & Neimeyer, R. A. (2010). Measuring meaning: Searching for and making sense of spousal loss in later life. *Death Studies, 34*, 804–834.

Corr, C. A. (1993). Coping with dying: Lessons we should and should not learn from the work of Elisabeth Kübler-Ross. *Death Studies, 17*, 69–83.

Currier, J. M., Neimeyer, R. A., & Berman, J. S. (2008). The effectiveness of psychotherapeutic interventions for the bereaved: A comprehensive quantitative review. *Psychological Bulletin, 134*, 648–661.

Datson, S. L., & Marwit, S. J. (1997). Personality constructs and perceived presence of deceased loved ones. *Death Studies, 21*, 131–146.

Doka, K., & Neimeyer, R. A. (2012). Orchestrating social support. In R. A. Neimeyer (Ed.), *Techniques of grief therapy: Creative practices for counseling the bereaved* (pp. 315–317). New York, NY: Routledge.

Downe-Wambolt, B., & Tamlyn, D. (1997). An international survey of death education trends in faculties of nursing and medicine. *Death Studies, 21*, 177–188.

Ecker, B. (2012). Overt statements for deep work in grief therapy. In R. A. Neimeyer (Ed.), *Techniques of grief therapy: Creative practices for counseling the bereaved* (pp. 152–154). New York, NY: Routledge.

Ecker, B., Ticic, R., & Hulley, L. (2012). *Unlocking the emotional brain.* New York, NY: Routledge.

Field, N. P., & Friedrichs, M. (2004). Continuing bonds in coping with the death of a husband. *Death Studies, 28*, 597–620.

Freud, S. (1957). Mourning and melancholia. In J. Strachey (Ed. & Trans.), *The complete psychological works of Sigmund Freud* (Vol. XIV, pp. 152–170). London, UK: Hogarth Press. (Original work published 1957)

Gamino, L. (2012). Opening the family photo album. In R. A. Neimeyer (Ed.), *Techniques of grief therapy* (pp. 231–233). New York, NY: Routledge.

Gamino, L. A., Sewell, K. W., Hogan, N. S., & Mason, S. L. (2009–2010). Who needs grief counseling? A report from the Scott & White Grief Sudy. *Omega, 60*, 199–223.

Gillies, J., Neimeyer, R. A., & Milman, E. (2014). The meaning of loss codebook: Construction of a system for analyzing meanings made in bereavement. *Death Studies, 38*, 1–10. doi:10.1080/07481187.2013.829367

Hedtke, L. (2012). *Bereavement support groups: Breathing life into stories of the dead.* Chagrin Falls, OH: Taos Institute Publications.

Holland, J. M., Currier, J. M., & Neimeyer, R. A. (2014). Validation of the Integration of Stressful Life Experiences Scale–Short Form in a bereaved sample. *Death Studies, 38*, 234–238. doi:10.1080/07481187.2013.829369

Holland, J. M., Currier, J. M., Coleman, R. A., & Neimeyer, R. A. (2010). The Integration of Stressful Life Experiences Scale (ISLES): Development and initial validation of a new measure. *International Journal of Stress Management, 17*, 325–352.

Holland, J. M., & Neimeyer, R. A. (2010). An examination of stage theory of grief among individuals bereaved by natural and violent causes: A meaning-oriented contribution. *Omega, 61*, 105–122.

Jordan, J. R. (2012). Guided imaginal conversations with the deceased. In R. A. Neimeyer (Ed.), *Techniques of grief therapy* (pp. 262–265). New York, NY: Routledge.

Klass, D., Silverman, P. R., & Nickman, S. (1996). *Continuing bonds: New understandings of grief.* Washington, DC: Taylor & Francis.

Kübler-Ross, E. (1969). *On death and dying.* New York, NY: Macmillan.

Lichtenthal, W. G., Currier, J. M., Neimeyer, R. A., & Keesee, N. J. (2010). Sense and significance: A mixed methods examination of meaning-making following the loss of one's child. *Journal of Clinical Psychology, 66*, 791–812.

Lindemann, E. (1944). Symptomatology and management of acute grief. *American Journal of Psychiatry, 101*, 141–148.

Meier, A. M., Carr, D. R., Currier, J. M., & Neimeyer, R. A. (2013). Attachment anxiety and avoidance in coping with bereavement: Two studies. *Journal of Social and Clinical Psychology, 32*(3), 315–334.

Neimeyer, R. A. (Ed.). (1994). *Death anxiety handbook: Research, instrumentation, and application*. New York, NY: Taylor & Francis.

Neimeyer, R. A. (2002). *Lessons of loss: A guide to coping*. Memphis, TN: Center for the Study of Loss and Transition.

Neimeyer, R. A. (2004). *Constructivist psychotherapy, Series 1: Systems of psychotherapy* [VHS video/DVD]. Washington, DC: American Psychological Association.

Neimeyer, R. A. (2009a). *Constructivist psychotherapy*. London, NY: Routledge.

Neimeyer, R. A. (2009b). Constructions of death and loss: A personal and professional evolution. In R. J. Butler (Ed.), *On reflection: Emphasizing the personal in personal construct psychology* (pp. 291–317). London, UK: Wiley.

Neimeyer, R. A. (2012a). Chair work. In R. A. Neimeyer (Ed.), *Techniques of grief therapy: Creative practices for counseling the bereaved* (pp. 266–273). New York, NY: Routledge.

Neimeyer, R. A. (2012b). Retelling the narrative of the death. In R. A. Neimeyer (Ed.), *Techniques of grief therapy: Creative practices for counseling the bereaved* (pp. 86–90). New York, NY: Routledge.

Neimeyer, R. A. (Ed.). (2012c). *Techniques of grief therapy: Creative practices for counseling the bereaved*. New York, NY: Routledge.

Neimeyer, R. A. (2013). The staging of grief: Toward an active model of mourning In S. Kreitler & H. Shanun-Klein (Eds.), *Studies in grief and bereavement*. Hauppauge, NY: Nova Science.

Neimeyer, R. A. (2014). Meaning in bereavement. In R. E. Anderson (Ed.), *World suffering and quality of life*. New York, NY: Springer Publishing Company.

Neimeyer, R. A., & Currier, J. M. (2009). Grief therapy: Evidence of efficacy and emerging directions. *Current Directions in Psychological Science, 18*, 252–256.

Neimeyer, R. A., Harris, D., Winokuer, H., & Thornton, G. (Eds.). (2011). *Grief and bereavement in contemporary society: Bridging research and practice*. New York, NY: Routledge.

Neimeyer, R. A., & Sands, D. C. (2011). Meaning reconstruction in bereavement: From principles to practice. In R. A. Neimeyer, H. Winokuer, D. Harris, & G. Thornton (Eds.), *Grief and bereavement in contemporary society: Bridging research and practice*. New York, NY: Routledge.

Neimeyer, R. A., Wittkowski, J., & Moser, R. P. (2004). Psychological research on death attitudes: An overview and evaluation. *Death Studies, 28*, 309–340.

Papa, A., Sewell, M. T., Garrison-Diehn, C., & Rummel, C. (2013). A randomized controlled trial assessing the feasibility of behavioral activation for pathological grief responding. *Behavior Therapy, 44*(4), 639–650. doi:http://dx.doi.org/10.1016/j.beth.2013.04.009

Parkes, C. M., & Prigerson, H. (2009). *Bereavement* (4th ed.). London, UK: Routledge.

Prigerson, H. G., Horowitz, M. J., Jacobs, S. C., Parkes, C. M., Aslan, M., Goodkin, K., . . . , Maciejewski, P. K. (2009). Prolonged grief disorder: Psychometric validation of criteria proposed for DSM-V and ICD-11. *PLoS Medicine, 6*(8), 1–12.

Rubin, S. S. (1999). The Two-Track Model of bereavement: Overview, retrospect and prospect. *Death Studies, 23*, 681–714.

Rubin, S. S., Malkinson, R., Koren, D., & Michaeli, E. (2009). The Two-Track Model of Bereavement Questionnaire (TTBQ): Development and validation of a relational measure. *Death Studies, 33*, 305–333.

Rubin, S. S., Malkinson, R., & Witztum, E. (2003). Trauma and bereavement: Conceptual and clinical issues revolving around relationships. *Death Studies, 27*, 667–690.

Rubin, S. S., Malkinson, R., & Witztum, E. (2011). *Working with the bereaved*. New York, NY: Routledge.

Schut, H. (2010). Grief counseling efficacy: Have we learned enough? *Bereavement Care, 29*, 8–9.

Shear, K., Boelen, P., & Neimeyer, R. A. (2011). Treating complicated grief: Converging approaches. In R. A. Neimeyer, D. Harris, H. Winokuer, & G. Thornton (Eds.), *Grief and bereavement in contemporary society: Bridging research and practice* (pp. 139–162). New York, NY: Routledge.

Stroebe, M., Gergen, M., Gergen, K., & Stroebe, W. (1992). Broken hearts or broken bonds: Love and death in historical perspective. *American Psychologist, 47*, 1205–1212.

Stroebe, M., & Schut, H. (1999). The Dual Process Model of coping with bereavement: Rationale and description. *Death Studies, 23*, 197–224.

Stroebe, M., & Schut, H. (2010). The Dual Process Model of Coping with Bereavement: A decade on. *Omega, 61*, 273–289.

Thompson, B. E., & Neimeyer, R. A. (Eds.). (2014). *Grief and the expressive arts: Practices for creating meaning.* New York, NY: Routledge.

Zech, E., & Arnold, C. (2011). Attachment and coping with bereavement. In R. A. Neimeyer, D. Harris, H. Winokuer, & G. Thornton (Eds.), *Grief and bereavement in contemporary society: Bridging research and practice* (pp. 23–35). New York, NY: Routledge.

Therese A. Rando _____ # 23

WHEN TRAUMA AND LOSS COLLIDE: THE EVOLUTION OF INTERVENTION FOR TRAUMATIC BEREAVEMENT

For better or worse, the topic of this chapter is quite near and dear to my heart. When I was 17 years old, my father, never sick a day in his life, suddenly dropped dead at home from a massive myocardial infarction. Fifty weeks later, my mother, who had successfully survived open heart surgery for which her chances had not been that good, died 10 days post-op after bleeding internally from an undiagnosed aneurysm. The bleeding, over the course of a number of hours, went unnoticed by the staff attending her at the world-class hospital in which she was a patient. In the letter of explanation written by her hospital physician to her referring physician, the fact that there was a difficult situation going on with another patient that had demanded the staff's attention was the reason cited as to why such a clear-cut, treatable but life-threatening, process—one that was explicitly documented and easily recognizable in her medical record—was totally overlooked. That left me, along with my younger sister and brother, orphaned—stunned by the two sudden deaths and trying to contend all by our young selves with the "craziness" of traumatic bereavement in a world that was now almost totally unrecognizable. Is it any wonder why, when I came to choose an area of focus within psychology, I honed in on those who struggled with issues with which I was so, unfortunately, familiar?

Yet, although personal experience brought me to this area, there were—again, unfortunately—other less-personal realities that drew me to concentrate on this phenomenon. Two vignettes legitimize the reasons that professional attention *must* be directed to traumatic bereavement.

On one hot summer day when she was 6 years old, Emily discovered her father's body hanging in their garage following a successful suicide attempt. It was a grisly scene, replete with horrific sights and smells that overwhelmed the little girl. Well aware of how devastating this could be to her, Emily's family took her to a succession of therapists before she assumed that role herself as an adult. Each therapist addressed with her issues such as the psychological impact of dealing with her father's decision to take his own life, the resulting abandonment she experienced, growing up fatherless, and grieving for all she had lost. Although Emily improved somewhat over the years, she continued to have frequent nightmares, some emotional numbness, fear of intimacy, an exaggerated startle response, and increased agitation in hot weather. She felt unable to embrace her life and experienced herself as stuck. It took fully 50 years of periodic therapy before one therapist asked the crucial question that led Emily onto the road to true healing: "Exactly what did you see when you found your father?"

Finally, someone had begun to tap into the grotesque circumstances associated with her father's death, not solely the deprivation it had caused.

Although, in this case, those specializing in bereavement had missed the boat in overlooking the trauma brought about by the circumstances of the death, it might just as easily have been a trauma expert who failed to recognize the loss issues. Or, there may have been those who eschewed using trauma at all to illuminate loss reactions, as was the case described in the following vignette:

It was spring 1990, and I was attending the course "Psychological Trauma" offered by the preeminent institutions of Harvard Medical School and the Massachusetts Mental Health Center Department of Psychiatry and Trauma Clinic. The faculty members were among the best and brightest in the trauma field. I was particularly thrilled to get the chance to speak with one of the most lauded architects of the two recent editions of the Diagnostic and Statistical Manual of Mental Disorders (American Psychiatric Association), *who was speaking on classification of posttraumatic reactions. I excitedly shared with him my observations about the PTSD (posttraumatic stress disorder) I repeatedly had observed in many mourners contending with the sudden, accidental deaths of their loved ones. I was shocked when he looked at me with disdain and told me that I was one of the people "diluting" the concept of PTSD. It was, he asserted, a diagnosis that was to be reserved for events "outside the range of usual human experience." To which I responded, "And how usual is it for a person to lose their mother (or father or child or any other beloved person) to a sudden death? To most of us, a particular loved one only dies once! That makes it outside of the range of my usual human experience to lose this person!"*

Although traumatically bereaved people have been with us forever, it is only in relatively recent times that proper clinical and empirical attention has been paid to their experience, to say nothing of their treatment needs. All too often, they were approached as if theirs had been an anticipated loss, and with the expectation that all they required were sufficient opportunities to ventilate. Although there certainly was recognition that specific types of bereavement left mourners with particular loss-related issues (for example, suicide engenders feelings of rejection, guilt, and blame), there was little to no awareness that the traumatic nature of the death often meant that the personal traumatization the mourner experienced rendered him or her unable—at least temporarily—to contend with those issues without significant problems, if indeed they could be dealt with at all. This explains why one so often still hears stories about traumatized mourners being expected to match profiles and trajectories suitable for those who have lost loved ones to anticipated, natural deaths. This happens on the large scale too, as when on 9/11 caring, but ignorant, volunteers attempted to "talk about and process the feelings" of affected persons at the World Trade Center, who were totally traumatized, in shock, and incapable of feeling feelings—they were numb—to say nothing of talking about or processing them.

In recent times, there has been a shift in that reality. In this chapter, I explore the evolution of intervention for traumatic bereavement. Following some definitions and conceptual clarifications, I briefly sketch a noncomprehensive timeline of that evolutionary process. Next, I specify what I perceive as the most important works in the area up until 2000, and then since that time. Finally, I conclude by identifying concerns facing the field today.

DEFINITIONS AND CONCEPTUAL CLARIFICATIONS

Traumatic bereavement is the state of having suffered the loss of a loved one when grief and mourning over the death are complicated or overpowered by the traumatic stress brought about by its circumstances (Rando, 2015).

Traumatic stress refers to distress that is caused by a person's experience of psychological trauma, in this case, the particular dying and death of the loved one. (Some use the term *posttraumatic stress* if the stressor has ended or if the stress reactions began after the traumatic event had ceased. To minimize confusion, in this chapter the generic term *traumatic stress* is used to refer to all types of reaction to psychological trauma, regardless of whether the stressor persists or when the reactions developed.) Traumatic stress can occur during and/or after the dying and death. Traumatic stress reactions can occur, internally and externally. Internally, traumatic stress may affect one's feelings, thoughts and thinking processes, mental images, strivings, desires, perceptions, defenses and attempts at coping, as well as one's body sensations and physical health. Externally, it can affect one's behaviors and social responses to others. Finally, traumatic stress can refer to general reactions (such as intrusions, flashbacks, anxiety, emotional numbness, irritability, avoidance, or relationship problems), as well as to any of a number of specific mental or physical disorders that can develop out of general traumatic stress reactions (such as disorders associated with anxiety, depression, substance abuse, dissociation, eating or impulse-control problems, and stress-related illness, among others). It is a mistake to believe that posttraumatic stress disorder is the sole way traumatic stress is manifested.

The traumatic deaths discussed here as giving rise to traumatic bereavement go beyond the traditional ones from *accident and disaster, suicide,* and *homicide.* They include as well *acute natural deaths,* with such deaths usually caused by catastrophic medical events (such as heart attack, stroke, sudden cardiac arrest, aneurysm, embolism, thrombosis, seizure, or hemorrhage); acute medical illness (such as an acute bacterial or viral infection); or acute syndromes (such as sudden infant death syndrome, sudden arrhythmia death syndrome, or sudden unexpected nocturnal death syndrome). As noted later in the chapter, the failure to include acute natural deaths as a type of traumatic death is worrisome.

By definition, traumatic bereavement inherently embodies trauma and its ensuing traumatic stress, as well as loss and its ensuing grief and mourning. Note that I distinguish between the terms "grief" and "mourning." *Grief* refers to the psychological, behavioral, social, and physical reactions to the perception of loss (Rando, 1993). *Mourning* refers to efforts to cope with that loss through engagement in six processes (the six "R" processes of mourning; Rando, 1993) that promote the personal readjustments and three reorientation operations (vis-à-vis the deceased loved one, the mourner, and the external world) that are required to accommodate the loss of a loved one (Rando, 2015). Technically, mourning inherently includes the experience of grief in its beginning processes. However, mourning goes beyond grief's mere reactivity to encompass as well additional undertakings in order to be able to make the necessary changes required for accommodation and adaptation to occur. In traumatic bereavement, as with all types of bereavements, mourners tend to receive more assistance in the beginning with their acute grief than with their later mourning processes. Adding to the challenge, from the beginning and all the way through, traumatic bereavement constitutes one of the highest risk factors for complicating grief, mourning, and adaptation (Rando, 1993, 2015).

There exist *four possible sources of trauma* in any individual's grief and mourning. First, it can come from its being a normal component of grief and mourning. Acute grief is a form of traumatic stress reaction and, as such, contains traumatic stress (Horowitz, 1976/1986; Rando, 2000). Second, trauma also can stem from the circumstances of the death, the very topic of this chapter. Third, trauma can arise because of relationship issues between the mourner and the deceased (for instance, the death is of someone on whom the mourner was excessively dependent). Fourth, the experience of trauma can come about because of mourner liabilities (such as the age or mental health vulnerabilities of that person). It must be remembered that traumatic bereavement from traumatic deaths is *not* the only source of traumatic stress after the loss of a loved one. Relationship and developmental issues, along with the mourner's attributes (such as attachment style or mental health), certainly may contribute to infusing the survivor's bereavement reaction with trauma. However, these latter two scenarios are not dealt with in this chapter.

FROM TWO DISPARATE AREAS TO ONE: PIVOTAL STEPS IN THE DEVELOPMENT OF TRAUMATIC BEREAVEMENT

The understanding of traumatic bereavement, with its intersection of trauma and loss, traces its roots back thousands of years to the studies of responses to trauma and to death. The antecedents of *traumatology*—the study of trauma—emanate from an ancient Egyptian physician's reports of hysterical reactions published in 1900 B.C.E. in *Kunyus Papyrus* (Figley, 1993). *Thanatology*—the study of dying, death, and bereavement—predates it significantly. References to death and reactions to it date back over 10,000 years and are found in the ancient myths of Sumeria, such as the myth of Gilgamesh the Wrestler, who was stricken with grief and set out to find immortal life (Pine, 1986).

As can be seen from the definitions of each field, there is absolutely nothing that should keep them disparate and much that would seem to be in common, particularly in situations of traumatic death. Yet, despite being conceptually, clinically, and often empirically associated, the fields of traumatology and thanatology traditionally remained relatively independent. This is actually quite surprising, as was observed by Simpson (1997), a pioneer in both fields:

> A relation between traumatology and thanatology may seem so obvious as to be a tautology, for almost all traumatic stressors encompass death or the threat of death. You may have grief without much trauma, but you can never have much trauma without grief. Ignoring the trauma component of grief, or the grief component of trauma, is surely negligent. (p. 6)

What this meant is that each field addressed the issues it had been trained to identify and treat. Consequently, after a death under traumatic circumstances, the traumatologists focused on trauma mastery and the thanatologists focused on accommodation of loss. Unfortunately, what the traumatically bereaved individual required was assistance with both. Although a few authors in each field recognized this important reality—for example, Eth and Pynoos (1985), Green (1993), and Lindy (1986) in traumatology and Raphael (1983, 1986), Redmond (1989), and Lord (1987/2006) in thanatology—the vast majority of authors, researchers, and practitioners in both fields insufficiently integrated treatment of posttraumatic stress and loss when working with mourners. There was little to no recognition that mourners were *both* traumatized *and* grief stricken.

The evolution of thought and practice regarding traumatic bereavement appears to have progressed through four major periods of focus. Although some of the studies and reports within a given period do not always run consecutively with those from another, the focus of each period seems to have grown out of the previous one to help lead us to where we are today. The first period, as noted previously, was characterized by the relative isolation of traumatology from thanatology. In essence, this was the *independent period*. Each field developed on its own, the chronologies of which are not in my purview here since our focus is on the integration of the two.

Next, there came the *personal disaster and sudden death period*, when there was an extension of thinking associated with traumatology to thanatology. The first part of the name (that is, personal disaster) derives from the title of Beverley Raphael's seminal article in 1981, which delineated that the same dynamics and issues found in extraordinary and/or mass casualty disasters—such as shock and denial, distress, helplessness, death and destruction, and images—could visit individuals in more personal or private cataclysmic events, such as death of a loved one, personal experience of major disaster, or severe, life-threatening accident or illness. This ushered in a time of great analysis of sudden death, characterized by clinical and empirical investigation into the effects of death that took place without warning or expectation. Among the more notable contributions of this time were Parkes and Weiss's (1983) identification of the unanticipated grief syndrome; Lundin's (1984a, 1984b) empirical demonstrations of the increased grief and morbidity of sudden death survivors; and Sanders's (1989) findings regarding the debilitating, anger-producing, and grief-prolonging effects of unexpected deaths. Earlier, Lehrman (1956) had delineated issues and clinical sequelae associated with untimely, often sudden, deaths and Glick, Weiss, and Parkes (1974) discovered how such deaths overwhelmed coping, interfered with full functioning, and caused many survivors to become so insecure that they resisted remarriage lest they suddenly become widowed again. Later on, Rando (1994, 1996) joined this group when she outlined complications in mourning traumatic—in particular, sudden—deaths and delineated specific intervention strategies for sudden, unanticipated deaths of all kinds. The emphasis for all of the authors in this period was on the impact of the personal traumatization brought about by sudden death.

The next focus that evolved was exploration of the effects of different types of sudden deaths. In this *specific traumatic death period*, personal traumatization was explicitly acknowledged, as was the loss-related consequences associated with the particular death. A partial listing of specific traumatic deaths that were put under the spotlight include the following, with space permitting only one author to be identified for each: Disaster deaths were studied by Raphael (1986); motor vehicle deaths were investigated by Lehman, Wortman, and Williams (1987); suicide was examined by Shneidman (1969, 1981); Redmond (1989) illuminated homicide bereavement; Pynoos and Nader (1990) researched children exposed to violence and traumatic death through a school sniper attack.

The *conceptual integration period*, which continues into the present, represents the time in which clinicians and researchers actively bridged the gap to join traumatology and thanatology. Among the many contributions, the following are notable: In 1975, Ann Burgess observed that after homicide, victim-oriented thought (the horror over manner of death) interferes with ego-oriented thought (the loss of a family member). Following this, Horowitz (1976/1986) identified bereavement as a specific precipitant of the stress response syndrome. In 1985, Eth and Pynoos specified the dual tasks of trauma mastery and grief resolution in childhood bereavement following violent death. In 1993, Rando explored the treatment of complicated mourning, which in large part focused on the issues and treatment requirements of bereavement following traumatic deaths. The Series in Trauma and Loss, published by Brunner/Mazel, was established in 1996 by Charles Figley and Therese Rando with the expressed intent to provide a vehicle specifically for integrating the two fields of traumatology and thanatology. A number of publications emanated from that endeavor. That same year, Doka (1996), on behalf of the Hospice Foundation of America, convened the first national teleconference on living with grief in the aftermath of sudden death and published a companion book to accompany it. This was followed 7 years later by a teleconference and companion book on living with grief after public tragedy, which inherently involves traumatic deaths (Lattanzi-Licht & Doka, 2003). Both the teleconferences and books underscored the potent trauma–loss connection.

In 1997, Kathleen Nader distinguished the independence as well as interaction of trauma and grief and observed that the lack of attention to such interaction can undermine treatment. In a 1998 survey study of trauma in the community, Breslau and colleagues identified sudden, unexpected death of a loved one as "the single most important trauma as a cause of PTSD" (Breslau et al., 1998, p. 628). That same year, Stroebe, Schut, and Stroebe (1998) did an in-depth comparative analysis of trauma and grief, recognizing overlap between the two phenomena yet finding limitations in adopting a general trauma framework for studying grief. In 2000, Malkinson, Rubin, and Witztum richly explored myriad clinical interfaces of bereavement and trauma. In 2002, John Harvey culminated years of integrating all manner of loss (including death) with trauma with his survey publication examining assaults on the self as a consequence of the loss and trauma experience (Harvey, 2002). In 2006, after many publications, significant research, and much provision of training, Cohen, Mannarino, and Deblinger published a treatment book devoted to trauma-focused therapy for childhood traumatic grief, in which the trauma and loss intersection is a main focus.

It should be noted that during this time period, a number of other authors wrote about "traumatic grief" (e.g., Jacobs, 1999; Shear et al., 2001). However, this was not the traumatic grief being addressed in this chapter, but rather it represented an earlier name for what is now termed prolonged grief disorder (PGD; Prigerson, Vanderwerker, & Maciejewski, 2008). Works that focus on "traumatic grief" associated with PGD are not incorporated in this review, which focuses only on traumatic bereavement as defined earlier.

Also during this period, there was a huge focus on violent death. Among others, Rynearson (see 2001, 2006, among many), Kaltman and Bonanno (2003), Neimeyer and colleagues (see, for example, Currier, Holland, & Neimeyer, 2006; Currier, Holland, Coleman, & Neimeyer, 2008; Neimeyer, 2002, among others), Kristensen, Weisaeth, and Heir (2012), and Stevenson and Cox (2008) explicated the critically adverse role that violence in death circumstances plays in the experience of those left behind, articulating in depth the negative sequelae of the trauma and loss combination.

Finally, during this time, there were numerous attempts to compare and contrast acute grief and traumatic stress. Some perceived more differences among the two (e.g., Nader, 1997; Raphael & Martinek, 1997) than others (e.g., Rando, 2000; Simpson, 1997). Illustrating how the differences that had been identified were "primarily in content and degree and not necessarily in process" Rando (2000, p.183) used these works, along with others, to lead to delineation of nine arguments for acute grief itself being a form of traumatic stress reaction.

THE "CLASSICS" IN THE FIELD: SIX FOUNDATIONAL CONCEPTS ASSOCIATED WITH THE TREATMENT OF TRAUMATIC BEREAVEMENT UP TO 2000

The authors identified in the previous section, along with many unmentioned others, all have contributed to the development of the traumatic bereavement field. Up until 2000, there are six major concepts that seem especially noteworthy, foundational, and never to be forgotten by anyone practicing with traumatized mourners. Such "classics" include:

Virtually anything authored by Beverley Raphael, but particularly her writing on the concept of "personal disaster" (1981) and explications of the "shock effects of sudden death" (1983) and "coping with catastrophe" (1986). Together, these works expose in great detail the personal phenomenology of the traumatized mourner, wherein, with no time to gradually anticipate and prepare for the loss, the full and total confrontation of it all at once overpowers the mourner, assaults his or her coping abilities, overwhelms adaptive capacities, and complicates mourning. Further, Raphael vividly explores the person's experience of striving to master the helplessness and other flooding emotions with which they are inundated, the intrusion of associated traumatic memories, and the resulting sense of personal threat and vulnerability. In each work, she specifies treatment requirements.

Parkes and Weiss's (1983) presentation of the "unanticipated grief syndrome." This demonstrates how the lack of anticipation in sudden death can be so disruptive in impact that uncomplicated recovery simply cannot be expected. Their description of the assaults perpetrated by the absence of forewarning—such as the bewilderment, anxiety, overwhelmed adaptive capacities and coping abilities, plus the inability to grasp the full implications of the loss and difficulty accepting that it happened despite intellectual recognition of its occurrence—are extremely useful not only for those involved with survivors caught up in this syndrome, but also for explicating the early experiences of *all* sudden death mourners.

Rynearson's (1987) identification of the significant differences between natural and unnatural death, and his identification of the three Vs (violence, violation, and volition) of unnatural dying. This gem forever disabused the myth that concepts of grief and mourning after natural dying could be extended to unnatural dying. He made it explicitly clear that the three Vs precipitate compensatory psychological responses (with violence spawning traumatic stress, violation stimulating victimization, and volition creating compulsive inquiry). He shows how such responses can and do occur independently of antecedent psychopathology or an ambivalent relationship with the deceased and that they represent the psychological consequences of overwhelming affect and defensive collapse in the wake of unnatural deaths.

The work of Pynoos and Nader (1990), both together, with others, and individually (Eth & Pynoos, 1985; Nader, 1997), pointed out both the independence and interaction between trauma and grief reactions following traumatic deaths. This work, initially conducted with children but extrapolated later by Nader (1997) and others to adults, clarified the importance of appreciating the effects of trauma, the effects of loss, and the effects of the amalgamation of both. The dual tasks of trauma mastery and grief resolution were identified. The authors clarified that relieving traumatic anxiety takes psychological priority over mourning.

The empirical research on traumatic death conducted by Lehman, Wortman, and Williams (1987; and in part confirmed later by Shirley Murphy and colleagues [see Murphy et al., 2003, among others]) demonstrate that following traumatic loss, long-lasting distress is extremely common. The data indicate that such long-term distress is not a sign of individual coping failure, but rather a common response to the situation, with the subjects (from 30% to 85% depending on the question) still actively dealing with and significantly distressed by the motor vehicle death of a spouse or child 4 to 7 years earlier. The study eviscerated arguments that difficulties coming to terms with such traumatic loss, at least from 4 to 7 years after the death, signals pathology in the mourner or poor coping on his or her part.

Specific types of traumatic death confront the mourner with particular challenges that demand informed and targeted treatment intervention. As much as all traumatic deaths share in common the generic demands for trauma mastery and loss accommodation, each type has its own particular issues requiring attention. Delineation of these is impractical here due to space constraints. Those treating mourners after all forms of traumatic death—acute natural death, accident, disaster, suicide, and homicide (including deaths from war and terrorism)—must be aware of the thanatology and mental health literatures pertinent to the issues that survivor faces (e.g., preventability concerns after an accident or extreme fearfulness after an unsolved homicide). Such issues include, among others, postdeath experiences, personal needs, social reactions, impediments to mourning, potential secondary victimization, disenfranchisement, and civil and criminal justice system involvements. Because traumatic deaths are so highly associated with youth, dynamics associated with the parental loss of a child will often be relevant. Obviously, each mourner will need to be assessed individually and understood and approached within the context of the factors influencing his or her mourning (Rando, 1993).

SOMEDAY TO BE "CLASSICS" IN THE FIELD: FIVE OF THE NEWEST, MOST VALUABLE AREAS OF CONTRIBUTION TO THE TREATMENT OF TRAUMATIC BEREAVEMENT SINCE 2000

This is an exciting time to be researching, treating, or writing about traumatic bereavement. Building on the contributions of those who have come before them, a number of authors are pushing the field to expand its conceptualizations, attend to important dimensions, and incorporate new types of interventions. In this section, I briefly address five areas of contribution which, I believe, form some of the most valuable work in the field today.

Rynearson's work with restorative retelling. With his 2001 opus, *Retelling Violent Death,* Edward Rynearson introduced the process of retelling violent dying. The purpose of this restorative process is to assist survivors whose factual or imagined retelling of their loved one's violent death has become prolonged or excessive, in other words, they are stuck in focusing on the death of their loved one. This could be the result of their own traumatic re-experiencing responses and/or demands for public retelling of that death (such as through media interest, criminal investigation, justice system involvement, and so forth). Such things can keep their attention aimed exclusively on the loved one's dying, which can interfere with spontaneous restorative retelling and the necessary normal transition to a focus on the whole person, not on his or her death. Further, it can crowd out memories of the relationship with that person and his or her life. Essentially, the focus becomes fixed on the dying of that person and not on that person's life. In effect, this can "rob" a mourner of his or her loved one. The therapeutic goal is for the mourner to reconnect with living memories through restorative retelling. This is accomplished by naming and retelling vital and life-affirming experiences that encompass and counterbalance the loved one's dying. In turn, the loved one is no longer completely "lost" to the horrific dying imagery, and the survivor is released from the trauma of helplessly "watching" the loved one die through repeated dying reenactments. For a variety of restorative retelling approaches and conceptually related interventions, see the chapters in Rynearson's book on violent death (2006).

Neimeyer and colleagues' work on violent death intensifying grief, causing greater narrative destruction, compromising sense making and meaning reconstruction, and complicating mourning (see, for example, Currier, Holland, & Neimeyer, 2006; Currier, Holland, Coleman, & Neimeyer, 2008; Neimeyer, 2002). In recent times, constructivist Robert Neimeyer has focused attention on the significant problems created for the mourner by a sudden death that is violent in nature. His work, independently and with others, has elucidated how the violence of the loss interferes with symbolizing and speaking about the death, impedes narrative emplotment, violates the assumptive world, complicates reconstruction of fractured personal meaning, engenders posttraumatic stress, and predisposes to complicated mourning. In his works, he consistently offers useful treatment recommendations and implications.

Rando's work on the conceptualization, phenomenon, and treatment of traumatic bereavement, for intervention by professionals (Pearlman, Wortman, Feuer, Farber, & Rando, 2014 [see below]; Rando, 2000) and self-help for traumatized mourners (Rando, 2000, 2015). Following up on her pre-2000 writings on sudden death, traumatic loss, and the necessity of integrating thanatology and traumatology, Therese Rando has in recent years proffered a number of clinical concepts related to traumatic bereavement. Among those generating the most interest are the 12 core strategies for treating traumatic bereavement; the three levels of association of acute grief and traumatic stress and their treatment implications; the 12 high-risk elements for traumatic bereavement; the four types of sudden death; the 17 challenges created by the personal traumatization of sudden death; the 14 challenges created by loss of a loved one under sudden death circumstances; the 16 particularly problematic aftereffects of sudden, traumatic death; the "window" in traumatic bereavement; the traumatic bereavement trajectory; the components identified by research as necessary to integrate with complicated mourning treatment strategies for effective intervention in traumatic bereavement; the protocol that is in development with Roger Solomon for use of EMDR (eye movement desensitization training) in the treatment of traumatic bereavement; and the 12 core self-help strategies for traumatized mourners (Rando, 2000, 2015).

A truly integrated, manualized, evidence-based treatment of traumatic bereavement is now available (Pearlman et al., 2014). A team of traumatologists and thanatologists have worked for over a decade to develop what appears to be the most comprehensive and research-based treatment for those contending with sudden, traumatic death. The treatment is composed of three core components: (1) resource building—this entails building the survivor's internal and interpersonal resources in six areas: self-capacities, coping skills, social support, bereavement-specific issues, meaning and spirituality, and values and personal goals; (2) trauma processing—this calls for processing the traumatic death both cognitively (through cognitive processing therapy and selected cognitive techniques) and emotionally (through imaginal and in vivo exposure techniques drawn from emotional processing theory); and (3) mourning—this involves enabling the survivor to move through the six "R" processes of mourning (Rando, 1993). Informational handouts, worksheets, and independent activities are offered to support the resource building, trauma processing, and mourning. A sample 25-session treatment plan is provided. The treatment provides a compilation of the "best of the best" theory and practice in traumatology, thanatology, and psychology.

Neurobiological and psychophysiological advancements are enabling increased understanding of how psychological trauma affects the brain, the body, emotions, and behavior. From a more sophisticated understanding of the neurobiology of both hyperarousal and freeze responses during traumatic events (Rothschild, 2000) to the identification of immunological and neuroimaging biomarkers of complicated grief (O'Connor, 2012) to diagnosis by functional magnetic resonance imaging of heightened amygdala reactivity after high-intensity trauma exposure during the 9/11 attacks (Ganzel, Casey, Glover, Voss, & Temple, 2007), we are becoming increasingly proficient at understanding the mechanisms and biological bases for trauma and grief responses. This obviously has profound implications for intervention in traumatic bereavement. One recent investigation of those bereaved by violent death led to the conclusion that presence of PTSD contributed to the development of one form of complicated grief by suppressing certain brain functions (the functioning of the medial prefrontal cortex and the anterior cingulate cortex [ACC], which facilitates the mourning process) and interfering with "normal" grief and acceptance of death (Nakajima, Ito, Shirai, & Konishi, 2012). This will continue to be an area of emerging importance for our field as such work has the potential to be helpful in developing effective preventive intervention and treatment.

FUTURE CONCERNS REGARDING TRAUMATIC BEREAVEMENT AND ITS TREATMENT

It can easily be seen just how far our thoughts about and approaches to traumatic bereavement have come over the years. Yet, at the time of the writing of this chapter, there are a number of concerns still to be addressed. From my perspective, these six are particularly important:

Acute natural deaths remain the "poor stepchild" of the traumatic deaths. This is the case despite the fact that many such deaths are quite traumatic (such as witnessing a loved one "bleeding out" in a hemorrhage, gasping for air in a heart attack, having a grand mal seizure, or being devoured by flesh-eating bacteria; finding a cherished baby dead in her crib from sudden infant death syndrome; or learning that your healthy teenager has collapsed and died from sudden arrhythmia death syndrome). Not all horrific deaths are stimulated external to the deceased.

Many clinicians jump into traumatic material way too soon. They act without proper assessment, stabilization, and, if necessary, building up of the mourner's resources. Premature intervention with an unprepared person can revictimize the mourner if he or she is pushed to confront traumatic material associated with the loved one's death before having the proper coping capacities to do so (e.g., knowing how to modulate emotion, soothe oneself, or ground oneself).

Although it is well accepted that the psychological priority of the ego is generally to deal with trauma before loss, it is imperative to avoid operating as if this were written in stone. As so well articulated by Fleming (2012), it behooves one to follow the mourner's lead as to whether to focus on trauma or loss first, or at any given point.

In *DSM-5 (American Psychiatric Association, 2013)*, for persistent complex bereavement disorder, a condition included "for further study," the specifier "with traumatic bereavement" is included only for homicide or suicide. This suggests that a person whose loved one died from a mutilating accident, a horrific acute natural death, or a devastating disaster would not qualify for the specifier. This does not make sense because the specifier refers to preoccupations regarding the traumatic nature of the death, which certainly are not relegated solely to survivors of homicide or suicide.

In much of the current research on traumatic bereavement, there appears to be the fallacy that PGD is "equivalent" to complicated grief (Rando, 2013). This is not true. PGD certainly is *one form* of complicated grief, and definitely a well-researched and empirically validated form, but by no means the only one (Rando et al., 2012). The notion that it is taken to represent all types of the complicated grief phenomenon is extremely problematic. Indeed, even its originators specify it as one form and not "the only, or even the primary, complication that may follow from bereavement" (Prigerson et al., 2008, p. 173). Unfortunately, a great number of researchers have used specific measures of PGD (such as the PG-13 (Prigerson et al., 2008) or the Inventory of Complicated Grief [Prigerson et al., 1995]) as a measure of complicated grief in general. This means that other forms are being overlooked, and, more important, that research findings based on the operationalization of complicated grief solely as a score on a PGD measure may well be invalid. Simple changes such as stating that "PGD is one form of complicated grief" or "as one example of complicated grief, we examined PGD" would clearly indicate that complicated grief can be manifested in a variety of other ways. The great equation myth of PGD representing *all* of complicated grief must be dispelled. Especially with regard to traumatic bereavement, this is mandatory. Consider the mourner who has full-blown PTSD as an indicator of his or her complicated mourning after a traumatic death, but who does not meet criteria for PGD (and I have had many such cases). It certainly would be egregiously wrong to suggest that there is no grief-related problem merely because this person does not have PGD.

Because of the impact of medical advances, along with the presence of certain technological developments and the exposures they bring, there will continue to be an increasing amount of sudden, traumatic death relative to natural death. As well, there may be more human-caused mass casualty events (such as 9/11 and other terrorist instances). All of these trends translate to an increase in the amount of traumatic bereavement. This means our work in this field is cut out for us. Yet, although the bad news is that traumatic deaths will increase, the good news is that we have evolved and have greater and more accurate understanding of traumatic bereavement and ways to treat it.

REFERENCES

American Psychiatric Association. (2013). *Diagnostic and statistical manual of mental disorders* (5th ed.). Arlington, VA: American Psychiatric Press.

Breslau, N., Kessler, R., Chilcoat, H., Schultz, L., Davis, G., & Andreski, P. (1998). Trauma and posttraumatic stress disorder in the community: The 1996 Detroit Area Survey of Trauma. *Archives of General Psychiatry, 55*, 626–632.

Burgess, A. (1975). Family reaction to homicide. *American Journal of Orthopsychiatry, 45*, 391–398.

Cohen, J., Mannarino, A., & Deblinger, E. (2006). *Treating trauma and traumatic grief in children and adolescents.* New York, NY: Guilford.

Currier, J., Holland, J., Coleman, R., & Neimeyer, R. (2008). Bereavement following violent death: An assault on life and meaning. In R. Stevenson & G. Cox (Eds.), *Perspectives on violence and violent death* (pp. 177–202). Amityville, NY: Baywood.

Currier, J., Holland, J., & Neimeyer, R. (2006). Sense-making, grief, and the experience of violent loss: Toward a meditational model. *Death Studies, 30*, 403–428.

Doka, K. (Ed.). (1996). *Living with grief after sudden loss: Suicide, homicide, accident, heart attack, stroke.* Washington, DC: Taylor & Francis.

Eth, S., & Pynoos, R. (1985). Interaction of trauma and grief in childhood. In S. Eth & R. Pynoos (Eds.), *Post-traumatic stress disorder in children* (pp. 171–186). Washington, DC: American Psychiatric Press.

Figley, C. R. (1993). Foreword. In J. Wilson & B. Raphael (Eds.), *International handbook of traumatic stress syndromes* (pp. xvii–xx). New York, NY: Plenum.

Fleming, S. (2012). Complicated grief and trauma: What to treat first? In R. Neimeyer (Ed.), *Techniques of grief therapy: Creative practices for counseling the bereaved* (pp. 83–85). New York, NY: Routledge.

Ganzel, B., Casey, B. J., Glover, G., Voss, H. U., & Temple, E. (2007). The aftermath of 9/11: Effect of intensity and recency of trauma on outcome. *Emotion, 7*(2), 227–238.

Glick, I. O., Weiss, R. S., & Parkes, C. M. (194). *The first year of bereavement.* New York, NY: Wiley.

Green, B. (1993). Identifying survivors at risk. Trauma and stressors across events. In J. Wilson & B. Raphael (Eds.), *International handbook of traumatic stress syndromes* (pp. 135–144). New York, NY: Plenum.

Harvey, J. (2002). *Perspectives on loss and trauma: Assaults on the self.* Thousand Oaks, CA: SAGE.

Horowitz, M. J. (1986). *Stress response syndromes* (2nd ed.). Northvale, NJ: Jason Aronson. (Original work published 1976)

Jacobs, S. (1999). *Traumatic grief: Diagnoses, treatment, and prevention.* Philadelphia, PA: Brunner/Mazel.

Kaltman, S., & Bonanno, G. (2003). Trauma and bereavement: Examining the impact of sudden and violent deaths. *Journal of Anxiety Disorders, 17*, 131–147.

Kristensen, P., Weisaeth, L., & Heir, T. (2012). Bereavement and mental health after sudden and violent losses: A review. *Psychiatry, 75*(1), 76–97.

Lattanzi-Licht, M., & Doka, K. (Eds.). (2003). *Living with grief: Coping with public tragedy.* New York, NY: Brunner-Routledge.

Lehman, D., Wortman, C., & Williams, A. (1987). Long-term effects of losing a spouse or child in a motor vehicle crash. *Journal of Personality and Social Psychology, 52*(1), 218–231.

Lehrman, S. (1956). Reactions to untimely death. *Psychiatric Quarterly, 30*, 564–578.

Lindy, J. (1986). An outline for the psychoanalytic psychotherapy of post-traumatic stress disorder. In C. Figley (Ed.), *Trauma and its wake: Traumatic stress theory, research, and intervention* (Vol. 2, pp. 195–212). New York, NY: Brunner/Mazel.

Lord, J. (2006). *No time for goodbyes: Coping with sorrow, anger, and injustice after a tragic death* (6th ed.). Burnsville, NC: Compassion Press. (Original work published 1987)

Lundin, T. (1984a). Long-term outcome of bereavement. *British Journal of Psychiatry, 145*, 424–428.

Lundin, T. (1984b). Morbidity following sudden and unexpected bereavement. *British Journal of Psychiatry, 144*, 84–88.

Malkinson, R., Rubin, S., & Witztum, E. (Eds.). (2000). *Traumatic and nontraumatic loss and bereavement: Clinical theory and practice.* Madison, CT: Psychosocial Press.

Murphy, S., Johnson, L., Wu, L., Fan, J., & Lohan, J. (2003). Bereaved parents' outcomes 4 to 6 months after their children's deaths by accident, suicide, or homicide: A comparative study demonstrating differences. *Death Studies, 27*, 39–61.

Nader, K. (1997). Childhood traumatic loss: The interaction of trauma and grief. In C. Figley, B. Bride, & N. Mazza (Eds.), *Death and trauma: The traumatology of grieving* (pp. 17–41). Washington, DC: Taylor & Francis.

Nakajima, S., Ito, M., Shirai, A., & Konishi, T. (2012). Complicated grief in those bereaved by violent death: The effects of post-traumatic stress disorder on complicated grief. *Dialogues in Clinical Neuroscience, 14*(2), 210–214.

Neimeyer, R. (2002). Traumatic loss and the reconstruction of meaning. *Journal of Palliative Medicine, 5*, 935–942.

O'Connor, M. (2012). Immunological and neuroimaging biomarkers of complicated grief. *Dialogues in Clinical Neuroscience, 14*(2), 141–148.

Parkes, C. M., & Weiss, R. S. (1983). *Recovery from bereavement.* New York, NY: Basic Books.

Pearlman, L., Wortman, C., Feuer, C., Farber, C., & Rando, T. (2014). *Treating traumatic bereavement: A practitioner's guide.* New York, NY: Guilford.

Pine, V. R. (1986). An agenda for adaptive anticipation of bereavement. In T. A. Rando (Ed.), *Loss and anticipatory grief* (pp. 39–60). Lexington, MA. Lexington Books.

Prigerson, H., Maciejewski, P., Reynolds, C., et al. (1995). Inventory of complicated grief: A scale to measure maladaptive symptoms of loss. *Psychiatry Research, 59,* 65–79.

Prigerson, H., Vanderwerker, L., & Maciejewski, P. (2008). A case for inclusion of prolonged grief disorder in DSM-V. In M. Stroebe, R. Hansson, H. Schut, & W. Stroebe (Eds.), *Handbook of bereavement research and practice: Advances in theory and interventions* (pp. 165–186). Washington, DC: American Psychological Association.

Pynoos, R., & Nader, K. (1990). Children's exposure to violence and traumatic death. *Annals of Psychiatry, 20*(6), 334–344.

Rando, T. A. (1993). *Treatment of complicated mourning.* Champaign, IL: Research Press.

Rando, T. A. (1994). Complications in mourning traumatic death. In I. Corless, B. Germino, & M. Pittman (Eds.), *Dying, death, and bereavement: Theoretical perspectives and other ways of knowing* (pp. 253–271). Boston, MA: Jones and Bartlett.

Rando, T. A. (1996). On treating those bereaved by sudden, unanticipated death. *In Session: Psychotherapy in Practice, 2*(4), 59–71.

Rando, T. A. (2000). On the experience of traumatic stress in anticipatory and postdeath mourning. In T. A. Rando (Ed.), *Clinical dimensions of anticipatory mourning: Theory and practice in working with the dying, their loved ones, and their caregivers* (pp. 155–221). Champaign, IL: Research Press.

Rando, T. A. (2013). On achieving clarity regarding complicated grief: Lessons from clinical practice. In M. Stroebe, H. Schut, & J. van den Bout (Eds.), *Complicated grief: Scientific foundations for health care professionals* (pp. 40–54). East Sussex, UK: Routledge.

Rando, T. A. (2015). *Coping with the sudden death of your loved one: A self-help handbook for traumatic bereavement.* Indianapolis, IN: Dog Ear Publishing.

Rando, T., Doka, K., Fleming, S., Franco, M., Lobb, E., Parkes, C., & Steele, R. (2012). A call to the field: Complicated grief in the DSM-5. *Omega, 65*(4), 251–255.

Raphael, B. (1981). Personal disaster. *Australian and New Zealand Journal of Psychiatry, 15,* 183–198.

Raphael, B. (1983). *The anatomy of bereavement.* New York, NY: Basic Books.

Raphael, B. (1986). *When disaster strikes: How individuals and communities cope with catastrophe.* New York, NY: Basic Books.

Raphael, B., & Martinek, N. (1997). Assessing traumatic bereavement and posttraumatic stress disorder. In J. Wilson & T. Keane (Eds.), *Assessing psychological trauma and* PTSD (pp. 373–395). New York, NY: Guilford.

Redmond, L. (1989). *Surviving: When someone you love was murdered.* Clearwater, FL: Psychological Consultation and Education Services.

Rothschild, B. (2000). *The body remembers: The psychophysiology of trauma and trauma treatment.* New York, NY: W. W. Norton.

Rynearson, E. (1987). Psychological adjustment to unnatural dying. In S. Zisook (Ed.), *Biopsychosocial aspects of bereavement* (pp. 77–93). Washington, DC: American Psychiatric Press.

Rynearson, E. (2001). *Retelling violent death.* Philadelphia, PA: Brunner/Routledge.

Rynearson, E. (Ed.). (2006). *Violent death: Resilience and intervention beyond the crisis.* New York, NY: Routledge.

Sanders, C. (1989). *Grief: The mourning after.* New York, NY: Wiley.

Shear, M. K., Frank, E., Foa, E. B., et al. (2001). Traumatic grief treatment: A pilot study. *American Journal of Psychiatry, 158,* 1506–1508.

Shneidman, E. S. (1969). Suicide, lethality, and the psychological autopsy. In E. S. Shneidman & M. Ortega (Eds.), *Aspects of depression.* Boston, MA: Little, Brown.

Shneidman, E. S. (1981). Postvention: The care of the bereaved. *Suicide and Life Threatening Behavior, 2*(4), 349–359.

Simpson, M. (1997). Traumatic bereavement and death-related PTSD. In C. Figley, B. Bridge, & N. Mazza (Eds.), *Death and trauma: The traumatology of grieving* (pp. 3–16). Washington, DC: Taylor & Francis.

Stevenson, R., & Cox, G. (Eds.). (2008). *Perspectives on violence and violent death.* Amityville, NY: Baywood.

Stroebe, M., Schut, H., & Stroebe, W. (1998). Trauma and grief: A comparative analysis. In J. Harvey (Ed.), *Perspectives on loss: A sourcebook.* Philadelphia, PA: Brunner/Mazel.

Judith M. Stillion

24

TO BE OR NOT TO BE: SUICIDE THEN AND NOW

In Chapter 2, I wrote about how I came to enter the field of death, dying, grief, and bereavement. Here I will relate what drew me to write two books on suicide.

Any psychology professor at any college or university will, within a year or 2 of beginning to teach, encounter suicidal young people. Many professors will not recognize them. Some will recognize them but not engage them. Others will confront them and refer to appropriate counseling centers. Still others will not only refer but also find ways to support those students. I tried to be one of the latter.

My background in counseling as well as my teaching in developmental psychology enabled me to recognize troubled adolescents, and my open-door policy helped many to feel that they could confide their situations to me. As I read the literature on suicide, I began to develop and norm the Suicide Attitude Vignette Experience (SAVE) Scales. This led to research on attitudes toward suicide. At the same time, I was confronted with the suicide of a fellow faculty member's wife as well as the suicide of a colleague's father. The final impetus came when I was asked to talk to a residence hall population following the attempted suicide of one of the residents. I realized that there was little in common in the suicidal behavior of these three people and nothing in the literature that explored suicides among people of different ages and life situations. My colleague, Eugene McDowell, and I decided to remedy that situation, and in 1986 we coauthored with a former student the book *Suicide Across the Life Span: Premature Exits*. In 1996, Gene and I coauthored a completely revised second edition, which dropped the subtitle of *Premature Exits*.

Obviously, one chapter cannot cover the complete territory about suicide that is covered in a full book. This chapter will therefore provide a brief history of suicide, describe the dimensions of the problem internationally and in the United States, and highlight approaches designed to aid in understanding, preventing, and intervening in suicidal behavior. The chapter after this one, written by Jack Jordan, will discuss postvention with suicide survivors. I will only note here that postvention can be, and often is, a primary kind of suicide prevention, especially when it is undertaken in schools and in the community.

A LITTLE HISTORY

Suicide is universal. It has occurred in every society of which we have a record. However, it has been viewed very differently at different times and in different cultures. For example, the act of suicide has variously been thought to be a rational or honorable act, evidence of insanity, a sin, a crime, or a failure to cope.

The ways in which societies have reacted to self-killing has also changed across times and cultures. Until the 20th century, the Catholic Church viewed it as a mortal sin and would not bury someone who took his or her life in hallowed ground. Some countries and many states in the United States passed laws against suicide and prosecuted those who attempted but did not complete it. Until recently, survivors of one who had died by suicide were stigmatized, and if one survived a suicidal attempt, he or she was looked at as weak or mentally ill. At best, such people were wracked by shame and guilt; at worst, they were deemed insane and, as a threat to themselves, were often institutionalized.

We can trace the beginning of a change in attitudes toward suicide to two remarkable books. The first was the publication of a treatise on the subject written by John Merian, a Frenchman, in 1763. In it, he claimed that suicide was neither a crime against society nor a sin against the faith, but rather a product of emotional illness (Merian, 1763). The second, *Le Suicide*, written by Emile Durkheim in 1897 ushered in the modern era of research on suicide. Durkheim, who is viewed as the father of modern sociology, examined suicide from a societal angle. He maintained that suicide occurs as a result of a lack of fit between a person and his or her society (Durkheim, 1951). He was the first to develop categories of suicide, which included *altruistic suicide* in which an individual dies to better his or her society in some way; *ritualistic suicide,* such as suttee; *anomic suicide* in which socially isolated people died by their own hand; and *fatalistic* suicide in which people became hopeless and helpless within their life circumstances. Some support for a sociological view of suicide can be found in the growing incidence of suicide throughout the 19th century as agrarian life gave way to the Industrial Revolution, resulting in close ties being broken and an urban way of life replacing the more familiar and closer village life.

As the incidence of suicide increased in first-world countries, individuals and governments began to take notice. As early as 1953, the Samaritan organization, founded by Reverend Chad Varah, began its suicide prevention work in Great Britain. From the outset, it engaged volunteers who were trained to understand depression and to recognize the warning signs and risk factors associated with suicide. These volunteers used the technique of active listening and were expected to take all talk of suicide seriously and focus on the person and his or her immediate situation. Today, the organization has grown to oversee more than 400 suicide prevention centers in 42 different countries. In the United Kingdom alone, it has 201 centers and receives a call over its 24-hour helplines every 6 seconds.

In the United States, the first suicide prevention center was established in Los Angeles in 1958 with a 5-year grant from the U.S. Public Health Service. Edwin Shneidman was the founding director. The center had three major goals: (1) to save lives, (2) to serve as a major public health agency for the community, and (3) to carry out research on suicide. This center quickly became the model for suicide prevention and intervention centers throughout the United States, and its success changed the way the nation viewed suicide and suicidal behavior. There was a shift away from seeing suicide as the act of a sinner or an insane person to seeing it as an act by a troubled person who was crying for help.

In 1966, Shneidman was asked to develop a national prevention program at the National Institute of Mental Health (NIMH). He then served as the first director of the Center for Studies of Suicide Prevention for a brief period. While he was director, the number of suicide prevention centers in the United States tripled. Today, there are more than 150 crisis centers in the United States that participate in the National Suicide Prevention Lifeline (www.sucidepreventionlifeline.org). It is important to note that Shneidman also founded the American Association for Suicidology and the journal *Suicide and Life-Threatening Behavior*. His work formed the foundation for today's study of suicidal behavior and still informs the clinical work with suicidal people and survivors of suicide (1983, 1993, 1996). He richly deserves the title of the Father of Suicidology in the United States.

DIMENSIONS OF THE PROBLEM

The frequency of suicide has continued to increase in the last half century. The World Health Organization (WHO) reports that suicide frequency has increased by 60% in the last 45 years (WHO, 2014). The organization estimates that nearly 1 million people die from suicide each year; a rate of 1 death every 40 seconds. Figure 24.1 shows the growth in suicide for 50 years ending in 2000. As the figure shows, males in nearly all nations complete suicide more frequently than do females, and the discrepancy between the genders has grown across time.

In the United States alone, there are approximately 750,000 suicide attempts each year, 1 every 40 seconds. An estimated 5 million persons living in the United States have attempted suicide. Each suicide intimately affects at least six others. The Centers for Disease Control estimates that based on more than 742,000 suicides that occurred between 1977 and 2001, there are 4,450,000 survivors living in the United States today. Suicide has remained the 10th leading cause of death in the United States for at least five decades.

The statistics on completed suicide tell only a part of the story. For every completed suicide, the American Foundation for Suicide Prevention estimates that there are approximately 12 people hospitalized for self-harm. This is a gross underestimate, however, as many attempts do not lead to hospitalization in the United States.

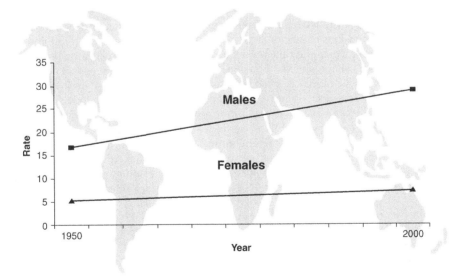

FIGURE 24.1 Worldwide suicide statistics: evolution of global suicide rates 1950–2000 (per 100,000).
Source: World Health Organization, (2002).

MYTHS ABOUT SUICIDE

At least some of the increase in suicide can be related to the myths that still surround it and result in inaction or wrong action. Because suicide has been cloaked in secrecy across millennia, many misconceptions have arisen. Thankfully, enough experience with suicidal people now exists to dispel some of the more common myths. Perhaps the greatest misconception is that people who talk about suicide won't kill themselves. Talk of suicide can be cast aside with the thought that "he or she is only seeking attention" or that "he or she is just depressed today but will be better tomorrow." Psychological autopsies after completed suicides have shown that discussing suicide and/or talking about death are warning signs to be taken seriously.

Another myth is that if people have attempted suicide before, they will not do it again. On the contrary, attempted suicide is a good predictor of future attempts.

A third myth is that if a person is suicidal, there is nothing anyone can do to help him or her. The truth is that the ambivalence inherent in suicidal behavior can be used to "talk the person out of it" temporarily and the success of cognitive behavioral therapy often combined with antidepressants makes a lie of this myth.

UNDERSTANDING AND PREVENTING SUICIDE

The first step in understanding a behavior is to define it. Edwin Shneidman defined "suicide" as follows: "Currently in the Western world, suicide is a conscious act of self-induced annihilation, best understood as a multidimensional malaise in a needful individual who defines an issue for which the suicide is perceived as the best solution" (Shneidman, 1985, p. 203).

But what makes up that "multidimensional malaise?" In our first book, we reviewed the research and clinical case studies reported in the literature about suicide (Stillion, McDowell, & May, 1986). This review, coupled with our own experience, led to the development of a model for understanding the multiple dimensions of suicide. In the second totally revised edition (Stillion & McDowell, 1996), we applied the model across the life span, illustrating how each risk factor could shape suicidal behavior differently at different ages. For example, suicide among children is often impulsive and dependent on environmental conditions (e.g., presence of guns or poisons at home), whereas suicide among elders is generally well planned and more heavily influenced by psychological conditions (e.g., feelings of helplessness and hopelessness).

The model contained four major categories of risk factors that should be taken into account when one is confronted with a suicidal person or counseling with a suicide survivor who is attempting to understand any death by suicide. If we were writing a third edition of the text, we would undoubtedly add a fifth category: spiritual risk factors, as new theories and research now exist that show that spiritual wellness is important to positive mental health (Peterson & Seligman, 2004). As Seligman explains, "After a half century of neglect, psychologists are again studying spirituality and religiosity in earnest, no longer able to ignore their importance to people of faith" (Seligman, 2011, p. 261). Spirituality does not refer to religious beliefs, although such beliefs may be a part of it. Rather it refers to having "strong and coherent beliefs about the higher meaning and purpose of the universe" that serve as a means of comfort to you and give your life meaning because of your attachment to something larger than yourself (Peterson & Seligman, 2004, p. 600). Our revised model appears in Figure 24.2.

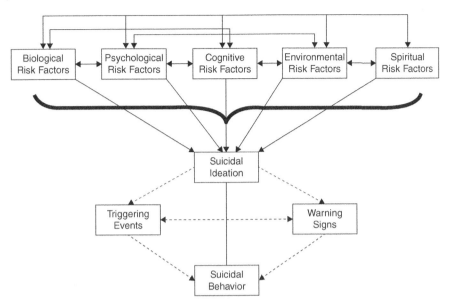

FIGURE 24.2 The suicide trajectory model.
Source: Adapted from Stillion, McDowell, and May (1989, p. 240).

The model depicts five major categories of risk factors: biological, psychological, cognitive, environmental, and spiritual. The closed lines depicted by the top-level arrows reflect the fact that each of these categories can and do interact with any and all of the others. When the combined weight of these risk factors, indicated by the brace, reaches the point where coping skills are overwhelmed, suicidal ideation may result. Suicidal ideation may range from occasional thoughts of suicide to obsessively thinking about it, even to the extent where the person may have devised a plan, including time, place, and method. There may or may not be triggering events and/or warning signs, indicated by the dotted arrows, which then may result in suicidal behavior. Those may be recognized only after the suicidal event. The entire model demonstrates the complexity of behavior that leads to suicide. It is this very complexity that causes many people and organizations to despair of ever successfully preventing suicide.

However, when a situation is complex, it is helpful to break it into its components. The model can serve as a template for responding to any given person. Discussing each risk factor with the suicidal person can pinpoint the elements feeding into the suicidal ideation he or she may be experiencing. For example, examining the environment in which the individual must function, including home, school, social ties, community, availability of weapons and poisons, and the like may suggest immediate remedial steps that could be taken to alleviate some risk (e.g., removing weapons from home). Exploring psychological strengths and past coping practices may provide clarity and allow for expanding on old and/or building new approaches. Probing current cognitive strengths (e.g., learning abilities as well as the mental messages the individual is routinely telling him or herself) may not only provide needed insights into the reason suicide is being considered but also suggest strategies for building up learning capabilities and breaking down negative self-talk. When possible, consideration of biological factors may lead to alternative approaches, such as drug therapy, nutritional counseling, and/or exercise programs for dealing with the individual. Spiritual considerations are also important to probe because suicidal individuals have frequently lost a sense of purpose in their lives and/or think that life has no meaning. Such existential ennui can lead to feelings of helplessness and hopelessness, which are serious indicators of suicidal ideation and behavior.

The most common treatment of overtly suicidal people in the recent past has been to treat them with antidepressants with or without talk therapy. However, it is much more powerful to consider cases holistically by exploring with them their current dimensions of environmental, psychological, cognitive, biological, and spiritual thinking.

The use of the suicide trajectory model is enriched if it is done within a life-span context. To illustrate, let's examine two suicidal people: one of them a 16-year-old girl named Jean; the other a 75-year-old man, David. The biological factors to be considered in Jean's case include the changing hormonal conditions that occur first at puberty and go on into early adulthood. These changes affect the brain as well as the body and may feed into a mood disorder. In David's case, biological factors might include neurotransmitter decline in the brain, general physical decline, onset of organic mental decline, and/or chronic illness accompanied by untreatable pain.

The psychological risk factors that should be considered in Jean's case might include a crisis in identity formation as well as fluctuating mood states. In addition, because adolescence is generally a period of exploration, there might be psychological changes because of experimentation with alcohol or drugs. In David's case, long-term substance abuse, if present, may be accompanied by personality changes. Loneliness is also a factor and the cumulative losses experienced by many elderly people may bring on feelings of uselessness and despair.

Cognitive risk factors to be explored with Jean might include her level of formal operational thinking; that is, does she have a fully mature concept of the finality, universality, and irreversibility of death. Egocentrism peaks in adolescence and may impede her ability to move beyond her current emotional state and/or to view the future realistically. In addition, adolescents tend to have an illusion of invulnerability, which may permit Jean to engage in high-risk behaviors while not thoroughly believing she can die from them. Cognitive factors in David's case might include a decline in fluid intelligence leading to more rigidity of thinking that makes suicide the best solution to life's problems as well as a higher acceptance of death.

Environmental factors to be explored differ with each individual. However, in Jean's case, the family of origin and peer pressures are still potent forces to be examined, whereas that is less true for David. In his case, the quality of social support of peers and children (if any) are more important elements.

In examining spiritual risk factors, Jean may be at risk because of the novelty associated with formal operations: the time in life when youth can first begin to think philosophically about the world. She may be struggling with new questions about fairness, injustice, and dishonesty that she may see around her. David, on the other hand, may or may not be able to depend on a well-thought-out worldview to inoculate him against the despair that sometimes accompanies the entropy that is a hallmark of aging.

PATTERNS OF SUICIDE

The World Health Organization presents data on suicide for more than 110 countries. In all countries reporting, males complete suicide more often than do females; more than five times as often in some countries. The roots of this male–female discrepancy may lie to some extent in biology. However, traditional socialization patterns and environmental factors undoubtedly also play a role (Stillion, 1995). Traditionally, males have been taught to be problem solvers. They have also been taught in many cultures not to show emotional weakness and to be stoic, confiding in few, if any, other people. Such socialization pressures in conjunction with difficult life circumstances can lead to suicidal ideation and to regarding the act of suicide as the best solution to their problems. Because their socialization does not permit them to be dependent and puts a premium on success, if they attempt the act, they may feel great need to complete it. Females, on the other hand, have higher rates of suicide attempts than do males; three times as high in countries like the United States. Their socialization may permit them to use suicide gestures and attempts as cries for outside help. The stigma of a failed suicide attempt is not as great for females and may even bring the desired effect: the attention of medical personnel and the larger community.

In addition, age and level of development are important variables to consider when attempting to prevent suicide. Suicide rates are very high among middle-aged and older populations in the United States. However, much more attention has been placed on the growing incidence of youth suicide for two reasons. First, the death of a teen represents more years of potential life lost (YPLL) than does the death of an adult or elderly person. Second, teen suicide has increased across the past half century. For example, in the United States, suicide among those aged 15 to 24 grew from 4.5 per 100,000 in 1950 to a high of 13.2 per 100,000 in 1990. Although it has since decreased to 10.5 per 100,000 in 2010 (the last year such statistics were available at this writing), it retains the attention of health organizations and it has spurred national and international efforts to respond to suicidal people. It is the 10th leading cause of death among 15-to-24-year-olds. Surprisingly, it is the second leading cause of death among 10-to-14-year-olds in the United States.

It is also important to understand that the rate of death by suicide changes depending on membership in a cohort group. Historically, suicide rates have been low in childhood, rise in adolescence and young adulthood, level off in middle age, especially for women, and rise again in old age, particularly for White males. However, in the late 1990s, these historical patterns began to change (Hu, Wilcox, Wissow, & Baker, 2008). A public health report dated 2010 notes that suicide among middle-aged people has substantially increased in frequency across the last two decades (Phillips, Robin, Nugent, & Idler, 2010). It is now the leading cause of death for people between the ages of 45 and 64 (18.6 per 100,000), which surpasses the rate of those 85 and older (17.6 per 100,000). Because the oldest cohorts have traditionally experienced the highest rate of suicide, this change in cohort rates is noteworthy, especially in light of the rate of suicide for adolescents, aged 15 to 24 (10.5 per 100,000).

Part of this increase among the middle-aged may be due to a cohort effect as it is the baby boom generation that is now in middle age, and it is that cohort that was responsible for the swift rise in adolescent suicide when they were in their teens and young-adult years. The authors note that a large cohort restricts opportunities across the life span and that may be affecting the current middle-aged group. In addition, lifestyle choices among this cohort (e.g., the use of drugs, higher rate of rejection of religion, higher divorce rates, etc.) might feed into the rising rate. An alternative explanation suggested by Phillips et al. (2010) is that the recent harsher economic conditions may lead to a higher level of depression among this cohort group. The authors warn that suicide rates may skyrocket in the near future as the baby boomers enter old age, a time in life that has historically seen high suicide rates, especially for White males.

Another pattern seen in suicide rates is that of marital status. At all ages in adulthood, married people have lower rates of suicide than do single, widowed, or divorced people.

SUICIDE PREVENTION

There are three levels of suicide prevention: primary, which centers on the family, school, and society; secondary, which is made up of intervention and treatment of overtly suicidal persons; and tertiary, which targets survivors of suicide, including the family and friends of someone who has committed suicide and is sometimes referred to as postvention (Stillion & McDowell, 1996, p. 199).

The suicide statistics in the United States and other developed countries tell the tale of failure to teach adequate coping skills in families and schools. Caring families can inoculate children against suicide in many ways. At the most basic level, families are the only place that can offer unconditional acceptance. Children need to know that there is one place where their worth is unquestioned, regardless of their accomplishments. This knowledge wards against feelings of hopelessness that can lead to suicidal behavior. Families are also the starting point for teaching coping skills. In recent years, resilience has been the subject of much research. Although research is somewhat limited, it has been shown that resilience can be taught (Brunwasser, Gillham, & Kim, 2009) and that it can be a defense against depression and suicidal ideation. An example of teaching resilience is encouraging humor within the home. Another example is teaching children that what appears to be failure can be viewed merely as feedback—a lesson to be learned and alternative, more successful techniques to be employed. Avoiding shaming and blaming when a child experiences failure or acts out unacceptably may lead to an opportunity to teach more positive and fruitful behaviors. Finally, families provide many opportunities to teach specific skills.

Parents don't necessarily need the help of professionals to help children deal with anxiety or depression. Indeed, by the time children reach their teen years, they have developed many coping mechanisms on their own. One study, done with gifted ninth graders, showed that those teens had 23 coping mechanisms that they employed to help themselves feel better (Stillion, 1985). These included exercising; eating; talking with friends; listening to music; writing out their feelings in diaries or in letters to friends; composing poetry; taking long walks; focusing on the pluses in their lives; and talking with parents, counselors, and other adults. The teens in this study had not thought of their behaviors as coping mechanisms but recognized them as such once they were labeled in that way. Parents can help children to become aware of using such behaviors when they are feeling low and to suggest other coping behaviors that might guard against depression and/or suicidal ideation. Teaching meditation techniques, systematic relaxation, the use of imagery, and positive self-talk are some other venues for inoculating children against feelings of helplessness.

The relatively new school of positive psychology offers many other suggestions that can serve to fortify children's coping abilities. First among them is to develop an attitude of gratitude. Such an attitude helps children focus beyond the latest hurt or failure by recognizing the positive in their lives. Simple exercises like having very young children relay at bedtime the one thing that happened that day that made them happy can be the beginning of creating a constant habit of gratitude. Learning to have an optimistic, rather than a pessimistic, stance toward life has been correlated with many positive outcomes, such as good health, longevity, even success in academics and vocations. And if you are not born with a tendency to be a cheerfully optimistic person, the best news is that optimism can be learned (Seligman, 1991)!

Other ways that parents can help to suicide-proof their children include having reasonable expectations of behavior and accomplishments; maintaining a warm, supportive, and nurturing environment; encouraging and modeling health interactions with people out of the family; enforcing clear boundaries; and being flexible in dealing with family problems (SAVE.org).

Suicide Prevention in Schools

Beyond the family, schools have powerful opportunities as well as the responsibility to help promote positive mental health among students. It is true that schools have been asked to do many things beyond teaching the basics. They serve as baby-sitters, especially in after-school hours; they are the first defense against hunger with their lunch (and sometimes breakfast) programs; they are required by law to report suspected child abuse and/or neglect; they provide counseling and socialization training; and they teach discipline and provide many other services. Regardless of their many burdens, however, they cannot ignore their duty to observe, identify, and react to students at risk. The 2011 Youth Risk Behavior Survey showed that more than one in seven high school students nationwide reported having seriously considered attempting suicide in the 12 months before the survey was taken and that 7.8%, or about 1 in 13, reported having attempted to take their lives in the same period.

One promising approach to teaching coping skills is resiliency training. Resiliency has been defined in many different ways. Basically, however, it is the ability to rebound from adversity (Henderson & Milstein, 2003). The resilient person not only adapts to a given stressful situation, but by adapting strengthens his or her coping mechanisms to meet ensuing stresses. Many programs have been and are being developed to teach resiliency.

One of the most promising school-based programs is the Penn Resiliency Program (PRP), which is designed for elementary and middle school students. In this program, students learn to detect inaccurate thoughts, challenge negative beliefs, solve problems, and deal with emotions. They also learn specific skills of assertiveness, negotiation, relaxation, and decision making. The program uses skits, role plays, short stories, and cartoons delivered in 12 90 minute or 18 to 24 60 minute sessions to teach these skills. This program differs from others in that it has conducted more than 13 controlled studies, including more than 2,000 children aged 8 to 15. Taken together, the findings of these studies show that the program prevents symptoms of depression and anxiety. Several follow-up studies show that the effects of the training endure even 2 years after the treatment. PRP is being used by some schools in Great Britain and Australia as well as by many schools in the United States.

Before we leave the role of schools in suicide prevention, we need to explore two other avenues used by many schools to deal with the subject: Suicide prevention guidelines for teachers and other school personnel and postvention work in the schools after a suicide has occurred.

Many states now have guidelines specifically designed to help teachers approach the topic with their classes. Such guidelines generally include facts about youth suicide, including national and statewide statistics. They also have curriculum materials that include information about the dimensions of the youth suicide problem, individual coping skills that can be taught, and referral options. In-service training guidelines for faculty and staff are also included that focus on prevention, intervention, and postvention procedures. Finally, guidelines for identifying suicidal students and ways to assess suicide risks as well as crisis response measures are available (Stillion & McDowell, 1996).

Most schools now have well-developed procedures for dealing with crisis situations. Youth suicide has been shown to have both cluster and copycat effects; that is, when one suicide occurs in a given school, it provides a modeling effect. If the follow-up of that suicide is not handled well, other troubled youth may follow the example and choose suicide as a way out of the angst they are feeling. The cluster effect has been documented in several places (e.g., Plano, Texas, where six adolescents died in 1 school year and Cary, North Carolina, where eight students died in a little over 1 year). For these reasons, completed suicide in a school should qualify as a crisis situation.

Both the copycat and the cluster phenomena have caused schools to develop postvention programs for dealing with students, especially those who may be at risk. A widely used set of guidelines for such programs was proposed by Wenckstern and Leenaars (1991). They proposed eight principles for postvention programs. These include the following:

- Begin as soon as possible after the tragedy
- Expect resistance from some but not all students
- Be willing to explore negative emotions toward the victim when the time is right
- Provide ongoing reality testing for students who consider themselves survivors
- Be ready to refer when necessary
- Avoid cliches and banal optimism
- Be prepared to spend significant amounts of time (particularly with self-identified disturbed students)
- Develop the postvention program within a comprehensive health care setting that also includes prevention and intervention

SOCIETY'S ROLE IN SUICIDE PREVENTION

Society's role in the prevention of suicide is both more global and more basic. Much has been written about the ways in which societies feed into suicidal behavior and statistics. Poverty; an environment conducive to drug and alcohol usage; unchecked aggression; prevalence of weapons, especially guns; widespread unemployment; and low aspirations are the breeding grounds for the depression, helplessness, and hopelessness that accompany suicidal behavior.

The World Health Organization through its affiliate, the International Association for Suicide Prevention (IASP), has a website (www.iasp.info/) that provides information on suicide prevention for physicians, teachers, media personnel, and many other groups. Many individual nations have worked to create plans for decreasing suicidal behavior. For example, Canada, Finland, Norway, and Australia have all adopted national strategies for suicide prevention. In 2012, the United States, following up on several earlier reports, published the *National Strategy for*

Suicide Prevention: Goals and Objectives for Suicide Prevention (Benjamin, 2012). The national strategy includes 13 goals and 60 objectives that were updated from the earlier reports to reflect advances in suicide prevention knowledge, research, and practice, as well as broader changes in society and health care delivery that have created new opportunities for suicide prevention. The 60 objectives include promotion of health, methods of treating high-risk individuals, care for people who have lost a loved one to suicide, as well as issues related to research, evaluation, and surveillance. The report takes a comprehensive public health perspective. It highlights promising practices. Cognitive behavioral therapy is one of those as well as the presence of crisis lines and continuity of care within a community. Promoting overall health and personal connectedness with others and with organizations within a community are two other approaches that seem promising. Finally, the report provides information about online resources that show referral on programs and interventions that work. Two of these are the National Registry of Evidence-based Programs and Practices (NREPP) and Best Practice Registry (BPR).

INTERVENTION

Although prevention strategies generally are long term in structure, intervention must be immediate if it is to succeed. Intervention entails recognizing warning signs, responding appropriately to the suicidal individual, and accessing long-term aid for him or her. The suicide trajectory model presented earlier recognizes the importance of both warning signs and triggering events. Although there can be many kinds of warning signs (some not recognized until after the event), some of the most common behavioral signs include talking about death, looking for a method (e.g., buying a gun), talking about being a burden, increasing use of alcohol or drugs, behaving recklessly, sleeping too much or too little, withdrawing from others, visiting or calling people to say goodbye, setting affairs in order, and giving away prized possessions. Emotional signs may include uncontrolled rage; extreme mood swings; acting anxious or agitated; feelings of being trapped, in unbearable pain, or isolated; and, most important, feeling helpless and hopeless in the current situation (Suicide Awareness Voices of Education, 2013). Sometimes caring people can be fooled into thinking a depressed person has "turned the corner" when he or she suddenly seems noticeably happier or calmer after a prolonged period of anxiety, depression, and/or agitation. The apparent calmness may indicate that the person has made the decision to attempt suicide.

When interacting with a person who seems actively suicidal, the common wisdom is to confront the person directly. Almost all suicide hotlines and most suicide websites contain common intervention strategies. Generally, they include advice to assess the level of lethality of the person. Such questions as "How bad are you feeling? Bad enough to consider harming yourself?" are appropriate as are follow-up questions such as "Have you considered how you might do it?," "When?," "Where?." An adolescent who is in the midst of a depressive episode after a break-up with his girlfriend but denies considering suicide and has no plan for it is obviously less at risk than a 45-year-old man who has lost his job and family, has a gun, and intends to use it the next day, which would have been his next wedding anniversary in the driveway of his ex-wife's home. In the first instance, the adolescent might consider seeking the support of a trained professional to get him through the worst of his depression. In the second instance, most untrained confidants as well as trained professionals would recognize the imminent danger and would know to stay with the person until he or she could be hospitalized for observation and treatment.

A LOOK AHEAD

Since suicide has existed throughout history, it is not likely to disappear in any imaginable future. However, the incidence of suicide can be lessened. Suicide is most likely to occur when people feel an overwhelming sense of helplessness in their life circumstances and hopelessness to change them. Societies that are serious about decreasing the frequency of suicide must address the conditions that lead to those feelings.

However, even if poverty were eradicated and unlimited opportunity were a reality for everyone, suicide would still exist. There is a biological basis for the depression that can contribute to suicide. In fact, biological changes are most likely present in every suicide as they are the "final common pathway" that is brought about by a person's life circumstances, lack of coping mechanisms, negative self-talk and cognitive rigidity, and spiritual aridity. A person may also be born with a biological inclination toward depression. Such people need far fewer stressors of any kind to consider suicide as an answer to their problems. This necessitates more research directed toward the biological basis of suicidal depression. In addition, outcomes-oriented research into cognitive behavioral approaches, resilience training, and other measures aimed at preventing suicide are needed. As communities come together and adopt a public health approach to suicide prevention and intervention, the statistics on suicide should decrease. Education for school and medical personnel as well as for the public should lead not only to better understanding of the nature of the suicidal mind but also to early identification of those at risk and subsequent treatment and follow-up. Caring societies in the 21st century cannot do less.

REFERENCES

Benjamin, R. U.S. Department of Health and Human Services, Office of the Surgeon General, & National Action Alliance for Suicide Prevention. (2012). *National strategy for suicide prevention: Goals and objectives for action.* Washington, DC: U.S. Department of Health and Human Services.

Brunwasser, S., Gillham, J., & Kim, E. (2009). A meta-analytic review of the Penn Resiliency Program's effect on depressive symptoms. *Journal of Consulting and Clinical Psychology, 77*(6), 1042–1054.

Durkheim, E. (1951). *Le suicide* (J. A. Spaulding & G. Simpson, Trans.). Glencoe, IL: Free Press. (Original work published 1897)

Henderson, N., & Milstein, M. (2003). *Resiliency in schools: Making it happen for students and educators.* Maxico, TX: Corwin Press.

Hu, G., Wilcox, H., Wissow, L., & Baker, S. (2008). Midlife suicide: An increasing problem in U.S. whites, 1999–2005. *American Journal of Preventive Medicine, 35*(6), 589–593.

Merian, J. (1763). Sur la crainte de la mort, sur le mepris de la mort, sur le suicide, memoire [About the fear of death, about contempt for death, about suicide, recollection]. In *Histoire de l'Academie Royale des Sciences et Belles-Lettres de Berlin* (Vol. 19).

Peterson, C., & Seligman, M. (2004). *Character strengths and virtues: A handbook and classification.* Washington, DC: Oxford University Press.

Penn Resiliency Program. (n.d.). Retrieved from www.ppc.sas.upenn.edu/prpsum.htm

Phillips, J., Robin, A., Nugent, C., & Idler, E. (2010). Understanding recent changes in suicide rates among the middle-aged: Period or cohort effects? *Public Health Report, 125*(5), 680–688.

Seligman, M. (1991). *Learned optimism: How to change your mind and your life.* New York, NY: Alfred A. Knopf.

Seligman, M. (2011). *Flourish: A visionary new understanding of happiness and well-being.* New York, NY: Free Press.

Shneidman, E. (1985). *Definition of suicide.* New York, NY: Wiley.

Shneidman, E. (1993). *Suicide as psychache: A clinical approach to self-destructive behavior.* Northvale, NJ: Jason Aronson.

Shneidman, E. (1996). *The suicidal mind.* New York, NY: Oxford University Press.

Stillion, J., McDowell, E., & May, J. (1989). *Suicide across the lifespan: Premature exits.* New York, NY: Taylor and Francis.

Stillion, J. (1995). Premature deaths among males. In D. Sabo & D. Gordon (Eds.), *Men's health and illness: Gender, power and the body.* Thousand Oaks, CA: SAGE.

Stillion, J., & McDowell, E. (1996). *Suicide across the lifespan* (2nd ed.). New York, NY: Taylor & Francis.

Suicide Awareness Voices of Education. (2013). www.save.org/index.cfm?fuseaction=home .viewpage&page_id=705f4071-99a7-f3f5-e2a64a5a8beaadd8

Wenckstern, S., & Leenaars, A. (1991) Suicide postvention: A case illustration in a secondary school. In A. A. Leenaars (Ed.), *Suicide prevention in the schools.* New York, NY: Hemisphere.

WHO (2014). World Health Statistics:2013. Geneva, Switzerland: WHO press.

John R. Jordan

25

GRIEF AFTER SUICIDE: THE EVOLUTION OF SUICIDE POSTVENTION

Like a tornado that sweeps through a community, a suicide can leave in its wake a wide swath of psychological wreckage: shock and confusion, horror, profound guilt, anger and blame, and, of course, sorrow. Suicide survivors (people who are grieving after the loss of someone important to them to suicide) are left to wonder "Why did they do this? Whose fault is it? Could we have done something to see it coming or prevent it? How could they do this to me/us?" And the survivors can be more than just the immediate family of the deceased—friends, neighbors, coworkers, and entire communities can be devastated when suicide happens.

In this chapter, I hope to accomplish several things. First, I would like to briefly describe my involvement in the field and then offer the reader some background on the impact of suicide, and the domain of postvention (the term coined by Edwin Shneidman for the efforts after a suicide to help the survivors and to mitigate its deleterious impact; Shneidman, 1972). I will identify many of the key figures and landmark intellectual events in the development of suicide postvention in the United States. Next, I will discuss current interventions for survivors across different therapeutic modalities, including organizational postvention, and group, family, and individual therapies. Last, I will discuss some future directions and developments that I believe are likely for the field of postvention in the 21st century.

PERSONAL EVOLUTION

I would like to explain briefly my own involvement with suicide prevention and postvention. Personally, I had a great uncle die by suicide in 1987, at the age of 87. Likewise, I had one patient die by suicide—a man who took his life about 3 months after stopping couples therapy and ending the marriage with his wife. Although initially disturbing and sad for me, neither event significantly influenced the course of my personal or professional life.

What did have a major impact was an event in my private practice. I had a number of survivors in my practice with whom I was meeting individually. One day, I had a realization that there was something that these individuals could offer to each other that I, as a mental health clinician and a "distant survivor," could not. So, I began a survivor support group that ran, in various formats, for more than 13 years. Over the course of that group, I was moved by the amount of suffering in the group, yet inspired by the tremendous resilience that survivors showed when they were provided a setting that offered nonjudgmental support, compassion, and hope.

From this experience, I began to specialize in working with suicide survivors. I also became actively involved with the American Foundation for Suicide Prevention (AFSP), helping them to develop a training for survivors (and professionals) who wanted to run bereavement support groups for survivors. More recently, I have helped AFSP and the American Association of Suicidology develop a training for mental health professionals about providing grief therapy for survivors. At this point, about 90% of my writing, research, clinical practice, and training activities are related to suicide postvention.

EVOLUTION OF THE RESPONSE TO A PUBLIC HEALTH PROBLEM

There is a cultural shift going on in the United States (and around the world) in which suicide is coming "out of the closet" and increasingly viewed as an important public health problem. As the tenth overall leading cause of death and third overall leading cause of death for adolescents, significant strides are being made to reduce the incidence of suicide in America (U.S. Department of Health & Human Services, Office of the Surgeon General & National Action Alliance for Suicide Prevention, 2012). Along with this shift, there is a growing appreciation of the psychological damage that suicide may cause to those left behind and therefore of the importance of postvention efforts after a suicide occurs. There is now compelling evidence that people exposed to suicide, particularly those who are emotionally close or biologically related to the deceased, are at elevated risk for suicide themselves (Qin, Agerbo, & Mortensen, 2002). Suicide-prevention leaders are recognizing that postvention is not just the morally correct and compassionate response to such a tragedy, but a crucial component of suicide prevention with a population of people known to be at elevated risk for suicide.

Beyond this elevated risk, there is also substantial evidence that survivors may experience high levels of psychiatric morbidity, social alienation, and stigmatization, and longer term mental health consequences (De Groot & Killen, 2013; Jordan, 2001; Jordan & McIntosh, 2011c; McIntosh & Jordan, 2011b). The literature on whether and in what ways bereavement after suicide is different from other types of death has been the source of some controversy and confusion, because the studies comparing populations bereaved by different causes of death have shown mixed results (Jordan, 2001; Sveen & Walby, 2008). In a recent review of the studies in question, Jordan and McIntosh concluded that suicide bereavement shares universal elements of grief after any type of loss (e.g., yearning for the deceased); elements of grief after sudden unexpected losses (e.g., shock and disbelief); and elements of grief after other sudden, violent deaths, such as homicide (e.g., PTSD; Jordan & McIntosh, 2011b). They also suggested that some elements of bereavement are likely to be more prominent after a suicide than after most other types of death. These include increased levels of guilt, stigmatization, anger, perceived abandonment by the deceased, and blaming. Also prominent is the difficulty in making sense of the suicide. For those who are blind-sided by the death, a suicide may seem inexplicable and incomprehensible ("he could never have done this"). In this sense, suicide may entail a powerful rupturing of the mourner's assumptive world, including the belief that we can fully know other people or that we can always keep those we love safe from harm. For other survivors, however, particularly when the deceased suffered from a serious psychiatric condition, the death may not have been unexpected or seen as out of character. Instead, such a "feared suicide" may elicit more prominent themes of helplessness, relief that the suffering is over, and guilt for feeling that relief.

INTERVENTIONS FOR SURVIVORS—HISTORY

The effort to help survivors has become a social/political movement, often driven by activists who found themselves bereaved, isolated, and with nowhere to turn for support. Many survivors also feel that the mental health system in America has failed both their loved one before the suicide, and now themselves. As such, much of the "resource infrastructure" available to the bereaved by suicide in the United States consists of services begun by, and often run by, survivors themselves. By far, the most common services are open, drop-in bereavement support groups that are facilitated by a survivor (Cerel, Padgett, Conwell, & Reed, 2009; Cerel, Padgett, & Reed, 2009). In addition to groups, other services may include annual memorial services, fund-raising efforts, outreach to new survivors, newsletters, community education, and the creation of other venues by which survivors can find and interact with one another. Examples of such survivor-initiated programs include Heartbeat, begun by LaRita Archibald in Colorado, Friends for Survivors begun by Marilyn Koenig in California, and The LINK Counseling Center begun by Iris Bolton in Georgia (Jordan & McIntosh, 2011a). Another striking example of a survivor–professional partnership is the Baton Rouge Crisis Intervention Center, begun by Dr. Frank Campbell. This center offers a full range of interventions for suicide survivors: professional therapy, peer-led support groups, and a ground-breaking outreach program called the LOSS Team. The latter consists of a mental health professional and a trained survivor volunteer who go with the police or medical examiner to visit newly bereaved families on the day of the death, often at the scene of the suicide (Campbell, 2011). This pattern of intimate involvement of survivors in providing help to other survivors has played a much larger role in developing suicide postvention services than in most other nations around the world.

Also central to the development of postvention in the United States have been three national organizations. The first is the American Association of Suicidology (AAS; Linn-Gust, 2011). AAS was founded in 1968 by clinical psychologist Edwin Shneidman, considered the father of modern suicidology. The organization is a multidisciplinary membership organization that creates a nexus for clinicians, researchers, and academics to exchange ideas, findings, and concerns. Within the annual AAS meeting, a "conference within a conference" called the Healing After Suicide Conference has been introduced, specifically for suicide survivors. This gathering has become a focal event for the postvention community, along with the newsletter published by AAS (*Surviving Suicide*), an online searchable database of support groups, and other activities sponsored by AAS. Also unique is an online support resource for clinicians who are survivors of either patient or family suicides. For more information about AAS and its postvention resources, see www.suicidology.org.

A second important national organization is the American Foundation for Suicide Prevention (Harpel, 2011). This group, originally founded in 1987 to raise funds for research into suicide prevention, has expanded its mission to become the largest U.S. organization concerned with the needs of suicide survivors. AFSP's services include International Survivors of Suicide Day, an event that gathers survivors at more than 300 sites within the United States and more than two dozen nations around the world. AFSP also trains survivor volunteers and mental health professionals in the skills necessary to facilitate bereavement support groups for survivors, provides informational home visits for newly bereaved survivors through its network of local chapters, and partners with AAS to offer a new training for mental health professionals focused on clinical work with suicide survivors. AFSP also sponsors "Out of the Darkness" fund-raising walks that serve as a venue for survivors to take positive action together to prevent suicide and help new survivors. Beyond postvention, AFSP sponsors several million dollars' worth of research into the causes and prevention of suicide and maintains an active advocacy effort on behalf of suicide prevention and postvention. For more information on AFSP, see www.afsp.org.

Third, the recently formed National Action Alliance for Suicide Prevention (NAASP) is a public–private partnership dedicated to reducing suicide in America. Among its activities have been the issuing of an updated U.S. National Strategy for Suicide Prevention (U.S. Department of Health & Human Services, Office of the Surgeon General & National Action Alliance for Suicide Prevention, 2012), and the formation of a Survivors of Suicide Loss Task Force. The task force is currently writing postvention guidelines for the United States. When completed, this groundbreaking document will provide recommendations for communities, tribes, states, and the nation as a whole for the development of comprehensive and effective postvention services. For more information on NAASP, see www.actionallianceforsuicideprevention.org/.

There have been several important milestones in the expansion of our theoretical understanding of the impact of suicide and the role of postvention. Arguably, the field of survivor studies can be traced back to the publication of Albert Cain's landmark book, *Survivors of Suicide* (1972). This pioneering publication was the first clinically oriented volume to describe some of the problematic reactions to a suicide experienced by many survivors. A second major contribution was the book *Suicide and Its Aftermath: Understanding and Counseling the Survivors* (Dunne, McIntosh, & Dunne-Maxim, 1987). This comprehensive volume offered chapters on the social context of suicide, personal accounts of survivors, the impact of patient suicide on professional caregivers, and interventions for both first responders (clergy, police, funeral directors, etc.) and mental health clinicians. A subsequent book by Mishara followed a similar track by examining the impact of suicide on individuals, families, helping professionals, and society as a whole (Mishara, 1995). A long hiatus followed, until the publication in 2011 of Jordan and McIntosh's broad update of the knowledge base about survivors and interventions to help them. This work surveyed the considerable body of new research produced in the last two decades on suicide bereavement in both adults and children, addressed key questions in the field (e.g., Is suicide bereavement different? What is a working definition of a survivor?), offered chapters on clinical work with individuals, families, groups, and organizations after a suicide, presented capsule summaries of 19 U.S. and international survivor support programs, and concluded with detailed recommendations for advancing both research and clinical/programmatic agendas within the field (Jordan & McIntosh, 2011a). Currently, this book stands as the most complete and up-to-date summary of the "state of the art" in suicide postvention.

INTERVENTIONS FOR SURVIVORS—CURRENT STANDING

Despite the widespread negative impact of suicide, little has been studied about the mitigation of its effects and assistance for those affected by this significant public health problem. Recent reviews of the literature on interventions for suicide survivors concur on the paucity of studies on interventions for survivors (Cerel, Padgett, Conwell, et al., 2009; Jordan & McMenamy, 2004; McDaid, Trowman, Golder, Hawton, & Sowden, 2008). Of the research that has been conducted (primarily on group or family interventions), the results have been mixed about the efficacy of the interventions, although most studies have found small positive effects for the treatments studied. Regrettably, most of the research has suffered from a number of methodological limitations that make evidence-based conclusions very tentative (McIntosh & Jordan, 2011a). There have also been a number of clinical descriptions of interventions published, using group, individual, and family methods (Jordan, 2008, 2009, 2011a, 2011b; Kaslow, Samples, Rhodes, & Gantt, 2011; Mitchell & Wesner, 2011).

Organizational Postvention

Suicide can have a shocking effect on organizations and groups—schools, workplaces, churches, and so forth. Historically, the tendency has been to simply ignore the "elephant in the room" after a suicide, avoiding public discussion of the event and its impact on members of the group. This is changing, however, as organizations recognize that a community-wide response is required after a suicide. This is true not only because suicide is disturbing to the equilibrium of the community, but also because within settings that are populated by adolescents and young adults (e.g., schools, the military), there is a danger of suicide contagion—the spread of suicidal behavior among other vulnerable young people in that setting (Gould, Greenberg, Velting, & Shaffer, 2006).

Postvention typically includes a multipronged response that begins with providing active support and education for the leadership of the community so that they in turn can respond appropriately and openly to the reactions of students or employees. Postvention also includes helping members of the community find safe and appropriate ways to express and share their grief, while also using the event as a "teachable moment" about the causes of suicide, resources that are available to suicidal persons, and suitable ways of reaching out to community members who might be suicidal themselves. Last, comprehensive postvention responses help the organization to develop well-thought-out plans for dealing with the longer term fallout from the suicide and the implementation of efforts to prevent suicide in the future. For more information about organizational postvention after suicide, see Berkowitz, McCauley, Schuurman, and Jordan (2011) and the excellent toolkit for schools developed by AFSP (http://www.afsp.org/content/search?SearchText=toolkit).

Support Groups

Support groups have become a major source of intervention for suicide survivors in the United States. Most groups are open, "drop-in" groups, often led by survivors. Sometimes they are run by a professional through a local organization (typically a hospice), and sometimes they are co-led by a hybrid team of a survivor volunteer and a professional. Unfortunately, there has been very little systematic research about the efficacy of participation in support groups, although anecdotal evidence suggests that for people who participate in groups, they are quite helpful (Cerel, Padgett, Conwell, et al., 2009; Feigelman, Jordan, McIntosh, & Feigelman, 2012).

Unlike formal, therapy groups, support groups do not typically focus on changing dysfunctional behaviors or attitudes among the participants. Rather, they make available an emotionally safe and nonjudgmental setting in which members can tell their story, receive empathic support, and exchange ideas about coping and resources. They also provide a venue in which "veteran" survivors help themselves by helping others who are new in their grief—a process of reempowerment that may counteract the helplessness often engendered by suicide. Last, support groups can reduce the tremendous isolation and estrangement that many survivors feel from their regular social networks, while offering hope for a restoration of one's life (Feigelman et al., 2012).

Although their number has been growing, finding an accessible support group still continues to be a major problem for many new survivors (McMenamy, Jordan, & Mitchell, 2008). In addition, the format of a support group may feel uncomfortable for many people, particularly men. Thus, other types of support resources are needed (Jordan, McIntosh, et al., 2011). One possibility is the growing number of online support groups and other forms of survivor-to-survivor interaction, which may better meet the needs of survivors (Beal, 2011). For more on suicide bereavement support groups, see Feigelman et al. (2012) and Jordan (2011a).

Family Interventions

Suicide impacts the entire family, in complex and sometimes devastating ways (Cerel, Jordan, & Duberstein, 2008). To begin with, suicide may be an outcome that is embedded in family conflict and distress. There is evidence that families with a suicide often display more dysfunction, abuse, substance abuse, and psychiatric disorder before the death than families without a suicide (Cerel et al., 2008). When the family has had significant problems before the death, issues of guilt and blame are likely to be at a high level after the death. The scapegoating that may follow a suicide can be toxic to family cohesion, sometimes leading to a permanent fracturing of the relationships in families. It is important to note that the majority of families with a suicide do not manifest excessive levels of family problems, other than the problems caused by a member with a psychiatric disorder. Emerging from societal ignorance about suicide, the popular public perception that a suicide is "proof" that the family is dysfunctional is simply wrong.

A suicide can contribute to tension within a family, even when members are not caught up in anger and blaming around the death. Any type of traumatic death tends to produce "coping asynchrony," a mismatch of individual family members' coping styles that may create relational strain. For example, parents who lose a child to suicide may employ very different ways of managing the intense pain associated with their grief. In a similar fashion, a deeply bereaved and traumatized parent may be considerably less emotionally present for their remaining children, sometimes for an extended period of time. Likewise, the family's collective assumptive world—its collective belief system about the predictability and controllability of events and the availability of members—may all be shattered by the suicide (Jordan, Kraus, & Ware, 1993).

Interventions to mitigate some of these negative effects for families bereaved by suicide have not been extensively studied, although family-oriented models of postvention have been proposed in the literature (Kaslow et al., 2011; Mitchell & Wesner, 2011). Several clinically based guidelines have also been offered (Dunne & Dunne-Maxim, 2004; Kaslow & Gilman Aronson, 2004; Parrish & Tunkle, 2003). In the only randomized controlled trial of a brief family intervention specifically designed to reduce complicated grief, de Groot found that her intervention helped to reduce blame and maladaptive grief reactions in participants, but did not reduce the incidence of complicated grief or depression (de Groot et al., 2007). In general, recommendations for family interventions call for the creation of a psychologically safe setting for family members to share their grief and support one another; provision of extensive psychoeducation of family members about suicide, grief, and posttraumatic stress disorder (PTSD); extension of help in dealing with the stigmatized social reactions of others; and assessment of developing psychiatric morbidity among members (depression, substance abuse, and suicidal ideation). It should also be noted that several family-focused and evidence-based bereavement interventions have been developed (Kissane & Hooghe, 2011; Sandler et al., 2003). Although not specifically developed for or tested with suicide survivors, these therapies could potentially be helpful after a suicide as well.

Individual Grief Therapy

Perhaps the most common form of intervention for suicide survivors is individual grief therapy, with a significant number of survivors seeking mental health consultation at some point in their recovery process (Dyregrov, Plyhn, Dieserud, & Oatley, 2012; McMenamy et al., 2008). As with family interventions, individual therapy has not been studied specifically in the context of suicide.[1] However, there are a number of reports of promising general treatments for complicated grief (Wittouck, Van Autreve, De Jaegere, Portzky, & van Heeringen, 2011). There have also been a number of clinical descriptions of individual treatment of survivors (Pearlman, Wortman, Feuer, Farber, Rando, 2014), with perhaps the most recent and comprehensive ones being offered by Jordan (Jordan, 2011b). Jordan has identified a number of "tasks of healing" that are relevant for most suicide survivors and can become the agenda for individual grief therapy with survivors (Jordan, 2009). These tasks include the following:

- *Containment of the trauma*—Suicide often produces PTSD-type symptoms in survivors (physiological arousal, "flashbacks," disruption of biorhythms, irritability, emotional numbing, etc.) that are both intrusive and highly distressing. These typically need to be addressed early in the treatment because the horror of the death and accompanying trauma symptoms make attending to grief work much more difficult. Effective trauma-reduction techniques may include eye movement desensitization and reprocessing (EMDR) and other forms of exposure therapies that help to habituate the trauma response (Pearlman et al., 2014).
- *Learning skills for dosing grief, finding sanctuary, and cultivating psychic analgesia*—Traumatic bereavement entails intense psychic pain, and a major task for survivors is to gain some regulatory control over that pain so that it can be absorbed in manageable pieces. Imparting these skills can empower the mourner to make the grief more "voluntary," with the time and place of experiencing the grief more under the control of the bereaved. These skills can include the development of self-soothing activities (meditation, massage, etc.) and distraction and avoidance skills (recognizing and avoiding unnecessary "triggers" associated with the loss, and cultivation of positive affective experiences that produce relief). These skills can then be alternated with exposure skills that are necessary for confronting the loss (visiting the grave, looking at photographs or videos, etc.). This alternation between moving toward and away from the loss fits well with the dual-process model of grieving proposed by Stroebe (Stroebe & Schut, 1999).
- *Creation of a complex, realistic, and compassionate narrative of the suicide through a personal psychological autopsy*—Suicide can be described as the "perfect storm"—a complex convergence of multiple factors in just the "wrong" way that allows suicide to happen (genetics, neurobiology, psychiatric disorder, life stressors, difficult access to treatment and easy access to a means for suicide, and decision making on the part of the deceased; Stillion & McDowell, 1996). Conversely, suicide is rarely, if ever, the result of just one event, problem, or

factor. Most survivors know little about what contributes to suicide. They tend to feel that the suicide could and should have been prevented, if someone had done something different—and for most survivors, that someone starts with themselves. Over time, survivors often need to conduct a kind of psychological autopsy to understand the state of mind of the deceased and to piece together a narrative of why the suicide happened and what role various people (including themselves) played in the suicide. The path to successful coping with this crucial "why" question often involves acquiring the capacity to "hold complexity" (Sands, Jordan, & Neimeyer, 2011). This means being able to see the many elements in the perfect storm, to realistically sort out what was and was not under the survivor's control, to accept the limitations on their ability to influence the outcome, and to forgive themselves for actions that, in hindsight, might have been taken differently.

- *Learning skills to manage changed social connections*—Suicide frequently disrupts the social bonds between people, both within the family and with the larger social network. Survivors have to deal with what has been called the "social incompetence" of parts of their social networks (Dyregrov et al., 2012). Survivors may sometimes encounter anger, blame, and outright shunning from some people in their family or community (Range, 1998). They may be the recipients of insensitive and intrusive comments from others ("Didn't you know they were depressed?" "What a selfish thing they did to you!"). Perhaps more commonly, survivors encounter avoidance behaviors from other people due to what can be called "social ambiguity"—avoidance behavior that is not necessarily the result of outright condemnation of the suicide or survivor, but more of awkwardness and confusion about how to appropriately interact with the survivor. Nonetheless, this social distancing can be experienced as abandonment and can greatly contribute to the isolation that suicide may generate. The management of these altered social connections becomes a new skill set that survivors are forced to learn in the midst of their need to mourn their loss, adding to the difficulty of navigating in a postsuicide interpersonal landscape.

- *Repair and transformation of the bond with the deceased*—Suicide almost always entails a rupturing of the relationship with the deceased. If it comes at the end of a long, downward trajectory of psychiatric illness, the rupturing may have begun long before the actual suicide. Conversely, the suicide may be a stunning event, one that is experienced as an utterly unforeseen abandonment and betrayal by the loved one. Thanatology has advanced in the last two decades by recognizing that many people continue a psychological relationship with their deceased loved one (Klass, Silverman, & Nickman, 1996; Stroebe, Schut, & Boerner, 2010). Just as relational repair might be needed if the deceased had emotionally injured the person while alive (e.g., a husband running off with another woman), this psychological healing work often needs to be accomplished between the mourner and their loved one after a suicide. This is a task for which a skilled grief therapist, equipped with the right clinical technique, at the right time, can be particularly helpful to a survivor (Jordan, 2012; Neimeyer, 2012).

- *Memorialization of the deceased*—Memorialization is a universal practice among human beings. However, this important process can be more difficult after a suicide, a type of death that is often stigmatized, disenfranchised, and experienced by the mourner as a personal rejection or a publically dishonorable action. A significant task for survivors is to find ways to remember and honor the *whole* life of the deceased, while putting the suicide in the context of that life. Just as we do not define people by their mode of death if they die of cancer or heart disease, we do not need to do that with suicide. Survivors often need support for reviewing and valuing the entire life of the deceased, rather than just their manner of death.

• *Restoration of functioning and reinvestment in life*—As with all bereavement, survivors have to "relearn the world" that may have been profoundly changed by the suicide (Attig, 2011). This involves transforming the attachment to the deceased and learning to find meaning, pleasure, and purpose in a changed but still satisfying way of life without the deceased.

A skilled grief therapist can be instrumental in helping a traumatized survivor work on all of these healing tasks. The core of all grief therapy is an empathically attuned and skillfully applied use of the therapeutic relationship as an attachment bond that helps the bereaved and traumatized individual to reregulate their physical, cognitive, and emotional life (Jordan, 2008, 2011b; Winokuer & Harris, 2012). Various techniques are evolving in thanatology that allow the survivor and clinician to work on each of these tasks of healing activities (Neimeyer, 2012; Pearlman et al., 2015). For example, a technique described by Jordan (2012) involves the use of a guided-imagery conversation with the deceased that includes visualizing them as completely physically and, in the case of suicide, psychologically healed. The deceased is imagined as an empathic and attuned listener, ready to hear whatever the mourner needs to tell them. The mourner can then proceed to talk with the loved one about any aspect of the ruptured relationship that remains problematic, as well as the impact of the suicide on the mourner. Although this technique can most obviously be helpful with repair of the bond with the deceased, it can also be useful for working through the traumatic aspects of the death, the elaboration of a narrative for the death, and memorialization of the deceased.

INTERVENTIONS FOR SURVIVORS—FUTURE DIRECTIONS

There are a number of promising directions in which survivor services are moving. There are also a number of recommendations that have been made for expanding survivor services in the United States that I will briefly summarize to conclude this chapter (Jordan, McIntosh, et al., 2011; McIntosh & Jordan, 2011a).

Closer Integration With Suicide-Prevention Efforts

Suicide bereavement has traditionally been the "caboose" in suicidology, even though much of the support for prevention efforts results from the fund-raising, political advocacy, and hard work of survivors. There is considerable evidence that exposure to suicide is both more widespread than generally understood (particularly if one includes exposure to suicide attempts) and that exposure carries with it many negative mental health consequences, including an elevated rate of suicidality. Despite this, the field of suicidology has generally failed to recognize that postvention services should be an integral part of suicide-prevention programs. One important development in this regard is the work of the Suicide Loss Task Force of the National Action Alliance for Suicide Prevention (see http://actionallianceforsuicideprevention.org/task-force/survivors-suicide-loss). This working group of experts in postvention expects to release national guidelines for suicide postvention in 2014, an action that should help to accelerate this awareness of the need for effective postvention.

Training of First Responders and Clinicians Who Work With Survivors

People who are traumatized by the suicide of their loved one are in a vulnerable psychological state of mind. For better or worse, the actions of caregivers who have early contact with survivors (police, emergency medical professionals, clergy, funeral directors, etc.) can have a lasting impact on the newly bereaved. Likewise, mental health professionals can play a pivotal role in the longer term healing process of survivors (Campbell, Simon, & Hales, 2006). Regrettably, the great majority of first responders and clinicians receive little or no training in how to respond to survivors. Indeed, many times these professional caregivers reflect the larger societal attitudes of fear and condemnation of anything connected with suicide. Recognition of the vital need for training in the provision of psychological first aid and grief therapy with survivors is growing, driven in part by survivors who have had damaging experiences with one or both groups of caregivers. An excellent example of a statewide program that provides this kind of discipline-specific training is the Connect Program in New Hampshire (see http://www.theconnectprogram.org/new-hampshire-suicide-prevention-resources-and-links). Likewise, a new, collaborative training developed by the American Association of Suicidology and the American Foundation for Suicide Prevention will provide a day-long training in grief therapy for suicide survivors for interested mental health professionals (see http://www.afsp.org/coping-with-suicide/education-training/aas-afsp-suicide-bereavement-clinician-training-program). AAS/AFSP will also develop a searchable, online database of clinicians who have completed the training so that survivors can have an accessible resource for finding a "survivor knowledgeable" therapist in their area.

Development of Culturally Competent Postvention Services

Suicide is no respecter of race, ethnicity, or religious affiliation. Anecdotal evidence suggests that there are commonalities in the psychological experience of survivors across different cultural groups. Still, the way in which grief is processed by diverse cultures, along with the differing social attitudes toward suicide, mean that postvention services that are culturally sensitive and specific need to be developed. In the United States, most postvention services have been designed by and tend to service Caucasian people of European descent. With a few notable exceptions, services for African Americans, Latinos, Asians, and other ethnic minorities in this country are yet to be developed. The expansion of such culturally competent programs must include the active input of people from the communities for whom the services are being established (Kaslow et al., 2011).

Expansion and Innovation of Postvention Services

Many new survivors report great difficulty locating services when the need arises (Jordan, Feigelman, McMenamy, & Mitchell, 2011; McMenamy et al., 2008). Even when survivors are able to find services, they may be very limited in nature and unsuitable for the emotional needs and desires of some survivors. For example, a twice-a-month, face-to-face bereavement support group may work well for some individuals, but will be actively rejected by others who feel they are too public, too psychologically threatening, or just not sufficient for their needs. This suggests a pressing need to create multiple pathways by which new survivors can find the support they need and multiple interventions once they find a provider of such services (Jordan, McIntosh, et al., 2011).

For example, the literature suggests that in the first year after bereavement, many survivors are too traumatized and depressed to seek out community services. Outreach teams of trained survivors and/or mental health professionals who visit new survivors in their homes can often provide both immediate, crisis-oriented support and also serve as a bridge to increase their willingness and capacity to find needed services (Cerel & Campbell, 2008). The Baton Rouge Crisis Center (Campbell, 2011), Grief Support Services of the Samaritans in Boston (Hurtig, Bullitt, & Kates, 2011), and the outreach program of the American Foundation for Suicide Prevention (Harpel, 2011) are all outstanding examples of this type of innovative service.

Other examples of groundbreaking services for survivors can be mentioned. Schwartz has described an innovative facilitated family retreat for survivor families (Schwartz, 2011). This intervention is a 1- or-2-day networking meeting of the immediate and extended family members of the deceased to share perspectives on the suicide, provide mutual support, and identify and deal with the effects of the suicide on the family. Beal has developed a pioneering Internet-based support service for survivors that includes multiple forms of message boards where survivors post their experience and receive feedback and support from other survivors, a memorial website to honor loved ones, and an e-newsletter (Beal, 2011). Beal's group also has begun holding face-to-face retreats for survivors who have met through the website. Last, programs are experimenting with the facilitation of other forms of survivor-to-survivor contact. These might include matching survivors one-on-one in person or on the Internet with another survivor with a similar experience (e.g., a bereaved mother with another bereaved mother). All of these pioneering efforts are built on the common principle of creating an emotionally safe venue where survivors can share their experience, learn from others, and receive inspiration and hope that surviving the death of a loved one to suicide is, indeed, possible.

CONCLUSION

Suicide is a major public health problem in the United States. This is true not only because of the direct loss of almost 40,000 lives a year to suicide, but also because of the tremendous damage suicide leaves in its wake. Historically, the survivors of suicide loss have been a highly disenfranchised group of mourners, being isolated and left to grieve and rebuild their lives on their own. This tragic set of circumstances is changing, however, as suicide survivors become more public in their grief and more active in their push to receive the services they need from their communities and the mental health system. With time, effort, and perseverance in the development of suicide-prevention and postvention programs, the hope is that the United States will be able to reduce the number suicide deaths in its soil and to provide effective, accessible, and compassionate help for those left to carry on when suicide occurs.

NOTE

1. At the time of this writing, there is underway a multisite randomized controlled trial of Shear's Complicated Grief Therapy with suicide survivors with complicated grief (Shear, Frank, Houck, & Reynolds, 2005).

REFERENCES

Attig, T. (2011). *How we grieve: Relearning the world* (rev. ed.). New York, NY: Oxford University Press.

Beal, K. C. (2011). Parents of suicides—Friends & families of suicides Internet community. In J. R. Jordan & J. L. McIntosh (Eds.), *Grief after suicide: Understanding the consequences and caring for the survivors* (pp. 381–388). New York, NY: Routledge/Taylor & Francis.

Berkowitz, L., McCauley, J., Schuurman, D. L., & Jordan, J. R. (2011). Organizational postvention after suicide death. In J. R. Jordan & J. L. McIntosh (Eds.), *Grief after suicide: Understanding the consequences and caring for the survivors* (pp. 157–178). New York, NY: Routledge/Taylor & Francis.

Cain, A. C. (1972). *Survivors of suicide*. Oxford, UK: Charles C Thomas.

Campbell, F. R. (2011). Baton Rouge Crisis Intervention Center's LOSS Team Active Postvention Model approach. In J. R. Jordan & J. L. McIntosh (Eds.), *Grief after suicide: Understanding the consequences and caring for the survivors* (pp. 327–332). New York, NY: Routledge/Taylor & Francis.

Campbell, F. R., Simon, R. I., & Hales, R. E. (2006). Aftermath of suicide: The clinician's role. *The American Psychiatric Publishing textbook of suicide assessment and management* (1st ed., pp. 459–476). Arlington, VA: American Psychiatric Publishing.

Cerel, J., & Campbell, F. R. (2008). Suicide survivors seeking mental health services: A preliminary examination of the role of an active postvention model. *Suicide and Life-Threatening Behavior, 38*(1), 30–34.

Cerel, J., Jordan, J. R., & Duberstein, P. R. (2008). The impact of suicide on the family. *Crisis: The Journal of Crisis Intervention and Suicide Prevention, 29*, 38–44.

Cerel, J., Padgett, J. H., Conwell, Y., & Reed, G. A., Jr. (2009). A call for research: The need to better understand the impact of support groups for suicide survivors. *Suicide and Life-Threatening Behavior, 39*(3), 269–281. doi:10.1521/suli.2009.39.3.269

Cerel, J., Padgett, J. H., & Reed, G. A., Jr. (2009). Support groups for suicide survivors: Results of a survey of group leaders. *Suicide and Life-Threatening Behavior, 39*(6), 588–598. doi:10.1521/suli.2009.39.6.588

De Groot, M., de Keijser, J., Neeleman, J., Kerkhof, A., Nolen, W., & Burger, H. (2007). Cognitive behaviour therapy to prevent complicated grief among relatives and spouses bereaved by suicide: Cluster randomised controlled trial. *British Medical Journal, 334*(7601), 994. doi:10.1136/bmj.39161.457431.55

De Groot, M., & Killen, B. J. (2013). Course of bereavement over 8–10 years in first degree relatives and spouses of people who committed suicide: Longitudinal community-based cohort study. *British Medical Journal Open, 347*. doi:10.1136/bmj.f5519

Dunne, E. J., & Dunne-Maxim, K. (2004). Working with families in the aftermath of suicide. In F. Walsh & M. McGoldrick (Eds.), *Living beyond loss: Death in the family* (2nd ed., pp. 272–284). New York, NY: W. W. Norton.

Dunne, E. J., McIntosh, J. L., & Dunne-Maxim, K. (1987). *Suicide and its aftermath: Understanding and counseling the survivors*. New York, NY: W. W. Norton.

Dyregrov, K., Plyhn, E., Dieserud, G., & Oatley, D. (2012). *After the suicide: Helping the bereaved to find a path from grief to recovery*. London, UK: Jessica Kingsley.

Feigelman, W., Jordan, J. R., McIntosh, J. L., & Feigelman, B. (2012). *Devastating losses: How parents cope eith the death of a child to suicide or drugs*. New York, NY: Springer.

Gould, M. S., Greenberg, T., Velting, D. M., & Shaffer, D. (2006). Youth suicide: A review. *Prevention Researcher, 13*(3), 3–7.

Harpel, J. L. (2011). American foundation for suicide prevention's survivor initiatives. In J. R. Jordan & J. L. McIntosh (Eds.), *Grief after suicide: Understanding the consequences and caring for the survivors* (pp. 417–424). New York, NY: Routledge/Taylor & Francis.

Hurtig, R., Bullitt, E., & Kates, K. (2011). Samaritans grief support services. In J. R. Jordan & J. L. McIntosh (Eds.), *Grief after suicide: Understanding the consequences and caring for the survivors* (pp. 341–348). New York, NY: Routledge/Taylor & Francis.

Jordan, J. R. (2001). Is suicide bereavement different? A reassessment of the literature. *Suicide and Life-Threatening Behavior, 31*(1), 91–102.

Jordan, J. R. (2008). Bereavement after suicide. *Psychiatric Annals, 38*(10), 679–685. doi:10.3928/00485713-20081001-05

Jordan, J. R. (2009). After suicide: Clinical work with survivors. In J. R. Jordan & J. L. McIntosh (Eds.), *Grief Matters: The Australian Journal of Grief and Bereavement, 12*(1), 4–9.

Jordan, J. R. (2011a). Group work with suicide survivors. In J. R. Jordan & J. L. McIntosh (Eds.), *Grief after suicide: Understanding the consequences and caring for the survivors* (pp. 283–300). New York, NY: Routledge/Taylor & Francis.

Jordan, J. R. (2011b). Principles of grief counseling with adult survivors. In J. R. Jordan & J. L. McIntosh (Eds.), *Grief after suicide: Understanding the consequences and caring for the survivors* (pp. 179–223). New York, NY: Routledge/Taylor & Francis.

Jordan, J. R. (2012). Guided imaginal conversations with the deceased. In R. A. Neimeyer (Ed.), *Techniques of grief therapy: Creative practices for counseling the bereaved* (pp. 262–265). New York, NY: Routledge.

Jordan, J. R., Feigelman, W., McMenamy, J., & Mitchell, A. M. (2011). Research on the needs of survivors. In J. R. Jordan & J. L. McIntosh (Eds.), *Grief after suicide: Understanding the consequences and caring for the survivors* (pp. 115–131). New York, NY: Routledge/Taylor & Francis.

Jordan, J. R., Kraus, D. R., & Ware, E. S. (1993). Observations on loss and family development. *Family Process, 32*(4), 425–440.

Jordan, J. R., & McIntosh, J. L. (2011a). *Grief after suicide: Understanding the consequences and caring for the survivors.* New York, NY: Routledge/Taylor & Francis.

Jordan, J. R., & McIntosh, J. L. (2011b). Is suicide bereavement different? A framework for rethinking the question. In J. R. Jordan & J. L. McIntosh (Eds.), *Grief after suicide: Understanding the consequences and caring for the survivors* (pp. 19–42). New York, NY: Routledge/Taylor & Francis.

Jordan, J. R., & McIntosh, J. L. (2011c). Suicide bereavement: Why study survivors of suicide loss? In J. R. Jordan & J. L. McIntosh (Eds.), *Grief after suicide: Understanding the consequences and caring for the survivors* (pp. 3–17). New York, NY: Routledge/Taylor & Francis.

Jordan, J. R., McIntosh, J. L., Bolton, I. M., Campbell, F. R., Harpel, J. L., & Linn-Gust, M. (2011). A call to action: Building clinical and programmatic support for suicide survivors. In J. R. Jordan & J. L. McIntosh (Eds.), *Grief after suicide: Understanding the consequences and caring for the survivors* (pp. 523–534). New York, NY: Routledge/Taylor & Francis.

Jordan, J. R., & McMenamy, J. (2004). Interventions for suicide survivors: A review of the literature. *Suicide and Life-Threatening Behavior, 34*(4), 337–349.

Kaslow, N. J., & Gilman Aronson, S. (2004). Recommendations for family interventions following a suicide. *Professional Psychology: Research and Practice, 35*, 240–247.

Kaslow, N. J., Samples, T. C., Rhodes, M., & Gantt, S. (2011). A family-oriented and culturally sensitive postvention approach with suicide survivors. In J. R. Jordan & J. L. McIntosh (Eds.), *Grief after suicide: Understanding the consequences and caring for the survivors* (pp. 301–323). New York, NY: Routledge/Taylor & Francis.

Kissane, D. W., & Hooghe, A. (2011). Family therapy for the bereaved. In J. R. Jordan & J. L. McIntosh (Eds.), *Grief and bereavement in contemporary society: Bridging research and practice* (pp. 287–302). New York, NY: Routledge/Taylor & Francis.

Klass, D., Silverman, P. R., & Nickman, S. L. (1996). *Continuing bonds: New understandings of grief.* Philadelphia, PA: Taylor & Francis.

Linn-Gust, M. (2011). American Association of Suicidology and survivors of suicide loss. In J. R. Jordan & J. L. McIntosh (Eds.), *Grief after suicide: Understanding the consequences and caring for the survivors* (pp. 413–415). New York, NY: Routledge/Taylor & Francis.

McDaid, C., Trowman, R., Golder, S., Hawton, K., & Sowden, A. (2008). Interventions for people bereaved through suicide: Systematic review. *British Journal of Psychiatry, 193*(6), 438–443.

McIntosh, J. L., & Jordan, J. R. (2011a). Going forward: A research agenda for suicide survivors. In J. R. Jordan & J. L. McIntosh (Eds.), *Grief after suicide: Understanding the consequences and caring for the survivors* (pp. 507–522). New York, NY: Routledge/Taylor & Francis.

McIntosh, J. L., & Jordan, J. R. (2011b). The impact of suicide on adults. In J. R. Jordan & J. L. McIntosh (Eds.), *Grief after suicide: Understanding the consequences and caring for the survivors* (pp. 43–79). New York, NY: Routledge/Taylor & Francis.

McMenamy, J. M., Jordan, J. R., & Mitchell, A. M. (2008). What do suicide survivors tell us they need? Results of a pilot study. *Suicide and Life-Threatening Behavior, 38*(4), 375–389. doi:10.1521/suli.2008.38.4.375

Mishara, B. L. (1995). *The impact of suicide.* New York, NY: Springer Publishing Company.

Mitchell, A. M., & Wesner, S. (2011). A bereavement crisis debriefing intervention for survivors after a suicide. In J. R. Jordan & J. L. McIntosh (Eds.), *Grief after suicide: Understanding the consequences and caring for the survivors* (pp. 397–402). New York, NY: Routledge/Taylor & Francis.

Neimeyer, R. A. (Ed.). (2012). *Techniques of grief therapy: Creative practices for counseling the bereaved.* New York, NY: Routledge.

Parrish, M., & Tunkle, J. (2003). Working with families following their child's suicide. *Family Therapy, 30*(2), 63–76.

Pearlman, L. A., Wortman, C. B., Feuer, C. A., Farber, C. H., & Rando, T. A. (2014). *Treating traumatic bereavement: A practitioner's guide.* New York, NY: Guilford.

Qin, P., Agerbo, E., & Mortensen, P. B. (2002). Suicide risk in relation to family history of completed suicide and psychiatric disorders: A nested case-control study based on longitudinal registers. *Lancet, 360*(9340), 1126–1130.

Range, L. M. (1998). When a loss is due to suicide: Unique aspects of bereavement. In J. H. Harvey (Ed.), *Perspectives on loss: A sourcebook* (pp. 213–220). Philadelphia, PA: Brunner/Mazel.

Sandler, I. N., Ayers, T. S., Wolchik, S. A., Tein, J.-Y., Kwok, O.-M., Haine, R. A., . . . Griffin, W. A. (2003). The Family Bereavement Program: Efficacy evaluation of a theory-based prevention program for parentally bereaved children and adolescents. *Journal of Consulting and Clinical Psychology, 71*(3), 587–600. doi:10.1037/0022-006x.71.3.587

Sands, D. C., Jordan, J. R., & Neimeyer, R. A. (2011). The meanings of suicide: A narrative approach to healing. In J. R. Jordan & J. L. McIntosh (Eds.), *Grief after suicide: Understanding the consequences and caring for the survivors* (pp. 249–282). New York, NY: Routledge/Taylor & Francis.

Schwartz, M. (2011). The retrospective profile and the facilitated family retreat. In J. R. Jordan & J. L. McIntosh (Eds.), *Grief after suicide: Understanding the consequences and caring for the survivors* (pp. 371–379). New York, NY: Routledge/Taylor & Francis.

Shear, K., Frank, E., Houck, P. R., & Reynolds, C. F., III. (2005). Treatment of complicated grief: A randomized controlled trial. *JAMA: Journal of the American Medical Association, 293*(21), 2601–2608. doi:10.1001/jama.293.21.2601

Shneidman, E. (1972). Foreword. In A. C. Cain (Ed.), *Survivors of suicide.* Oxford, UK: Charles C Thomas.

Stillion, J. M., & McDowell, E. E. (1996). *Suicide across the life span: Premature exits* (2nd ed.). Philadelphia, PA: Taylor & Francis.

Stroebe, M., & Schut, H. (1999). The dual process model of coping with bereavement: Rationale and description. *Death Studies, 23*(3), 197–224. doi:10.1080/074811899201046

Stroebe, M., Schut, H., & Boerner, K. (2010). Continuing bonds in adaptation to bereavement: Toward theoretical integration. *Clinical Psychology Review, 30*(2), 259–268. doi: 10.1016/j.cpr.2009.11.007

Sveen, C.-A., & Walby, F. A. (2008). Suicide survivors' mental health and grief reactions: A systematic review of controlled studies. *Suicide and Life-Threatening Behavior, 38*(1), 13–29.

U.S. Department of Health & Human Services, Office of the Surgeon General & National Action Alliance for Suicide Prevention. (2012). *National strategy for suicide prevention: Goals and objectives for action.* Washington, DC: Author.

Winokuer, H. R., & Harris, D. L. (2012). *Principles and practices of grief counseling.* New York, NY: Springer Publishing Company.

Wittouck, C., Van Autreve, S., De Jaegere, E., Portzky, G., & van Heeringen, K. (2011). The prevention and treatment of complicated grief: A meta-analysis. *Clinical Psychology Review, 31*(1), 69–78. doi:S0272-7358(10)00149-2 [pii]10.1016/j.cpr.2010.09.005

Colin Murray Parkes

26

RESPONDING TO GRIEF AND TRAUMA IN THE AFTERMATH OF DISASTER

Human beings are multicellular organisms whose cells are being born and are dying in an organized fashion throughout the life of each individual. We are, you might say, a community whose overall death takes place when the organization breaks down to the point where the mass death of the remaining cells takes place. Viewed in this way, every death is a disaster for the community of attached cells that makes up a human being. Our central nervous system is the link that joins and cares for and about our whole being. We naturally resist death and do our best to delay it as long as possible or until our appetite for life becomes depleted.

But our central nervous system is also an organ of communication and links us with others, to some of whom we become attached. Another factor affecting our resistance to death is the assumption that our life will benefit those to whom we are attached. When that is lost, when, for instance, we believe ourselves to be a burden to them or that our survival threatens theirs, we soon lose our will to live and may even desire our own death. For we are also social animals, part of something more important than ourselves, and find it easier to accept the prospect of our own death if others, to whom we are attached, survive us in the families and wider communities in which we live. Families and communities, we hope, are immortal. Or are they?

Disasters are events that threaten not only the lives of individuals but those of the families and larger social units of which we are a part. At such times, we become aware of our commitment to a greater whole. We may even sacrifice our own chances of survival for the sake of others. It is in all our interests to prevent disasters wherever possible and to ensure that those that do take place give rise to the minimum possible damage.

Although the term "disaster" is defined as "anything ruinous or distressing that befalls" (SOED, 1970) it will be confined here to situations giving rise to numerous and untimely deaths of individuals over a relatively short space of time. Within this definition, disasters vary greatly; they may be small, medium, or large in scale; narrow (local), medium (national), or wide (international) in spread; man-made or accidental ("acts of God") and associated with varying degrees of destruction of homes, occupational and other attachments and resources. In some, the disaster is soon over, whereas in others aftershocks or other threats remain a major source of fear and anxiety.

There are some disasters in which secondary consequences are almost as traumatic as the primary. For example, contaminated water supplies, blocked roads, release of toxic or irradiated materials, or community unrest may cause more deaths and trauma, hamper rescue operations, and deter helpers from outside the affected area.

Most disasters are unexpected, which usually means that we are unprepared for them. Expectedness does not equate precisely with predictability, and there are many disasters that cast their shadows before. In "tornado alley" people may not know *when* the next twister is coming, but they *are* better prepared than those who live elsewhere. Earthquakes, hurricanes, floods, bushfires, avalanches, and epidemics are of sufficient frequency in particular locations that disasters can often be avoided or minimized.

Wealthy people can choose to live in low-risk areas, whereas many disasters kill or injure people who have been forced by poverty to live in areas of risk. Man-made disasters, including those caused by wars and other deadly conflicts, are also more frequent in poorer countries, and we shall see that they easily create cycles of violence that escalate beyond the confines of the communities in which they arise. This last consideration makes it all the more important that we pay attention to disasters wherever they take place.

In this chapter, we examine how communities can be prepared for and respond to disasters in ways that take these risks into account and mitigate them. Given the wide range of problems to which disasters can give rise, it may be useful to summarize some of those that research has shown to constitute a risk to mental health and to suggest possible solutions to those problems that will be discussed in more detail below. The empirical factors that have been found to increase risk, the particular problems to which they may give rise, and possible solutions to each problem are listed in Table 26.1. Several of them are not peculiar to disasters and lie within the expertise of every well-trained responder. They will not be discussed further here. The rest will be discussed in the order in which they arise.

As in the management of all emergent problems, it is necessary to consider first the balance between needs and resources. Although most members of the caring professions think that they are fully stretched most of the time and never have enough funds and staff to provide an ideal service, we rally round at times of trouble and "go that extra mile." Disasters can stretch that reserve to the limit, particularly in parts of the world that are already underresourced.

The Inverse Care Law states that the care given is inversely proportional to the need (Hart, 1971). It is no coincidence that much of the research on the consequences of disasters has been carried out in "developed countries," where the risk is low, resources are plentiful, and emotional reactions to those disasters that do occur correspondingly great. In poorer countries, where disasters and other causes of death are untimely, both financial and professional medical care are scanty and deaths before old age frequent. Children are exposed to death at home from an early age, and familiarity with death and, in many places, religious beliefs foster acceptance of death and other stressful events. This does not mean that people do not feel grief, frustration, or misery; they may indeed feel and be more helpless than those brought up in the "West." All that is clear is that we should not assume that our "solutions" are the same as theirs, and we should take the time and trouble to find out. As General Kagame remarked after the genocide in Rwanda evoked a response from many NGOs (nongovernmental organizations) from the West, "They come here knowing almost nothing, understanding almost nothing, and they judge and criticize and tell you what you should do. A big part of the misunderstanding is that they expect us to be a normal country, like the ones where they are from. They do not understand that we are operating in a very different context" (Grant, 2010, p. 6). This does not absolve us of the responsibility to

TABLE 26.1 Risks, Problems, and Possible Solutions

RISK FACTOR	PROBLEM	SOLUTION
Type of Disaster		
Large local	Local services overwhelmed	National disaster response
Very large national	National services overwhelmed	International disaster response
Large local homelessness	Loss of communality	Relocate community together; community development programs
Witness or imagine horrific deaths	Posttraumatic stress disorder (PTSD)	Cognitive therapies & eye movement desensitization and reprocessing (EMDR)
Continuing danger	Chronic fear/anxiety	Relocate to safe area
Multiple losses of livelihood & unemployment	Loss of self-esteem/depression/ alcohol & drug abuse	Restore or retrain
Multiple injured/mutilated	Loss of self-esteem/depression/ alcohol & drug abuse	Rehabilitation and mutual help groups
Man-made—accidental death	Anger/rage/depression	Family liaison officer (FLO) Seek justice + counseling
Man-made—terrorism	Media, leadership, and communal overreaction	Education, resist polarization, support leaders, media liaison
Man-made—threats to kill leader(s)	Fear impairs judgment of leader	Protection and support to leader and family
Man-made—threaten or use weapons of mass destruction	Risk of mass destruction	Urgent response by international community
Man-made—civil war	Community divided, NGOs at risk, Security Council unable to agree on intervention	Mediation by neutral agents to support depolarization/ reconciliation
Personal/Communal Vulnerability		
Children	Loss of trust in parent's protection; PTSD	Support for children and parents; group counseling
Elderly	Loss of will to live, helplessness	Individual and social supports; reassurance of worth
Communal poverty, poor education	Learned helplessness and depression/bitterness	Provide resources to strengthen empowerment & mutual respect
Endemic passivity & obedience	Reliance on autocratic leaders	Education for empowerment
Separation anxiety disorder	Persistent Complex Bereavement Disorder	Complicated grief therapy
Previous depression	Major depression	Cognitive behavior therapy or antidepressant medication
Social Supports Lacking		
Families dysfunctional	Lack of mutual support	Family-focused grief therapy
Social units ruptured or overwhelmed	Social isolation	Support groups and community development program

give help to those outside our own religious and cultural environment, but it does suggest that we should take the trouble to learn about and respect their norms, their beliefs, and their ways of coping with death and disaster. Parkes, Laungani and Young's multicontributor book was first published in 1997 to meet these needs, and a new edition is in press (Parkes, Laungani, & Young, 1997/2014), but there is a great need for cross-cultural studies to investigate why some individuals and communities cope with disasters better than others.

The Inverse Care Law also applies at the other end of the social scale. It is a paradox that the leaders on whom we most depend are assumed to be brave, strong, wise, and immune to the traumas and losses that afflict the rest of us. This assumption makes it difficult for them to ask for and for us to give the support that all human beings may need at times of trouble. Failure to acknowledge this is one of the causes of failures of leadership, civil disorder, and even war. But the situation is not hopeless; for instance, Gersons and Nijdam (2014) provide a support service in the Netherlands to politicians and their families under protection from threats of assassination. They now find themselves consulted by other politicians regarding a wider range of threats and forming relationships that may well prove valuable should terrorist attacks take place.

Taking all of these variables into consideration, it is not surprising that those who are at greatest risk are the very old and the very young, the socially isolated and the disorganized, rather than mutually supportive families and communities.

PREPARATION FOR DISASTERS

Every hospital has its disaster plan and training programs that prepare health care staff for emergencies and disasters. These are mainly concerned with saving lives and pay little or no attention to the psychosocial and spiritual needs of the affected population. This is a pity, for disasters constitute a risk to mental health and to the integration of families and societies. What's more, there are some disasters, such as large aircraft crashes, from which there may be no survivors, and the role of the emergency services involves little more than "picking up the pieces" and breaking bad news. Professionals and volunteers who have received proper training, including taking part in disaster exercises, will be very much better prepared and in a position to take a lead in the organization and psychological support of affected individuals, families, and communities.

But preparation for disasters is not limited to the inclusion of counselors, psychologists, and priests in hospital disaster plans. As part of the programs of death awareness described in Chapters 15 and 16 on death education, it is important to recognize that we are none of us immune from disasters; sooner or later they will come our way. Knowing roughly what to expect and what to do about them gives confidence and reduces helplessness. It is a public health responsibility to appoint and train a few individuals to be ready to take leadership roles and to ensure that reserve funds can be easily mobilized to provide a rapid response to a wide range of such needs.

It is also worth noting that the violence that easily escalates into deadly attacks and terrorism is rooted in the social units in which it arises. Long-standing insecurity fuelled by prejudices and myths underlie hostility that is channeled into subversive extremism (Parkes, CM 2014a). Schools and universities have important roles to play in counteracting the magnet of violence into which many young people are drawn. This has particular salience in areas of endemic social insecurity and violence (Glees, 2014; Parkes, J 2007, 2014).

Despite the wide range of disasters, there are commonalities, and many of them follow a sequence from impact, to recoil, to aftermath and, one hopes, to recovery. Each of these phases requires its own response.

THE IMPACT PHASE—PSYCHOLOGICAL FIRST AID

This is the period during which attempts to assess needs and save lives take priority. Emergency services will normally set up a Disaster Center as soon as possible, and this should act as a hub for information, recording of casualties and damage, as well as offers of support. There is no time for democratic debate, and those involved must expect and follow a military chain of command. The disaster center should, but may not, provide space for the psychological support services that need to be integrated and in close liaison with the hub, if they are to plan an effective response.

Readers will be forgiven if, at this point, they feel discouraged: the problem is " just too big." That is certainly the way I felt when, as a young psychiatrist with a special interest in bereavement, I first visited Aberfan, in South Wales. A week earlier, an avalanche of coal waste from the mine that had been dumped over a stream liquefied and thundered down the hill to sweep away the village school and destroy a line of houses: 144 people died, 116 of them children.

The images on television stirred us all. Miners in hard hats dug desperately, while relatives waited in silent misery, and bodies were carried to a local chapel. When I arrived in Aberfan, I found that I was not the only volunteer. I was told that, within hours of those images of disaster appearing on television, so many people had flocked to the small village that the single road in and out had become blocked, and the police had had to force a way through a mass of stationary cars to enable the ambulances and other rescue vehicles to get through.

What was it that drew us? In my case, I had been nagged by a friend to go. I was reluctant: They were not my children, and I had no experience of disasters. Wales seemed to be a different country and, although I have some Welsh blood in me, that was not sufficient for me to be closely attached to the Welsh. But my friend pointed out that I had published papers on bereavement and might be able to help the stricken community. He had himself come from a coal-mining community, and he knew what they must be suffering. He tapped some duty of care that made me feel I had to go. I mention all this because it is important to understand why people volunteer or keep away. In Aberfan, pictures in the media had brought home the grief and aroused feelings of attachment to our fellow human beings of which we were hardy aware.

I did not want to go in uninvited, so I phoned the community physician, who was pleased to accept my help and offered to introduce me to key people in the village. I soon discovered that it was not grief but numbness that was the predominant reaction to the disaster. Before long, I too had shut down on feelings that threatened to overwhelm me. I kept a "good face," and it was only on the way home that I started to cry. I had to stop the car three times. My wife opened the door. "How was it?" she said. I could not speak.

Everyone I met in Aberfan felt the same, helpless and ashamed. Why should we survive in the face of such desolation and despair? What could we do that would bring some kind of meaning out of the chaos that we faced?

Forty-eight years later, I can look back on this and the other disasters that followed, and realize that this feeling need not outweigh the fact that, little by little, we do make a difference. We may never know how great a difference, but individuals and communities do recover. As we have seen elsewhere in this book, people can grow through grieving. Having worked in Aberfan, Rwanda, and other places impacted by disaster, I have realized that it is not only individuals but communities that can mature. They will be permanently changed by the disaster, but the long-term consequences are not all necessarily bad.

But even that awareness will not reduce the impact of a disaster. Every therapist and counselor will have had the experience of clients who flood us with problems. No sooner do we try to answer one question when they interrupt us with another. In the wake of disasters, it is not one client flooding us with problems but a multitude. Before long, we begin to feel as if we too are being drowned; the avalanche is carrying us away. And perhaps that gives us a glimpse of how the survivors feel—overwhelmed.

There is a useful way to handle these situations. We have to recognize that the only way to cope with the avalanche is to decide which problem is the most important at this moment in time, and to focus on that while leaving the rest until later. In other words we have to hang in there, take stock, decide which problem to tackle first, and get on with the job. Recognizing the importance of this simple sequence does not solve all the problems, but it does help us to regain some sense of control. It can also enable us to help our clients to do the same.

The primary aim then, for others and ourselves, is to overcome feelings of helplessness. This can be achieved by obtaining and providing clear and accurate information as soon as it becomes available. Facile reassurance will only confuse, but it is sometimes wise to break bad news into "bite-sized chunks" and invite questions rather than snowing survivors with more "bitter truth" than they can take in. The invitation passes control to the recipient, for people do not ask questions until they are ready for the answers; at the same time, it tells them that we are not afraid to be asked; and that, in itself, reflects our expectation that they too can cope with the news, however bad it may be.

Perhaps the most important thing is not what we say but how we say it. Nonverbal communication is more important than verbal because it communicates emotion, and we must rely on our empathy to gauge the visual message that feels right for each situation. Some will need the touch of a hand and a smile, whereas others will need to be "taken seriously." Clients easily detect insincerity, and because fear is infectious, only those who are confident about their ability to stay calm are suitable for this work. Such confidence can best be obtained by experience, and for that reason alone, it is best to select experienced counselors to work in disaster areas. Confidence can also be obtained by training that includes role-play and other experiential techniques.

Members of the emergency services and other rescuers are at particular risk of "burn-out" and need similar support. There is a tendency for rescuers to keep going long after they would normally take a rest. But rescue operations go on long after they can be expected to achieve success. In Aberfan, nobody was brought out alive after the first hour, but digging was still in progress a week later. It is important, therefore, for those in authority to take charge and insist that rescuers are supported with refreshments and reassurance, and that rest periods are necessary if they are to keep going.

As for us caregivers, for our own sake as well as that of the survivors, we need to work as part of a team. Disasters attract would-be supporters, sometimes in large numbers, and it is essential that they be assessed and those thought suitable assigned to one or more teams, depending on the needs and the resources available. And, because disasters are stressful for the carers as well as the cared-for, we need to look after ourselves and each other, take rest breaks, and meet together to provide the same kind of mutual support to the team that we are providing to the rescuers and the survivors.

Fortunately, the skills that we have learned from helping individual clients and families in a clinical setting are not fundamentally different from the skills that help individuals and families following disasters. Bereavement support has been discussed in other chapters of this book, where it is recognized that bereavement gives rise to many kinds of losses in addition to the loss of a loved person. Homes, income, jobs, and much else may be lost after ordinary bereavements. In the same way, disasters give rise to a wide range of traumas and losses, some of which have been listed previously.

Of particular importance in disaster areas are pervading feelings of anxiety and fear. Those living in disaster areas may have to cope with witnessing the violent deaths of others, including those they love, and may themselves have been injured or exposed to dangers that still exist. Although panic is rare, it sometimes occurs when people believe themselves to be trapped. More often the immediate response to disaster is a defensive disengagement or "numbness" that protects people from the emotional impact and disorganization of thinking that would otherwise emerge. Even so, anxiety and fear are only an inch away and will have given rise to an *alarm response* that triggers deep-seated bodily reactions resulting from stimulations of the sympathetic and inhibition of the parasympathetic nervous systems. In the environment in which man evolved, these reactions improved our chance of survival. Hyperalertness, increased muscle tension, sweating, and rapid heartbeat ensured that we could survive by fighting or fleeing from danger. In our current environment, these responses are seldom useful; indeed, people who are already anxious may misinterpret their physical responses as symptoms of illness and become even more alarmed. Health care workers have an important role to play in reassuring people of the normality of such "symptoms" and teaching methods of relaxation. Tiredness and exhaustion impair thinking and performance, and may be aggravated by insomnia.

Is there a place for medication in the wake of disasters? The most popular drugs are alcohol and tobacco, which are self-prescribed and do help to take the edge off the horror, facilitating social activities and relaxation. But they work so well that they easily lead to escalation and abuse. Alcohol may help break down inhibitions against the expression of grief, but it also unlocks aggression, impairs judgment, interferes with sleep patterns, and damages health. It is particularly dangerous when used by drivers, leaders, and youngsters with deadly weapons.

The effects of most tranquillizers are similar to alcohol but have the advantage that they are controlled by an independent other person, a doctor. Most doctors agree that sedatives have their place as short-term aids to sleep, as do tranquillizers to reduce alarm, but they are also aware that every care should be taken to avoid dependence, and the combination of tranquilizers *and* alcohol can be dangerous. It seems that "medicalization" has its uses but can easily be abused.

Those who are unprepared for the disaster tend to overreact. For instance, people on the periphery of the disaster often assume that they are at the center, and this "illusion of centrality" may result in some individuals expecting and getting a disproportionate amount of support, whereas others get none. Overreaction is particularly hazardous following disasters for which someone, rightly or wrongly, is held to blame.

RECOIL—PLANNING AND IMPLEMENTATION—POSTTRAUMATIC REACTIONS

Once the situation is clear, under control, and the immediate danger is past, life is less chaotic. It is now possible for both survivors and helpers to take stock and begin to face the often massive changes that are imminent in their lives. Wounds have been dressed, bodies have been removed, those who have lost their homes are in temporary accommodation, and power supplies have been restored. It is now possible for psychosocial services to get their act together, mobilizing resources of money and staff, providing a crash program of disaster training, organizing a service that can respond to requests for help, and beginning to screen volunteers and professional staff for the disaster team.

Given that, in many societies, mental health services are in short supply and those that are required may be too expensive for people who have lost jobs, homes, and family members to pay for, it is important that government and nongovernmental funds be made available and volunteer services mobilized to meet the needs that are emerging. As we have seen, most disasters attract public sympathy, and it is not usually difficult to raise funds. National and international bodies such as the Red Cross, the United Nations Children's Fund (UNICEF), and Save the Children are well used to working in disaster areas.

Disaster teams are social services and, although it is useful to make use of psychiatrists and clinical psychologists as consultants, leadership should be the responsibility of nonmedical staff with training and experience of working in disaster areas. In Britain, these are usually social workers, although some areas have specialized disaster officers with responsibility for advanced planning and preparation for disasters as well as heading up a disaster team when needed. The size and composition of the team(s) will depend on the magnitude and nature of the disaster as well as the resources available. People often volunteer because they have had personal losses and have learned what helps. Most will have come through their own grief, but it is important to select out any with unresolved problems of their own.

It is not uncommon for professionals to distrust voluntary organizations, but there are some, such as Cruse Bereavement Care in Britain, which provide advanced-level training in disaster support for experienced volunteers who have already been carefully selected, trained, and supervised in bereavement and trauma care.

Self-help groups can also play a useful role in offering mutual support and empowerment for their members, but they can be vulnerable to the influence of angry or paranoid members, particularly if these individuals then take leadership roles. In some places, such as immigrant communities in Palestine and elsewhere, entire neighborhoods have experienced loss of homes, homelands, and loved ones. They too provide mutual support to their members, but they are also vulnerable to the influence of angry and discontented leaders who may motivate young men to join armed gangs or terrorist groups (Merari, 2010).

Because every disaster is different, one or more training days are needed soon after a disaster to introduce the team(s) to each other, reassure them about the support they will get, and prepare them for the problems they are likely to meet. In most cases, more than one team will be needed, and they should meet together with the team leader on a regular basis, usually daily. Records should be kept of all interventions and discussed in supervision (which can be individual or in small groups).

It is also helpful to hold a conference to which a wider range of involved persons, such as members of health care teams and voluntary agencies, can be invited in order to monitor progress, identify problems, and listen to speakers, such as psychiatrists, forensic pathologists, lawyers, and clergy, with relevant knowledge of particular issues.

During the recoil stage, feelings of numbness will usually decline, grief will peak, and other emotions will break through. Occasionally, however, the numbness continues and may be associated with a dissociative disorder in which people lose their memory for the traumatic event (amnesia) or shut down other areas of mental functioning, such as hearing, seeing, feeling (anaesthesiae of limbs), or movement (paralyses). Sufferers may enter a fugue state. For example, a young policeman was first on the scene following a multiple collision on a motorway. He witnessed horrific mutilation of passengers but followed correct procedures and exerted a rigid control of his feelings until seniors arrived and took over. At this point, he wandered away from the accident and was found 2 days later, lost and unaware of his own identity. Taken to a local psychiatric unit, he was treated with kindness and respect by the staff. With no more treatment than a minor tranquilizer, his memory soon returned, and he was able to return home. In other cases, treatment may include abreaction in which the patient is helped by hypnosis or medication to relive the traumatic event in the safe setting of a psychiatric unit. This treatment often brings about a dramatic cure. Professionals and other caregivers have to maintain their calm control of emotions for the sake of their clients and, although this may not present a serious problem, they may be surprised to find that memories return in the form of posttraumatic dreams or flashbacks some time later.

In my own case, I experienced just such a flashback 10 years after the Aberfan disaster. As part of a training program, I was in a role play in which I played the part of a husband who was returning home from hospital after the death of his wife. Arriving home I was met by my "sister" with the words "How was it?" These were the words my wife had used on my first return from Aberfan, and I reacted, as I had then, in freezing immobility; I could not speak. My "sister," with instant empathy, threw her arms around me, and we both burst into tears. The audience was most impressed.

Flashbacks of this kind are not uncommon in disaster areas and can be a symptom of PTSD. This cannot be diagnosed until it has been present for over a month, but that does not mean that it cannot be prevented by giving attention and support to those with incipient symptoms in the recoil stage of a disaster. The symptoms are most likely to occur if people have been exposed to actual or threatened death, serious injury, or sexual violence, but they can also arise in the relatives of people who have witnessed such violence or learned of its occurrence in a close family member.

The sufferer from PTSD is haunted by intrusive painful memories, "flashbacks" or dreams of the event that are triggered by reminders of the disaster. These are so painful that people will do their best to avoid any situation or person who might trigger the memories. Thus they may shut themselves up at home and refuse to go out, forbid their relatives and friends from mentioning the disaster, or distract themselves by trivial activities. It is a paradox that, in order to avoid reminders, the sufferer has to keep them "at the back of his mind" all the time. Small wonder that they remain jumpy, irritable and hyperalert, sleep poorly, and withdraw from emotional attachments. Some are at risk of suicide.

Because grieving involves remembering the dead, posttraumatic symptoms may prevent bereaved people from expressing or sharing their grief. This implies that people whose PTSD has been successfully treated may still benefit from the support of a bereavement volunteer (BV).

Given a safe place and the support of family, friends, or BVs, symptoms will usually decline, and psychiatric treatment will seldom be required. If, however, they persist and prevent people from returning to work or carrying out other responsibilities, it is important that the sufferer be referred to a competent therapist. Fortunately, current treatments, including cognitive therapy and EMDR, are very effective methods of intervention.

Doctors, police, ambulance persons, and members of other rescue services are not immune from PTSD; in fact, those "experiencing repeated or extreme exposure to aversive details of the traumatic event(s) (e.g., first responders collecting human remains . . .)" are at special risk and may need extra support (American Psychiatric Association, 2013, p. 271).

Tears are not the only expression of emotion that erupts in recoil from a disaster. Anger is a natural reaction to loss and to the many frustrations that are frequent in disaster areas. In the environment of evolution, it would have helped people to survive by assertiveness and preparation for fighting. Like the alarm response, it gives rise to increased muscle tension, rapid heartbeat, and an increase in blood pressure, which, if it persists, may endanger health. In our present environment, it occasionally causes opponents to give way but at the cost of antagonizing others. Suppressing anger does not prevent its physiological effects and may cause cardiac problems. Like fear, anger is infectious, and this makes it particularly dangerous in both leaders and followers during the recoil phase after man-made disasters. In these circumstances, it can undermine clear thinking and decision making just when these are most needed (Parkes, CM 2014b). Even when anger is justified, it can also be disproportionate and misdirected against family and would-be supporters, who may then back off just when they are most needed. It is hard to bear the brunt of unfair treatment.

Events, such as terrorist attacks and assassinations, can affect entire nations and their leaders. They are perceived or misperceived through the eyes of the press and other media who may choose words and show images that aggravate the anger. Leaders are similarly affected and may feed fears and prejudice in order to take advantage of the public support evoked by fear. These responses may give rise to overreaction and an escalation of violence that then becomes disproportionate and/or cyclical (International Work Group on Death, Dying and Bereavement, 2013). For example, popular media blamed the assassination of the president of Rwanda on the Tutsi ethnic group. This triggered a genocidal terror that killed about 700,000 and brought about a successful invasion by a Tutsi emigrant army (Hall & Parkes, 2014).

Although there are some disasters in which victims come from far and wide, most involve one or more communities in which multiple losses have taken place. Some of these destroy families by death *and* communities by destruction of homes and public services. Although many of us take our communities for granted much of the time, like families, they become more important at times of trouble. Rapid restoration of power, water, and food distribution will prevent further disaster. Whenever populations have to be relocated, even in temporary accommodation, it is important to ensure that communities are not split up.

This was very evident in the response to the Buffalo Creek disaster (West Virginia), in which 125 people died and 151 homes were destroyed when a dam burst and water inundated three linear villages. Survivors from the villages were dispersed more or less at random across no fewer than 13 trailer parks, thereby destroying the communities just when they most needed to support their members. Two years after the disaster, Kai Erickson reported high levels of insecurity, anxiety, and depression and that "the loss of communality in Buffalo Creek has meant that people are alone and without very much in the way of emotional shelter.... There is no one to warn you ... care for you, ... rescue you ... or mourn for you ... and in the long run—the community can no longer ... edit reality in such a way that it seems manageable" (Erickson, 1979, p. 189). In the similar Aberfan disaster, 144 died (116 of them children), and 21 homes were destroyed. Grief and anger caused conflicts, three public meetings broke up in fistfights during the first year, and distrust of leaders led to a paralysis of decision making. But the community remained intact and, as we shall see, it too recovered.

AFTERMATH—COMMUNITY CARE AND RECOVERY

By this time, rescue operations are at an end, security has been largely restored, and the more transient emotional responses are declining. It will now become apparent that, following most disasters, the majority of affected persons are resilient enough to cope without the need for much help from outside their family and friendship networks. But there are some disasters in which these networks break down.

Whenever destruction has been widespread, populations relocated, and/or sources of income lost, it is important to reestablish community, involve all in planning for the future, and implement a recovery program. Judicial inquiries and the distribution of disaster funds play a part, but they need to be transparent, easily accessible, and seen to be fair.

Mistakes were made after the Aberfan disaster by paternalistic attempts to manage funds and make plans without community involvement. This aggravated pre-existing distrust of authorities and fed paranoid attitudes that further divided the community. But these mistakes were rectified, and the more the local community was trusted, the more trustworthy they became. Anger did not cease, rather it became channeled into worthwhile causes where it would do good.

For instance, the Coal Board claimed that they had made safe the remaining tips of slurry on the mountainside above the village, but, as one woman said, "It's like having your child's murderer dead on your doorstep. You never know when it's coming to life again." A local "Tip Removal Committee" was formed, which organized a public protest outside the office of the Secretary of State in Cardiff. At a crucial point in the dialogue between the committee and the Minister when it seemed that nothing had been achieved, a signal was given, and the protesters entered the building and dumped coal slurry on the Minister's carpet. The Minister left in tears, and the following week announced a new plan to "landscape" the tips.

After most disasters, including Aberfan, there is a minority who will need intervention from outside the family if lasting psychiatric or social problems are to be prevented. One or more psychiatrists and trauma psychologists may be needed to liaise with the disaster team and the psychiatric services.

A large number of research studies agree that some disasters are more traumatic than others, some individuals more vulnerable than others, and some families more supportive than others (Reviewed in Parkes & Prigerson, 2010, chapters 10–12). Awareness of these influences makes possible an outreach program that is not a psychiatric service and aims to reduce the need for psychiatric help by recognizing the problems before they become clinical and giving or steering survivors toward appropriate and effective help.

When people are already mentally ill, it will facilitate early diagnosis and treatment. For that reason alone it is important for the disaster teams to be familiar with those mental disorders that are most likely to arise or be aggravated by disasters. These include PTSD (see above), persistent complex bereavement disorder (PCBD; see Chapter 23), and major depression, all of which are associated with an increased risk of suicide. Because effective treatments are available for each of these disorders, it is important that they be diagnosed when present and treated without delay. Sadly, distrust of psychiatric services often prevents people from getting the help that they need, sometimes with fatal consequences (e.g., suicide). This said, as we have seen, there are many precursors of psychiatric conditions that are likely to respond to alternative sources of help.

Depression is a normal accompaniment of feelings of helplessness that are widespread following disasters. It is maintained by lack of self-esteem, by loss of status, social isolation, and by shame and self-reproach, all of which increase the risk that the depression will escalate. These feelings often result from expressions of pity and encouragement of dependence, such as "I'll look after you," or the equally unhelpful injunction to "pull yourself together" as if depression were a choice. Depression and helplessness are undeserved and consequences of the special circumstances and irreversible losses to which sufferers have been subjected. By the same token, they will be reversed by anything that increases self-esteem, restores status, enriches social life, and reduces self-blame. It follows that the most important thing we have to offer to the depressed is our respect for their true value and worth. By treating them as equals, asking their advice and rewarding their efforts, with approval and regard, we try to create a relationship of collaboration rather than dependence.

The same applies to depressed communities. Experts from outside the community and support from "on high" may have been desperately needed in the acute stages of a disaster, but it is important that the outsiders do not take advantage of their status to colonize or foster dependency.

A good example of an international response to a national disaster was that undertaken by UNICEF in Rwanda. Rwanda is one of the poorest countries in the world, with a population of 6 million and only three Rwandese psychiatrists. There was no way in which the government could afford sufficient mental health practitioners to provide the support that was needed by the survivors of the genocide. UNICEF appointed an American psychologist, Leila Gupta, to plan and head a trauma recovery program. She worked closely with three Rwandese professionals—a psychologist, a child psychologist, and a school teacher—to recruit a batch of Rwandese "trauma advisers." Each of them trained another batch, and they eventually recruited and trained 6,193 "social agents," who provided support to over 145,000 children and family units all over Rwanda. They also used the local radio to run a series of regular programs on mental health issues and established a national trauma center in the city of Kigali for more specialist help. They invited mental health specialists, of whom I was one, to take part in their training, provide training materials, and help with broadcasts. We were all too aware of the danger of cultural imperialism and liaised closely with Rwandese psychologists and a psychiatrist to ensure that the teaching was compatible with Rwandese cultural norms (Parkes & Hill, 2014).

RECOVERY—WITHDRAWAL OF EXTERNAL SERVICES

Funding bodies must realize that the need for supportive services does not suddenly come to an end 1 year after a disaster. Indeed, the first anniversary usually gives rise to an exacerbation of distress that may temporally increase the need for support. This said, once the anniversary is over, things often improve, and it becomes possible to taper off the work of the disaster team.

Although the first anniversary in Aberfan was very painful, a carefully planned conference entitled "The Way Ahead" was held a few weeks later to which trusted leaders from each of the main groupings in the village and local authority were invited. During the morning, a sociologist, a psychiatrist, and a community development officer gave their slant on the current situation, explaining how disasters inevitably affect feelings, behavior, and organizations. They emphasized the extent to which the responses to this disaster were natural and expectable. As one woman said after the meeting, "It was the first time I had stood aside from my anger and seen it as normal."

The chairman, Professor Leaper, from the department of Social Administration at the University of Exeter, ended the morning by explaining that most of the professionals from outside the village would be withdrawn during the coming year. Our work was nearly done, and we were happy to leave it to the community to plan the way ahead. During the afternoon, the participants were divided into groups deliberately chosen to represent the diverse social groups to which they belonged. By the end of the meeting, a turning point had been reached and, in an atmosphere of enthusiasm, the plenary session agreed to form a community association to further the process that had been initiated.

During the succeeding year, the community came together in an impressive way and 6 years later hosted a similar conference on "community development" to which they invited representatives from all of the Welsh mining valleys. As the headmistress of the school said, "The disaster was caused by apathy, and it is up to Aberfan never to become apathetic again."

Man-made disasters, and the Aberfan disaster was one, do not occur in a vacuum. Aberfan was a mining community depending on a dangerous industry that was in decline. Economic depression had given rise to psychological depression even before the disaster. Professor Leaper, in his foreword to the book that summarizes community development in the Welsh mining valleys, wrote, "From the center of the dark pool of near despair after the disaster at Aberfan have spread out ever-widening ripples of involvement, interest and action to the present outer circle of a 'socio-economic strategy for the Valleys' in 1975 and beyond . . . it is an irony that it took a disaster to bring us together and to stir us into action" (Ballard & Jones, 1975, p. 6).

During the 5 years that followed the disaster, the birth rate in Aberfan rose by comparison with other villages in the valley, to the point where the number of extra babies born slightly exceeded the number who had died in the disaster. It was not the bereaved mothers who were responsible; most of them were now beyond reproductive age, but the community as a whole (Parkes & Williams, 1975).

It would be naive to pretend that "The Year of the Valleys" was the end of the story of Aberfan. Later years were to see the closure of the mine; the ex-migration of many of the inhabitants; and the persistence, in many of the survivors of the disaster, of PTSD which, at the time of the disaster, had not been described and for which no treatments had been discovered. On follow-up 45 years later, 19 from a sample of 41 (46%) reported PTSD *at some time* after the disaster compared with 20% of controls from a neighboring village. Twelve survivors (29%) reported current symptoms of PTSD (Morgan et al., 2003). The authors conclude that exposure to disaster in childhood can increase vulnerability to PTSD throughout life. Other psychiatric disorders were not more frequent in the disaster-exposed group.

The disaster in Aberfan was medium-sized in scale and local in spread. The Rwandan genocide was large in scale and national in spread, with international repercussions. Recovery took longer, yet it did take place. When I first visited Kigali, Rwanda, a year after the massacres, I wrote, "In Rwanda the rule of law has broken down. People no longer sleep securely in their beds at night. Neither their own government nor the United Nations was able to protect them from the most appalling horror imaginable. They know that it could happen again and it probably will" (Parkes, CM 1996, p. 110).

The city was still under curfew, and sporadic violence continued. United Nations observers knew of daily violations of human rights, but there was no judicial system, and reporting them to the secretary general made little difference. Twenty years later, Rwanda is one of the most peaceful and rapidly developing states in Africa. The reasons for this recovery have been analyzed and summed up as follows.

> Rwanda is winning. The world has taken pity on one of its smallest, weakest, and most desperate countries and is attempting to love it to life; the Rwandans are finding new, more positive myths to replace the old negative ones; and a tough, suspicious, warrior leader (General Paul Kagame) has discovered how to charm, and work with women, politicians, industrialists and bankers. Psychologists may have played a small part, by providing psychological first aid when it was most needed, setting up secure bases from which people could begin to explore ways out of the monstrous pit into which they had fallen, by encouraging people to take stock and talk about their distress, and helping them to regain sufficient confidence and self-respect to look forward rather than over their shoulders. The world, as embodied in its many-headed institutions and leaders, has opened the door to its own success, finance, and know-how; bringing hope to a hopeless case. And, although his human rights record is not good, pragmatic Paul Kagame has proved that he can be a brilliant strategist at home as well as in battle. In the great continent of Africa, the success of Rwanda is viewed with interest, and others are beginning to follow their example. (Parkes & Hill, 2014)

IMPLICATIONS FOR FUTURE DEVELOPMENTS

It seems that, given the right help, individuals, families, and communities can survive disasters and, in the process, become more mature and caring. They do not go back to being what they were before the disaster. Neither can the professionals who choose to work with them. When in the course of time they come to the end of their contracts in a disaster area, few of them want to return to "ordinary" jobs. It is important for management staff to recognize that fact and to assist them in finding rewarding posts in which they can make use of the lessons that they have learned.

Most of the individuals who provide psychosocial services in disaster areas have been trained for one-to-one counseling or psychotherapy with individuals; some have been trained to work with groups, and others with larger organizations and systems. Each has an important contribution to make, but there is a regrettable tendency for each to work in his or her own boxes and use different theoretical models.

In this chapter, a pattern seems to be emerging of special relevance to a volume that draws on a wide range of perspectives. Perhaps the way is opening for a new kind of specialism that draws on well-found knowledge from family dynamics, organizational systems, spirituality, and other areas that may be unfamiliar to most of us. Those who have had the privilege of working in disaster areas have important contributions to make to this new nascent field.

REFERENCES

American Psychiatric Association. (2013). *Diagnostic and statistical manual of mental disorders* (5th ed.). Arlington, VA: America Psychiatric Press.

Ballard, P. H., & Jones, E. (1975). *The valleys call: A self-examination by the people of the South Wales valleys during the year of the valleys 1974.* Ferndale, Rhondda: Ron Jones.

Erikson, K.T. (1979) *In the Wake of the Flood* Allen and Unwin, London.

Gersons, B. P. R., & Nijdam, M. J. (2014). Supporting leaders under threat, and their protection. In C. M. Parkes (Ed.), *Responses to terrorism: Can psycho-social approaches break the cycle of violence?* (pp. 181–189). London, UK: Routledge.

Glees, A. (2014). Islamist terrorism and British universities. In C. M. Parkes (Ed.), *Responses to terrorism: Can psycho-social approaches break the cycle of violence?* (pp. 144–150). London, UK: Routledge.

Grant, R. (2010, July 22). Paul Kagame: Rwanda's redeemer or ruthless dictator? *The Telegraph.* Retrieved from http://rwandarwabanyarwanda.over-blog.com/article-paul-kagame-rwanda-s-redeemer-or-ruthless-dictator-54300233.html

Hall, P., & Parkes, C. M. (2014). The assassination and genocide in Rwanda. In C. M. Parkes (Ed.), *Responses to terrorism: Can psycho-social approaches break the cycle of violence?* (pp. 118–132). London, UK: Routledge.

Hart, J. T. (1971). The inverse care law. *Lancet, 1*(7696), 405–412.

International Work Group on Death, Dying and Bereavement. (2013). Armed conflict: A model for understanding and intervention. *Death Studies, 37*(1), 61–88. doi: 10.1080/07481187.2012.655647

Merari, A. (2010). *Driven to death: Psychological and social aspects of suicidal terrorism.* Oxford, UK: Oxford University Press.

Morgan, L., Scourfield, J., Williams, D., Jasper, A. & Lewis, G. (2003) The Aberfan Disaster: Thirty three year follow-up of survivors. *The British Journal of Psychiatry* 182: 532–536 doi: 10.1192/02-417

Parkes, C. M. (1996). Genocide in Rwanda: Personal reflections. *Mortality, 1*(1), 95–110.

Parkes, C. M. (2014a). On the Psychology of Extremism. In C. M. Parkes (Ed.), *Responses to Terrorism: Can psycho-social approaches break the cycle of violence?* (pp. 9–28). London, UK: Routledge.

Parkes, C. M. (2014b). Responses to Terrorism that feed Cycles of Violence: A model. In C. M. Parkes (Ed.), *Responses to Terrorism: Can psycho-social approaches break the cycle of violence?* (pp. 77–100). London, UK: Routledge.

Parkes, C. M., & Hill, P. (2014). After the genocide: The peace process in Rwanda. In C. M. Parkes (Ed.), *Responses to terrorism: Can psycho-social approaches break the cycle of violence?* (pp. 208–229). London, UK: Routledge.

Parkes, C. M., Laungani, P., & Young, W. (Eds.). (2014). *Death and bereavement across cultures* (2nd ed.) London, UK: Routledge. (First edition published 1997.)

Parkes, C. M., & Prigerson, H. G. (2010). *Bereavement: Studies of grief in adult life* (4th ed.). London, UK: Routledge.

Parkes, C. M., & Williams, R. M. (1975). Psychosocial effects of disaster: Birth rate in Aberfan. *British Medical Journal, 2*, 303–304.

Parkes, J. (2007). Resisting the magnet: A study of South African children's engagements with neighborhood violence. In R. G. Stevenson & G. R. Cox (Eds.), *Perspectives on violence and violent death.* Amityville, NY: Baywood.

Parkes, J. (2014). Countering violence: The role of the school. In C. M. Parkes (Ed.), *Responses to terrorism: Can psycho-social approaches break the cycle of violence?* (pp. 135–143). London, UK: Routledge.

The Shorter Oxford English Dictionary on Historical Principles (3rd edition). (1970). Little, W., Fowler, H. W., Coulson, H. Revised & edited by C. T. Onions. Clarendon Press, Oxford.

Mary L. S. Vachon **27**

CARE OF THE CAREGIVER: PROFESSIONALS AND FAMILY MEMBERS

My first childhood memory is the day after my brother Richard's death. Each of my parents had major deaths in their childhood. My father's father died when he was 12 and his mother when he was 17. My mother's father died at the age of 45 when she was 12; four of her uncles, all of whom lived in their neighborhood then died at 45, all leaving young families. My father's step-brother, Leo, an integral part of our family, was killed going to babysit for friends when he was 22 and I was 10, and my grandmother died when I was 15. Death, chronic grief, meaning-making, premonitions regarding death and stories of the distress and compassion of the caregivers involved in these deaths were an integral part of my childhood.

PROFESSIONAL HISTORY

My professional interest in the field started in my early years as a student nurse at Massachusetts General Hospital, School of Nursing (MGH). We met regularly with a psychologist to discuss our experiences as student nurses, so I assumed that it was normal to be able to discuss the experiences one had in one's initial role as a nurse, being exposed to trauma, death, and loss. As a third-year student nurse, I heard Dr. Tom Hackett speak of Dr. Erich Lindemann's (1944) research with the Coconut Grove fire. He spoke of anticipatory grief, delayed grief, and chronic grief. The next day I was able to immediately make use of the concept of delayed grief to give meaning to what appeared to be a heart attack in my "ICU (intensive care unit) case," but was actually a delayed reaction to her husband's death 16 years ago that day. I decided to go into psychiatry to learn how to talk with people.

My work in the field of cancer, bereavement, and occupational stress in oncology and palliative care began in 1971 when my colleagues and I were invited to begin to work with the nurses at Princess Margaret Hospital, a cancer hospital in Toronto. The nurses were upset that the doctors weren't being helpful to them in dealing with the death of a young patient, but the doctor was crying in his office. We were invited to investigate the stress of staff working with cancer patients and to develop programs of intervention for staff members (Rochester, Vachon, & Lyall, 1974; Vachon, Lyall, & Freeman, 1978). Simultaneously, we began to accept referrals of cancer patients and their family members who were experiencing stress leading to a series of research studies on adaptation to cancer and intervention with persons with cancer and adaptation to bereavement and intervention with newly bereaved women. From the 1970s through 2000, I was employed in teaching hospitals and did research and clinical work with people dealing with cancer and bereavement as well as research and writing regarding occupational stress in health care providers. Today my primary role is as a psychotherapist working with people with cancer and bereavement, and I continue to write in the field.

My introduction to the hospice/palliative care movement began in 1974 when my colleague Dr. Alan Lyall met a young urologist, Dr. Balfour Mount, who had a vision of opening a unit at the Royal Victoria Hospital in Montreal, Quebec, to care for the terminally ill. The unit was to be based on the philosophy of St. Christopher's Hospice. Quebec is a French-speaking province. "Hospice" translated as "'poor house" in French, so Dr. Mount looked for a new term and developed the concept of "palliative care." To palliate is to "alleviate (disease) without curing." Dr. Lyall suggested to Dr. Mount that as our team had already studied the stress of staff at Princess Margaret Hospital, we might study the stress of the staff of the newly developing Royal Victoria Hospital.

OVERVIEW

The experience of caring for another, or others, whether as a professional, volunteer, or family member, can be both stressful and very rewarding. This chapter reviews very briefly the major constructs used in the field of occupational stress: stress and distress, burnout and job engagement, and compassion fatigue and compassion satisfaction (CS) and will identify some key findings for professionals, volunteers, and family caregivers. The reader interested in more detail is referred to previous reviews of this literature (Vachon, 1995, 2010, 2011; Vachon, Huggard, & Huggard, in press). The focus in this chapter will be on what is known about what helps caregivers deal with their personal and job stress, current exciting interventions being done in the field of caregiving, and reflections on major challenges and hopes for future developments in the field. Insofar as possible, due to space limitations, the chapter will refer to recent review articles.

STRESS AND DISTRESS

Definition of Terms

"Stress" is defined as "the nonspecific response of the body to any demand made upon it" (Selye, 1974, p. 27). Stress is not something to avoid. Complete freedom from stress is death. Distress is defined as "damaging or unpleasant stress" (Selye, 1974, p. 1).

The European Agency for Safety and Health at Work (2000) has stated, "There is increasing consensus around defining work-related stress in terms of the 'interactions' between employee and (exposure to hazards in) their work environment. Within this model stress can be said to be experienced when the demands from the work environment exceed the employee's ability to cope with them."

Stress and Distress in Professional Staff

In our early work, dying patients were not the major problem; difficulties with the work situation and staff communication problems were mentioned as often as were difficulties watching patients suffer and die (Vachon et al., 1978). This finding has been fairly consistent since those early days (Vachon, 1987, 1995, 2011).

Stress and distress in caregivers is often measured using the Goldberg General Health Questionnaire (GHQ; Goldberg, 1978). It is often referred to as

psychiatric disturbance. In a literature review (Vachon, 2010), psychiatric disturbance in oncology and palliative care staff ranged from a low of 9.5% of support
staff and 10.5% of allied health staff in Ontario cancer centers to 12% of Japanese
palliative care physicians to between a quarter and one third of the sample in the
other studies of oncologists and palliative care specialists. Previous reviews have
generally found stress in palliative care to be less than that in other specialties
(Vachon, 1995, 2011).

Data from an international convenience sample of almost 600 people
(Vachon, 1987) found that major stressors identified by those working in palliative care ($N = 60$) were communication problems with "others" in the system,
role ambiguity, team communication problems, administrative communication
problems, and role conflict. The 81 caregivers in oncology were different from
the other specialty areas in that they had equal numbers of stressors in the areas
of patients and families, occupational role, and environmental stressors, such as
team communication problems.

Stress in Volunteers

Claxton-Oldfield and Claxton-Oldfield (2008) reviewed the literature on stress in
hospice volunteers and found those who left were more apt to have higher anxiety, high death anxiety, and lower purpose-in-life scores. Some volunteers left
their roles because of the attitude of nurses toward the volunteers or because of
feeling underused. Stress or burnout seldom contributed to volunteers leaving
their roles. Volunteers identified four main areas of stress, which they catego-
rized as role ambiguity, status ambiguity, stress related to patients and families,
and stress related to their own personal lives.

Stress and Distress in Family Caregivers

Being a family caregiver may "have physical, psychological, social and financial
consequences for carers, which outlast their period of care and may influence
their bereavement" (Payne & Grande, 2013, p. 579). They may be challenged by
witnessing the last period of the patient's life "with the potential for vicarious
distress and suffering, from the direct physical and emotional demands of being
a carer or from their own emotional and social changes in bereavement" (Payne &
Grande, 2013, p. 579).

A meta-analysis of 43 studies compared cancer patients' anxiety and depression 2 to 10 years after diagnosis with normal controls and with family caregivers (Mitchell, Ferguson, Gill, Paul, & Symonds, 2013). Neither the prevalence of
depression (26.7% vs. 26.3%) nor the prevalence of anxiety (28.0% vs. 40.1%) differed significantly between cancer patients and their spouses. The authors suggest that anxiety, rather than depression, should be a focus of intervention in
patients and families dealing with cancer.

Hudson (2013) says that family caregiving should not be pathologized but
contends it would be a breach of care if the more than 40% of family carers who
appear to meet the criteria for psychological distress are not given the care they
require. Carer resources, rather than patient diagnosis or illness severity, are the
primary predictors of caregiver burden and other caregiver outcomes. The quality of social support was more important than the size of the social support network (Hudson, 2013).

BURNOUT AND JOB ENGAGEMENT

Burnout is understood to be a form of mental distress manifested in "normal" people who did not suffer from prior psychopathology and who experience decreased work performance resulting from negative attitudes and behaviors (Maslach & Leiter, 2008). Burnout is a psychological syndrome in response to chronic interpersonal stressors on the job (Maslach, Schaufeli, & Leiter, 2001). The three key dimensions are (1) overwhelming emotional exhaustion (EE)—the basic *individual stress dimension* of burnout; (2) feelings of cynicism and detachment from the job, depersonalization (DP)—the *interpersonal context* dimension of burnout (referring to a negative, callous, or excessively detached response to various aspects of the job); and (3) a sense of ineffectiveness and lack of personal accomplishment (PA)—the *self-evaluation dimension* of burnout (referring to feelings of incompetence and a lack of achievement and productivity at work [Maslach & Leiter, 2008]).

Six areas of work life encompass the major organizational antecedents of burnout: workload, control, reward, community, fairness, and values (Maslach et al., 2001). Emotion–work variables (e.g., requirement to display or suppress emotions on the job, or requirements to be emotionally empathic) account for additional variance in burnout scores over and above job stressors (Maslach et al., 2001). Elsewhere, the literature in palliative care and oncology is reviewed using this framework (Vachon, 2011; Vachon et al., in press).

Job engagement is defined as a persistent, positive-affective-motivational state of fulfillment in employees that is characterized by vigor, dedication, and absorption (Maslach, 2003). Job engagement includes energy, involvement, and efficacy. Engagement includes a sustainable workload, feelings of choice and control, appropriate recognition and reward, a supportive work community, fairness and justice, and meaningful and valued work. It is characterized by high levels of activation and pleasure (Maslach, 2003).

Prevalence of Burnout

A review of 10 studies (Peterson et al., 2008; total $N = 2,357$) identified a range of 8% to 51% of oncology staff suffering from severe burnout on at least one of the burnout components, with overall EE and DP prevalence rates of 36% and 34%, respectively, only slightly higher than Maslach's and Jackson's norms. The considerable heterogeneity in burnout rates across studies was attributed to the multiprofessional nature of respondents and the international nature of the samples that come from different health care systems. In contrast, a survey of volunteer emergency medical service volunteers showed an alarming percentage of participants scored high on emotional exhaustion (92%) and depersonalization (99%); however, 75% also reported high levels of personal accomplishment (Essex & Scott, 2008).

Factors Associated With Burnout

Factors associated with burnout include feeling insufficiently trained in communication and management skills, not having sufficient time to communicate with patients, insufficient confidence in psychological care of patients, being overloaded, dealing with death and dying, inadequate preparation, staff conflict, low prestige of one's specialty, not being religious, no or lower spirituality, not having the personality characteristic of *hardiness*, diminished self-awareness and not engaging in self-care activities (Vachon, 2010, 2011; Vachon et al., in press).

For trauma therapists, younger age, having no special trauma training, having an increased percentage of individuals on the caseload with posttraumatic stress disorder (PTSD), being an inpatient practitioner, and not using evidence-based practices significantly predicted burnout (Craig & Sprang, 2010).

COMPASSION FATIGUE, EMPATHY, AND COMPASSION SATISFACTION

Compassion fatigue is described as the "'cost of caring' for others in emotional pain that has led helping professionals to abandon their work with traumatized persons" (Figley, 1995, p. 7). Compassion fatigue is a combination of secondary traumatic stress and burnout, as well as previous severe early traumatic experiences that may leave one with an increased vulnerability when exposed to another's pain and suffering. This can be complicated because it is often early adverse experiences that motivate people to pursue careers in the health care and helping professions (Baranowsky & Schmidt, 2013).

CS measures the positive aspect of work. CS has been defined as "the pleasure you derive from being able to do your work well" (Stamm, 2009, p. 12). It stands in sharp contrast to compassion fatigue, which pertains to the negative effects arising from one's work. The research on compassion fatigue and CS and the controversies in the field are discussed elsewhere (Vachon et al., in press).

WHAT ARE CAREGIVERS ALREADY DOING THAT WORKS?

Coping Strategies

Caregivers often derive considerable satisfaction from their jobs. This can be defined as job engagement or CS. The construct of CS is similar to the top coping mechanism Vachon (1987) found. When caregivers were asked what "kept them going" in their work, the most common response was "a sense of competence, control and pleasure in one's work." Caregivers frequently commented, "I like my work. I'm good at it and I have been doing it long enough to have some control over my work environment." The words would also be reflective of job engagement. In that study, younger caregivers had more stressors, more manifestations of stress, and fewer coping strategies. The same holds true in more recent studies (Lemaire, Wallace, & Jovanovic, 2013).

A study of employee assistance professionals (EA) providing crisis intervention and disaster management (Jacobson, 2006) showed a low to moderate risk for compassion fatigue and burnout. EA professionals who used more positive coping skills reported higher potential for CS and lower risk for burnout. The most effective coping method reported by participants was talking to others about the stress (i.e., peers, colleagues, family members), followed by physical exercise and then prayer and spirituality.

EA professionals who reported using more passive coping skills (expressing or venting negative feelings; learning to live with work-related stress; engaging in activities, such as watching TV, reading, etc., to think about the stress less; and using humor) scored higher on risk for burnout. Finally, EA professionals who used more negative coping skills (i.e., using alcohol and drugs to feel better, denying the situation, criticizing oneself, giving up on trying to cope with work-related stress, and blaming oneself for the stress) scored higher on risk for compassion fatigue, higher on risk for burnout, and lower on potential for CS.

Lemaire et al. (2013) report that physicians in Alberta, Canada ($N = 1,178$) who kept their work stress to themselves, concentrated on what to do next, and kept going on as if nothing has happened had higher burnout. The authors suggested that those strategies reflected denial and avoidance responses that didn't involve dealing with the source of the stress in a constructive manner. "The coping strategies that were associated with lower levels of burnout include: taking a time out (which doctors rarely do), using humor, talking to colleagues, and making a plan of action and working through it, which tend to reflect more active coping strategies" (Lemaire et al., 2013, p. 236). Outside of work, talking to one's spouse, spending time with one's family, taking a break from work, exercise, finding a quiet time for oneself, and leaving work at work were all associated with decreased stress or burnout (Lemaire et al., 2013). These coping strategies stand in contrast to those of the overcoper whom Baranowsky and Schmidt say is at increased risk of compassion fatigue.

> Overcopers may regard themselves as high achievers in their careers as a means of establishing a buffer for their lives and job struggles and to ward off, at all costs, their feelings of failure. Frequently overcopers will push beyond pain even when life and work demands have become unmanageable, because of the belief that their career identity as viewed by others is more important than their own individual needs. In their world, stopping to rest and reflect is a weakness; high performance at any cost is the expectation. (Baranowsky & Schmidt, 2013, p. 207)

Self-care

Residents studied by Shanafelt et al. (2005) who had a broader repertoire of coping styles, including meditation and spirituality, were more empathic. The caregivers studied by Vachon (1987) reported not only the sense of competence, control, and pleasure in one's work, but also a personal philosophy of illness, death, and one's role in caring for dying persons and their families as well as lifestyle-management techniques, including engaging in physical activities and diversions, organizing non-job-related social interactions, taking time off, attending to one's need for good nutrition and adequate sleep, and meditation and relaxation exercises. Volunteers found that outside interests, a supportive social network, taking a break from volunteering, and having a clear idea of their role within the system were helpful coping strategies (Claxton-Oldfield & Claxton-Oldfield, 2008). We cannot be compassionate to others if we are not first compassionate to ourselves. In practicing self-compassion, we as caregivers need to practice holistic self-care and wellness strategies to bring compassion to others (Kearney, Weininger, Vachon, Mount, & Harrison, 2009).

Exquisite Empathy

Harrison and Westwood (2009) studied protective practices that mitigated vicarious trauma among mental health therapists, including professionals working in palliative care. One theme stood out—"exquisite empathy." Empathic engagement with traumatized clients appeared to be a protective practice for clinicians working with them. Exquisite empathy "required a sophisticated balance on the part of the clinician as s/he simultaneously maintains clear and consistent boundaries, expanded perspective, and highly present, intimate, and heartfelt interpersonal connection in the therapeutic relationship with clients, without fusing, or losing sight of the clinician's own perspective" (Harrison & Westwood, 2009, p. 214). Trauma therapists who engaged in exquisite empathy were "invigorated rather than depleted by their intimate professional connections with traumatized clients" (Harrison & Westwood, 2009, p. 213) and protected against compassion fatigue and burnout.

The therapists studied by Harrison and Westwood had a "secure base" through the self-compassion that they practiced. The idea that trauma therapists can be both invigorated and protected in their work has been referred to as bidirectionality. The practice of exquisite empathy is facilitated by clinician self-awareness (Harrison & Westwood, 2009; Kearney et al., 2009).

Resilience

Resilience in professional caregivers is defined as "the ability to maintain personal and professional well-being in the face of on-going work stress and adversity" (McCann et al., 2013, p. 60). Developing and fostering resilient environments and individuals within the health professions is emerging as a way to reduce negative, and increase positive, outcomes of stress in health professionals. McCann et al. conducted a literature review of five professions: nursing, social work, psychology, counseling, and medicine. They investigated behavioral and cognitive strategies in personal and professional spheres. Summarizing their findings across the disciplines, they found that being female and maintaining a work–life balance were found to relate consistently to resilience across the five disciplines. Four other factors related to resilience in four of the five disciplines: laughter/humor, self-reflection/insight, beliefs/spirituality, and professional identity.

Resilience in Family Caregivers

The widows Bonanno and his colleagues studied had often been caregivers for their husbands before the husband's death. Prebereavement, they had relatively high scores related to the ability to adapt well to loss (e.g., acceptance of death, belief in a just world, instrumental support; Bonanno, 2004). Bonanno defines *resilience* as reflecting the ability to maintain a stable equilibrium. The difference between the resilient individuals and the other participants was that their experiences were transient rather than enduring and did not interfere with their ability to continue to function in other areas of their lives, including the capacity for positive affect.

Fauth, Zarit, and Femia (2008) reported on a study of 229 caregivers for persons with dementia. They defined resilience in caregiving as maintaining low levels of burden despite high demands for care. The study identified those who were "resilient," as well as a comparison group experiencing high care demands and high burden. Variables, such as demographic characteristics, care receiver characteristics, risk factors (e.g., daily exposure to behavioral and psychological symptoms of dementia and global feelings of stress), and protective characteristics (e.g., social support), were used to predict membership into the resilient caregiver group.

Spirituality

Spirituality has been found to be helpful to caregivers in coping with work stress as well as perhaps being in a "better place" from which to meet the challenges of the work situation. Huggard, Stamm, and Pearlman (2013) found greater CS in those who reported greater spirituality. However, earlier Huggard (2008) found a positive correlation between religion and vicarious traumatization. High scores on the "relationship with a higher power" subscale were related to high scores on the compassion fatigue subscale. He also demonstrated a negative and significant correlation between spirituality and burnout. Other authors have also found those with little or no spirituality were at increased risk of burnout, as were young males (Vachon et al., in press).

CURRENT INTERVENTIONS

Interventions to decrease stress, distress, burnout, and compassion fatigue and promote job engagement and CS involve the creation of a healthy work environment as well as individuals, whether professionals, volunteers, and even family caregivers, realizing the importance of developing self-awareness and self-care practices and integrating these practices into their lives. Physicians who engage in self-care and have some form of spiritual practice are more empathic (Shanafelt et al., 2005) and are less prone to burnout (Kearney et al., 2009) and compassion fatigue (Huggard et al., 2013; Vachon et al., in press).

Shanafelt and Dyrbye (2012) emphasize that recovery from burnout is possible, with prospective studies in medical students and residents suggesting that approximately 12% to 27% recover over the following 12 months. However, recovery requires deliberate and sustained effort to identify and address the factors contributing to burnout. A review of burnout interventions identified 25 relevant studies (Awa, Plaumann, & Walter, 2010). Most (80%) programs led to reduced burnout. Person-directed interventions reduced burnout in the short term (6 months or less), whereas a combination of person- and organization-directed interventions had longer lasting effects (>12 months). The Joint Committee on Accreditation in the United States has mandated that all hospitals have a program to address physician well-being, separate from disciplinary processes (Vachon & Butow, in press).

It will not be sufficient to intervene on just one level. The Registered Nurses of Ontario (2013) recently published *Developing and Sustaining Interprofessional Health Care: Optimizing Patients/Clients, Organizational, and System Outcomes*. The document provides key concepts of the Healthy Work Environments Framework, which include system-based, organizational, and individual/team recommendations. The document identifies levels of evidence for the suggestions given, which provides starting points for future research.

Educational Interventions

As already noted, stress and burnout were more prevalent in physicians who did not feel they had adequate communication skills and had difficulty with psychosocial communication. Reviews of the impact of communication skills training on burnout have reached varied conclusions, with the most recent one finding inadequate evidence to support a positive impact (Moore, Rivera Mercado, Grez Artigues, & Lawrie, 2013).

Phelps, Lloyd, Creamer, and Forbes (2009) propose a primary, secondary, and tertiary model of intervention for carers in the aftermath of trauma. They suggest that much of the focus to date has been on identifying stress symptoms that arise in such workers. There is now enough evidence to develop programs of intervention that would (a) minimize the risk of carers developing problems and (b) early on identify those who are at risk and begin intervention. Increased awareness of the early signs of stress and regular self-screening will be helpful. Early intervention could include self-care, organizational or social support, and stress management that might prevent more serious problems. Cognitive behavioral therapy might be beneficial for those who have developed stress-related conditions. As noted earlier, the use of evidence-based practices was found to decrease compassion fatigue and burnout in trauma therapists (Craig & Sprang, 2010).

Family Interventions

In an editorial in *Palliative Medicine* devoted to family caregivers, Hudson (2013) notes,

> Current indications are that palliative care providers should assist carers by targeting social support and resources and provide education that focuses on coping strategies and preparation for the carer role. . . . Carers typically want to know what the role entails, how to manage symptoms, signs of imminent death and resources and strategies to sustain their own well-being. (Hudson, 2013, p. 581)

Recent evidence shows that telephone and video-phone support may be as effective as face-to-face intervention in some circumstances (Hudson, 2013). Hudson suggests that a realistic objective in family intervention would be to reduce the psychosocial burden on the primary family carer. Such changes would also need to be taken into the community setting where generalist carers are dealing with dying persons and their families. Legitimizing family caregivers as "care recipients" could facilitate making needed resources available and allow health care workers to have time for family member interventions.

Accelerated Recovery Program for Compassion Fatigue

The Accelerated Recovery Program (ARP) for Compassion Fatigue was established in 1997 as "a five-session individual treatment model for treating professional care providers who had become overwhelmed by the demands of their work" (Baranowsky & Schmidt, 2013, p. 211). The idea was that secondary exposure to serious illness, trauma, or injury resulted in a wound in caregivers that required further intervention. The program expanded beyond individuals to large groups, and trainers were trained internationally to offer psychoeducational intervention to large groups, including health care professionals, emergency responders, funeral home personnel, and Red Cross members.

"The stages of the treatment process focus on issues such as the therapeutic alliance between clinician and patient, clinicians' quantitative assessment of their own distress, anxiety-management skills, the importance of narrative regarding personal and work-related experiences, and issues related to the exposure and resolution of secondary traumatic stress (STS). A key component of this training is cognitive restructuring for self-care and integration of new concepts and skills. In addition, the ARP provides an aftercare resiliency plan emphasizing resiliency skills, self-management and self-care skills, connection with others, skills acquisition, and conflict resolution" (Baranowsky & Schmidt, 2013, p. 211).

In the ARP, self-reflective and self-care skills are taught to establish a nonanxious presence and self-validated caregiving. "Non-anxious presence is the ability to sit comfortably with the emotional strain on exposure to patient distress and remain a compassionate witness" (Baranowsky & Schmidt, 2013, pp. 211–212). This model may involve a paradigm shift for physicians from being a hero to being a healer. "It is within this 'healer' paradigm that maintaining a non-anxious presence can make sense for physicians. Here they can learn that being non-anxious can be healing *in and of itself* to a patient possibly facing the most terrifying time in his or her life. Through this practice physicians may also learn a more spiritual lesson: that healing and being successful as a healer does not necessarily mean the cure of disease" (Baranowsky & Schmidt, 2013, p. 212). Self-reflection and self-care lead to increased ability to attend to one's own needs or those of others feeling replenished. This leads to improved self-validated caregiving, and nonanxious presence while caring for others and self.

Meaning-Centered and Mindfulness-Based Interventions

Very important, systematic research is being done at Quebec by Lise Fillion and her colleagues, including Melanie Vachon (no relation to the author). Fillion and her colleagues are working with meaning-centered interventions combined with mindfulness meditation in palliative care as well as recent work being done in intensive care units. The work is based in part on the Being With Dying Program earlier developed by Roshi Joan Halifax and her colleagues, updated most recently in Halifax (2013). In a synopsis of their work, Fillion et al. (2013) note their goal in their research and cite their multiple previous references.

> In the current context of labour shortages and limited access to palliative care, a major challenge arises in making organizational choices that take into account the evolution in the working community, new occupational requirements, as well as the improved management of workplaces and well-being of personnel. The researchers' primary objective is to improve the conditions in which palliative care is provided by validating a conceptual framework that results in a better understanding of the work satisfaction and well-being of nurses in this field. The results of this study will offer decision-makers a choice of models of services to be favoured and a better understanding of the aspects to be considered before implementing training services or programs for caregivers and managers. (Fillion, Truchon, & L'Heureux, 2013; this research report is in French but an English translation is given, p. 1)

The recommendation of complementing meaning-centered interventions (MCI) with mindfulness is in line with the Being With Dying intervention (BWD; Halifax, 2013). The BWD program is an 8-day residential program based on scientific data that

> encompasses ethical, spiritual, psychological, existential and social aspects of care of the dying. It includes mindful and compassionate approaches to end-of-life care, compassion-based ethics and communication strategies in EOLC [End-of-Life Care], clinician self-care and contemplative interventions appropriate for clinicians/caregivers and dying people. The program builds on reflective practices that can regulate attention and emotion, cultivate compassion, aid in the development of a meta-cognitive perspective, promote calm and resilience, reduce stress, and foster emotional balance, embodiment and compassion. The training also emphasizes basic neuroscience research in relation to the clinical, contemplative and conceptual content of the training. (Halifax, 2013, p. 467)

The premise of BWD, which is based on the development of mindfulness and receptive attention through contemplative practice, is that cultivating stability of mind and emotions enables clinicians to respond to others and themselves with compassion. The program provides skills, attitudes, behaviors, and tools to change how caregivers work with the dying and bereaved. Roshi Joan and her colleagues developed the G.R.A.C.E. process used in the program to prime compassion in clinicians for compassion-based clinician–patient interactions. The acronym G.R.A.C.E. stands for:

- Gather your attention
- Recall your intention
- Attune by checking in with yourself, then the patient
- Consider what will really serve your patient by being truly present with your patient and letting insights arise
- Engage, enact ethically, and then end the interaction

The program was developed to help prevent burnout and secondary trauma in caregivers, including doctors, nurses, human rights activists, and others working in stressful situations. The practice offers "a simple and efficient way to open to the experience of the suffering of others, to stay centered, and to develop the capacity to respond with compassion" (Halifax, 2014). Roshi Joan defines compassion as

> the capacity to be attentive to the experience of others, to wish the best for others, and to sense what will truly serve others. Ironically, in a time when we hear the phrase "compassion fatigue" with increasing frequency, compassion as we are defining it does not lead to fatigue. In fact, it can actually become a wellspring of resilience as we allow our natural impulse to care for another to become a source of nourishment rather than depletion. (Halifax, 2014, blog, n.p.)

She notes that compassion makes it possible for us to help others in a more skillful and effective way. Recent research studies show that compassion helps us as well by reducing physiological stress and promoting physical and emotional well-being (Halifax, 2014).

Stress Vaccine

Very exciting work is being done by colleagues in Toronto who were recently awarded the International 2013 Ted Freedman Award for Innovation in Education for the Stress Vaccine. Maunder et al. (2010) began their work to bolster the resilience of health care workers during the 2003 severe acute respiratory syndrome (SARS) epidemic in Toronto. During the epidemic, 44 people died of the disease in Canada, including two nurses and a doctor, with most of the deaths occurring in Toronto. Observations made during and after the 2003 outbreak of SARS suggested that an emerging infectious disease causes stress in health care settings because of fear of contagion, concern for family health, job stress, interpersonal isolation, quarantine, and perceived stigma. Maunder et al. (2010) designed a program to improve resilience in the face of the epidemic. They used the definition of resilience as overcoming stress or adversity or, more precisely, as having a good outcome after an adverse experience. The initial idea was to develop a program that could be used before a pandemic, which would reduce the adverse stress-related aspects of pandemic exposure, hence the name "Stress Vaccine." This program has now been adapted for hospital-wide use and testing is underway to determine its efficacy in other populations. Their training aimed to ensure that staff were well prepared for the pandemic or other stressful aspects of heath care work. The goals were "to (i) increase confidence in being well-supported by the hospital and well prepared for the pandemic and (ii) enhance adaptive strategies of coping (increasing problem solving and seeking support and decreasing escape-avoidance)" (Maunder et al., 2010, p. 2). The intervention was based on social learning theory to improve self-efficacy. Finally, because many aspects of infectious disease are interpersonal, as are many other aspects of health care work, the final goal was to reduce interpersonal problems at the personal and organizational levels. Improvements were obtained in three of the four targeted domains of psychological function: pandemic self-efficacy, confidence in support and training, and interpersonal problems (Maunder et al., 2010).

The intervention was then adapted to be used more broadly in the hospital and is now being tested in other settings. The Stress Vaccine–Hospital Edition is a highly individualized, interactive, e-learning training program that helps hospital workers to develop resilience to workplace stress. It works via

- attention to *interpersonal* determinants of stress and resilience and
- increasing *reflection*, reducing reactivity (i.e., use the *slow* parts of your brain to think about what is going on in your mind and in the minds of others).

There are 10 computerized sessions that take 20 to 30 minutes and staff can proceed at their own pace. The sessions include the following:

- Self-assessment with feedback
- Coping, interpersonal problems and challenges, empathy
- Didactic teaching about interpersonal interactions, reflective thought, and coping
- Skills practice—relaxation training
- Interactive simulations of stressful situations + reflection +/− coaching

The multiple modalities include simulated interpersonal interactions that use video enactments of stressful scenarios, which are combined with personalized "dialogue" with the computer to reflect on difficulties that are encountered and discover new options. Learning also occurs via (1) identification of one's own interpersonal style and preferences using validated questionnaires with feedback, (2) guided reflection about recent difficult interactions—identifying patterns and applying insights about ones own style, (3) practicing relaxation exercises, (4) role-playing responses to interpersonal challenges, (5) guided self-evaluation of the empathic quality of responses to challenge, and (6) the comments of videotaped peer coaches. Following multiple paths to the same goals, health care workers learn to increase their capacity to reflect, thus improving tolerance for the ambiguity, uncertainty, and conflict, that are core contributers to workplace stress.

MAJOR CHALLENGES AND HOPES FOR THE FUTURE

Some of the most exciting work being done at this point is the integration of neuroscience into trying to change occupational stress in health care providers and volunteers. When I look at my very early research, the stressors identified have not really changed. Staff in the 1970s complained of overwork and difficulty dealing with the psychosocial issues of patients and families, particularly those facing death, as well as problems communicating with one another. These continue to be major stressors.

Current interventions, such as the Stress Vaccine, the Being With Dying Program, and the work of Lise Fillion and her colleagues, are using skills training and drawing on new findings in neuroscience aimed at building resilience and exploring the benefits of compassion for self and others. Some of these findings of neuroscience show, for example, that compassion can activate parts of the brain associated with love and reward, whereas empathy, particularly if there is empathic strain, can lead to feelings of exhaustion and burnout (Singer & Bolz, 2013). The free downloadable e-book by Singer and Bolz (2013) is an incredible resource that explores a variety of ways in which neuroscience and mindfulness meditation can be integrated into personal and organizational settings to improve health and resilience and make the world a better and kinder place.

Really changing occupational stress will involve organizational and systems change, but it will also challenge caregivers to learn how to care for themselves and to integrate self-care and self-compassion into their daily lives recognizing that it is in giving that we receive, but also acknowledging that the heart first pumps blood to itself (Kearney et al., 2009).

REFERENCES

Awa, W. L., Plaumann, M., & Walter, U. (2010). Burnout prevention: A review of intervention programs. *Patient Education and Counseling, 78*(2), 184–190.

Baranowsky, A., & Schmidt, D. (2013). Overcopers: Medical doctor vulnerability to compassion fatigue. In C. R., Figley, P. K. Huggard, & C. Rees (Eds.), *First do no self-harm* (pp. 203–215). New York, NY: Oxford University Press.

Bonanno, G. A. (2004). Loss, trauma, and human resilience. *American Psychologist, 59*(1), 20–28.

Claxton-Oldfield, S., & Claxton-Oldfield, J. (2008). Keeping hospice palliative care volunteers on board: Dealing with issues of volunteer attrition, stress, and retention. *Indian Journal of Palliative Care, 14*(1), 30–37.

Craig, C. D., & Sprang, G. (2010). Compassion satisfaction, compassion fatigue, and burnout in a national sample of trauma treatment therapists. *Anxiety, Stress, & Coping, 23*(3), 319–339.

Essex, B., & Scott, L.B. (2008). Chronic stress and associated coping strategies among volunteer EMS personnel. *Prehospital Emergency Care, 12*, 69–75.

European Agency for Safety and Health at Work. (2000). *Safety at work*. Retrieved from http://agency.osha.eu.int/publications/factsheets/8/en/facts8_en.pdf

Fauth, E., Zarit, S., & Femia, E. (2008). Stress and well-being in a caregiving population: Predicting resilience in family caregivers. *The Gerontologist, 48*, 680.

Figley, C. (1995). *Compassion fatigue: Coping with secondary traumatic stress disorder in those who treat the traumatized*. New York, NY: Brunner-Routledge.

Fillion, L., Truchon, M., L'Heureux, M., Dallaire, C., Langlois, L., Bellemare, M., & Dupuis, R. (2013). *To improve services and care at the end of life: Understanding the impact of workplace satisfaction and well-being of nurses* (Rapport R-794). Montréal, Quebec, Canada: IRSST. Retrieved from http://www.irsst.qc.ca/-projet-vers-l-amelioration-des-services-et-des-soins-de-fin-de-vie-mieux-comprendre-l-impact-du-milieu-de-travail-sur-la-satis faction-et-le-bien-etre-des-0099-6050.html

Goldberg, D. (1978). *Manual of the general health questionnaire*. Windsor, UK: NFER Nelson.

Halifax, J. (2013). Being with dying: Experiences in end-of-life-care. In T. Singer & M. Bolz (Eds.), *Compassion: Bridging practice and science ebook* (pp. 108–120). Munich, Germany: Max Planck Society.

Halifax, J. (2014, February 12). *G.R.A.C.E.: Training in cultivating compassion in interactions with others* [Web log post]. Santa Fe, NM: Upaya Zen Center. https://www.upaya.org/2014/02/practicing-g-r-c-e-bring-compassion-interactions-others-roshi-joan-halifax/

Harrison, R., & Westwood, M. (2009). Preventing vicarious traumatization of mental health therapists: Identitiying protective practices. *Psychotherapy, Theory, Research, Practical Training, 46*(2), 203–219.

Hudson, P. (2013). Improving support for family carers: Key implications for research, policy and practice (Editorial). *Palliative Medicine, 27*(7), 581–582.

Huggard, P. K. (2008). *Managing compassion fatigue: Implications for medical education* (Unpublished doctoral dissertation). University of Auckland, Auckland, New Zealand.

Huggard, P. K., Stamm, B. H., & Pearlman, L. A. (2013). Physician stress: Compassion satisfaction, compassion fatigue and vicarious traumatization. In C. R. Figley, P. K. Huggard, & C. Rees (Eds.), *First do no self-harm* (pp. 127–145). New York, NY: Oxford University Press.

Jacobson, J. M. (2006). Compassion fatigue, compassion satisfaction, and burnout: Reactions among employee assistance professionals providing workplace crisis intervention and disaster management services. *Journal of Workplace Behavioral Health, 21*(3/4), 133–152.

Kearney, M. K., Weininger, R. B., Vachon, M. L. S., Mount, B. M., & Harrison, R. L. (2009). Self-care of physicians caring for patients at the end of life: "Being Connected . . . A Key to My Survival." *Journal of the American Medical Association, 301*, 1155–1164.

Lemaire, J., Wallace, J. E., & Jovanovic, A. (2013). Stress and coping: Generational and gender similarities and differences. In C. R. Figley, P. K. Huggard, & C. Rees (Eds.), *First do no self-harm* (pp. 216–246). New York, NY: Oxford University Press.

Lindemann, E. (1944). The symptomatology and management of acute grief. *American Journal of Psychiatry, 101*, 141–148.

Maslach, C. (2003). Job burnout: New directions in research and interventions. *Current Directions in Psychological Science, 13*, 189–192.

Maslach, C., & Leiter, M. P. (2008). Early predictors of job burnout and engagement. *Journal of Applied Psychology, 93*, 498–512.

Maslach, C., Schaufeli, W. B., & Leiter, M. P. (2001). Job burnout. *Annual Review of Psychology, 52*, 397–422.

Maunder, R. G., Lancee, W. J., Mael, R., Vincent, L., Peladeau, N., Beduz, M. A., . . . Leszcz, M. (2010). Computer-assisted resilience training to prepare healthcare workers for pandemic influenza: A randomized trial of the optimal dose of training. *Bio Med Central Health Services Research, 10*, 72. Retrieved from http://www.biomedcentral.com/1472-6963/10/72

McCann, C. M., Beddoe, E., McCormick, K., Huggard, P., Kedge, S., Adamson, C., & Huggard, J. (2013). Resilience in the health professions: A review of recent literature. *International Journal of Wellbeing, 3*(1), 60–81.

Mitchell, A. J., Ferguson, D. W., Gill, J., Paul, J., & Symonds, P. (2013). Depression and anxiety in long-term cancer survivors compared with spouses and healthy controls: A systematic review and meta-analysis. *Lancet Oncology, 14*, 721–32.

Moore, P. M., Rivera Mercado, S., Grez Artigues, M., & Lawrie, T. A. (2013). Communication skills training for healthcare professionals working with people who have cancer (review) *Cochrane Library, 3*. Retrieved from http://www.thecochranelibrary.com

Payne, S., & Grande, G. (2013). Towards better support for family career: A richer understanding (Editorial). *Palliative Medicine, 27*(7), 579–580.

Peterson, U., Demerouti, E., Bergstrom, G., Samuelsson, M., Asberg, M., & Nygren, A. (2008). Burnout and physical and mental health among Swedish healthcare workers. *Journal of Advanced Nursing, 62*, 84–95.

Phelps, A., Lloyd, D., Creamer, M., & Forbes, D. (2009). Caring for carers in the aftermath of trauma. *Journal of Aggression, Maltreatment & Trauma, 18*, 313–330.

Registered Nurses' Association of Ontario. (2013). *Developing and sustaining interprofessional health care: Optimizing patients/clients, organizational, and system outcomes.* Toronto, Canada: Author.

Rochester, S. R., Vachon, M. L. S., & Lyall, W. A. L. (1974). Immediacy in language: A channel to the care of the dying patient. *Journal of Community Psychology, 2*(1), 75–76.

Selye, H. (1974). *Stress without distress.* Philadelphia, PA: Lippincott.

Shanafelt, T., & Dyrbye, L. (2012). Oncologist burnout: Causes, consequences and responses. *Journal of Clinical Oncology, 30*(11), 1235–1241.

Shanafelt, T. D., West, C., Zhao, X., Novotny, P., Kolars, J., Habermann, T., & Sloan, J. (2005). Relationship between increased personal well-being and enhanced empathy among internal medicine residents. *Journal of General Internal Medicine, 20*, 559–564.

Singer, T., & Bolz, M. (2013). *Compassion: Bridging practice and science* (e-book). Munich, Germany: Max Planck Society.

Stamm, B. (2009). The concise manual for the Professional Quality of Life Scale: The ProQOL. Pocatello, ID: ProQOL.org.

Vachon, M. L. S. (1987). *Occupational stress in the care of the critically ill, dying and bereaved.* Washington, DC: Hemisphere.

Vachon, M. L. S. (1995). Staff stress in palliative/hospice care: A review. *Palliative Medicine, 9,* 91–122.

Vachon, M. L. S. (2010). Oncology staff stress and related interventions. In J. C. Holland, W. S. Breitbart, P. B. Jacobsen, M. S. Lederberg, M. J. Loscalzo, & R. McCorkle (Eds.), *Psycho-oncology* (2nd ed., pp. 575–581). New York, NY: Oxford University Press.

Vachon, M. L. S. (2011). Four decades of selected research in hospice/palliative care: Have the stressors changed? In I. Renzenbrink (Ed.), *Caregiver stress and staff support in illness, dying, and bereavement* (pp. 1–24). Oxford, UK: Oxford University Press.

Vachon, M. L. S., Lyall, W. A. L., & Freeman, S. J. J. (1978). Measurement and management of stress in health professionals working with advanced cancer patients. *Death Education, 1,* 365375.

Vachon, M. L. S., & Butow, P. N. (in press). Oncology staff stress and related interventions. In J. C. Holland, W. S. Breitbart, P. Butow, P. B. Jacobsen, M. J. Loscalzo, & R. McCorkle (Eds.), *Psycho-oncology* (3rd ed.).

Vachon, M. L. S., Huggard, P. K., & Huggard, J. (in press). Reflections on occupational stress in palliative care nursing: Is it changing? In B. R. Ferrell & N. Coyle (Eds.), *Oxford textbook of palliative nursing* (4th ed.). New York, NY: Oxford University Press.

AFTERWORD

As we draw this book to a close, we want to express our gratitude for

- the vision, insight, courage, and persistence of all who have contributed to the remarkable unfolding of the contemporary death, dying, and bereavement movement
- the few who pioneered when death was hidden from everyday life and the aftermath of war and threat of nuclear holocaust rendered many silent and helpless
- thought leaders who founded and shaped the interdisciplinary field of thanatology, developing an expanding body of knowledge and capturing considerable wisdom about death, dying, and bereavement
- institutional innovators who established hospices, palliative care services, home care programs, informed-consent regulations, advanced-directives procedures, ethical review services, bereavement services, counseling centers, private practices, mutual support groups, contemporary funeral service, suicide-prevention centers, and death education programs to meet needs of the dying, the bereaved, and the general public
- practitioners in many fields who developed a broad spectrum of end-of-life care, counseling, and therapy practices to meet the unique needs of dying, grieving, and traumatized individuals, their families, and broader communities
- our distinguished authors who joined with us in telling eyewitness and participant stories of the beginning and evolution of the movement and shared their wisdom about what must not be forgotten, the state of the art in their areas of expertise, and insights about the path ahead in the continuing evolution of the movement

We have indeed come a very long way together. However, as with other social movements in our time, including civil rights, women's rights, LGBT (lesbian, gay, bisexual, and transgender) rights, antiwar, and environmental movements, the conditions that originally prompted the movement in death, dying, and bereavement have by no means disappeared. The work of the movement is by no means finished. Increasingly familiar and new faces of death still challenge us to find better ways of living in response individually and collectively. We have come far enough to be confident that the movement has the footing and staying power to continue after many of us are gone. It is a multigenerational effort, and those new to the field need have no fear that there is nothing more to be accomplished.

Here we want to look ahead together and share some of our fondest hopes and concerns about the future of the movement:

- Promoting understanding that the multidimensional experiences of facing mortality, dying, and bereavement provide fertile ground for study from the perspectives of many disciplines
- Encouraging scholarship in a broader spectrum of disciplines, enabling establishment of interdisciplinary undergraduate major and minor and graduate programs in thanatology, comparable to scholarship and programs in gerontology (so many scholars still work in isolation at their home institutions)
- Encouraging granting agencies and foundations to allocate sustained funding for research and program development in thanatology
- Recognizing the value of qualitative research; resisting the temptation to think that if it cannot be counted, it does not count; appreciating that in counseling and clinical professions attunement to the stories and needs of unique individuals and families is key; and acknowledging that the stories told by the dying and bereaved and their caregivers comprise core evidence for evidence-based practice
- Lobbying for curriculum reform in colleges and universities, especially in medical and nursing schools, mental health and counseling professions, and journalism, to bring the best thinking in the field to the attention of those who most need it in working with the dying and the bereaved and informing the general public
- Supporting broader death education in public school systems and through public health agencies and programming, recognizing that broad public understanding is the foundation for more effective public-health-based response to the needs of dying, grieving, and traumatized individuals, families, and communities
- Promoting dialogue and collaboration among scholars, researchers, clinicians, and counselors to promote continued refinement of understanding and caregiving practices
- Increasing the number of physicians who refer the dying and their families to hospice or palliative care services and the frequency and timeliness of their referrals to improve the average stay from a mere few days to much longer and more appropriate lengths of service
- Promoting and funding implementation of a palliative approach to care of all with life-threatening conditions, not only cancer patients, at the end of life
- Continuing the global expansion of provision of hospice and palliative care services, recognizing the need for cultural sensitivity in working with diverse populations
- Resisting persistent budgetary and institutional pressures to reduce hospice and palliative care to pain and symptom control, neglecting the broader spectrum of needs of the dying and their families
- Sustaining appreciation of core values in the provision of hospice and palliative care, including a team-based versus hierarchical approach, whole person care, family support and bereavement care, and the extensive use of community volunteers
- Continuing recognition of the values of dialogue between health care providers and those in their care, informed-consent regulations, rights to refuse or insist on withdrawal of medical treatment, and advanced directives to respect personal autonomy and promote dignity in dying

- Expanding the implementation of a narrative approach to ethical care of the dying and the bereaved, both in end-of-life decision making and in all caregiving interactions
- Expanding the availability of suicide prevention, intervention, and postvention services, recognizing that suicide is normatively irrational and undertaken in crisis
- Recognizing the possibility of rational suicide and continuing public dialogue and debate about cautious, carefully safeguarded regulation of physician-assisted suicide, including close monitoring of existing programs
- Resisting tendencies to treat grieving as pathology and recognizing it as a natural reaction and adaptive response to bereavement
- Recognizing that we grieve in all dimensions of our being, socially and spiritually as well as psychologically, and that families and communities also grieve collectively
- Appreciating the value of grief counseling for those who seek it or who respond positively when asked if they would like to meet with a counselor, resisting any temptation to think that everyone needs it
- Appreciating the wide variety of counseling techniques and practices that can serve the bereaved in relearning the worlds of their experience
- Extending the availability of counseling services to underserved populations and globally
- Continuing best practices in referring those who are struggling with especially challenging bereavements and trauma to grief therapists and traumatologists trained to help them
- Continued affirmation of the value of mutual support groups for the bereaved
- Promoting further research into resilience-based and positive psychology-based understandings of and approaches to relearning the world in bereavement
- Extending understanding and provision of support for non-death-related losses
- Widely disseminating understanding of the bereavement and trauma needs of individuals, families, and communities following disaster and preparing communities for the likely increase in the numbers and extent of such disasters as climate change takes hold

Shakespeare said, "What's past is prologue." We have shared with you the best thinking of the past and of contemporary minds. The prologue is over. Now, we need the best minds and creative energies of new theorists, researchers, educators, medical personnel, ethicists, counselors, and therapists to move this field into the future. Just as our authors have shared their stories, knowledge, and concerns with you, the reader, we trust that you will take on the challenges of the present and, continuing to build on what has been done, create new knowledge, support continuing institutional evolution, refine and create new practices, and find ways to pass the best of the death, dying, and bereavement movement on to ensuing generations.

Judith M. Stillion and Thomas Attig

INDEX

Made in United States
North Haven, CT
08 April 2024

51054670R00241